Gaps and Actions in Health Improvement from Hong Kong and Beyond

Ben Yuk Fai Fong · William Chi Wai Wong
Editors

Gaps and Actions in Health Improvement from Hong Kong and Beyond

All for Health

Springer

Editors
Ben Yuk Fai Fong
Hong Kong Polytechnic University
Kowloon, China

William Chi Wai Wong
University of Hong Kong
Hong Kong, China

ISBN 978-981-99-4490-3 ISBN 978-981-99-4491-0 (eBook)
https://doi.org/10.1007/978-981-99-4491-0

This Springer imprint is published by the registered company Springer Nature Singapore Pte Ltd.
The registered company address is: 152 Beach Road, #21-01/04 Gateway East, Singapore 189721, Singapore

Foreword

Some 45 years ago, a globally shared dream of "health for all" was adopted in the Declaration of Alma-Ata. This ambitious book asks not only the question of why are we not yet there, but more importantly asks what else we have to do to get there. Along the way, the authors recognise the changing contexts, the evolving knowledge base and the lessons we have learned.

The adoption by world leaders of the 2030 Sustainable Development Agenda, and as part of the goal of Universal Health Coverage, reflects what the world has learned and how the world has changed. These updated global aspirations reflect our more recently articulated understanding of the social determinants of health as well as re-affirmation of primary health care as the foundation for good health and good health systems.

Our understanding of the social nature of ill-health and our own failings have been further reinforced by the COVID-19 pandemic. In all countries, we have seen existing health inequalities exacerbated, with the burden of ill-health falling on the disadvantaged or vulnerable population groups, since as the elderly, migrants or ethnic minorities, those in insecure employment. We have seen health activities and health care deferred, be it physical activity or non-communicable disease care. We have seen our gaps in health literacy and community engagement lead to vaccine hesitancy. We have come to recognise more clearly that there is no health without mental health. At the same time, we have seen digital health offers new possibilities for solving problems of access to care.

This volume offers insights about how the gaps in the health system can be filled and what it would take to ensure our actions for health improvement can be more successful. The book adopts both a life course approach to cover people across the life span as well as a continuum of care approach, ranging from primary prevention through structural interventions through to rehabilitation and palliation. There is focus on the macro-environment, such as cities, as well as micro settings, such as workplaces. The question of equity and the importance of culture and social environment are prominent before the reader.

I congratulate the editors for bringing together such a large partnership of authors and offering materials which are not only deeply relevant for Hong Kong and also holds lessons for the region and globally.

Professor Vivian Lin
Executive Associate Dean, Faculty of Medicine; Former Director of Health Systems, WHO Regional Office for the Western Pacific
The University of Hong Kong
Hong Kong, China

Preface

The 1978 Alma-Ata Declaration of "Health For All by Year 2000" initiated by the World Health Organization mapped the road for primary health care as health is essential for all people and for human progress in terms of economic development and social justice. However, 45 years have gone and most societies and countries have yet achieved "health for all", despite so much has been changed in technology, disease pattern and population ageing in the world. It is timely to review what has been accomplished and identify the gaps in health improvements in the population. Everyone should work harder in promoting community health and improving service delivery. Development and implementation of "All for Health" strategies shall steer stakeholders in the right direction towards the amicable goals of universal health coverage. The book consists of four sections of review of "Health for All in 2000"; gaps and actions in Health Improvements; the All for Health Strategies; and Health in All Policies (HiAP). The chapters review and discuss the issues in a general coverage, illustrated by both Asian and international examples and research by the authors. Contributors are academics and practitioners from diversified professional backgrounds of medical, nursing, allied health, dietetics, social sciences, life sciences, education, business, administration and public policy. The contents serve as a reference to university studies in primary care, public health and related disciplines, and are also useful to policymakers, researchers, community and public health practitioners, health executives and interns.

Kowloon, China — Ben Yuk Fai Fong
Hong Kong, China — William Chi Wai Wong

Acknowledgements

The editors wish to thank the colleagues of the Centre for Ageing and Healthcare Management Research (CAHMR) at the College of Professional and Continuing Education of the Hong Kong Polytechnic University (PolyU) for the support to the book. A few members of CAHMR have contributed the book chapters. The editors also appreciate the involvement of professional and academic colleagues for writing up the manuscripts in their busy schedules. Efforts made by all chapter authors in the preparation and refinement of the manuscripts are acknowledged in the highest honours and appreciation. We are also indebted to Tommy Ng and Nicolette Lee for their meticulous review and proof-reading of the manuscripts. We also appreciate the support from Professor Vivian Lin, Executive Associate Dean of Faculty of Medicine at The University of Hong Kong who has kindly written the Foreword for the book. The Editors would like to thank Alexandra Campbell and Rajasekar Ganesan of Springer for their advice and help in the planning and development of the book.

Ben Yuk Fai Fong
William Chi Wai Wong

Acknowledgements

The editors wish to thank the colleagues of the Centre for Ageing and Healthcare Management Research (CAHMR) at the College of Professional and Continuing Education of the Hong Kong Polytechnic University (PolyU) for the support to the book. A few members of CAHMR have contributed the book chapters. The editors also appreciate the involvement of professional and academic colleagues for writing up the manuscripts in their busy schedules. Efforts made by all chapter authors in the preparation and refinement of the manuscripts are acknowledged in the highest honours and appreciation. We are also indebted to Tommy Ng and Nicolette Lee for their meticulous review and proof-reading of the manuscripts. We also appreciate the support from Professor Vivian Lin, Executive Associate Dean of Faculty of Medicine at The University of Hong Kong who has kindly written the Foreword for the book. The Editors would like to thank Alexandra Campbell and Rajasekar Ganesan of Springer for their advice and help in the planning and development of the book.

Ben Yuk Fai Fong
William Chi Wai Wong

Contents

Editors and Contributors

About the Editors

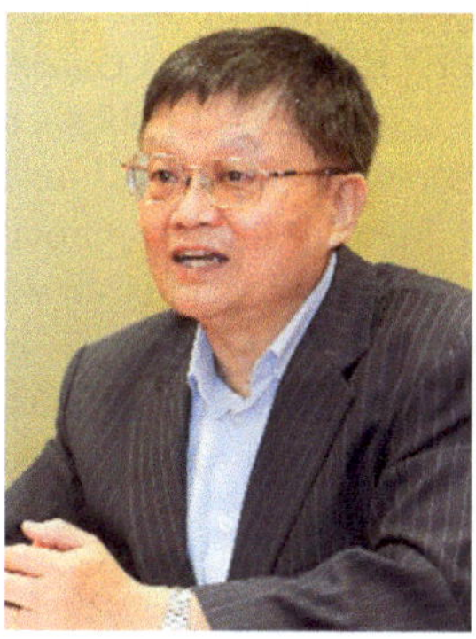

Dr. Ben Yuk Fai Fong is a Specialist in Community Medicine, holding Honorary Clinical Associate Professorship at the two local medical schools and a school of Chinese Medicine in Hong Kong, China. He is currently the Professor of Practice (Health Studies) and Associate Division Head of the Division of Science, Engineering and Health Studies, and Centre Director of the Centre for Ageing and Healthcare Management Research of the College of Professional and Continuing Education at the Hong Kong Polytechnic University and an Adjunct Professor in Public Health & Tropical Medicine in the College of Public Health, Medical and Veterinary Sciences at James Cook University, Australia. He is the President of Hong Kong College of Community Health Practitioners and has contributed to publications, including The Routledge Handbook of Public Health and the Community (as lead editor, 2021), Primary Care Revisited: Interdisciplinary Perspectives for a New Era (as lead editor, 2020), a training manual for general practitioners in China published by the People's Medical Publishing House in Beijing (as co-editor, 2020), over 30 health books in Chinese, and 60 journal papers. https://directory.speed-polyu.edu.hk/staff-directory/en/speed/spd-speed-acadiv-sehs-acastf/ben-fong.

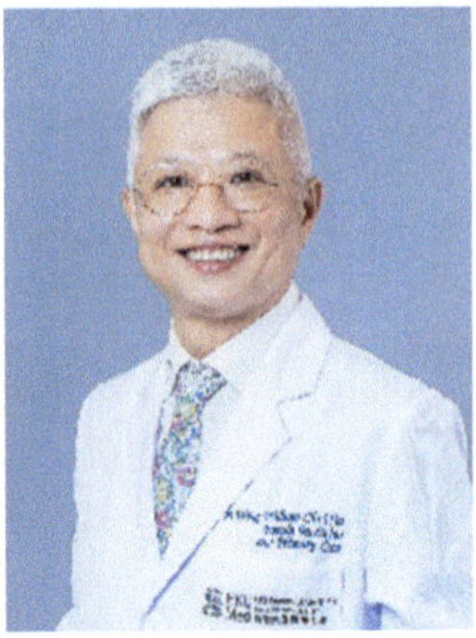

Dr. William Chi Wai Wong is a Family Medicine Specialist as well as an educator and untiring advocate in Family Medicine and Primary Care. He has worked extensively in hospitals and local communities in the UK, Australia, China and Hong Kong for the last 25 years. In 2010, he joined the University of Hong Kong as Clinical Associate Professor, currently Chairperson & Chief of Research in the Department of Family Medicine and Primary Care with honorary consultant appointments in the Department of Family Medicine at HKU–Shenzhen Hospital and Hospital Authority of Hong Kong. A well-recognised world leader in Family Medicine, he is actively engaged with the WHO and WONCA—contributed to the Strategic and Technical Advisory Committee on HIV, Viral Hepatitis and Sexually Transmitted Infections as well as a number of WHO guidelines on HIV/ sexual health issues. He is the principal architect of the first *Primary Care Guideline on CHB Management in China (2021)* published by Chinese Medical Association. In 2014, he found the WONCA Health Equity Special Interest Group addressing the social dimension of health and ensuring equitable access to high-quality health services in primary care. With over 180 peer-reviewed publications, his contributions to research have led to international recognition with >60 invited lectures and as an editor of four academic/ general books on primary care.

Contributors

Derrick Kit-Sing Au CUHK Centre for Bioethics, The Chinese University of Hong Kong, Hong Kong, China

David Briggs University of New England, Armidale, NSW, Australia

Mark Brommeyer College of Business, Government and Law, Flinders University, Adelaide, SA, Australia

Wendy F. M. Chan HKCC, The Hong Kong Polytechnic University, Hong Kong, China

Yim Fan Chan Hong Kong College of Paediatric Nursing, Hong Kong, China

Yumi Y. T. Chan Hong Kong College of Community Health Practitioners, Hong Kong, China

Karen K. M. Cheung School of Nursing and Health Studies, Hong Kong Metropolitan University, Hong Kong, China

Wang-Kin Chiu Division of Science, Engineering and Health Studies, College of Professional and Continuing Education, The Hong Kong Polytechnic University, Hong Kong, China

Yuk-sik Chong Hong Kong Institute of Asia-Pacific Studies, The Chinese University of Hong Kong, Hong Kong, China

Holy Lai Man Chu T.W.G.Hs. Yow Kam Yuen College, Hong Kong, China

Po Po Chung School of Nursing and Health Studies, Hong Kong Metropolitan University, Hong Kong, China

Roger Yat-Nork Chung JC School of Public Health and Primary Care, CUHK Centre for Bioethics and CUHK Institute of Health Equity, The Chinese University of Hong Kong, Hong Kong, China

Thomas M. C. Dao Department of Family Medicine and Primary Health Care, Kowloon West Cluster, Hospital Authority, Hong Kong, China

Bowen Dong Faculty of Business, City University of Macau, Macau, China

Bean S. N. Fu Department of Family Medicine and Primary Health Care, Kowloon West Cluster, Hospital Authority, Hong Kong, China

Billy S. H. Ho School of Professional Education and Executive Development, The Hong Kong Polytechnic University, Hong Kong, China

Wing Tung Percy Ho Hong Kong College of Community Health Practitioners, Hong Kong, China

Helen S. M. Hsu The Hong Kong Federation of Youth Groups, Hong Kong, China

Shixin Huang Department of Sociology and Social Policy, Lingnan University, Hong Kong, China

Sze Ki Lai School of Nursing and Health Studies, Hong Kong Metropolitan University, Hong Kong, China

Peter T. K. Lau Jockey Club School of Public Health and Primary Care, The Chinese University of Hong Kong, Hong Kong, China

Sin Ping Law School of Nursing and Health Studies, Hong Kong Metropolitan University, Hong Kong, China

Vincent T. S. Law College of Professional and Continuing Education, The Hong Kong Polytechnic University, Hong Kong, China

Janet Lok Chun Lee Department of Rehabilitation Sciences, The Hong Kong Polytechnic University, Hong Kong, China

John Lee United Christian Nethersole Community Health Service, Hong Kong, China

Linda Yin King Lee School of Nursing and Health Studies, Hong Kong Metropolitan University, Hong Kong, China

Alan K. T. Leung School of Professional Education and Executive Development, The Hong Kong Polytechnic University, Hong Kong, China

Carman K. M. Leung The Hong Kong Polytechnic University, Hong Kong, China

Tiffany Cheng Han Leung Faculty of Business, City University of Macau, Macau, China

Will L. H. Leung Jockey Club School of Public Health and Primary Care, The Chinese University of Hong Kong, Hong Kong, China

Leon Wai Li Hong Kong College of Community Health Practitioners, Hong Kong, China

Zhanming Liang College of Public Health, Medical and Veterinary Science, James Cook University, Queensland, Australia

Mei Kuen Li School of Nursing and Health Studies, Hong Kong Metropolitan University, Hong Kong, China

Siu Yin Li School of Nursing and Health Studies, Hong Kong Metropolitan University, Hong Kong, China

Haoyu Liu Faculty of Business, City University of Macau, Macau, China

Chor Ming Lum Institute of Ageing, The Chinese University of Hong Kong, Hong Kong, China

Fanny Y. F. Ng The Hong Kong Federation of Youth Groups, Hong Kong, China

Fowie S. F. Ng Tung Wah College, Hong Kong, China

Tommy K. C. Ng College of Professional and Continuing Education, The Hong Kong Polytechnic University, Hong Kong, China

Francesca Quattri Department of Population Health Sciences, University of Leicester, Leicester, UK

Bun Sheng Department of Medicine and Geriatrics, Princess Margaret Hospital, Hong Kong, China

Simpson S. C. Tam School of Clinical Medicine, University of Cambridge, Cambridge, UK

Candy Yuen Yee Tsoi Hong Kong College of Midwives, Hong Kong, China

Po-san Wan Hong Kong Institute of Asia-Pacific Studies, The Chinese University of Hong Kong, Hong Kong, China

Pui Yu Chesney Wong Department of Surgery, Queen Mary Hospital, Hong Kong, China

Sarah S. S. Wong School of Nursing and Health Studies, Hong Kong Metropolitan University, Hong Kong, China

Suet Lai Wong School of Nursing and Health Studies, Hong Kong Metropolitan University, Hong Kong, China

Daphne M. Y. Wu The University of Hong Kong, Hong Kong, China

Ruixin Xing School of Business, Macau University of Science and Technology, Macau, China

Sui Yu Yau School of Nursing and Health Studies, Hong Kong Metropolitan University, Hong Kong, China

Hilary H. L. Yee Department of Rehabilitation Sciences, The Hong Kong Polytechnic University, Hong Kong, China

Pi-Ying Yen School of Business, Macau University of Science and Technology, Macau, China

Cynthia S. C. Yip Hong Kong Chu Hai College of Higher Education, Hong Kong, China

Shi Xiang You Faculty of Business, City University of Macau, Macau, China

Victor W. T. Zheng Hong Kong Institute of Asia-Pacific Studies, The Chinese University of Hong Kong, Hong Kong, China

Part I
Review of "Health for all by 2000"

Chapter 1
Achievements in HFA2000 Since 1978

Carman K. M. Leung and Wang-Kin Chiu

Abstract Primary care is commonly considered the bottom layer of the healthcare system. In practice, it is the primary and first, as well as the continuing contact for people with healthcare providers who offer fundamental and comprehensive health and nursing care and interventions. Educational programmes are provided for the public to maintain health and prevent them from being ill. In 1978, the World Health Organization (WHO) and member countries declared "Health for all by the year 2000" (the HFA) in Alma-Ata, advocating that all citizens could not only reach the level of health defined by the WHO but also be economically productive in 2000. The project has been underway for more than four decades. While various governments have implemented a range of strategies and policies to accomplish the target, some have yielded substantial achievements. This chapter will discuss the HFA-related measurements in detail and review the achievements in various countries, as well as how to evaluate their performance and effectiveness for health improvement of the population.

Keywords Health for All · Primary health care · Health in All Policies · Water sanitation · Maternal and child health

C. K. M. Leung (✉)
The Hong Kong Polytechnic University, Hong Kong, China
e-mail: kmcarman.leung@polyu.edu.hk

W.-K. Chiu
Division of Science, Engineering and Health Studies, College of Professional and Continuing Education, The Hong Kong Polytechnic University, Hong Kong, China
e-mail: oscar.chiu@cpce-polyu.edu.hk

B. Y. F. Fong and W. C. W. Wong (eds.), *Gaps and Actions in Health Improvement from Hong Kong and Beyond*,
https://doi.org/10.1007/978-981-99-4491-0_1

Background of Primary Health Care and Health for All Strategy

Primary health care (PHC) is a fundamental level of the healthcare system which provides a series of services including basic treatments and health education, to ensure people receive a high quality of comprehensive care (World Health Organization, 2021a). In the early years, there was no standard interpretation of the term PHC, so different norms exist in different countries (Donaldson et al., 1996; Kronenberg et al., 2017). Primary health care is defined by Starfield (1992) as "initial contact, accessibility, longitudinally, and comprehensiveness". McMurray and Clendon (2015) considered that PHC is a department that must collaborate with other departments, and physicians assist people in achieving health in a fair and equitable manner. Although the definition of PHC differs by nation, it is undeniable that it offers the community with holistic health care.

Until 1977, the 30th World Health Assembly advocated "Health for All by 2000" (HFA) as the key health target for governments and World Health Organization (WHO) in the future decades. In the following year, the World Health Organization and United Nations International Children's Emergency Fund (UNICEF) co-chaired the International Conference on Primary Health Care and issued the Alma-Ata Declaration (Declaration), which laid the framework for the development of primary health care. This declaration sets forth worldwide guidelines for the improvement and promotion of PHC (World Health Organization, 1978). It is made up of four dimensions and eight components. All of them enable countries to develop and implement primary healthcare measures from the beginning, such as disease prevention and control, mothers and children care, improving safe drinking water and basic sanitation facilities, or medical professionals providing diagnosis, treatment, and rehabilitation services, and to encourage research and development, technical support, and training through international exchange of information, gradually reaching the right to primary health care for all people (World Health Organization, 1978).

The strategy has been signed by a total of 134 member states and 67 international organisations. Given the inequities in health across countries, especially in developing countries, the declaration works to ensure and promote everybody's health as a fundamental human right and a universal social aim by the year 2000, so that everyone can live a socially and economically productive life without barriers to health (Fong et al., 2020; World Health Organization, 1978). Throughout the project, the World Health Organization performed frequent monitoring and evaluations of different nations to determine their performance (World Health Organization, 1993). Looking back, this strategy has been in place for over 40 years, and the aims of various elements of work have yielded specific outcomes in both developed and developing countries, allowing people to live healthier lives and receive better medical care.

Health in All Policies Since 1978

The spirit of Alma-Ata, encompassing the significance of efforts from different sectors for health promotion, was emphasised in the Ottawa Charter for Health Promotion (World Health Organization, 2012). The Ottawa conference was held in 1986 with over 200 participants, including various stakeholders such as politicians, academicians, health workers, and government representatives, coming from 38 countries to share and reflect on the experiences of health promotion, during which "healthy public policies" were identified as an important area for the promotion of health and well-being. The Alma-Ata Declaration in 1978 and the Ottawa Charter in 1986 formed the international roots for the principles of the "Health in All Policies" (HiAP) approach, emphasising the critical roles of sectors other than health in the achievement of health for all (Ståhl, 2018). According to the definition by WHO, Health in All Policies is an approach to systematically consider the health and health-system implications of decisions, with the objective of improving population health and health equity. Collectively, "Health in All Policies" is a term or slogan built on the rationale that health is influenced by a variety of factors beyond the direct control of the healthcare sector (Puska, 2007; World Health Organization, 2014). Examples include education, environments, and lifestyles, which are not only individual choices, but also in strong linkages with social, cultural, and economic determinants. In fact, these determinants are influenced not only by health services or health policies, but can also be affected positively or negatively by various policy areas and decisions made in other sectors. Based on the principles of Health in All Policies, the WHO global health promotion conferences continued the prior work initialised by the Alma-Ata Declaration to establish it as an approach for horizontal health policy on a global level.

The Finland Experience

The experience from Finland in the implementation of Health in All Policies has been reported (Ståhl, 2018). The Benchmarking System for Health Promotion Capacity Building has been introduced and utilised as a primary source of information for the progress monitoring and evaluation of Health in All Policies. While Health in All Policies was identified as an approach requiring long-term commitment and vision, the findings also suggested the importance of having data on health and health determinants, as well as analysing the linkages between health outcomes, health determinants, and policies across different areas, in order to achieve continuity and sustainability when implementing Health in All Policies and carrying out intersectoral work. In addition, the Finnish initiatives which involved different sectors and policies, such as nutrition interventions at the national level with policy changes in health, agriculture, and commerce sectors, have led to significant improvement in public health (Puska & Ståhl, 2010). Policy measures implemented in relation to nutrition and public health included the introduction of comprehensive primary health care (health centres) in the 1970s for which the national public health law was designed with a major focus on prevention of diseases.

During the 1980s and 1990s, there had been legislations on salt labelling and contents. These measures were also in line with the global trend of increasing worldwide initiatives and interventions for reducing salt intake (Fong et al., 2021; Santos et al., 2021). Furthermore, during the 2000s, the Finnish initiatives also included the implementation of governmental policy programmes on healthy diet and physical activity. These efforts had led to intersectoral work in Finland which resulted in public health improvements and reduction in the mortality rate associated with cardiovascular diseases. For example, more than 90% of the population in the 1970s had the habit of using butter on bread while the percentage had dropped significantly to 5% in 2009 (Puska & Ståhl, 2010). The change was also accompanied with decreasing salt and fat intake, as well as increasing consumption of fruits and vegetables. The work in Finland not just brought about public health improvements, but also paved the way for the Health in All Policies programmes initiated in 2006 during the Finnish European Union (EU) presidency, with a policy-related strategy encompassing disease prevention and health promotion projects. The basic idea of considering health determinants influenced by different sectors such as education, environment, traffic, housing, and economy, are emphasised with an ultimate goal of improving evidence-based policymaking.

Community Engagement

Community involvement is a key component to achieving the goals of Health in All Policies. While healthy communities are essential to healthy living, promotion of good health and well-being in cities is complicated by the fact that they face unique challenges due to variations in economic bases, concentrated poverty, housing quality and resources, as well as exposure to different levels of environmental factors such as pollutions. Therefore, "healthy public policy", advocated by WHO since 1988, has been important for providing a broad framework to understand the factors contributing to both individual and population health while focusing on intersectoral work beyond the healthcare sector when making public policy. According to a recent survey, health officials of large cities identified "Health in All Policies" as a top priority (Hearne et al., 2015). In addition to Finland, since 2006, implementation of Health in All Policies has flourished in the United States (Wernham & Teutsch, 2015). Several major cities in the United States, including Seattle, Los Angeles, San Francisco, Boston, and Washington, have adopted the Health in All Policies approach and implemented programmes and activities focusing on health public policy. Moreover, a growing amount of research exploring the social, economic, and environmental influences on health and diseases further provides the rationales and paves the way for Health in All Policies. Examples of achievements include *Healthy People 2020* (Koh et al., 2014). For the first time, a broad set of indicators based on different determinants such as availability of healthful food, income, as well as housing quality and affordability, has been included in establishing the targets and measures of federal government's 10-year national health improvement.

Training and Systems Thinking in HiAP

While Health in All Policies serves as a crucial framework for the promotion of public health and well-being, it should be noted that evidence-based guidelines for ethical policies are important for making effective policy decisions. Systematic efforts of experts with broad partnership are necessary for identifying and prioritising the items on the Health in All Policies agenda. Notably, implementation of intersectoral health policies is not easy. Improvement of health literacy of the public and policy-makers, supported with innovative uses of the media and technology, are essential for enhancing the understanding on health implications of policies (Ollila, 2011; Puska & Ståhl, 2010). Intersectoral collaborations are significant in the implementation of Health in All Policies. Therefore, Health in All Policies requires a multidisciplinary team for organisation and facilitation. Subject matter experts, professionals with scientific skills, communicators, teachers, researchers, academic and educational institutions are all having critical roles. It is noteworthy that the adoption of systems-thinking approaches is expected to facilitate college and community education for the promotion of population health and sustainable development (Chiu et al., 2022). Under these circumstances, new training programmes offering opportunities for intersectoral collaboration and education incorporated with a systems-thinking mindset are highly desirable for developing the essential skills.

Health in All Strategies

Safe Drinking Water and Basic Sanitation Facilities

Water is an extremely important substance for humans, based on the fact that the human body is about 70 percent composed of water. It promotes thermoregulation and serves as a transporter for nutrients to various parts of the body (Jéquier & Constant, 2010). Bodily functions cannot operate effectively if the body is dehydrated. Humans are unable to produce water and must obtain it from a variety of sources. Drinking water is the simplest method. Over seventy percent of water covers the surface of earth, however, less than three percent of freshwater resources are available, and most are brackish and undrinkable (Dinka, 2018; Youssef et al., 2014). As shown in a study that examined worldwide water consumption from the 1950s to the 1990s, it rose by around thrice. Water was more commonly spent in agriculture in the 1950s, while industrial and domestic water accounted for a minor proportion (Nishijima et al.,

2013). The demand for domestic water is rising as the world's population increases. Some countries with high levels of economic development, such as Saudi Arabia, the United States, and the United Arab Emirates, have begun to develop saltwater desalination technology to filter and purify seawater into domestic water in order to meet people's demand for fresh water (Islam et al., 2018).

It is a pity that some developing countries, such as South Africa, lack the required technologies to address the problem of water scarcity. As a result, they depend greatly on rainfall as a freshwater resource (Islam et al., 2018). Furthermore, as many countries' industries developed in the twentieth century, so their consumption of water rose (Nishijima et al., 2013). Simultaneously, a large amount of untreated sewage is dumped into the sea, which is one of the major causes of declining water quality (Flörke et al., 2013; Pandey, 2006). As a result of some developing countries' lack of sanitary facilities to improve water quality or the impact of climate change, they have the challenges accessing fresh drinking water (Pandey, 2006). Because of water contamination, humans do not have access to safe water for lengthy periods, less than half of the worldwide population had access to safe water or sanitation facilities (Nagpal & Radin, 2014). As a result of their usage of polluted water sources and shared sanitation facilities in filthy environments, people developed intestinal related diseases, like diarrhoea (Baker et al., 2016; Just et al., 2018).

Until 1978, one of the strategies in the HFA was to ensure that all people have access to safe water and basic sanitation (World Health Organization, 1978). They have implemented a battery of strategies to promote safe water and sanitation for more than a decade, including constructing water infrastructure, promoting health education, improving operation and maintenance, and enhancing international coordination and cooperation. Degree of accessibility is the most significant way for determining how many individuals have access to pure water resources. The proportion of families being accessible to sufficient water for drinking and disinfecting the immediate area around their homes is one measurement which was implemented (World Health Organization, 1981). According to the 1993 report, these actions enabled more than 1.5 billion people to have access to adequate and safe water sources, while nearly half of them also had acceptable sanitation (World Health Organization, 1993). Also, the Joint Monitoring Programme (JMP) on Water Supply, Sanitation, and Hygiene established by WHO and the UNICEF in 1990, has tracked progress towards global water and sanitation targets in which the major goal is to assist developing nations in developing national surveillance capabilities in order to inform regulators about the quality of the water and sanitation sector through annual reports (United Nations, 2015c). With just 61 percent of the world population having access to securely managed drinking water and less than 30 percent utilising safely managed sanitation services by 2000, the World Health Organization failed to reach the goal of providing safe water and basic sanitation to all according to the HFA's strategy (United Nations Children's Fund, & World Health Organization, 2019). Although HFA's strategy is no longer applicable, this goal is still being worked on because the United Nations General Assembly adopted the 2030 Agenda for Sustainable Development in 2015, which includes 17 Sustainable Development Goals (SDGs), the sixth of which is

"Clean Water and Sanitation", which not only aims to ensure safety water and sanitation for all human beings but also pay attention to the ecosystem, for example, water quality and wastewater (Sadoff et al., 2020; United Nations, 2015b).

Maternal and Child Health and Family Planning

Human development can be divided into five stages, each with its own set of nutritional requirements (Balasundaram & Avulakunta, 2021; Barnard, 2020). The nutritional status of young children is a significant consideration while analysing their physical growth and development (World Health Organization, 1981). Socioeconomic status is an indicator that measures their background, ability to obtain resources on a financial basis, and reputation in the community. Multiple research and articles consistently indicate that those in high socioeconomic status have fewer possibilities to be confronted with health risks. In contrast, those with lower socioeconomic status are more likely to suffer from diseases (Baker, 2014; Wang & Geng, 2019). One of the factors that impact health is dietary consumption. Low income is often correlated with poor dietary intake. They tend to buy relatively cheap yet nutritionally inadequate foods. Malnutrition among youngsters is the long-term consequence of insufficient consumption of healthy food. Developmental delays will occur concurrently (Anderson et al., 2021; Henry, 2019). Malnutrition is a major risk factor of heavy disease burden for populations in developing countries or third-world countries (Budzulak et al., 2022; Mullero, 2005). Sadly, the issue of malnutrition linked to poverty in developing countries is still existing and the major concern on population health is not yet resolved. Over 300,000 young children die each year as a result of malnutrition and lack of medical facilities (Mullero, 2005). The UN is still dedicated to improving the situation as it stands. Hence, they aim at zero hunger while attempting towards eliminating malnutrition as one of their Sustainable Development Goals (SDGs).

Indeed, one of the factors for the negative impact on health quality in developing countries is a lack of medical equipment. Women having pregnancy rates are significantly greater than in developed countries, due to their need for local children as a working population to support their families, as well as their poor levels of education and lack of contraception, which result in higher fertility rates (Nargund, 2009; World Health Organization, 1993). Unfortunately, despite their high fertility rate, the birth rate is low since over 99 percent of maternal fatalities occur in developing countries because many women have complications during pregnancy and birth with inadequate access to medical professionals (United Nations, 2008). Also, some pregnant women are treated only by people with no or little medical training during their pregnancy, and as a result, some of them suffer urinary tract infections, which can be harmful for pregnant women and newborns (Getaneh et al., 2021; World Health Organization, 1993).

The second WHO evaluation presented statistical data on prenatal care services delivered by trained personnel in both developing and developed countries between

1985 and 1991, following the release and implementation of the HFA strategy. The coverage rate in developing countries has increased from 50% to more than 60%. In developed countries, coverage had reached 99 percent (World Health Organization, 1993). An article discovered that women with higher education had later fertility rates in developed countries (Nargund, 2009). Some developing countries, such as Egypt, Guinea, and others, have implemented safe motherhood programmes and actions for pregnant women in order to improve maternal health services and increase knowledge about foetal care, based on the fact that improving mothers' education can improve birth rates, and reduce infant and child mortality (Cleland & Van Ginneken, 1988; Dursun et al., 2017; World Health Organization, 1993). An article has pointed out that the annual mortality rate for children under five fell below 10 million for the first time in 2006. It can be seen that education has a certain relationship with reducing child mortality (United Nations Children's Fund, 2007; Veneman, 2007).

Concluding Remarks

We cannot doubt that the HFA strategy had some positive impacts, especially in developing countries, notwithstanding the World Health Organization's failure to achieve the target of health for all in the year 2000. In order to improve medical care and living conditions and enable inhabitants to live with dignity, some governmental and non-governmental organisations have aided them. The task has not been completed while the HFA strategy has been successfully executed. Given the fact that 2 billion people would still lack safe drinking water until the year 2020, they may have to consume polluted water for their daily needs (World Health Organization, 2021b). The Sustainable Development Goals could be regarded as the HFA strategy's follow-up approach. A set of 17 measures to improve people's quality of life, the environment, and the economy were included in the "The 2030 Agenda for Sustainable Development" that the United Nations introduced in 2015. 193 United Nations member states at the time committed to achieve these aims. The UN Secretary General presents a report titled "SDG Progress Report" each year to evaluate the strategy's progression and effectiveness (United Nations, 2015a). As can be seen, the half-century primary objective for a better future for every life or economy on earth—remains the same irrespective of whether it is the HFA strategy or the SDGs.

References

Anderson, E., Wei, R., Liu, B., Plummer, R., Kelahan, H., Tamez, M., … & Mattei, J. (2021). Improving healthy food choices in low-income settings in the United States using behavioral economic-based adaptations to choice architecture. *Frontiers in Nutrition, 8*, 734991. https://doi.org/10.3389/fnut.2021.734991

Baker, E. H. (2014). Socioeconomic status, definition. *The Wiley Blackwell Encyclopedia of Health, Illness, Behavior, and Society*, 2210–2214. https://doi.org/10.1002/9781118410868.wbehibs395

Baker, K. K., O'Reilly, C. E., Levine, M. M., Kotloff, K. L., Nataro, J. P., Ayers, T. L., ... & Mintz, E. D. (2016). Sanitation and hygiene-specific risk factors for moderate-to-severe diarrhea in young children in the global enteric multicenter study, 2007–2011: Case-control study. *PLoS Medicine, 13*(5), Article e1002010. https://doi.org/10.1371/journal.pmed.1002010

Balasundaram, P., & Avulakunta, I. D. (2021). *Human growth and development.* In StatPearls. StatPearls Publishing, Treasure Island (FL); 2021. PMID: 33620844.

Barnard, N. D. (2020). *Nutritional requirements throughout the life cycle.* Nutrition Guide for Clinicians. https://nutritionguide.pcrm.org/nutritionguide/view/Nutrition_Guide_for_Clinicians/1342043/all/Nutritional_Requirements_throughout_the_Life_Cycle

Budzulak, J., Majewska, K. A., & Kędzia, A. (2022). Malnutrition as the cause of growth retardation among children in developed countries. *Annals of Agricultural and Environmental Medicine, 29*(3), 336. https://doi.org/10.26444/aaem/148010

Cleland, J. G., & Van Ginneken, J. K. (1988). Maternal education and child survival in developing countries: The search for pathways of influence. *Social Science & Medicine, 27*(12), 1357–1368. https://doi.org/10.1016/0277-9536(88)90201-8

Chiu, W. K., Fong, B. Y., & Ho, W. Y. (2022). The importance of environmental sustainability for healthy ageing and the incorporation of systems thinking in education for a sustainable environment. *Asia Pacific Journal of Health Management, 17*(1), 84–89. https://doi.org/10.24083/apjhm.v17i1.1589

Dinka, M. O. (2018). Safe drinking water: Concepts, benefits, principles and standards. In M. Glavan (Ed.), *Water challenges of an urbanizing world* (pp. 163–181). Intechopen. https://doi.org/10.5772/intechopen.71352

Donaldson, M. S., Yordy, K. D., Lohr, K. N., & Vanselow, N. A. (1996). *Primary care: America's health in a new era.* The National Academies Press. https://doi.org/10.17226/5152

Dursun, B., Cesur, R., & Kelly, I. R. (2017). The value of mandating maternal education in a developing country. *National Bureau of Economic Research Working Paper*. https://doi.org/10.3386/w23492

Flörke, M., Kynast, E., Bärlund, I., Eisner, S., Wimmer, F., & Alcamo, J. (2013). Domestic and industrial water uses of the past 60 years as a mirror of socio-economic development: A global simulation study. *Global Environmental Change, 23*(1), 144–156. https://doi.org/10.1016/j.gloenvcha.2012.10.018

Fong, B. Y. F., Chiu, W. K., Chan, W. F., & Lam, T. Y. (2021). A review study of a green diet and healthy ageing. *International Journal of Environmental Research and Public Health, 18*(15), Article 8024. https://doi.org/10.3390/ijerph18158024

Fong, B. Y. F., Law, V. T. S., & Lee, A. (2020). *Primary care revisited: Interdisciplinary perspectives for a new era.* Springer. https://doi.org/10.1007/978-981-15-2521-6

Getaneh, T., Negesse, A., Dessie, G., Desta, M., & Tigabu, A. (2021). Prevalence of urinary tract infection and its associated factors among pregnant women in Ethiopia: A systematic review and meta-analysis. *BioMed Research International, 2021*, Article 6551526. https://doi.org/10.1155/2021/6551526

Hearne, S., Castrucci, B. C., Leider, J. P., Rhoades, E. K., Russo, P., & Bass, V. (2015). The future of urban health: Needs, barriers, opportunities, and policy advancement at large urban health departments. *Journal of Public Health Management and Practice, 21*(1), S4–S13. https://doi.org/10.1097/PHH.0000000000000166

Henry, C. J. (2019). What children eat in developing countries: Diet in the etiology of undernutrition? *Nurturing a Healthy Generation of Children: Research Gaps and Opportunities, 91*, 43–53. https://doi.org/10.1159/000493693

Islam, M. S., Sultana, A., Saadat, A. H. M., Shammi, M., & Uddin, M. K. (2018). Desalination technologies for developing countries: A review. *Journal of Scientific Research, 10*(1), 77–97. https://doi.org/10.3329/jsr.v10i1.33179

Jéquier, E., & Constant, F. (2010). Water as an essential nutrient: The physiological basis of hydration. *European Journal of Clinical Nutrition, 64*(2), 115–123. https://doi.org/10.1038/ejcn.2009.111

Just, M. R., Carden, S. W., Li, S., Baker, K. K., Gambhir, M., & Fung, I. C. H. (2018). The impact of shared sanitation facilities on diarrheal diseases with and without an environmental reservoir: A modeling study. *Pathogens and Global Health, 112*(4), 195–202. https://doi.org/10.1080/20477724.2018.1478927

Koh, H. K., Blakey, C. R., & Roper, A. Y. (2014). Healthy People 2020: A report card on the health of the nation. *JAMA, 311*(24), 2475–2476. https://doi.org/10.1001/jama.2014.6446

Kronenberg, C., Doran, T., Goddard, M., Kendrick, T., Gilbody, S., Dare, C. R., Aylott, L., & Jacobs, R. (2017). Identifying primary care quality indicators for people with serious mental illness: A systematic review. *British Journal of General Practice, 67*(661), e519–e530. https://doi.org/10.3399/bjgp17X691721.

McMurray, A., & Clendon, J. (2015). *Community health and wellness: Primary health care in practice* (5th ed.). Churchill Livingstone/Elsevier.

Mullero, K. (2005). Malnutrition and health in developing countries. *Canadian Medical Association Journal, 173*(3), 279–286. https://doi.org/10.1503/cmaj.050342

Nagpal, T., & Radin, M. (2014). Water and sanitation for all. *The SAIS Review of International Affairs, 34*(2), 83–91. https://doi.org/10.1353/sais.2014.0029

Nargund, G. (2009). Declining birth rate in developed countries: A radical policy re-think is required. *Facts, Views & Vision in ObGyn, 1*(3), 191–193. https://fvvo.eu/assets/67/05-Nargund.pdf

Nishijima, S., Eckroad, S., Marian, A., Choi, K., Kim, W. S., Terai, M., … & Izumi, M. (2013). Superconductivity and the environment: A roadmap. *Superconductor Science and Technology, 26*(11), Article 113001. https://doi.org/10.1088/0953-2048/26/11/113001

Ollila, E. (2011). Health in all policies: From rhetoric to action. *Scandinavian Journal of Public Health, 39*(6), 11–18. https://doi.org/10.1177/1403494810379895

Pandey, S. (2006). Water pollution and health. *Kathmandu University Medical Journal, 4*(13), 128–134. http://www.kumj.com.np/issue/13/128-134.pdf

Puska, P. (2007). Health in all policies. *European Journal of Public Health, 17*(4), 328. https://doi.org/10.1093/eurpub/ckm048

Puska, P., & Ståhl, T. (2010). Health in all policies—the Finnish initiative: Background, principles, and current issues. *Annual Review of Public Health, 31*, 315–328. https://doi.org/10.1146/annurev.publhealth.012809.103658

Sadoff, C. W., Borgomeo, E., & Uhlenbrook, S. (2020). Rethinking water for SDG 6. *Nature Sustainability, 3*(5), 346–347. https://doi.org/10.1038/s41893-020-0530-9

Santos, J. A., Tekle, D., Rosewarne, E., Flexner, N., Cobb, L., Al-Jawaldeh, A., … & Trieu, K. (2021). A systematic review of salt reduction initiatives around the world: A midterm evaluation of progress towards the 2025 global non-communicable diseases salt reduction target. *Advances in Nutrition, 12*(5), 1768-1780. https://doi.org/10.1093/advances/nmab008

Ståhl, T. (2018). Health in all policies: From rhetoric to implementation and evaluation—the finnish experience. *Scandinavian Journal of Public Health, 46*(20), 38–46. https://doi.org/10.1177/1403494817743895

Starfield, B. (1992). *Primary care: Concept, evaluation, and policy*. Oxford University Press.

United Nations. (2008, September 19). *Nearly all maternal deaths occur in developing countries, UNICEF report finds*. https://news.un.org/en/story/2008/09/273572-nearly-all-maternal-deaths-occur-developing-countries-unicef-report-finds

United Nations. (2015a). *The United Nations World water development report 2015a—Water for a sustainable world*. https://unesdoc.unesco.org/ark:/48223/pf0000231823

United Nations. (2015b). *Transforming our world: The 2030 agenda for sustainable development*. https://sdgs.un.org/2030agenda

United Nations. (2015c). *WHO/UNICEF Joint monitoring program for water supply and sanitation (JMP)—2015c Update*. https://washdata.org/sites/default/files/2022-03/jmp-2022-regional-snapshot-Africa.pdf

United Nations Children's Fund. (2007). *The state of the world's children 2008: Child survival*. https://www.unicef.org/media/84861/file/SOWC-2008.pdf

United Nations Children's Fund, & World Health Organization. (2019). *Progress on drinking water, sanitation and hygiene 2000–2017: Special focus on inequalities*. https://www.unicef.org/media/55276/file/Progress%20on%20drinking%20water,%20sanitation%20and%20hygiene%202019%20.pdf
Veneman, A. M. (2007). Education is key to reducing child mortality: The link between maternal health and education. *UN chronicle, 44*(4), 33–34. https://doi.org/10.18356/8ba72cc6-en
Wang, J., & Geng, L. (2019). Effects of socioeconomic status on physical and psychological health: Lifestyle as a mediator. *International Journal of Environmental Research and Public Health, 16*(2), 281. https://doi.org/10.3390/ijerph16020281
Wernham, A., & Teutsch, S. M. (2015). Health in all policies for big cities. *Journal of Public Health Management and Practice, 21*(1), S56–S65. https://doi.org/10.1097/PHH.0000000000000130
World Health Organization. (1993). *Implementation of the global strategy for health for all by the year 2000, second evaluation: Eight report on the world health situation. v. 7, Western Pacific Region*. https://apps.who.int/iris/handle/10665/206943
World Health Organization. (1978). *Primary health care: Report of the International Conference on primary health care, Alma-Ata, USSR, 6–12 September 1978 / jointly sponsored by the World Health Organization and the United Nations Children's Fund*. https://apps.who.int/iris/handle/10665/39228
World Health Organization. (1981). *Development of indicators for monitoring progress towards health for all by the year 2000*. World Health Organization.
World Health Organization. (2012). *Ottawa charter for health promotion*. https://www.who.int/publications/i/item/ottawa-charter-for-health-promotion
World Health Organization. (2014). *Health in all policies: Helsinki statement. Framework for country action*. https://www.who.int/publications/i/item/9789241506908
World Health Organization. (2021a). *Primary health care: Overview*. https://www.who.int/health-topics/primary-health-care#tab=tab_1
World Health Organization. (2021b). *Progress on household drinking water, sanitation and hygiene 2000–2020: Five years into the SDGs*. https://www.who.int/publications/i/item/9789240030848
Youssef, P. G., Al-Dadah, R. K., & Mahmoud, S. M. (2014). Comparative analysis of desalination technologies. *Energy Procedia, 61*, 2604–2607. https://doi.org/10.1016/j.egypro.2014.12.258

Chapter 2
Implementation of Sustainable Development Goal 3 Since 2015

Tommy K. C. Ng

Abstract Health for all is a vital strategy that aims to close the health gaps within countries. People with lower socioeconomic status are more likely to have poorer health while those who are in the higher socioeconomic status have better health. Rural and urban populations have unequal healthcare utilisation, leading to health disparity in the community. It is important to minimise such gaps and inequity in any country to achieve the goal of health for all. The sustainable development goal (SDG) 3 aims to ensure healthy lives and promote well-being for all at all ages. Targets of SDG 3 set the objectives to improve and optimise the health in a country by reducing mortality rate of non-communicable diseases and achieving universal health coverage. The ultimate purpose of these targets is to attain health for all. This chapter will introduce SDG 3 and overview the impacts of implementation of SDG 3 in Demark, Hong Kong and South Africa. The impacts of implementation of SDG 3 targets will be evaluated by reviewing the literatures.

Keywords Sustainability Development Goal 3 · Health inequality · Health disparity · Universal health coverage

Introduction

Health is a fundamental human right for everyone in the world and it is directly related to the right of living a standard life and the right to attain standards of physical and mental health (McHale, 2010). Ensuring health for all people is a fundamental need around the world, irrespective of age, income level, race or gender. To achieve the concept of health for all, the United Nations had developed and adopted 17 Sustainable Development Goals (SDGs) with more than 165 targets in 2015 (United Nations, 2015). The SDGs pursue a world free of hunger or poverty, but should be achieved

T. K. C. Ng (✉)
College of Professional and Continuing Education, The Hong Kong Polytechnic University, Hong Kong, China
e-mail: tommy.ng@cpce-polyu.edu.hk

B. Y. F. Fong and W. C. W. Wong (eds.), *Gaps and Actions in Health Improvement from Hong Kong and Beyond*,
https://doi.org/10.1007/978-981-99-4491-0_2

with equitable and universal access of education and healthcare, as well as affordable, clean, and sustainable energy, water and sanitation. The SDGs are accepted by and applicable to all member states of the United Nations, including developed and developing countries, and the targets are expected to be fully implemented by 2030, so SDGs can demonstrate an enormous impact to the world. Ensuring healthy lives and promoting well-being for all of all ages is the main objective of Sustainable Development Goal 3 (SDG 3) (World Health Organization, 2017). SDG 3 has thirteen targets with specific indicators in reducing the global maternal mortality ratio, ending the epidemics of AIDS, tuberculosis, and other communicable diseases, reducing mortality from non-communicable diseases, and achieving universal health coverage. Apart from targeting physical health, promoting mental health and well-being is one of the targets of SDG 3. To achieve the targets of SDG 3, it is suggested to reduce the maternal mortality, incidence of some communicable diseases, suicide mortality rate, mortality rate attributed to cardiovascular disease, cancer, diabetes or respiratory disease, and enhance the coverage of essential health services. This chapter reviews the implementation of SDG 3 in different countries and evaluate the effectiveness and impacts of implementation since 2015.

Implementation of SDG 3 in Different Countries and Cities

Denmark

Denmark, one of the Nordic countries, provides an easy and equal access to healthcare. The Danish healthcare system has become almost entirely tax-funded by renovating hospitals, reducing acute hospitals and expansion of outpatient care (Schmidt et al., 2019). Based on the targets of SDG 3, Denmark has developed the Danish indicators and suggestions to achieve the targets (Statistics Denmark and the 2030-Panel, 2020). To fight communicable diseases, the Danish indicators focus on the number of hospital-acquired infections and the proportion of deaths that can be attributed to influenza. Hospital-acquired infections are associated with extended hospital stays and increased morbidity and mortality (Condell et al., 2016). In 2017, the Central Unit for Infectious Hygiene in Denmark released the first National Infection Hygiene Guidelines on general precautions in the healthcare sector, for managing hospital-acquired infections (Central Enhed for Infektionshygiejne, 2017). The guidelines highlight the importance of infection control, including hand hygiene, handling of utensils, management of patient excretion and other general precautions. In addition, urinary tract infection is one of the most prevalent hospital-acquired infections in Denmark (Condell et al., 2016; Gregersen et al., 2021), and so the Central Unit for Infectious Hygiene published a guideline about prevention of urinary tract infection for healthcare professional in 2019 (Central Enhed for Infektionshygiejne, 2019). It demonstrates that national guidelines for the prevention and management of communicable diseases have attributed to achieving the targets of SDG 3.

For non-communicable diseases, increasing the survival rate of cancer patients is one of the Danish targets of SDG 3. The incidence and mortality rate of colorectal cancer in Denmark was ranked the fifth and thirty-third respectively in the world in 2020 (International Agency for Research on Cancer, 2022). For early detection of cancers, Denmark has offered free national screening programmes for cervical, breast, and colorectal cancer (Danish Health Authority, 2021). Colorectal cancer screening programme was launched in 2014 for all Danish citizens aged 50 or above (Nielsen et al., 2021). The programme was free of charge so financial barriers should not be the concern for eligible Danish citizens. Moreover, the screening programme was rated well by comparing the performance indicators from the European Guidelines (Njor et al., 2018). The invitation coverage of the screening programme was close to 100% based on the residents' address, while the participation rate was more than 60%. In addition, Denmark had launched a national breast cancer screening programme in 2010 with the aim to reduce breast cancer mortality (Lynge et al., 2017, 2020). Invitations were sent to women by postal mail and the coverage was at least 75% in two studies (Larsen et al., 2018; Lynge et al., 2017). The screening programme was found to be effective in the reduction of breast cancer mortality which was declining (Lynge et al., 2017).

The mission of the Danish healthcare system is health for all (Danish Health Authority, 2020). Denmark was ranked seventeenth in the universal health coverage service coverage index in 2019 (World Health Organization, 2022). The index measures health services coverage for child health, infectious diseases, non-communicable diseases and capacity and accessibility of services. On the other hand, Denmark was above average in the universal health coverage effective index, a validated index measuring effective coverage of healthcare system (Lozano et al., 2020). Both indexes reflect the effective coverage of healthcare services in Denmark. Healthcare in Denmark is almost entirely covered by the public sector, based on the principles of free and equal access to healthcare for all citizens (Ministry of Health, 2017). Danish citizens have two options for their health services. They can either access free medical coverage by the general practitioners in the public sector and specialists in private sector if they have referrals from the general practitioners; or they can have access to any general practitioners or specialists in private practice without a referral but they may need to pay on their own. Therefore, 99% of the Danish citizens are covered by the former option (Ministry of Health, 2017). The financing scheme and social health insurance of Denmark are found to be positively associated with the performance of universal health coverage of SDG 3 (Wagstaff & Neelsen, 2020).

Hong Kong

Life expectancy in Hong Kong has been leading the world since 2013, with the expectation of life being 82.2 years and 88.1 years for males and females respectively in 2019 (Census & Statistics Department, 2020; Ni et al., 2021). These figures are projected to increase to 88.4 and 93.9 years in 2069 respectively, while the fertility rates are projected to decrease from 1,051 per 1,000 women in 2019 to 955 per 1,000 women in 2039 (Census & Statistics Department, 2020). With the rising life expectancy and declining fertility rates, the ageing population in Hong Kong is expected to cause a heavy burden to the healthcare system because of high prevalence of comorbidity and disabilities among older people. To address the problems, there is no set of solutions but preventive healthcare, lifelong learning and other practical measures can ameliorate the impacts arising from the increasing ageing population (Larkin & Larkin, 2022).

In Hong Kong, various strategies and regulations pertaining to the targets of SDG 3 were established to combat the ageing population (Fong et al., 2021). For target 3.3 of SDG 3, which is about prevention of communicable diseases, Hong Kong has been managing well in tackling human immunodeficiency virus (HIV) and tuberculosis. The number of HIV reports was decreased from 725 in 2015 to 447 in 2021 (Centre for Health Protection, 2022). The Hong Kong Advisory Council on AIDS has developed five strategies to set the priority of action for prevention, care and control of HIV/AIDS since 1994 (Hong Kong Advisory Council on AIDS, 2017). Education regarding HIV knowledge and training to improve the awareness and knowledge about HIV infection are delivered to students and healthcare professionals. Improving the universal testing is also one of the priority areas of action against HIV. Moreover, the situation of tuberculosis in Hong Kong is under control (Tam et al., 2018). Early detection, effective treatment and management of tuberculosis infection are promulgated to control the incidence of tuberculosis. Nevertheless, the incidence rate of tuberculosis remains high for residents aged 75 or above (Statistics Unit of Tuberculosis & Chest Unit, 2021; Tam et al., 2018). Difficulties in diagnosing tuberculosis among older adults have been evaluated by studies of chronic conditions because older adults have concurrent comorbidities associated with tuberculosis (Negin et al., 2015; Yoo et al., 2021). To achieve the SDG 3 target of ending tuberculosis in Hong Kong, a clear timeline and protocol targeting older adults is necessary in the future because there is no concrete supportive guideline for tackling tuberculosis in the elderly.

Hong Kong developed two strategic frameworks to control the non-communicable diseases in 2008 and 2018 (Department of Health, 2008, 2018). The frameworks provide indicators and targets for different stakeholders according to the recommendations from World Health Organization, with an objective to reduce premature mortality. To address the incidence and mortality of non-communicable diseases, early detection by screening and education are found to be effective. Hong Kong residents aged 61 to 75 were subsidised by the colorectal cancer screening programme to receive screening service in the private sector from September 2016. Subsequently, the programme included eligible persons aged 50 to 75 from August 2018. Although service providers and receivers had a positive attitude towards the screening programme, insufficient technical support and misunderstanding of details of the programme were found to be the barriers (Chan et al., 2020). Besides, a reference framework for diabetes care in providing continuous, comprehensive and evidence-based care for adults in primary care settings in the community was first published in 2010 (Health Bureau, 2021). It is updated regularly and facilitates early detection and better management of diabetic patients.

Access to quality essential healthcare services, safe and affordable medicines and vaccines for all are essential for achieving universal health coverage, which is one of the targets of SDG 3. In Hong Kong, the healthcare system constitutes of public and private sectors, offering different healthcare options for citizens. The public healthcare services ensure that no one is denied adequate medical treatment due to lack of means. The costs of public medical services are relatively low (HK$180 and HK$75 for each attendance at the accident and emergency department and admission fee of in-patient service, respectively), and low-income patients and some chronically ill patients can have the fees waived. The "close to free" public services allow all eligible residents to enjoy the affordable and quality medical services heavily subsidised by the government through taxation. Additionally, safe, accessible and affordable medicines and vaccines are provided to the population. Over 880 general drugs and 410 special drugs are available at standard fees under the Drug Formulary. Children and older adults can have free vaccination under Hong Kong Childhood Immunisation Programme and Elderly Vaccination Subsidy Scheme, respectively (Centre for Health Protection, 2021; Family Health Service, 2021).

South Africa

With underfunding of public health and underdeveloped healthcare systems in sub-Saharan African countries, availability, accessibility, affordability and quality of healthcare fall behind and have been negatively influenced. The burden of communicable and non-communicable diseases in Africa is an enormous challenge to the respective health systems (Frank et al., 2019; Gouda et al., 2019). The leading cause of disease burden in sub-Saharan African countries was HIV (Dwyer-Lindgren et al., 2019). According to Frank et al. (2019), more than 62% of the global new HIV infections and 74% HIV deaths were found in sub-Saharan Africa in 2017. Nevertheless, increased urbanisation and changes in population lifestyle in many sub-Saharan African countries have led to an epidemiological shift from acute to chronic diseases (Hamid et al., 2019). On the other hand, the total years of healthy life lost to premature death and disability due to non-communicable diseases had increased by more than two-thirds between 1990 and 2017 (Gouda et al., 2019), indicating a rising burden from non-communicable diseases in sub-Saharan African countries.

South Africa, one of the most developed and urbanised sub-Saharan African countries, is also facing a heavy burden of both communicable and non-communicable diseases. There were estimated to be more than 7 million people living with HIV in South Africa, which accounted for nearly one-fifth of all HIV cases in the world in 2017 (Marinda et al., 2020). The incidence rate of HIV in the age group of 15 to 49 was 1.4% in 2011–2012 and expected to decline to 0.29% in 2035 after the initiation of antiretroviral treatment and increase in use of condoms in non-marital relationships (Johnson et al., 2016). To minimise the burden of HIV, the Joint United

Nations Programme on HIV/AIDS had suggested to achieve the 90–90-90 target, which means (1) 90% of all people living with HIV will know their HIV status, (2) 90% of all people with diagnosed HIV infection will receive sustained antiretroviral therapy and (3) 90% of all people receiving antiretroviral therapy will have viral suppression, by 2020 (Joint United Nations Programme on HIV/AIDS, 2014). In 2015, the achievement of 90–90-90 target was only 85.5%, 56.9% and 78.4% in South Africa and the situation remained a huge challenge (Johnson et al., 2017). Furthermore, some areas in South Africa had significant progress on not only reaching the 90–90-90 target but also ending the AIDS epidemic worldwide (Grobler et al., 2017; Huerga et al., 2018; Marinda et al., 2020). South Africa had adopted Universal Test and Treatment strategy recommended by the World Health Organization, and launched the provision of antiretroviral therapy in 2016 for citizens infected by HIV (Marinda et al., 2020; National Department of Health, 2020). To achieve the 90–90-90 target, policymakers and stakeholders play an essential role to enhance the accessibility of HIV testing and antiretroviral therapy. Apart from high burden of HIV in South Africa, tuberculosis is also causing heavy burden to the health system. The estimated prevalence of tuberculosis in South Africa in 2018 was 737 per 100,000 population while it contributed 3% of tuberculosis cases globally (National Department of Health, 2021). A national strategic plan on HIV, tuberculosis and sexually transmitted infection had been launched in South Africa since 2000. The number of cases of multidrug-resistant tuberculosis in South Africa was ranked second in the world. In 1994, South Africa had established National Tuberculosis Programme by integrating tuberculosis service to primary healthcare services. However, tuberculosis cases were increased from 1994 to 2012 because of the emergence of the HIV epidemic and weak primary healthcare systems (Churchyard et al., 2014). In view of the epidemics of HIV and tuberculosis, South Africa had revised the national strategic plans on HIV, tuberculosis and sexually transmitted infection since 2012 in order to reduce the incidence and mortality of tuberculosis. Advanced screening and treatment for tuberculosis were introduced in South Africa so that early detection and treatment could be improved.

Non-communicable diseases are becoming a rising burden to many low- and middle-income countries. South Africa has prioritised the management of non-communicable diseases (Hamid et al., 2019). It had also established tobacco control act since 1993 and revised the regulations several times (Ndinda et al., 2018). Tobacco smoking, especially in the younger generation, had reduced by more than 20% between 1999 and 2009 (Ndinda et al., 2018). The increase in tobacco taxes in South Africa had led to a reduced tobacco consumption (Chelwa et al., 2017; Delobelle et al., 2016). Likewise, the mortality of lung cancer in South Africa from 2010 to 2025 is expected to decrease (Winkler et al., 2015). Tobacco regulation in South Africa can effectively reduce the tobacco consumption and therefore diminish the risks of non-communicable diseases.

Universal health coverage entails accessibility, affordability and quality of healthcare services (Marten et al., 2014). The inequitable access of healthcare services has pushed the poorest people in South Africa to have lower utilisation of health services. The government of South Africa is reforming the healthcare system by developing a national health insurance programme, which is designed to pool funds to provide accessible, affordable and quality personal health services for all South Africans (Fusheini & Eyles, 2016). Under the programme, vulnerable groups will have the priority to access and obtain care. Direct payments have been eliminated and so the individuals do not need to pay for user charges, co-payments or direct out-of-pocket payments to accredited health service providers (Fusheini & Eyles, 2016). The affordability of healthcare has thus been enhanced. For the accessibility and quality of healthcare services, the Ideal Clinic Realisation and Maintenance programme has been implemented in South Africa with the aim of transforming all primary healthcare facilities in South Africa and improving its quality (Muthathi et al., 2020, 2021). After the introduction of the programme, the standard and accessibility of the primary healthcare services as well as the availability of medicine have been improved (Muthelo et al., 2021). Therefore, South Africa is making a huge progress towards achieving universal health coverage.

Conclusion

SDGs provide a framework for all countries and cities in order to achieve better life for people in the world. SDG 3 focuses on the health and wellness. It includes different targets and indicators to combat non-communicable diseases and communicable diseases, reduce injuries and death from traffic accidents and achieve universal health coverage. The implementation of SDG 3 varies in different countries and cities like Denmark, Hong Kong and South Africa as described above. In Denmark, the implementation of free national screening programme for several cancers allows citizens to detect cancer earlier. The coverage and participation of the screening programme are satisfactory and can increase the survival rate of cancer patients. In addition, the coverage of healthcare services in Denmark is effective, reflecting its performance in universal health coverage. The implementation of health strategies in Denmark can effectively ensure healthy lives. In Hong Kong, some preventive measures, including screening programmes, had been adopted to address the communicable and non-communicable diseases. However, more concrete support from the government, such as guidelines and technical support, should be provided in order to maximise the effectiveness of preventive measures. The underdeveloped healthcare system in South Africa is improving after the implementation of SDG 3 because SDG 3 provides a clear direction and motivation for the government to reduce the burden of communicable and non-communicable diseases. Furthermore, the coverage of health services in South Africa is improving and more equitable, accessible, affordable and quality services can be offered to citizens.

Financial barriers of a country can be one of the reasons that lead to the differences in achieving SDG 3 targets. Poverty can influence the effectiveness of the implementation of SDGs, especially SDG 3 (Filho et al., 2021). Hence, it is challenging for countries with limited financial resources and healthcare manpower to implement SDG 3. Low-income countries may not be able to achieve some of the SDG 3 targets in 2030 or even later (Yovo, 2022). Therefore, operational research is necessary to guide public healthcare interventions, particularly in low-income countries. Although some countries may be struggling to achieve SDG 3 by 2030, it provides a direction and guidance for all countries to improve the quality of health and to achieve health for all.

References

Census and Statistics Department. (2020). *Hong Kong population projections 2020–2069*. https://www.censtatd.gov.hk/en/data/stat_report/product/B1120015/att/B112001508 2020XXXXB0100.pdf

Central Enhed for Infektionshygiejne. (2017). *om generelle forholdsregler i sundhedssektoren* [on general measures in the health sector]. https://hygiejne.ssi.dk/-/media/arkiv/subsites/infektionshygiejne/retningslinjer/nir/nir-generelle.pdf?la=da

Central Enhed for Infektionshygiejne. (2019). *forebyggelse af urinvejsinfektion i forbindelse med urinvejsdrænage og inkontinenshjælpemidler* [prevention of urinary route infection in connection with urinary route drains and incontinence aids]. https://hygiejne.ssi.dk/-/media/arkiv/subsites/infektionshygiejne/retningslinjer/nir/nir-urinvejsinfektion.pdf?la=da

Centre for Health Protection. (2021). *Vaccination schemes—Persons aged 50 years or above (seasonal influenza vaccine)/persons aged 65 years or above (pneumococcal vaccine)*. https://www.chp.gov.hk/en/features/18881.html

Centre for Health Protection. (2022). *Factsheet on HIV/AIDS situation in Hong Kong [2021]*. https://www.aids.gov.hk/english/surveillance/sur_report/hiv_fc2021e.pdf

Chan, F., Wu, J., Ng, S., Ng, S., Wong, M. C. S., & Ching, J. (2020). *Evaluation of the colorectal cancer screening pilot program in Hong Kong: Awareness, knowledge, attitude, perception, practice and satisfaction of stakeholders*. https://rfs1.fhb.gov.hk/search/#/fundedsearch/projectdetail?id=1904&lang=en

Chelwa, G., van Walbeek, C., & Blecher, E. (2017). Evaluating South Africa's tobacco control policy using a synthetic control method. *Tobacco Control, 26*(5), 509–517. https://doi.org/10.1136/tobaccocontrol-2016-053011

Churchyard, G. J., Mametja, L. D., Mvusi, L., Ndjeka, N., Pillay, Y., Hesseling, A. C., ... & Babatunde, S. (2014). Tuberculosis control in South Africa: successes, challenges and recommendations: Tuberculosis control-Progress towards the Millennium Development Goals. *South African Medical Journal, 104*(3), 244–248. https://doi.org/10.7196/SAMJ.7689

Condell, O., Gubbels, S., Nielsen, J., Espenhain, L., Frimodt-Møller, N., Engberg, J., ... & Kristensen, B. (2016). Automated surveillance system for hospital-acquired urinary tract infections in Denmark. *Journal of Hospital Infection, 93*(3), 290–296. https://doi.org/10.1016/j.jhin.2016.04.001

Danish Health Authority. (2020). *Strategy mission and values*. https://www.sst.dk/en/English/About-us/Strategy-and-aims/Strategy-mission-and-values

Danish Health Authority. (2021). *National screening programme*. https://www.sst.dk/en/English/Responsibilities-and-tasks/Health-promotion/National-screening-programme

Delobelle, P., Sanders, D., Puoane, T., & Freudenberg, N. (2016). Reducing the role of the food, tobacco, and alcohol industries in noncommunicable disease risk in South Africa. *Health Education & Behavior, 43*(1), 70S-81S. https://doi.org/10.1177/1090198115610568

Department of Health. (2008). *Promoting health in Hong Kong: A strategic framework for prevention and control of non-communicable diseases*. https://www.change4health.gov.hk/filemanager/common/image/strategic_framework/promoting_health/promoting_health_e.pdf

Department of Health. (2018). *Towards 2025: Strategy and action plan to prevent and control non-communicable diseases in Hong Kong.* https://www.chp.gov.hk/files/pdf/saptowards2025_fullreport_en.pdf

Dwyer-Lindgren, L., Cork, M. A., Sligar, A., Steuben, K. M., Wilson, K. F., Provost, N. R., ... & Hay, S. I. (2019). Mapping HIV prevalence in sub-Saharan Africa between 2000 and 2017. *Nature, 570*(7760), 189-193. https://doi.org/10.1038/s41586-019-1200-9

Family Health Service. (2021). *Schedule of Hong Kong childhood immunisation programme.* https://www.fhs.gov.hk/english/main_ser/child_health/child_health_recommend.html

Filho, W. L., Lovren, V. O., Will, M., Salvia, A. L., & Frankenberger, F. (2021). Poverty: A central barrier to the implementation of the UN sustainable development goals. *Environmental Science & Policy, 125*, 96–104. https://doi.org/10.1016/j.envsci.2021.08.020

Fong, B. Y. F., Law, V. T. S., Leung, T. C. H., Lo, M. F., Ng, T. K. C., & Yee, H. H. L. (2021). Sustainable development goal 3: Health and well-being of ageing in Hong Kong. *Routledge.* https://doi.org/10.4324/9781003220169

Frank, T. D., Carter, A., Jahagirdar, D., Biehl, M. H., Douwes-Schultz, D., Larson, S. L., ... & Hosseinzadeh, M. (2019). Global, regional, and national incidence, prevalence, and mortality of HIV, 1980–2017, and forecasts to 2030, for 195 countries and territories: A systematic analysis for the Global Burden of Diseases, Injuries, and Risk Factors Study 2017. *The Lancet HIV, 6*(12), e831–e859. https://doi.org/10.1016/S2352-3018(19)30196-1

Fusheini, A., & Eyles, J. (2016). Achieving universal health coverage in South Africa through a district health system approach: Conflicting ideologies of health care provision. *BMC Health Services Research, 16*, Article 558. https://doi.org/10.1186/s12913-016-1797-4

Gouda, H. N., Charlson, F., Sorsdahl, K., Ahmadzada, S., Ferrari, A. J., Erskine, H., ... & Whiteford, H. (2019). Burden of non-communicable diseases in sub-Saharan Africa, 1990–2017: Results from the Global Burden of Disease Study 2017. *The Lancet Global Health, 7*(10), e1375–e1387. https://doi.org/10.1016/S2214-109X(19)30374-2

Gregersen, M., Mellemkjær, A., Foss, C. H., & Blandfort, S. (2021). Use of single-bed rooms may decrease the incidence of hospital-acquired infections in geriatric patients: A retrospective cohort study in Central Denmark region. *Journal of Health Services Research & Policy, 26*(4), 282–288. https://doi.org/10.1177/1355819621994866

Grobler, A., Cawood, C., Khanyile, D., Puren, A., & Kharsany, A. B. (2017). Progress of UNAIDS 90–90-90 targets in a district in KwaZulu-Natal, South Africa, with high HIV burden, in the HIPSS study: A household-based complex multilevel community survey. *The Lancet HIV, 4*(11), e505–e513. https://doi.org/10.1016/S2352-3018(17)30122-4

Hamid, S., Groot, W., & Pavlova, M. (2019). Trends in cardiovascular diseases and associated risks in sub-Saharan Africa: A review of the evidence for Ghana, Nigeria, South Africa. *Sudan and Tanzania. the Aging Male, 22*(3), 169–176. https://doi.org/10.1080/13685538.2019.1582621

Health Bureau. (2021). *Hong Kong Reference framework for diabetes care for adults in primary care settings.* https://www.healthbureau.gov.hk/pho/rfs/src/pdfviewer/web/pdf/diabetescare/en/15_en_RF_DM_full.pdf

Hong Kong Advisory Council on AIDS. (2017). *Recommended HIV/AIDS strategies for Hong Kong (2017–2021).* http://www.aca.gov.hk/english/strategies/pdf/strategies17-21.pdf

Huerga, H., Van Cutsem, G., Farhat, J. B., Puren, A., Bouhenia, M., Wiesner, L., ... & Etard, J. F. (2018). Progress towards the UNAIDS 90–90-90 goals by age and gender in a rural area of KwaZulu-Natal, South Africa: A household-based community cross-sectional survey. *BMC Public Health, 18*, Article 303. https://doi.org/10.1186/s12889-018-5208-0

International Agency for Research on Cancer. (2022). *Cancer today: Data visualization tools for exploring the global cancer burden in 2020.* https://gco.iarc.fr/today/home

Johnson, L. F., Chiu, C., Myer, L., Davies, M. A., Dorrington, R. E., Bekker, L. G., ... & Meyer-Rath, G. (2016). Prospects for HIV control in South Africa: A model-based analysis. *Global Health Action, 9*(1), Article 30314. http://doi.org/10.3402/gha.v9.30314

Johnson, L. F., Dorrington, R. E., & Moolla, H. (2017). Progress towards the 2020 targets for HIV diagnosis and antiretroviral treatment in South Africa. *Southern African Journal of HIV Medicine, 18*(1), Article a694. https://doi.org/10.4102/sajhivmed.v18i1.694

Joint United Nations Programme on HIV/AIDS. (2014). *90–90–90 An ambitious treatment target to help end the AIDS epidemic*. https://www.unaids.org/sites/default/files/media_asset/90-90-90_en.pdf

Larkin, R. & Larkin, J. (2022). Addressing the challenges of ageing: A global perspective on policies and practices. In S. Dhakal, A. Nankervis & J. Burgess (Eds.), *Ageing Asia and the Pacific in changing times: Implications for sustainable development* (pp. 17–32). Springer. https://doi.org/10.1007/978-981-16-6663-6_2

Larsen, S. H., Virgilsen, L. F., Kristiansen, B. K., Andersen, B., & Vedsted, P. (2018). Strong association between cervical and breast cancer screening behaviour among Danish women; A register-based cohort study. *Preventive Medicine Reports, 12*, 349–354. https://doi.org/10.1016/j.pmedr.2018.10.017

Lozano, R., Fullman, N., Mumford, J. E., Knight, M., Barthelemy, C. M., Abbafati, C., … & Cárdenas, R. (2020). Measuring universal health coverage based on an index of effective coverage of health services in 204 countries and territories, 1990–2019: A systematic analysis for the Global Burden of Disease Study 2019. *The Lancet, 396*(10258), 1250–1284. https://doi.org/10.1016/S0140-6736(20)30750-9

Lynge, E., Bak, M., von Euler-Chelpin, M., Kroman, N., Lernevall, A., Mogensen, N. B., ... & Vejborg, I. (2017). Outcome of breast cancer screening in Denmark. *BMC Cancer, 17*, Article 897. https://doi.org/10.1186/s12885-017-3929-6

Lynge, E., Beau, A. B., von Euler-Chelpin, M., Napolitano, G., Njor, S., Olsen, A. H., … & Vejborg, I. (2020). Breast cancer mortality and overdiagnosis after implementation of population-based screening in Denmark. *Breast Cancer Research and Treatment, 184*(3), 891–899. https://doi.org/10.1007/s10549-020-05896-9

Marinda, E., Simbayi, L., Zuma, K., Zungu, N., Moyo, S., Kondlo, L., … & Briggs-Hagen, M. (2020). Towards achieving the 90–90–90 HIV targets: Results from the South African 2017 national HIV survey. *BMC Public Health, 20*, Article 1375. https://doi.org/10.1186/s12889-020-09457-z

Marten, R., McIntyre, D., Travassos, C., Shishkin, S., Longde, W., Reddy, S., & Vega, J. (2014). An assessment of progress towards universal health coverage in Brazil, Russia, India, China, and South Africa (BRICS). *The Lancet, 384*(9960), 2164–2171. https://doi.org/10.1016/S0140-6736(14)60075-1

McHale, J. (2010). Fundamental rights and health care. In E. Mossialos, G. Permanand, R. Baeten, & T. K. Hervey (Eds.), *Health systems governance in Europe: The role of European Union law and policy* (pp. 282–314). Cambridge University Press. https://doi.org/10.1017/CBO9780511750496.007

Ministry of Health. (2017). *Healthcare in Denmark—An overview*. https://www.healthcaredenmark.dk/media/ykedbhsl/healthcare-dk.pdf

Muthathi, I. S., Kawonga, M., & Rispel, L. C. (2021). Using social network analysis to examine intergovernmental relations in the implementation of the Ideal Clinic Realisation and Maintenance programme in two South African provinces. *PLoS ONE, 16*(5), Article e0251472. https://doi.org/10.1371/journal.pone.0251472

Muthathi, I. S., Levin, J., & Rispel, L. C. (2020). Decision space and participation of primary healthcare facility managers in the Ideal clinic realisation and maintenance programme in two South African provinces. *Health Policy and Planning, 35*(3), 302–312. https://doi.org/10.1093/heapol/czz166

Muthelo, L., Moradi, F., Phukubye, T. A., Mbombi, M. O., Malema, R. N., & Mabila, L. N. (2021). Implementing the ideal clinic program at selected primary healthcare facilities in South Africa. *International Journal of Environmental Research and Public Health, 18*(15), Article 7762. https://doi.org/10.3390/ijerph18157762

National Department of Health. (2020). *2019 ART clinical guidelines for the management of HIV in adults, pregnancy, adolescents, children, infants and neonates*. https://www.health.gov.za/wp-content/uploads/2020/11/2019-art-guideline.pdf

National Department of Health. (2021). *The first national TB prevalence survey—South Africa 2018*. https://www.nicd.ac.za/wp-content/uploads/2021/02/TB-Prevalence-survey-report_A4_SA_TPS-Short_Feb-2021.pdf

Ndinda, C., Ndhlovu, T. P., Juma, P., Asiki, G., & Kyobutungi, C. (2018). The evolution of non-communicable diseases policies in post-apartheid South Africa. *BMC Public Health, 18*, Article 956. https://doi.org/10.1186/s12889-018-5832-8

Negin, J., Abimbola, S., & Marais, B. J. (2015). Tuberculosis among older adults–time to take notice. *International Journal of Infectious Diseases, 32*, 135–137. https://doi.org/10.1016/j.ijid.2014.11.018

Ni, M. Y., Canudas-Romo, V., Shi, J., Flores, F. P., Chow, M. S., Yao, X. I., … & Leung, G. M. (2021). Understanding longevity in Hong Kong: A comparative study with long-living, high-income countries. *The Lancet Public Health, 6*(12), e919–e931. https://doi.org/10.1016/S2468-2667(21)00208-5

Nielsen, J. B., Berg-Beckhoff, G., & Leppin, A. (2021). To do or not to do–a survey study on factors associated with participating in the Danish screening program for colorectal cancer. *BMC Health Services Research, 21*, Article 43. https://doi.org/10.1186/s12913-020-06023-6

Njor, S. H., Friis-Hansen, L., Andersen, B., Søndergaard, B., Linnemann, D., Jørgensen, J. C. R., … & Rasmussen, M. (2018). Three years of colorectal cancer screening in Denmark. *Cancer Epidemiology, 57*, 39–44. https://doi.org/10.1016/j.canep.2018.09.003

Schmidt, M., Schmidt, S. A. J., Adelborg, K., Sundbøll, J., Laugesen, K., Ehrenstein, V., & Sørensen, H. T. (2019). The Danish health care system and epidemiological research: From health care contacts to database records. *Clinical Epidemiology, 11*, 563–591. https://doi.org/10.2147/CLEP.S179083

Statistics Denmark and the 2030-Panel. (2020). *197 Danish indicators for a more sustainable world*. https://www.dst.dk/-/media/Kontorer/01-Befolkning/SDG/Vores-Maal/OurGoals_report_English_til_web.pdf

Statistics Unit of Tuberculosis & Chest Unit. (2021). *2019 annual report*. https://www.info.gov.hk/tb_chest/doc/Annual_Report_2019.pdf

Tam, G., Yang, H., & Meyers, T. (2018). Mixed methods study on elimination of tuberculosis in Hong Kong. *Hong Kong Medical Journal, 24*(4), 400–407. https://doi.org/10.12809/hkmj177141

United Nations. (2015). *Transforming our world: The 2030 agenda for sustainable development*. https://sdgs.un.org/sites/default/files/publications/21252030%20Agenda%20for%20Sustainable%20Development%20web.pdf

Wagstaff, A., & Neelsen, S. (2020). A comprehensive assessment of universal health coverage in 111 countries: A retrospective observational study. *The Lancet Global Health, 8*(1), e39–e49. https://doi.org/10.1016/S2214-109X(19)30463-2

Winkler, V., Mangolo, N. J., & Becher, H. (2015). Lung cancer in South Africa: A forecast to 2025 based on smoking prevalence data. *BMJ Open, 5*(3), Article e006993. https://doi.org/10.1136/bmjopen-2014-006993

World Health Organization. (2017). *Sustainable development goals (SDGs)*. https://www.who.int/health-topics/sustainable-development-goals#tab=tab_1

World Health Organization. (2022). *UHC service coverage index (SDG 3.8.1)*. https://www.who.int/data/maternal-newborn-child-adolescent-ageing/indicator-explorer-new/mca/uhc-service-coverage-index-(sdg-3.8.1).

Yoo, J. E., Kim, D., Choi, H., Kang, Y. A., Han, K., Lee, H., & Shin, D. W. (2021). Anemia, sarcopenia, physical activity, and the risk of tuberculosis in the older population: A nationwide cohort study. *Therapeutic Advances in Chronic Disease, 12*(1), 1–13. https://doi.org/10.1177/20406223211015959

Yovo, E. (2022). Challenges on the road to achieving the SDG 3.2 targets in resource-limited settings. *The Lancet Global Health, 10*(2), e157–e158. https://doi.org/10.1016/S2214-109X(21)00597-0

Chapter 3
Difficulties and Barriers in Accomplishment of HFA 2000

Hilary H. L. Yee and Vincent T. S. Law

Abstract Aiming at attaining the highest level of health possible for all people, "Health for All by the year 2000" is a valuable and insightful mechanism to promote health equity across the globe. It also affirms the importance of primary healthcare provision within a national healthcare system. There are some significant improvements in world's health such as decreasing child mortality and, better prevention and control of HIV/AIDS. Yet gaps in the quality of health and delivery of healthcare across racial, ethnic, gender, and socioeconomic groups still exist in different countries, resulting in health inequalities. The inequalities in the distribution of healthcare resources between and within wealthy and poor countries are the major barriers to achieving health for all. Causes of health inequalities vary with countries, but political and economic instability are barriers that especially affect how developing and less developed countries can improve their healthcare system. Even countries with advanced healthcare systems, the prevalence of chronic diseases and mental health problem are on the rise. Rapid ageing population and the outbreak of COVID-19 are exacerbating more health concerns for the future. Based on examples from regions and countries, barriers and difficulties in accomplishing health for all include finance insufficiency, healthcare system weaknesses, and cultural differences.

Keywords Health for All · Health inequalities · Barriers · Finance insufficiency · Healthcare systems · Cultural differences

---

H. H. L. Yee (✉)
Department of Rehabilitation Sciences, The Hong Kong Polytechnic University, Hong Kong, China
e-mail: hiulam.yee@polyu.edu.hk

V. T. S. Law
College of Professional and Continuing Education, The Hong Kong Polytechnic University, Hong Kong, China
e-mail: vincent.law@cpce-polyu.edu.hk

B. Y. F. Fong and W. C. W. Wong (eds.), *Gaps and Actions in Health Improvement from Hong Kong and Beyond*,
https://doi.org/10.1007/978-981-99-4491-0_3

Introduction

Being free from diseases and illnesses is fundamental for everyone around the world to obtain a good quality of life. The Alma Ata Declaration signed by 134 national governments and 67 international organisations in 1978 showed promising healthcare improvements to all, particularly the vulnerable population groups like women, children, and older adults. Since "Health for All" (HFA) has served as a global policy, implying that health is to bring to everyone within a country or region, with the removal of barriers such as malnutrition, contaminated drinking water, and unhygienic housing (Mahler, 2016).

Health Indicators Initiatives

WHO has developed different framework with goals, targets, and indicators to guide member states in achieving HFA. For global monitoring purposes, some baseline indicators are developed by the WHO, and other intergovernmental and nongovernmental organisations such as the OECD, the World Bank, United Nations Children's Fund (UNICEF), and World Resources Institute. The use of indicators is well-established in measuring different areas, for instance, poverty gap ratio as assessing extreme poverty, infant mortality rate as an indicator of child mortality, and death rates with malaria as one of the indicators of infectious disease.

Signed by 189 UN member states, the Millennium Development Goals (MDGs) aimed to combat disease, hunger, poverty, and inequalities by 2015. A total of 48 indicators had helped to evaluate the health-related outcomes in the MDGs. The World Health Statistics 2015 evaluated the performance of health-related targets in MDGs with respective indicators (WHO, 2015). For instance, the worldwide under-five mortality rate and maternal mortality ratio declined by 49% and 45%, respectively between 1990 and 2015. These indicators showed outstanding progress in child survival and the MDG of reducing child mortality has been met. In addition, malaria incidence rates per 1000 persons and mortality rates in children aged < 5 years declined by 30% and 53%. At global level, the MDG target of reversing the incidence of malaria has also been met.

The use of indicators helps to track essential health-related statistics accelerate health promotion movements. It has helped to lowering infant and child mortality and morbidity rates, improving life expectancy at birth, lowering out-of-pocket health expenditure, and endorsing universal health coverage (Liu et al., 2015; Pandey, 2018; Wagstaff et al., 2018). More people in developing countries can get some key health services such as immunisation, family planning, HIV treatment, and malaria prevention (World Health Organization, 2017). Fewer people are now being pushed into extreme poverty because of healthcare expenditure (World Health Organization, 2017).

Health Inequalities

The Sustainable Development Goals (SDGs) with 17 new goals and 232 unique indicators is a follow-up to the MDGs. It has a more comprehensive global governance framework and targets on marginalised and vulnerable groups (United Nations Sustainable Development Goals, 2019). Despite ongoing efforts to improve health for all, wide health gaps between developing and developed regions have remained the biggest barrier. There are still at least half of the world's population, mainly from developing countries, lack access to essential health services and social protection (United Nations Sustainable Development Goals, 2019; World Health Organization, 2017). For instance, it is estimated that 28 million and 12 million of children younger than five will die before 2030 in sub-Saharan Africa and Southern Asia, respectively (UNICEF, 2021). Ebola virus outbreaks in West Africa show convincing evidence of how inadequate healthcare systems and poorly resourced governments in developing countries failed to respond to early infections or control the spread (Bausch & Schwarz, 2014).

The largest inequality between developing and developed regions is the availability of financial resources. While the developing regions are still working on meeting basic healthcare needs, wealthy countries have already developed more advanced healthcare technology. For instance, developing countries lack the financial support to develop effective vaccines or to purchase them (Tchole et al., 2020). During the coronavirus disease 2019 (COVID-19) pandemic, vaccine has been perceived as one of the most feasible and effective ways to contain the spread of the coronavirus (Gao et al., 2020). However, higher-income countries which represent only 16% of the world's population had purchased more than half of all COVID-19 vaccine doses (Sheikh et al., 2021). More than 80% of vaccine doses were provided to people in high-income and upper-middle-income countries, while only 2% of people in low-income countries received one dose (United Nations, 2021). This disproportionate access to vaccines resulted in higher vaccine coverage and subsequently lower mortality rate in these wealthier nations (Hoxha et al., 2022). The developing countries rely on vaccines donated by wealthy countries, reflecting an inequality of vaccine distribution, and a widening gap between the rich and poor nations (Sheikh et al., 2021).

The promising start of Alma Ata Declaration in 1978 has continued an upsurge in implementation of HFA initiatives in many parts of the world. However, difficulties and barriers still persist, making the idealistic vision for HFA movement difficult to achieve over decades. Gaps in quality of health are seen not just between, but also within regions and countries. The COVID-19 pandemic has revealed widening disparities in infection and recovery rate by race, ethnicity, socioeconomic status, and place of residence, exposing weaknesses in almost all health systems globally (Perry et al., 2021). Through examples from different regions and countries, this chapter will discuss about the current difficulties and barriers in achieving the HFA initiatives.

Barriers and Challenges

Insufficient Financing in Healthcare Systems

Financial resources are essential input to health systems in order to pay for health workers, medical supplies and health facilities (Chang et al., 2019). Health financing is identified as the core function of healthcare systems. Expanding effective access to healthcare services relies on sufficient financial resources to fund health systems. Otherwise, overreliance on out-of-pocket expenditure may result, and hence lead to financial disruption and poverty in the household arising from high cost of healthcare (Chang et al., 2019).

To increase the proportion of the finance available for health and to manage it in an effective manner are core concerns of HFA initiatives. Countries have adopted different health financing reforms in order to expand equitable access to quality health services (Sparkes et al., 2019). Most high-income and developed countries have a sufficiently developed economy that enables them to allocate financial resources for well-structured healthcare systems. For instance, healthcare spending in the United States (US) grew 4.6% in 2018, accounting for 17.7% of nation's GDP (Nunn et al., 2020).

In contrast, developing countries have a much lower gross domestic product (GDP) to allow resources for health. Many developing countries with poor resources still rely on donor-supported health equity funds from the WHO, United Nations, Global Fund, and UNICEF to support their health financing and delivery systems (Chang et al., 2019). Such countries that mainly rely on external funding fail to reform their health system financing mechanisms through mobilising revenues, pooling resources, and purchasing services (Onwujekwe et al., 2020). Limited financial support results in poor conditions of the hospitals, lack of new medical facilities and devices, and the limited number of healthcare professionals prevent people from accessing health services and thus forgo treatment.

In the past two decades, financing for global health has increased steadily and spending is projected to increase to 15 trillion US dollars by 2050 (Chang et al., 2019). However, severe disparities in per capita health spending among countries remain, with high-income countries spending 130 times more on health per capita than low-income countries (Chang et al., 2019). The per capita health spending in Southeast Asia and sub-Saharan Africa is expected to remain the lowest by 2050 due to the absence of sustained investments in health (Chang et al., 2019). For instance, Laos and Cambodia, both resource-poor countries in Southeast Asia, rely largely on donor-supported health equity funds and unreliable external aids.

Lack of Health Insurance Protection

Achieving universal health coverage without financial hardship has long been aimed. People living in low and middle-income countries are not protected from financial consequences of paying for health services. Their countries tend to have fragmented health systems and feature high out-of-pocket spending. They struggle to provide financial risk protections and equitable access to healthcare (Yip, 2019). In Ethiopia, only 16% of total healthcare financing source came from the government and only 2% covered by employers or private institutions (Demissie & Gutema, 2020). In addition, Laos, Myanmar, and Cambodia have healthcare systems characterised by high out-of-pocket spending and pre-payment schemes are limited to civil servants and small-scale community-based insurance schemes (Phanphairoj & Loa, 2017; Yip, 2019). Their high out-of-pocket expenditure and limited financial risk protection features create significant barriers in achieving HFA (Yip, 2019).

However, healthcare systems in developed and wealthy countries are not flawless. Developed countries have higher health spending, but this does not necessarily contribute to equal access to healthcare, quality of care, or health outcomes. Inequalities in the access to health services can be escalated when the increase in total health expenditure is contingent upon private healthcare and out-of-pocket expenditure (Kim et al., 2017). The healthcare system in the US largely rely on private health insurance and private healthcare providers, and prices vary widely for the same service (Nunn et al., 2020). There is a growing population who does not have any health insurance and the proportion is expected to reach 10.6% of the population by 2028 (Keehan et al., 2020). Even those who are insured face substantial cost-related obstacles to care, and people in the US pay much more healthcare cost than those in other countries without enjoying better health outcomes (Crowley et al., 2020). Other underlying factors include high administrative cost and racial inequalities have escalated the situation on not being protected from financial hardship in health. This makes the US difficult to fulfil HFA despite being the most advanced economy in the world (Crowley et al., 2020; Yearby, 2018).

Unlike the predominantly private health system in the US, Hong Kong adopts a two-tiered health system, also known as the dual track system, where public healthcare is financed by general tax revenue and the private sector is paid by out-of-pocket payments and insurance. Because of heavily subsidised public healthcare services, costs of treatment are incredibly affordable and Hong Kong residents are protected from any financial risks. However, private clinics operate based on market demand and often charge higher fees. Currently, there is no mandatory health insurance requirement in Hong Kong. Private insurance companies typically negotiate rates with individual clinics, or patients have the option to pay out of pocket. Nevertheless, self-payment is only feasible for individuals with sufficient financial resources, leading to limited accessibility of healthcare services for those with limited financial means (Schoeb, 2016). To encourage private sector utilisation, the Hong Kong government introduced the Voluntary Health Insurance Scheme (VHIS) in 2019 (Food & Health Bureau, 2019). However, the scheme suffers from limited coverage.

VHIS policies primarily focus on a specific range of medical services and treatments, primarily emphasising inpatient services. As a result, individuals with complex or chronic health conditions requiring extensive medical care may find their needs inadequately addressed under VHIS. The lack of comprehensive insurance coverage in Hong Kong leads to disparities and inequalities within the healthcare system. Individuals who cannot afford insurance may face a long waiting time to access public sector services. Alternatively, seeking care in the private sector may lead to financial burdens as they are required to cover medical expenses out of their own pockets or find alternative means of financing. This situation disproportionately affects individuals with lower incomes, creating barriers that hinder their access to essential healthcare services.

South Korea is one of the few Asian countries that adopt a single-payer system in healthcare and provide national health insurance for its population (Yip, 2019). Since 2000, the South Korean government has consolidated all health insurance funds into a single-payer system. This has the advantages over multi-payer systems in terms of the efficiency for cost control, and subsidised healthcare for low-income group (Bichay, 2020; Cheng et al., 2018). The National Health Insurance Corporation covers almost all Korean citizens and the government decides on the level of cost sharing (Cheng et al., 2018). South Korea enjoys lower health spending per capita than other high-income countries like the United States, Germany, and the United Kingdom. However, Korea's benefit package is not comprehensive because it focuses on curative care such as emergency care, diagnosis and treatment, pharmaceuticals and dental care, instead of covering a sufficient fraction of expensive services like MRI scan (Yip, 2019). The extra bill from out-of-pocket payments accounted for around 37% of the total patient bill (Organisation for Economic Co-operation & Development, 2018). The incomplete coverage of costly inpatient care services results in out-of-pocket payment and high co-payment. South Korea also faces the challenge of being the fastest ageing country in the world (United Nations, 2019). Due to its hospital-centric and curative care-based healthcare delivery system, it was reflected that economic hardship among elderly people caused a higher unmet healthcare needs rate compared to younger age group in South Korea (Kim et al., 2018). The current service delivery and financing system will add pressure to healthcare quality as it is expensive, but not cost-effective, for ageing population with increasing chronic health conditions and comorbidities (Kim et al., 2022).

Limited Access and Support to Technology

With rapid evolution of communication technology, various forms of digital health, in particular telemedicine, mobile health, and web-based interventions have improved healthcare outcomes. For instance, electronic health records not only document patients' health history, but also helps to identify and determine prevalence of diseases and corresponding care needs. The development of an information feedback mechanism can move healthcare delivery towards results-based practice and improve the effective use of resources (Wyber et al., 2015). Using cloud computing and the big data approach in e-health technology such as hospital information systems, electronic medical records, and internet-based telemedicine are common in healthcare sectors in developed countries like Canada, Germany, and the United Kingdom (Meri et al., 2019; Wyber et al., 2015; Zayyad et al., 2018).

Yet, 17% of population in low- and middle-income countries are without basic mobile broadband coverage (United Nations, 2022). They face challenges of gaining access to communication devices such as computers and web-based applications. Issues like interruptions and connectivity to the internet, poor quality video and audio are also commonly found (Tiwari et al., 2023). Although low to middle countries have improved their national digital health strategies, most of them still lack digital health equipment, information and data exchange standards, as well as data privacy and protection (Iyamu et al., 2022; Meri et al., 2019; Zayyad et al., 2018). In addition, health practitioners have limited technical training and experience on implementing digital health technology. Healthcare workforce is found not being equipped with necessary skills in data manipulation, data analysis, and strategic decisions about health technologies. Lack of trust and willingness to learn new digital skills among some frontline workers are also barriers to integrate technology in health sector (Iyamu et al., 2022).

These abovementioned barriers have led to difficulty in producing quality data for effective health policies and integrating technology in healthcare services (Koumamba et al., 2021). Overall, the healthcare technology development gap between rich and poor countries remains large. Without adequate health technology support, it is difficult for poor or low-income countries to catch up with HFA by improving the effectiveness and efficiency of healthcare delivery.

Different Cultures and Perceptions of Health Needs

The influence of culture, religions, and beliefs can significantly affect the perceptions of health and illness, as well as the subsequent healthcare seeking behaviours and health outcomes. They can also influence one's diet, modesty, and even preferred gender of healthcare providers (Swihart et al., 2018). Knowledge and understanding of these religious and cultural beliefs can improve patient-provider communication, resulting in culturally sensitive care and better quality of healthcare outcomes (Swihart et al., 2018). However, religions and spirituality are often overlooked by the modern biomedical Western medical practitioners as invalid concerns, creating challenges to provide culturally competent healthcare (Kahissay et al., 2017).

Healthcare knowledge and awareness can be hindered by the beliefs and perceptions of illness between indigenous and non-indigenous communities. Illness is traditionally perceived to have supernatural and spiritual causes among indigenous people (Jidong et al., 2021; Kahissay et al., 2017). A study examined the wide range of perceptions regarding the causation of illness in five Tehuledere communities in Ethiopia and found that many of the Tehuledere people believe illness was caused by supernatural forces (Kahissay et al., 2017). The indigenous religion of the people in the study emphasised the importance of God/Allah in their day-to-day life to secure health and well-being, and they believed that they would not be rewarded by good health if they did not honour natural spirits (Kahissay et al., 2017). Another study reveals that Nigerians regarded mental health conditions as a spiritual curse beyond the individual, such as ancestors or magic possession (Jidong et al., 2021). Participants in the study believed a person could hire "false" ritualists purposely to trigger mental health conditions on another person. Therefore, people are inclined towards spiritual healing than Western medical care.

Although different religious groups co-exist in the community, beliefs imposed by cultural practices affect preferences of healthcare services. Even individuals sharing the same cultural background may hold different religious views, thus affecting their health status. For instance, people in Vietnam generally adhere to a combination of Buddhism, Confucianism, Taoism, and folk religion (Phanphairoj & Loa, 2017). Family is an important component in the Vietnam society due to the philosophical principles of Confucianism and Taoism. Confucian principles make the Vietnamese mostly respect and follow the decisions made by senior family members (Phanphairoj & Loa, 2017). Similarly, traditional Hmong family relies on the decisions related to any immediate family issues, even health screenings, made by the father or husband. It was found that Hmong Americans had lower rate of hepatitis B screening as they did not want to be labelled as unclean and wanted to protect family's reputation (Fang & Stewart, 2018). This shows that community-based health screening interventions among Hmong Americans will need to pay more attention to the Hmong's cultural practice, in which the fathers usually make decisions.

Migration between and within countries has increased the prevalence of language barriers, resulting in unequal access to healthcare and health outcomes (Al Shamsi et al., 2020; Ali & Watson, 2018). Migrants, including refugees, with diverse linguistic and cultural backgrounds may arrive with complex physical and mental health issues, adding more pressure on receiving appropriate healthcare (Saito et al., 2021). As language barrier contributes to difficulty in understanding medical instructions, people who do not speak local languages have lower satisfaction with healthcare and poorer health outcomes (Al Shamsi et al., 2020; Floyd & Sakellariou, 2017; Squires, 2017). Miscommunication between patients and healthcare providers may threaten patient's safety, and causes poor patient assessment or even misdiagnosis (de Moissac & Brown, 2019; Van Rosse et al., 2016). Bilingual or multilingual healthcare staff can act as interpreters for patients. Studies found that using professional interpreters increased care relationships and improved cost-effectiveness (Brandl et al., 2020; Jaeger et al., 2019; Jungner et al., 2019). A study conducted in Australia found that 50% of general practitioners sought help from bilingual staff and used online translation apps to communicate with patients of refugee backgrounds with limited English proficiency (Saito et al., 2021). However, bilingual staff may not be proficient in translating the medical terminology. Additional waiting and consultation time for arranging interpreters are identified issues that need to be addressed (Saito et al., 2021).

Concluding Remarks

It has been more than 44 years since Health for All was recommended in the Alma Ata Declaration, but the world is still far from achieving the goal. Despite decades of work by multilateral organisations like the WHO, NGOs, and national governments in strengthening global health, gaps in the quality of health and delivery of healthcare remain between developed countries and developing countries. There are several difficulties and blockades identified in the accomplishment of HFA around the world, no matter in low-, middle-, or high-income countries.

Financial difficulty is the biggest barrier for low- and middle-income countries to achieve HFA as they mainly rely on external funding to maintain their health financing. They, in general, have fragmented systems which feature high out-of-pocket payment and lack of the protection of health insurance. Much of the progress in HFA is therefore noted in developed countries due to their stable income that support their healthcare systems. Having insufficient financial source to reform health system financing through mobilising revenue, pooling resources, and purchasing services, lower-income countries lagged behind from utilising health information technology. Without adequate health-related data, it is difficult to identify the prevalence of diseases and healthcare needs, thus difficult to make progress towards HFA.

There is no perfect healthcare system even in developed countries. New challenges such as increasing prevalence of non-communicable diseases and continuing ageing population have posed pressure to eliminate the gap of healthcare inequalities. Different healthcare systems have their strengths but also weaknesses such as limited health insurance coverage and inadequate personalised care. The COVID-19 pandemic reveals the loopholes in the health systems of many developed countries, as they are incapable of responding to emergencies. It has also further exposed the long-standing gaps in public health and weak global health security.

Insufficient attention on religious and cultural differences can put people from diverse cultural backgrounds at higher risk of poor health status within a community. Migrants and refugees who do not conform to existing social norms in their living community receive poorer health outcomes when compared to the local people. Therefore, culturally competent healthcare services are needed in order to minimise the health gap and facilitate the accomplishment of HFA.

Lessons of COVID-19 Pandemic and the Way to HFA

The COVID-19 pandemic has severely affected the ongoing global health programmes and disrupted the progress in achieving HFA. Governments are urged to reflect on their current health governance and financing, health service delivery, public health security, and community engagement to strengthening resilience of the health system. Systems failures during the COVID-19 pandemic have reflected the importance of having stronger investments in UHC components. Achieving

UHC ensures people have access to necessary health services without relying on out-of-pocket spending on health.

Country capacities are varied and those with higher income may have stronger ability to protect people against financial risk. Given that health inequalities exist within countries, governments need to revisit their thresholds of health financing to achieve HFA and build resilient and equitable health systems (Fong, 2021). The strong relationship between GDP and health spending within a country suggests that supporting economic development in low-income countries is an important approach to improving equity in health financing. Additional research is still needed to identify effective policies, such as strengthening supply chains, reducing governments' corruption that can lead to more efficient use of health financing, and working towards UHC and HFA.

The COVID-19 pandemic demands essential and close international collaborations for sharing coronavirus-related research and vaccines to combat health crisis among countries. International cooperation is increasingly being challenged by political forces and geopolitics. As a result, local or national efforts have been constrained to influence better healthcare for people. Countries should have a shared responsibility to help create a well-organised global strategy for overcoming difficulties and barriers in achieving HFA. To accomplish HFA and rebuild a more sustainable health status of global citizens after COVID-19, countries need to work together through public–private partnerships, and innovative sustainable development strategies in healthcare. There is a great need for developed countries and multilateral organisations to continuously provide financial aids, technical assistance, and logistic support for developing countries to make progress on HFA. Developed countries should also revisit their national health policy in order to identify their internal health gaps. Improving health outcomes depends on international cooperation and collaboration by all partners, leaving no one behind.

References

Al Shamsi, H., Almutairi, A. G., Al Mashrafi, S., & Al Kalbani, T. (2020). Implications of language barriers for healthcare: A systematic review. *Oman Medical Journal, 35*(2), Article e122. https://doi.org/10.5001/omj.2020.40

Ali, P. A., & Watson, R. (2018). Language barriers and their impact on provision of care to patients with limited English proficiency: Nurses' perspectives. *Journal of Clinical Nursing, 27*(5–6), e1152–e1160. https://doi.org/10.1111/jocn.14204

Bausch, D. G., & Schwarz, L. (2014). Outbreak of Ebola virus disease in Guinea: Where ecology meets economy. *PLoS Neglected Tropical Diseases, 8*(7), Article e3056. https://doi.org/10.1371/journal.pntd.0003056.g002

Bichay, N. (2020). Health insurance as a state institution: The effect of single-payer insurance on expenditures in OECD countries. *Social Science & Medicine, 265*, Article 113454. https://doi.org/10.1016/j.socscimed.2020.113454

Brandl, E. J., Schreiter, S., & Schouler-Ocak, M. (2020). Are trained medical interpreters worth the cost? A review of the current literature on cost and cost-effectiveness. *Journal of Immigrant and Minority Health, 22*(1), 175–181. https://doi.org/10.1007/s10903-019-00915-4

Chang, A. Y., Cowling, K., Micah, A. E., Chapin, A., Chen, C. S., Ikilezi, G., … & Qorbani, M. (2019). Past, present, and future of global health financing: A review of development assistance, government, out-of-pocket, and other private spending on health for 195 countries, 1995–2050. *The Lancet, 393*(10187), 2233–2260. https://doi.org/10.1016/S0140-6736(19)30841-4

Cheng, S. H., Jin, H. H., Yang, B. M., & Blank, R. H. (2018). Health expenditure growth under single-payer systems: Comparing South Korea and Taiwan. *Value in Health Regional Issues, 15*, 149–154. https://doi.org/10.1016/j.vhri.2018.03.002

Cheung, J. T., Wong, S., Chan, D. C., Zhang, D., Luk, L. H., Chau, P. Y., … & Yeoh, E. K. (2020). Can voucher scheme enhance primary care provision for older adults: Cross-sectional study in Hong Kong. *BMC Geriatrics, 20*, Article 442. https://doi.org/10.1186/s12877-020-01851-x

Crowley, R., Daniel, H., Cooney, T. G., Engel, L. S., & Health and Public Policy Committee of the American College of Physicians. (2020). Envisioning a better US health care system for all: Coverage and cost of care. *Annals of Internal Medicine, 172*(2_Supplement), S7–S32. https://doi.org/10.7326/M19-2415

Demissie, B., & Gutema Negeri, K. (2020). Effect of community-based health insurance on utilization of outpatient health care services in Southern Ethiopia: A comparative cross-sectional study. *Risk Management and Healthcare Policy, 13*, 141–153. https://doi.org/10.2147/RMHP.S215836

de Moissac, D., & Bowen, S. (2019). Impact of language barriers on quality of care and patient safety for official language minority Francophones in Canada. *Journal of Patient Experience, 6*(1), 24–32. https://doi.org/10.1177/2374373518769008

Fang, D. M., & Stewart, S. L. (2018). Social–cultural, traditional beliefs, and health system barriers of hepatitis B screening among Hmong Americans: A case study. *Cancer, 124*, 1576–1582. https://doi.org/10.1002/cncr.31096

Floyd, A., & Sakellariou, D. (2017). Healthcare access for refugee women with limited literacy: Layers of disadvantage. *International Journal for Equity in Health, 16*, Article 195. https://doi.org/10.1186/s12939-017-0694-8

Food and Health Bureau. (2019). *Voluntary health insurance scheme certified plan policy Template.*https://www.vhis.gov.hk/doc/en/information_centre/e_standard_plan_template.pdf

Fong, B. Y. F. (2021). Equitable healthcare systems. *Medicine and Law, 40*(4), 547–558.

Gao, Q., Bao, L., Mao, H., Wang, L., Xu, K., Yang, M., … & Qin, C. (2020). Development of an inactivated vaccine candidate for SARS-CoV-2. *Science, 369*(6499), 77–81. https://doi.org/10.1126/science.abc1932

Hoxha, I., Agahi, R., Bimbashi, A., Aliu, M., Raka, L., Bajraktari, I., … & Adams, L. C. (2022). Higher COVID-19 vaccination rates are associated with lower COVID-19 mortality: A global analysis. *Vaccines, 11*(1), 74. https://doi.org/10.3390/vaccines11010074

Iyamu, I., Gómez-Ramírez, O., Xu, A. X., Chang, H. J., Watt, S., Mckee, G., & Gilbert, M. (2022). Challenges in the development of digital public health interventions and mapped solutions: Findings from a scoping review. *Digital Health, 8*, 20552076221102255. https://doi.org/10.1177/20552076221102255

Jaeger, F. N., Pellaud, N., Laville, B., & Klauser, P. (2019). The migration-related language barrier and professional interpreter use in primary health care in Switzerland. *BMC Health Services Research, 19*, Article 429. https://doi.org/10.1186/s12913-019-4164-4

Jidong, D. E., Bailey, D., Sodi, T., Gibson, L., Sawadogo, N., Ikhile, D., … & Mbah, M. (2021). Nigerian cultural beliefs about mental health conditions and traditional healing: A qualitative study. *The Journal of Mental Health Training, Education and Practice, 16*(4), 285–299. https://doi.org/10.1108/JMHTEP-08-2020-0057

Jungner, J. G., Tiselius, E., Blomgren, K., Lützén, K., & Pergert, P. (2019). Language barriers and the use of professional interpreters: A national multisite cross-sectional survey in pediatric oncology care. *Acta Oncologica, 58*(7), 1015–1020. https://doi.org/10.1080/0284186X.2019.1594362

Kahissay, M. H., Fenta, T. G., & Boon, H. (2017). Beliefs and perception of ill-health causation: A socio-cultural qualitative study in rural North-Eastern Ethiopia. *BMC Public Health, 17*, Article 124. https://doi.org/10.1186/s12889-017-4052-y

Keehan, S. P., Cuckler, G. A., Poisal, J. A., Sisko, A. M., Smith, S. D., Madison, A. J., ... & Hardesty, J. C. (2020). National health expenditure projections, 2019–28: Expected rebound in prices drives rising spending growth: National health expenditure projections for the period 2019–2028. *Health Affairs, 39*(4), 704–714. https://doi.org/10.1377/hlthaff.2020.00094

Kim, H., Jeon, B., Frisina Doetter, L., Tamiya, N., & Hashimoto, H. (2022). Same same but different? Comparing institutional performance in the long-term care systems of Japan and South Korea. *Social Policy & Administration, 56*(1), 148–162. https://doi.org/10.1111/spol.12761

Kim, T. J., Vonneilich, N., Lüdecke, D., & von dem Knesebeck, O. (2017). Income, financial barriers to health care and public health expenditure: A multilevel analysis of 28 countries. *Social Science & Medicine, 176*, 158–165. https://doi.org/10.1016/j.socscimed.2017.01.044

Kim, Y. S., Lee, J., Moon, Y., Kim, K. J., Lee, K., Choi, J., & Han, S. H. (2018). Unmet healthcare needs of elderly people in Korea. *BMC Geriatrics, 18*, Article 98. https://doi.org/10.1186/s12877-018-0786-3

Koumamba, A. P., Bisvigou, U. J., Ngoungou, E. B., & Gayo D. (2021). Health information systems in developing countries: Case of African countries. *BMC Medical Informatics and Decision Making, 21*, Article 232. https://doi.org/10.1186/s12911-021-01597-5

Liu, L., Oza, S., Hogan, D., Perin, J., Rudan, I., Lawn, J. E., ... & Black, R. E. (2015). Global, regional, and national causes of child mortality in 2000–13, with projections to inform post-2015 priorities: An updated systematic analysis. *The Lancet, 385*(9966), 430–440. https://doi.org/10.1016/S0140-6736(14)61698-6

Mahler, H. (2016). The meaning of "health for all by the year 2000." *American Journal of Public Health, 106*(1), 36–38. https://doi.org/10.2105/AJPH.2016.106136

Meri, A., Hasan, M. K., Danaee, M., Jaber, M., Safei, N., Dauwed, M., ... & Al-bsheish, M. (2019). Modelling the utilization of cloud health information systems in the Iraqi public healthcare sector. *Telematics and Informatics, 36*, 132–146. https://doi.org/10.1016/j.tele.2018.12.001

Nunn, R., Parsons, J., & Shambaugh, J. (2020). *A dozen facts about the economics of the US healthcare system.* The Hamilton Project. https://www.brookings.edu/wp-content/uploads/2020/03/HealthCare_Facts_WEB_FINAL.pdf

Organisation for Economic Co-operation and Development. (2018). *Out-of-pocket expenditure on health.* http://www.oecd-ilibrary.org/social-issues-migration-health/out-of-pocket-expenditure-on-health_oopexphtl-table-en.

Onwujekwe, O., Mbachu, C., Ezenwaka, U., Arize, I., & Ezumah, N. (2020). Characteristics and effects of multiple and mixed funding flows to public healthcare facilities on financing outcomes: A case study from Nigeria. *Frontiers in Public Health, 7*, Article 403. https://doi.org/10.3389/fpubh.2019.00403

Pandey, K. R. (2018). From health for all to universal health coverage: Alma Ata is still relevant. *Global Health, 14*, Article 62. https://doi.org/10.1186/s12992-018-0381-6

Perry, B. L., Aronson, B., & Pescosolido, B. A. (2021). Pandemic precarity: COVID-19 is exposing and exacerbating inequalities in the American heartland. *Proceedings of the National Academy of Sciences, 118*(8), Article e2020685118. https://doi.org/10.1073/pnas.2020685118

Phanphairoj, K., & Loa, R. (2017). Comparison of the determinants of the health service system and the health status of the people in the Greater Mekong Subregion (GMS). *Current Psychiatry Reviews, 13*(4), 246–251. https://doi.org/10.2174/1573400513666170720145042

Saito, S., Harris, M. F., Long, K. M., Lewis, V., Casey, S., Hogg, W., ... & Russell, G. (2021). Response to language barriers with patients from refugee background in general practice in Australia: findings from the OPTIMISE study. *BMC Health Services Research, 21*, Article 921. https://doi.org/10.1186/s12913-021-06884-5

Schoeb, V. (2016). Healthcare service in Hong Kong and its challenges. The role of health professionals within a social model of health. *China Perspectives, 2016*(2016/4), 51–58. https://doi.org/10.4000/chinaperspectives.7118

Sheikh, A. B., Pal, S., Javed, N., & Shekhar, R. (2021). COVID-19 vaccination in developing nations: Challenges and opportunities for innovation. *Infectious Disease Reports, 13*(2), 429–436. https://doi.org/10.3390/idr13020041

Sparkes, S. P., Bump, J. B., Özçelik, E. A., Kutzin, J., & Reich, M. R. (2019). Political economy analysis for health financing reform. *Health Systems & Reform, 5*(3), 183–194. https://doi.org/10.1080/23288604.2019.1633874

Squires, A. (2017). Evidence-based approaches to breaking down language barriers. *Nursing, 47*(9), 34–40. https://doi.org/10.1097%2F01.NURSE.0000522002.60278.ca

Swihart, D. L., Yarrarapu, S. N. S., & Martin, R. L. (2018). *Cultural religious competence in clinical practice.* In StatPearls [Internet]. Treasure Island (FL): StatPearls Publishing; 2022 Jan-. PMID: 29630268.

Tiwari, B. B., Kulkarni, A., Zhang, H., Khan, M. M., & Zhang, D. S. (2023). Utilization of telehealth services in low-and middle-income countries amid the COVID-19 pandemic: A narrative summary. *Global Health Action, 16*(1), 2179163. https://doi.org/10.1080/16549716.2023.2179163

Tchole, A. I. M., Li, Z. W., Wei, J. T., Ye, R. Z., Wang, W. J., Du, W. Y., ... & Cheeloo EcoHealth Consortium. (2020). Epidemic and control of COVID-19 in Niger: Quantitative analyses in a least developed country. *Journal of Global Health, 10*(2), Article 020513. https://doi.org/10.7189%2Fjogh.10.020513

UNICEF. (2021). *Levels and trends in child mortality.* https://data.unicef.org/resources/levels-and-trends-in-child-mortality/

United Nations. (2019). *World population ageing 2019: Highlights.* https://www.un.org/en/development/desa/population/publications/pdf/ageing/WorldPopulationAgeing2019-Highlights.pdf

United Nations. (2021). *Low-income countries have received just 0.2 per cent of all COVID-19 shots given.* https://news.un.org/en/story/2021/04/1089392

United Nations. (2022). The sustainable development goals report 2022. https://unstats.un.org/sdgs/report/2022/The-Sustainable-Development-Goals-Report-2022.pdf

United Nations Sustainable Development Goals. (2019). *The sustainable development goals report 2019.* https://unstats.un.org/sdgs/report/2019/The-Sustainable-Development-Goals-Report-2019.pdf

Van Rosse, F., de Bruijne, M., Suurmond, J., Essink-Bot, M. L., & Wagner, C. (2016). Language barriers and patient safety risks in hospital care: A mixed methods study. *International Journal of Nursing Studies, 54*, 45–53. https://doi.org/10.1016/j.ijnurstu.2015.03.012

Wagstaff, A., Flores, G., Smitz, M. F., Hsu, J., Chepynoga, K., & Eozenou, P. (2018). Progress on impoverishing health spending in 122 countries: A retrospective observational study. *The Lancet Global Health, 6*(2), e180–e192. https://doi.org/10.1016/S2214-109X(17)30486-2

World Health Organization. (2015). World health statistics. https://www.who.int/docs/default-source/gho-documents/world-health-statistic-reports/world-health-statistics-2015.pdf

World Health Organization. (2017). *World Bank and WHO: Half the world lacks access to essential health services, 100 million still pushed into extreme poverty because of health expenses.* https://www.who.int/news/item/13-12-2017-world-bank-and-who-half-the-world-lacks-access-to-essential-health-services-100-million-still-pushed-into-extreme-poverty-because-of-health-expenses#:~:text=At%20least%20half%20of%20the,out%20of%20their%20own%20pockets.

Wyber, R., Vaillancourt, S., Perry, W., Mannava, P., Folaranmi, T., & Celi, L. A. (2015). Big data in global health: Improving health in low-and middle-income countries. *Bulletin of the World Health Organization, 93*, 203–208. https://www.ncbi.nlm.nih.gov/pmc/articles/PMC4339829/

Yearby, R. (2018). Racial disparities in health status and access to healthcare: The continuation of inequality in the United States due to structural racism. *American Journal of Economics and Sociology, 77*(3–4), 1113–1152. https://doi.org/10.1111/ajes.12230

Yip, W. (2019). Healthcare system challenges in Asia. In J. H. Hamilton, A. Dixit, S. Edwards, & K, Judd (Eds.), *Oxford research encyclopedia of economics and finance.* https://doi.org/10.1093/acrefore/9780190625979.013.245

Zayyad, M. A., & Toycan, M. (2018). Factors affecting sustainable adoption of e-health technology in developing countries: An exploratory survey of Nigerian hospitals from the perspective of healthcare professionals. *PeerJ, 6*, e4436. https://doi.org/10.7717/peerj.4436

Chapter 4
A Systems Approach to Achieving Health for All in the Community

Ben Yuk Fai Fong and Wang-Kin Chiu

Abstract Health systems embrace the input and output, or outcome, of the health of a society or country. Performance of governments in population health is linked to the capacity and capability of respective health system in the policy, strategy, development, implementation, monitoring and financing healthcare in the community at the three levels of health services in preventive, curative and rehabilitative care. Most systems, often embedded with unpredictable behaviours, are not built with the capacity to understand or assess strengths, weaknesses or constraints in parts of or the whole health system. A systems approach will strengthen health systems and provide a framework for improvement and enhancement of the performance and efficiency. It helps to review the complexity, characteristics and relationships of the entire health system, which is constantly changing for obvious reasons. Systems thinking facilitates the design, implementation and evaluation of strategic and innovative plans, from simple to complicated interventions, for the successful and effective operations in services delivery in the equitable manner to the population. The adoption of the systems thinking approach will enable policymakers, academics and practitioners with scientifically sound plans to attain health improvement in the community. The WHO's framework of health system building blocks effectively describes six subsystems of an overall health system architecture. The chapter will review the systems approach and explore its feasibility and practicality in healthcare, particularly in achieving Health for All in the community.

Keywords Health systems · Policy · Health for all · Systems approach · Systems thinking

---

B. Y. F. Fong (✉) · W.-K. Chiu
College of Professional and Continuing Education, The Hong Kong Polytechnic University, Hong Kong, China
e-mail: byffong@gmail.com

W.-K. Chiu
e-mail: oscar.chiu@cpce-polyu.edu.hk

B. Y. F. Fong and W. C. W. Wong (eds.), *Gaps and Actions in Health Improvement from Hong Kong and Beyond*,
https://doi.org/10.1007/978-981-99-4491-0_4

Introduction

Health systems embrace the input and output, or outcome, of the health of a society or country. Performance of governments in population health is linked to the capacity and capability of respective health system in the policy, strategy, development, implementation, monitoring and financing healthcare in the community at the three levels of health services in preventive, curative and rehabilitative care. Most systems, often embedded with unpredictable behaviours, are not built with the capacity to understand or assess strengths, weaknesses or constraints in parts of or the whole health system. A systems approach will strengthen health systems and provide a framework for improving and enhancing the performance and efficiency. It helps to review the complexity, characteristics and relationships of the entire health system, which is constantly changing for obvious reasons. Systems thinking, applicable to both rural and urban community health systems, facilitates the design, implementation and evaluation of strategic and innovative plans, from simple to complicated interventions, for the successful and effective operations in services delivery in the equitable manner to the population. The adoption of the systems thinking approach will enable policymakers, academics and practitioners with scientifically sound plans to attain health improvement in the community. The WHO's framework of health system building blocks effectively describes six subsystems of an overall health system architecture (de Savigny & Adam, 2009).

Health Systems

Healthcare is essential for living and is a right of individuals. Without health, people cannot do anything, not even the simple activities in daily life. However, healthcare is a very expensive business because it is provided by people, particularly professionals who are highly paid in most economies. A system is an assemblage of entities comprising a whole with each and every component interacting with one another. The constituting elements are interacting, interrelated or interdependent, forming a complex structure. Health systems are formal structures established by the government, healthcare professionals and stakeholders to deliver services by health institutions and service providers with the objectives of improving, maintaining or restoring the health of individuals in the population. Services include prevention and control of diseases, health promotion, healthcare workforce planning and financing (World Health Organization, n.d.). Social, economic or environmental conditions in which people live are also components of the health systems that embrace the input and output, or outcome, of the health of a community or country. Capacity and capability of health systems in the policy, strategy, research and development, implementation, information, management, law and regulations and financing healthcare in the population are concerned with the three levels of health services in preventive, curative and rehabilitative care. The performance of health systems is the result of transdisciplinary actions by healthcare professionals, and will influence the determinants of health and steer health-improving activities. Hence, health systems are extremely important to mankind and have appeared so during the COVID-19 pandemic when the systems in many countries were not controlling the emergency of new cases or mortality.

Health systems are often determined by the historical, economic, social, political and technological factors. They are commonly evaluated by the quality of care, efficiency of financing, effectiveness of programmes, acceptability of services and equity of provision in the community. All governments have a major role in health systems because government policies determine the kind of delivery system for the community and its spectrum of services through direct or indirect financing of the system. They also regulate the modes of care, standards of services and the professionals providing care. There are different kinds of health systems, arising from the political systems and funding mechanisms. Such systems are designed to serve the specific and local needs of the society or country. They are not duplicated in other places. No systems are perfect but they must be functional, practical and, more importantly in the current world, sustainable both financially and professionally because most countries are facing with the increasing ageing population, technology advancement leading to sophisticated services and increasing expectation and demands among people. At the same time, like most systems, health systems are embedded with unpredictable behaviours as human bodies are sometimes full of wonders that do not follow scientific rules. There are vast variations in diseases and their management that cannot be similarly applied to all single individuals in a set protocol. This explains why clinical and public health practices cannot be taken over by machines although artificial intelligence has been playing an adjunct role in medicine and healthcare. Nonetheless, health systems are not usually built with the capacity to appreciate the strengths, shortcomings or constraints in the components, functional structures or the entire system. This explains the underdevelopment of primary care in most countries, forty-five years after the Declaration of Alma-Ata in 1978 to advocate "Health for all by the year 2000" at the International Conference on Primary Health Care of the World Health Organization (WHO) (World Health Organization, 1978).

Health for All

The historical Declaration of Alma-Ata (the Declaration) is a significant milestone in the history of public health. It defined primary health care (PHC) as follows (World Health Organization, 1978):

> Primary health care is essential health care based on practical, scientifically sound and socially acceptable methods and technology made universally accessible to individuals and families in the community through their full participation and a cost that the community and country can afford to maintain at every stage of their development in the spirit of self-reliance and self-determination. . . It is the first level of contact of individuals, the family

and community with the national health system bringing health care as close as possible to where people live and work, and constitutes the first element of a continuing health care process.

The Declaration set the framework and principles for all countries to develop and promote primary care, the key to "Health for All (HFA) by the year 2000". It was later further adopted in the achievement of universal health coverage and equity in healthcare contained in the sustainable development goals (SDGs) (World Health Organization, 2018). "Primary Health Care: Now More Than Ever" was the title of the World Health Report 2008 (World Health Organization, 2008).

The concepts of primary healthcare include equity, access, empowerment, community self-determination and intersectoral collaboration. It plays a core role in healthcare for the population and is a health system on its own right involving various stakeholders in the government, profession and the community, including government agencies, academics, primary care and social services professionals, non-government, community and professional organisations and the people. The system provides health education, health promotion, health protection, disease prevention, lifestyle modification, long-term care, as well as curative and rehabilitative in a person-centred, comprehensive and holistic model (Peters, 2014). Sustainability is the ultimate goal for the health and wellness of all people on earth. It has never been such a burning issue in the history of mankind, being affected by increasing ageing populations, competition for resources for economic and technological development as well as healthcare demands, climate and environment changes resulting from urbanisation and industrial growth, political instability as effects from globalisation in recent decades. The COVID-19 pandemic is a wake-up call to all countries without any exception. Health For All aims to set the goals and values for all governments to promulgate policies and action plans for sustainable health systems in facing global challenges such as the pandemics in recent times.

Systems Approach and Healthcare

Systems approach, or systems thinking, involves the use of structured, evidence-based systems-engineering approaches, which have been found to be successful when applied in industries, but not widely adopted in healthcare. Systems thinking is like a diagnostic tool in medical practice in which appropriate and corresponding treatment follows a full examination and a thorough diagnosis. Hence, the systems approach examines problems thoroughly with better questions before making conclusions or follow-up actions. In the changing world, informed choices or options for effective solutions are required. Operators and managers engaged in systems thinking should possess the quality of curiosity, clarity, compassion, choice, commitment and courage (Goodman, 2018).

The word system is derived from the Greek sunistánai, meaning "to cause to stand together" (Peters, 2014). Goodman (2018) suggests four characteristics in problems that are ideal for a systems thinking intervention: (i) The problem is important; (ii) It is a chronic, not short-term or one-time issue; (iii) It is a familiar event with a known history; and (iv) It has not been successfully solved before. The core step is to understand the problem and major issues of the system from three angles: events, patterns and structure, to get all viewpoints from different perspectives. These are quite similar to the three components of Donabedian model of quality: structure, process and outcome (Berwick & Fox, 2016). Behaviour of health systems is affected by the structure and feedback in the system. A high degree of interconnectivity of subsystems is noted. Continuing change is regarded a characteristic of sustainable systems because systems will eventually collapse if they do not change as the wider systems shall do. However, systems are normally adaptive and they often respond differently to the same input. This explains why some simple interventions do not work in some settings while they function very well in other places (de Savigny & Adam, 2009).

It has been noted that there is up to 30 per cent waste of expenditure in healthcare as health systems are very complex and the processes of care are often broken. Kaplan et al. (2013) suggest that the systems approach can be applied to healthcare to bring about improvements in quality of care, patient safety, client experience and overall health outcomes through the integration of people, processes, policies and organisations to achieve better health at lower costs. There is a large untapped potential from systems thinking, which is applicable for all levels of the health system. There are four general stages in the approach: (i) Identification—to identify the numerous elements and processes involved in healthcare to individuals and the whole population; (ii) Description—to describe how the elements and processes operate independently and interdependently; (iii) Alteration—to make changes to the design of organisations, structures, functional units, processes or policies to strike outcomes with continuous improvement and to promote learning at all levels of the system; and (iv) Implementation—to execute the integration of the new design to enhance the manners in which people, processes, equipment, facilities and organisations work together with the aim to attain better quality care at lower resources (Kaplan et al., 2013).

Causal loop diagrams (CLDs), production system methods, human-factors engineering and management systems, such as Six Sigma, lean, production system methods and Total Quality Management, are used to understand the problems and with the objective to improve operations. They help organisations to continuously identify problems and improve the operations in the appropriate and effective utilisation of resources, and in assurance of safety, quality and reliability of service delivery through the knowledge and analysis of how humans interact with processes in healthcare and technologies (Kaplan et al., 2013). Systems approach requires not only technological supports and devices as in the industries, but also the paradigm shift in professional culture, committed leadership and governance, community awareness and engagement, transdisciplinary co-ordination and teamwork, and appropriate investment of social and financial resources to the health systems in the implementation of changes through collective actions. Very often, a simple description of a problem would stimulate the dialogue for discussion, leading to a new way to see and understand the problem (Goodman, 2018).

WHO's Framework of Health System Building Blocks and Systems Thinking

The adoption of the systems thinking approach will enable policymakers, academics and practitioners with scientifically sound plans to attain health improvement in the community. De Savigny and Adam (2009) proposed a framework of health system building blocks that effectively describes six subsystems of an overall health system architecture. The six building blocks are:

(i) service delivery—to deliver effective, safe, quality health interventions with minimum waste of resources;
(ii) health workforce—sufficient competent, responsive, productive and efficient workforce to achieve the best possible health outcomes;
(iii) information—well-functioning health information systems to ensure reliable and timely information on health determinants, health system performance and health status;
(iv) medical products, vaccines and technologies—to ensure equitable access to these items of assured quality, safety, efficacy and cost-effectiveness;
(v) financing—to raise adequate funds to ensure needed services;
(vi) leadership and governance—to ensure strategic policy frameworks, appropriate regulations and incentives and to attend to system design and accountability.

In essence, the building blocks promote and facilitate access and coverage of health services of quality and safety with the aims to achieve improved health, responsiveness, social and financial risk protection and improved efficiency in health systems. There are many challenges, including synergies, to the systems and subsystems arising from the complex dynamics involving people, organisations and stakeholders and from the interactions among building blocks. Interventions and changes to the building blocks can be simple, incremental or complex, with system-level interventions targeting one or more building blocks. It is imperative to understand and strengthen the relationships among the building blocks and to develop sensitive but simple measurements for continually monitoring changes within the blocks, subsystems and the whole system.

In systems thinking, evaluation must go beyond the conventional 'input-blackbox-output' paradigm. The assessment should be focused on achieving health goals that are projected and expected from strengthening of health systems. Redesigning sophisticated interventions and anticipating the potential effects are applied in system-wide interventions. Among the six building blocks, it is found that information and governance are the most ignored. This has created problems to the system where malfunction can result from missing information. Incompetent governance will affect the operations of the other building blocks and thus it will compromise, or jeopardise, the optimal performance of the whole system. Solutions include strong leadership, broader stakeholder networks, innovative systems organisation and good systems knowledge (de Savigny & Adam, 2009).

Ten steps to systems thinking have been proposed by the WHO (de Savigny & Adam, 2009):

1. Convene stakeholders—Leaders to identify and convene stakeholders for each building block, including designers and executors of interventions, and the users and community representatives;
2. Collectively brainstorm—Small design team to deliberate on the system-wide effects and dynamics of interventions;
3. Conceptualise effects—To conceptualise how the interventions will affect health and the system;
4. Adapt and redesign—To adapt and redesign the intervention for optimal synergies and positive effects;
5. Determine indicators for evaluation;
6. Choose methods of evaluation;
7. Select design for evaluation;
8. Develop plan and timeline of evaluation;
9. Set the budget; and
10. Source funding.

Steps 5 to 10 help to evaluate the interventions and implementation in terms of the processes, contexts, effects and resources input.

Feasibility of Systems Thinking in Healthcare

Healthcare Systems are complex, consisting of numerous dynamic interactions involving organisational structures, specific tasks, technology, professionals and supporting people in physical, artificial, social and cultural environments, and responding to uncontrollable external factors. Change in one part can lead to unexpected effects elsewhere, and unpredictable changes in different parts such as service demand, staff capacity and other resources as well as organisational and goal conflicts of efficiency. Outputs are determined by the constantly changing interactions between the components of the system and the wider environment. Hence, application of a systems approach in healthcare aims to improve overall system functioning and not that of one single or individual component within the system like a general practice, a hospital ward, the emergency department, a pharmacy, an elderly day centre or a nursing home. Moreover, healthcare experts have different perspectives and other principles in the analysis of incidents and assessment of variability in demand, capacity and resources, as well as the subsequent design and implementation of solutions or changes. Practically, people do what makes sense to them in the field, usually based on the current conditions. This approach is adopted to cope with unplanned or unexpected system conditions. Such behaviour is referred to as experience that may result in inefficiency or even "human errors", and should not be developed into the organisational work culture (McNab et al., 2020) whereas the systems thinking approach is scientific and evidence-based.

Scientific research entails observation and experimentation leading to a model, whether physical or statistical to interpret the relationships between variables, or components in the case of a system. A mental, or conceptual, model often occurs in people's mind about how things fit together regarding the happening in events, whether it is an epidemic, a war or some social, biological or physical processes. This notion of event connections is used in conducting and interpreting research, or even professional practice when an intervention is made with due expectation of results. Systems thinking is designed to examine with data how things are connected to each other within the whole entity with explicit models, calibrated against real data. Healthcare leaders, planners, managers and researchers often encounter situations whereby interventions are effective at a small scale or in a research setting as a pilot project but not replicable at a large scale in population health programmes. In recent years, systems thinking methods and tools are being employed to interpret epidemics and major public health events or projects. A scientific habit of mind is being nurtured to better understand and continuously explore the nature of things, such as the improvement of people health and ageing and global health (Peters, 2014).

The systems thinking approach will strengthen health systems and provide a framework for improvement and enhancement of the performance and efficiency. It helps to review the complexity, characteristics and relationships of the entire health system, which is constantly changing for obvious reasons. Systems thinking facilitates the design, implementation and evaluation of strategic and innovative plans, from simple to complicated interventions, for the successful and effective operations in services delivery in the equitable manner to the population (de Savigny & Adam, 2009; Mutale et al., 2016). Systems approaches has the potential in designing healthcare operations for high performance through the understanding of healthcare structures, processes and outcomes, adopting measurement, feedback and control tools for continuous improvement, managing complex processes with the application of modelling and simulation tools, and discovering novel knowledge by data mining, predictive modelling and artificial intelligence (Kaplan et al., 2013).

There are barriers preventing the application of the systems approaches in healthcare. Contemporary culture of healthcare in most countries focuses on works by individual clinicians rather than performance of the systems, characterised by the standard blame reaction to errors and medical incidents. Such organisational cultures, embedded with punitive responses towards any failure, do not facilitate transparency, standardisation or scientific input required by a systems approach. Moreover, the absence of a supportive leadership is detrimental to successful implementation and sustainable solutions. Leaders, policymakers and top executives have the means and tools to promote systems concepts, including raising the visibility, prioritising the application, aligning staff expectations and sharing the vision. They should also ensure the provision of appropriate and adequate resources to attain the agreed targets (Kaplan et al., 2013).

Systems Thinking for Urban and Rural Community Health

Systems thinking is a holistic approach for identifying the underlying root causes and the interconnections between the health system and other systems. It is a functional approach for refining system design or redesign with relevant interventions and has been widely adopted for the strengthening of healthcare systems for both the urban and rural communities, as well as in health management, research and clinical practice (Chiu & Fong, 2022a).

In recent years, there have been increasing examples of adopting a systems thinking approach to understand system dynamics in healthcare and for the strengthening of health systems in the contexts of both urban and rural communities. Rwashana et al. (2014) conducted an empirical study which applied a systems thinking approach to understand the factors of neonatal mortality based on the case study of Kampala district in Uganda. Interviews were conducted with village health workers, community leaders, healthcare policymakers, as well as frontline healthcare workers from both public and private health centres and facilities. CLD was used as the systems thinking tool to visualise the underlying causes of neonatal mortality and further explore the dynamics arising from the neonatal health complexity and non-linearity, as well as the interconnections between different health systems factors. Recently, increasing attention has also been paid on the connections between urban environments and health. Adopting a systems thinking epistemological approach, the links between health issues and urban systems were analysed for the broadening of systemic knowledge of urban systems and health, as well as the identification of the impact potential of local urban governance on community health (Cristiano & Zilio, 2021). Sarriot et al. (2014) have studied the application of systems thinking in a complex urban health system which focused on sustainability evaluation using a case study in Northern Bangladesh. Both implicit and explicit systems thinking approaches were proposed for strengthening the sustainability of local health systems processes. Furthermore, systems thinking has also been applied in the integration of health into urban planning policy and decision-making. In the study by Pineo et al. (2020), the health-promotion value of urban health indicator (UHI) tools in urban planning policy was investigated with a thematic analysis. The results of the analysis, as informed by collaborative rationality and systems theories, were utilised for the development of CLDs of producers and users' mental models.

Meanwhile, there are reported examples of advancing the application of systems thinking in health in the context of rural health system development. Zhang et al. (2014) reported the investigation on the evolution of rural finance schemes in China as a case study of the complex process of health system development. The research team has further suggested that the realisation of complex adaptive systems concepts in the understanding of system behaviours is important for analysing the possible responses to different policy interventions. In addition, challenges to health systems in low-income countries have also given rise to increasing applications of systems thinking. In the context of rural community, there are particular concerns over the challenges to a health system such as inequalities in access to health services and high transport costs associated with long distance from health centres and limited access to ambulance services in many rural health facilities. Design and implementation of intervention measures to address these challenges are imperative, in particular for the people residing in distant rural regions. Adopting a systems approach, the Better Health Outcomes through Mentoring and Assessment (BHOMA) project was designed in response to the challenges in Zambia. Mutale et al. (2013) have further conducted a qualitative study to analyse the status of the six WHO building blocks for the strengthening of healthcare systems in three BHOMA districts. Focus group discussions were held with community members and the findings have further illustrated the prospect of systems thinking approach in the performance assessment of health system strengthening interventions. Last but not least, it is noteworthy that systems thinking approach is an important skill that students should learn and understand its versatile applications. Cultivating the next generations with a systems thinking mind-set is important for nurturing our future leaders and scientists in the community for advancing transdisciplinary research and collaborations towards a sustainable future (Chiu et al., 2022), with the prominent goal of providing the community with a sustainable healthy environment by addressing global challenges such as rising environmental pollutions, worldwide ageing populations, climate change and pandemic impact (Chiu & Fong, 2022b; Filip et al., 2022; Fong et al., 2021).

Achieving Health for All in the Community

The WHO has formulated a health system framework in terms of six building blocks of the systems. These blocks are found to be useful for assessing the process of strengthening the health system in a developing country. They help to identify opportunities for improvement and systems-based initiatives. The success of the changes requires special attention to patients and the community. Such principle has allowed the system to achieve the ultimate goal of serving the people in their role as patients or residents in the community through the continuing enhancement of population health and care experience. It has also been noted that the indicators of the WHO building blocks and the sustainable development goal (SDG) targets can be applied in parallel without contradiction (Manyazewal, 2017).

More importantly, innovation, data analytics and evidence in policies are adopted in systems thinking. All countries should aim to build up the capacity to apply a systems approach as there is a gross lack of transdiciplinary skills, training, experience and research in this area in healthcare. The related subjects should be taught widely in schools of public health and health management, and as electives in all programmes of health disciplines. Communities of practice, networks, professional organisations and journals of systems thinking should be promoted worldwide to tap the great potential of systems approach in making health systems more dynamic, efficient and sustainable with the goal to achieve health for all in the community. Public health leaders should be committed to adopt a whole system approach in community-centred public health to minimise health inequalities in the world (Manyazewal, 2017; Stansfield, 2020).

The Community Health Model—Five A's and Five C's

Community Health is about holistic care (comprehensiveness, continuity) at our doorstep, being the first point of contact for consultation, in the locality where people live and work. It is everyone's business. The services focus on the physical and mental well-being of the residents in a specific geographic community with the objectives to bring the greatest health benefits to the greatest number of people in need, to reduce the risk factors and prevalence of acute and chronic conditions, to alleviate the disease burden and injury occurrence and to promote, protect and preserve the health and safety of individuals and the environment. Local governments are the catalysts that drive community changes through the models, which help to increase the understanding of the inter-relationship of stressors, risk factors, social determinants, disease burden, coping or intervention policies, health outcome and longevity, based on factors like demography of population, culture of individuals in the community, economic situations, available funds and resources, and community needs, expectations and engagement. Community development models can be needs-based, goal-oriented or asset-based, and consist of five components, including socioecological framework, interpersonal, organisational, environmental and public policy factors. There is no one-size-fits-all model. The authors propose the Five A's and Five C's for the key characteristics of a community health model:

- Availability—The supply of healthcare services is adequate to provide enough opportunity to access healthcare for the community. Availability is determined by financial, social, cultural, and organisational factors that affect the utilisation of services.
- Acceptability—Acceptability is concerned about the quality of healthcare and is reflected by the interactions among the providers, users, the community and the healthcare system. It also refers to the beliefs, expectations and perceptions of the anticipated care with the services rendered, where there are mutual trust and service satisfaction, leading to the provision of patient-centred care.
- Accessibility—Being accessible means the timely use of the needed healthcare services to attain the best possible outcomes for the users in the community. Accessibility means equity in healthcare that aims to minimise health disparities. Universal health coverage is strongly advocated by the World Health Organization. Barriers to accessibility include lack of financial means, insurance, service provision, manpower, as influenced by political, economic, geographic, social or cultural factors.
- Affordability—Affordability is the ability to purchase or acquire healthcare goods or service, often with consideration of finite resources and value of the service.

It is a reflection of an individual, an organisation or a community to purchase without unnecessary or unacceptable sacrifices. Conversely, the person should have sufficient finance to pay for the direct cost of healthcare in view of the individual's needs and wants.

- Achievability—Objectives and expected outcomes of healthcare must be attainable and achieved in all health systems in providing quality and timely primary, secondary and tertiary care to the community. The service targets are established by evidence and consensus with reference to the SDGs and the environmental, social and governance (ESG) frameworks.
- Comprehensiveness—Comprehensive care to the community include health promotion, prevention, treatment and rehabilitation as a continuum of care for individuals and families, to meet their personal and specific healthcare needs in the community context. This is also known as the holistic or whole-person care in the physical, emotional, social and spiritual aspects.
- Continuity—Continuity of care is attained by both the providers and users and must be examined from the perspective of either patients or providers. Moreover, healthcare needs are commonly met by multidisciplinary teams of professionals. This model of service delivery can assure the continuity of services, but not necessarily personal care.
- Co-ordination—Care co-ordination is essential in the provision of services by multidisciplinary healthcare professionals. Nurses or community health practitioners often play the role of case managers to ensure the timely and appropriate services to the users. They need up-to-date information, clear role delineation and structural supports to deliver the services at the right time to the right people.
- Client-orientation—Respect for people is an integral part of any community. Client-orientation is advocated in all health systems to ensure the quality, safety, timeliness, effectiveness, efficiency and equity of care in the context of community empowerment because healthcare is basically a people business with the objective to maintain good health and excellent bodily and mental condition of individuals.
- Cross-discipline—Healthcare provision draws the services and expertise from different disciplines and specialties in health, with a multidisciplinary or transdisciplinary approach to achieving the best possible outcomes for the individuals in the community. A systems thinking approach is important for a sustainable healthcare system. Healthcare teamwork, and interpersonal processes, communication and collaboration have found to be crucial in knowledge and skill sharing among members of transdisciplinary healthcare teams.

All governments must be working in close partnership with the community to achieve the goals of Health for All and SDG 3.

References

Berwick, D., & Fox, D. M. (2016). Evaluating the quality of medical care: Donabedian's classic article 50 years later. *Milbank Quarterly, 94*(2), 237–241. https://doi.org/10.1111/1468-0009.12189

Chiu, W. K., & Fong, B. Y. F. (2022a). Systems thinking for sustainable healthcare systems. In B. Y. F. Fong, *Systems thinking and sustainable healthcare delivery*, pp. 1–17. Routledge.

Chiu, W. K., & Fong, B. Y. F. (2022b). Chemical Pollution and Healthy Ageing: The prominent need for a cleaner environment. In V. T. S. Law & B. Y. F. Fong (Eds.), *Ageing with dignity in Hong Kong and Asia: Holistic and humanistic care* (pp. 277–287). Springer Nature Singapore. https://doi.org/10.1007/978-981-19-3061-4_19

Chiu, W. K., Fong, B. Y. F., & Ho, W. Y. (2022). The importance of environmental sustainability for healthy ageing and the incorporation of systems thinking in education for a sustainable environment. *Asia Pacific Journal of Health Management, 17*(1), 84–89. https://doi.org/10.24083/apjhm.v17i1.1589

Cristiano, S., & Zilio, S. (2021). Whose health in whose city? A systems thinking approach to support and evaluate plans, policies, and strategies for lasting urban health. *Sustainability, 13*(21), 12225. https://doi.org/10.3390/su132112225

de Savigny, D., & Adam, T. (2009). *Systems thinking for health systems strengthening.* World Health Organization. https://apps.who.int/iris/handle/10665/44204

Filip, R., Gheorghita Puscaselu, R., Anchidin-Norocel, L., Dimian, M., & Savage, W. K. (2022). Global challenges to public health care systems during the COVID-19 Pandemic: A review of pandemic measures and problems. *Journal of Personalized Medicine, 12*(8), 1295. https://doi.org/10.3390/jpm12081295

Fong, B. Y. F., Chiu, W. K., Chan, W. F. M., & Lam, T. Y. (2021). A review study of a green diet and healthy ageing. *International Journal of Environmental Research and Public Health, 18*(15), 8024. https://doi.org/10.3390/ijerph18158024

Goodman, M. (2018). *Systems thinking: What, why, when, where, and how?* The Systems Thinker. https://thesystemsthinker.com/systems-thinking-what-why-when-where-and-how/

Kaplan, G., Bo-Linn, G., Carayon, P., Pronovost, P., Rouse, W., Reid, P., & Saunders, R. (2013). Bringing a systems approach to health. *NAM Perspectives.* https://doi.org/10.31478/201307a

Manyazewal, T. (2017). Using the World Health Organization health system building blocks through survey of healthcare professionals to determine the performance of public healthcare facilities. *Archives of Public Health, 75*, Article 50. https://doi.org/10.1186/s13690-017-0221-9

McNab, D., McKay, J., Shorrock, S., Luty, S., & Bowie, P. (2020). Development and application of 'systems thinking' principles for quality improvement. *BMJ Open Quality, 9*(1), Article e000714. https://doi.org/10.1136/bmjoq-2019-000714

Mutale, W., Balabanova, D., Chintu, N., Mwanamwenge, M. T., & Ayles, H. (2016). Application of system thinking concepts in health system strengthening in low-income settings: A proposed conceptual framework for the evaluation of a complex health system intervention: The case of the BHOMA intervention in Zambia. *Journal of Evaluation in Clinical Practice, 22*(1), 112–121. https://doi.org/10.1111/jep.12160

Mutale, W., Bond, V., Mwanamwenge, M. T., Mlewa, S., Balabanova, D., Spicer, N., & Ayles, H. (2013). Systems thinking in practice: The current status of the six WHO building blocks for health system strengthening in three BHOMA intervention districts of Zambia: A baseline qualitative study. *BMC Health Services Research, 13*, Article 291. https://doi.org/10.1186/1472-6963-13-291

Peters, D. H. (2014). The application of systems thinking in health: Why use systems thinking? *Health Research Policy and Systems, 12*, Article 51. https://doi.org/10.1186/1478-4505-12-51

Pineo, H., Zimmermann, N., & Davies, M. (2020). Integrating health into the complex urban planning policy and decision-making context: A systems thinking analysis. *Palgrave Communications, 6*, Article 21. https://doi.org/10.1057/s41599-020-0398-3

Rwashana, A. S., Nakubulwa, S., Nakakeeto-Kijjambu, M., & Adam, T. (2014). Advancing the application of systems thinking in health: Understanding the dynamics of neonatal mortality in Uganda. *Health Research Policy and Systems, 12*, Article 36. https://doi.org/10.1186/1478-4505-12-36

Sarriot, E. G., Kouletio, M., Jahan, S., Rasul, I., & Musha, A. K. M. (2014). Advancing the application of systems thinking in health: Sustainability evaluation as learning and sense-making in a complex urban health system in Northern Bangladesh. *Health Research Policy and Systems, 12*, Article 45. https://doi.org/10.1186/1478-4505-12-45

Stansfield, J., South, J., & Mapplethorpe, T. (2020). What are the elements of a whole system approach to community-centred public health? A qualitative study with public health leaders in England's local authority areas. *BMJ Open, 10*(8), Article e036044. https://doi.org/10.1136/bmjopen-2019-036044

World Health Organization. (n.d.). *Health system govenance.* https://www.who.int/health-topics/health-systems-governance#tab=tab_1

World Health Organization. (1978). *Declaration of Alma-Ata.* https://www.who.int/teams/social-determinants-of-health/declaration-of-alma-ata

World Health Organization. (2008). *The world health report 2008: Primary health care now more than ever*. https://apps.who.int/iris/handle/10665/43949

World Health Organization. (2018). *Declaration of Astana.* https://www.who.int/docs/default-source/primary-health/declaration/gcphc-declaration.pdf

Zhang, X., Bloom, G., Xu, X., Chen, L., Liang, X., & Wolcott, S. J. (2014). Advancing the application of systems thinking in health: Managing rural China health system development in complex and dynamic contexts. *Health Research Policy and Systems, 12*, Article 44. https://doi.org/10.1186/1478-4505-12-44

Chapter 5
Global Implementation of Primary Health Care

Yumi Y. T. Chan and William Chi Wai Wong

Abstract Primary health care (PHC) is the key to "Health for All", the paradigm shift in thinking about health as stated in the Declaration of Alma-Ata in 1978. The Ottawa Charter for Health Promotion in 1986 advocated five key areas of public health actions: healthy public policies, supportive environments, personal skills, community action, as well as reorientation of healthcare services. In 2005, the Bangkok Charter for Health Promotion in a Globalized World was signed. It identified major challenges, actions, and commitments required for formulating policies to address the factors of health in a globalised world by approaching the empowered community. Social justice and equality in national and global development were advocated in universal health coverage. Thirty years later, PHC was regained the spotlight in the World Health Report 2008, including putting people at the centre of health, and responding better and faster to the changing world and growing community expectations. This chapter examines the movement of PHC in the last four decades with respect to health promotion and repeat calls to promoting PHC in making social and behavioural changes to improve population health in all countries and societies. PHC practices in the global and local perspectives are illustrated in the context of various models of implementation and their social impacts in the community.

Keywords Primary health care · Community health · Public health · Population health

Y. Y. T. Chan (✉)
Hong Kong College of Community Health Practitioners, Hong Kong, China
e-mail: yuktingchan9@gmail.com

W. C. W. Wong
Department of Family Medicine and Primary Care, University of Hong Kong, Hong Kong, China
e-mail: wongwcw@hku.hk

B. Y. F. Fong and W. C. W. Wong (eds.), *Gaps and Actions in Health Improvement from Hong Kong and Beyond*,
https://doi.org/10.1007/978-981-99-4491-0_5

Introduction

Primary health care (PHC) is the first point of contact between patients and their healthcare provisions. It is significant for the healthcare system and the overall social and economic development of a society. There is good evidence that those with a comprehensive PHC would have better population health. The Ottawa Charter for Health Promotion instigated public health actions in five key areas in 1986, including healthy public policies, supportive environments, personal skills, community action, and reorientation of healthcare services (World Health Organization, n.d.). In 2008, PHC was underpinned in the World Health Report that advocated putting the needs of individuals at the forefront of health and responding more quickly to global change and rising community expectations (World Health Organization, 2008). The Organisation for Economic Co-operation and Development (OECD) mentioned that the more comprehensive the PHC, the lower the cost of providing health benefits to the general public (Organisation for Economic Co-operation and Development, n.d.). PHC generally refers to the first level of contact for the individuals and families with the healthcare system. It is the first point of care that delivers a continuum of care and provides healthcare services as close as possible to where the population work and live. PHC provides rehabilitative and curative management, and copes with the main and common health issues in the community (Freeman et al., 2021; Poitras et al., 2022). It also delivers primary prevention services to the community, including, diseases prevention, consultation, health promotion, health protection, and health education.

Global Primary Healthcare Movement

The Alma-Ata Declaration was embraced at the International Conference on Primary Health Care in 1978. It came into being a key milestone of PHC and public health in the twentieth century. The Alma-Ata Declaration identified the principles and practices of PHC central to the achievement of the goal of health for all populations. The Conference strongly reiterated that the meaning of health was not simply the absence of infirmity due to disease or illness but was a state of total physical, mental, and social well-being. Health was a fundamental human right. The achievement of the greatest possible level of health would be the most significant worldwide social goal. To attain the goal, action and collaboration of many other economic and social parties were required in addition to the health sector. In October 2018, the Alma-Ata Declaration was ratified at the Global Conference on PHC in Astana, Kazakhstan (World Health Organization, n.d.).

Ottawa of Canada hosted the inaugural international conference on health promotion in 1986. The major goal was to meet the growing demand for a cutting-edge global public health movement. The needs of other places with similar problems were also considered, even though the needs of industrialised nations were the main focus of discussion. It expanded upon the gains made by the World Health Assembly on intersectoral action for health, the WHO's Targets for Health for All declaration, and the Alma-Ata Declaration on PHC. Five main public health initiatives were listed in the Ottawa Charter for Health Promotion as needed to attain Health for All by the year 2000 and beyond (World Health Organization, n.d.). Then, in 2005, there was the Bangkok Charter for Health Promotion in a Globalised World, which outlined the key obstacles, steps, and pledges needed to develop policies addressing health determinants in a globalised society by engaging the voice of the community. Moreover, it determined the effective interventions which facilitated in moving forward into a healthier world and required strong political action, widespread participation, and sustained advocacy. The charter stated four key commitments that health promotion to the public should be central to the global development agenda, a key focus of communities and civil society, a core responsibility for all of the government, as well as a requirement for good corporate practice (Poitras et al., 2022).

In 2018, Astana of Kazakhstan held the Global Conference on PHC that endorsed a new declaration. This Declaration of Astana reiterated political commitment to PHC from governments, non-governmental organisations (NGOs), professional associations, academia, and global health development organisations. It used to notify the high-level conference of the UN General Assembly on universal health coverage (UHC) in 2019. The Declaration was also an opportunity to recall the 1978 Alma-Ata statement on primary health care and look back on how far the PHC had come and what the PHC was doing. It underscored the important role of PHC around the world. The purpose of this Declaration was to refocus efforts on PHC so that everyone everywhere could achieve the highest possible levels of health. There are four key commitments for health promotion in the Declaration, including aligning stakeholder support with national policies, building sustainable PHC that adapts to local conditions, empowering individuals and communities, and making daring political alternatives for health through all sectors (World Health Organization, 2019).

Global Situation of Implementation of Primary Health Care

Operational Framework for Primary Health Care

Currently, for many countries, substantial transformation of the approaches in which policies related to health and movement and action are implemented, funded, and prioritised is probably essential for the consolidation of PHC over a broad range of activities, services, policies, and strategies. In order to advance UHC and the health-related Sustainable Development Goals (SDGs), governments and international partners dedicated themselves in the Astana Declaration of 2018 to directing health systems towards PHC (Walraven, 2019). To advance towards Health for All, without distinction of any type, the bold vision and pledges enshrined in the Astana Declaration must be translated into practical actions. Additionally, to achieve the desired results for the reorientation of the healthcare system, strong leadership and concise political commitment at all levels and parties are needed to implement all PHC levers (World Health Organization, 2020).

The three key components of PHC consist of multisectoral policy and actions; integrated healthcare services with highlighting on PHC and functions of public health; and, empowered people as well as the communities. These components should probably be interdependent, mutually reinforcing, and inter-related as they spread on the building blocks of the health system to accelerate progress on PHC. Apart from these three components, WHO has mentioned 14 primary healthcare levers for accelerating progress on PHC, including digital technologies for health, engagement with private sector providers, engagement of community and other stakeholders, funding and allocation of resources, governance and policy frameworks, monitoring and evaluation, medications and other health products, models of care, PHC-oriented research, purchasing and payment systems, primary healthcare workforce, physical infrastructure, political commitment and leadership, systems for improving the quality of care. The above operational framework for PHC provides more in-depth information for every component and proposed activities and interventions. It facilitates in guiding different countries' efforts to strengthen PHC-oriented health systems (World Health Organization, 2020). The Lancet Global Health Commission on financing PHC has stressed it is utterly important to spend more on PHC and to improve financial arrangements to drive and equip PHC to react effectively to advancing health needs of the population (Hanson et al., 2022).

Implementation of Primary Health Care in Asia, Europe, America, and Africa

Globally, the implementation of PHC has been shaped by a variety of factors, including social and financial situations, as well as political will and investment in the infrastructure and workforce development. There is a wide range of social and economic circumstances over various countries and regions. While several countries have made significant progress towards implementing PHC systems, others still face formidable obstacles. The cost of PHC can be a significant burden and barrier for the government as well as the people, particularly those from low-income households (Rogers et al., 2021). Besides, health workforce is one of the major factors that may have affected PHC implementation worldwide. Many countries are facing significant shortages of health workers, particularly in rural and remote areas. Furthermore, these areas have limited healthcare infrastructure. All these attributes can limit access to care and lead to a lack of quality care (Li & Chen, 2022).

Financing

PHC requires adequate financing input to ensure that quality care is accessible to all. Finance-related aspects of PHC include funding sources, health insurance, investment in workforce, and cost-effectiveness.

Cuba has a well-developed PHC system that is fully funded by the government. This system has been successful in improving health outcomes and reducing healthcare costs. In 2015, 42.6% of Cuba's health budget was allocated to primary care, according to documents from the Ministry of Public Health (MINSAP). The government invests heavily in the education and training of healthcare workers, and the PHC system is designed to be community-based, with a focus on prevention and early intervention (Gonzalez et al., 2018). Likewise, the healthcare system in China places importance on managing risks and preventing diseases, as well as minimising the use of advanced facilities that may not be necessary. The Chinese PHC system is primarily publicly funded with the government providing subsidies to PHC clinics and hospitals. In order to reduce expenses of the healthcare system, primary care groups in China are changing their approach to outpatient care by prioritising community health centres instead of hospitals. This is because services at community health centres are 20% cheaper than those provided by hospitals. Additionally, patients are encouraged to seek care at community health centres because their out-of-pocket expenses (about 10% of the total cost) are significantly lower than what they would have to pay at hospitals (around 30% of the total cost). This is due to the higher insurance coverage and lower service fees at community health centres (Li et al., 2020; Wan et al., 2021). Although the primary health care (PHC) system in China is mainly supported by public funding, people are also accountable for paying for certain primary healthcare services out of their own pockets. Thus, implementation of PHC is often influenced by financial factors.

In Pakistan, approximately 42% of the population does not have health insurance. Uninsured individuals are less inclined to seek preventive or primary care services, for example, children who are uninsured may not receive vaccinations, leading to unfavourable health outcomes. People without health insurance often delay seeking medical service when they are sick or injured. In contrast, those with health insurance are more likely to receive necessary care for illnesses and injuries promptly (Hassan, 2022). On the hand, Africa carries 25% of the global disease burden, but their health expenditure accounts for less than 1% of the world. The limited health budget restricts the development and implementation of PHC services in Africa and those countries with low PHC budget (Mash et al., 2018).

Social

The implementation of PHC requires consideration of social aspects to ensure that health services are accessible, acceptable, and equitable. In Australia, implementation of PHC is focused on cultural appropriateness. Indigenous Primary Health Care (IPHC) services are designed to be culturally appropriate and responsive to the needs of indigenous communities. The IPHC services employ indigenous healthcare workers and incorporate traditional healing practices, which have been successful in improving health outcomes and reducing healthcare disparities. Jongen et al. (2019) have identified four overarching strategies for indigenous PHC workforce strengthening in Australia, including Strengthening Workforce Stability, Having Strong Leadership, Growing Capacity, and Working Well Together. These factors can exist on different levels, like the macro, community, organisational, and individual levels.

Canada has established Primary Care Networks (PCNs), which are decentralised entities responsible for supporting the provision of PHC services. They are funded through capitation and operate as partnerships between the healthcare administration system of the province and family physicians. In Canada, the key of PHC implementation is to be accessible to all Canadians, regardless of their socioeconomic status. The PHC services are provided through interdisciplinary teams of physicians, nurses, and other healthcare providers, to ensure that patients receive comprehensive and coordinated care (Leslie et al., 2020). In addition, PHC services include health education programmes, which aim to promote healthy behaviours and prevent the spread of diseases. These help to increase public perception about primary health and awareness in the utilisation of PHC services. However, in countries such as Thailand, India, Nigeria, and those countries with low-income and minority populations, people are having insufficient perception about PHC (Muhammed et al., 2013; Sivanandan et al., 2020).

Health Workforce

Inadequate healthcare workers affect the provision of services, and thus can restrict the access to PHC and may result in low quality of health care (Li et al., 2022). Patients may experience long waiting time and rushed consultations when a PHC setting has insufficient number of healthcare providers. It may also result in incomplete assessments and documentation, which can lead to missed diagnoses and insufficient treatment strategies. Moreover, workforce shortage may lead to unevenly high workload, high turnover rate, and insufficient specialised skills of PHC providers. This may make it more likely to commit mistakes or miss important details, resulting in lower quality patient care, such as inadequate follow-up care and inaccurate dosing of medication. It may further contribute to a high turnover rate of workers because of overwork and understaffing. The PHC providers may then experience burnout, leading to turnover and a loss of experienced and skilled staff. This staffing situation can result in the lack of continuity of care, which can negatively impact the health outcomes and quality of PHC (Leong et al., 2021; Wu et al., 2022).

In numerous regions, a shortage of primary healthcare workers is a major issue, particularly in rural and remote regions. Countries in sub-Saharan Africa have a severe shortage of healthcare workers, with low numbers of doctors, nurses, and other healthcare professionals per capita. Although the African continent carries 25% of the world's disease burden, it has only 3% of the world's healthcare workers. Nonetheless, over the past 25 years, chronic diseases, both communicable and non-communicable, such as HIV/AIDS, heart disease, stroke, and diabetes, have become significant contributors to the disease burden (Mash et al., 2018). In Pakistan, approximately half of the population lacks access to PHC services (Hassan, 2022). In 2019, the population of Pakistan was 223.3 million. However, the total number of community health workers was only 18,009 (World Health Organization, 2023; World Population Review, 2023). On the other hand, although the United States has a relatively high number of healthcare providers compared to many other countries, there are shortages of PHC providers in certain areas in the country, particularly in rural and low-income communities (Agency for Healthcare Research and Quality, n.d.). As stated in the 2011 report by the Health Resources and Services Administration (HRSA), there was an estimated shortage of 17,722 primary care providers in America (Larson et al., 2020). Japan is also a country experiencing a shortage of physicians, particularly in primary care, and there are more physicians working in urban areas than in rural areas. To solve this problem, the education system has taken steps to increase the enrolment of medical students and several universities have introduced the Chiiki-Waku system. This system offers selective admission for students from medically underserved areas. Under this system, medical students receive scholarships but are required to work in a rural area for a certain period after graduation (Yuda, 2022).

Improvement of Population Health Through Social and Behavioural Changes

The Health Promotion and Programs Branch of Health Canada stated that reducing health disparities between population groups and preserving and improving the general population's health are the two key objectives of a population health approach. The authors defined population health improvement as a variety of initiatives to enhance health outcomes. The American Hospital Association argued that effective programmes for improving population health are implemented to raise the awareness of evidence-based preventive health services and behaviours as well as those programmes that enhance the standard of care, patient safety, and care coordination are essential for population health. Finding a standard definition for "population health improvement" is problematic. However, it is potentially a great beginning to create more education and studies in the future (Katz et al., 2018; Shahzad et al., 2019).

Social Changes

Social aspects in terms of live and work of people may affect their health. Therefore, PHC interventions may be a great consideration for population health improvement. According to the WHO, social determinants of health refer to the "conditions in which people are born, grow, work, live and age, and the wider set of forces and systems shaping the conditions of daily life". Disciplines including health policy, social services, and public health have mainly been addressing socioeconomic determinants. In primary care, there are effective screening methods for particular psychosocial disorders including substance misuse and intimate partner violence (DeVoe et al., 2016; Katz et al., 2018). Additionally, there is a rising recognition of how crucial it is for family doctors to comprehend the living circumstances that patients encounter after leaving the doctor's office or the hospital. In primary care settings, more and more attempts have been made in recent years to screen for a wider range of social determinants, such as unemployment, insufficient food and nutrition, housing problem, and illiteracy. People with these issues could be referred to community services, such as job training centres, food pantries, housing programmes, and general educational development programmes. Quality primary care is significant in improving population health through social changes and the primary care settings are good places to examine and address social determinants of health. For instance, addressing inequalities of income and inadequate basic needs can reduce harmful health effects that are related to specific social aspects (Andermann, 2016; Council on Community Pediatrics, 2016).

Behavioural Changes

The maintenance and improvement of population health have been linked to behavioural changes that promote health. According to the WHO, disease-related fatalities account for roughly 70–80% of deaths in rich nations and 40–50% of deaths in poor countries. Adopting healthy lifestyles and engagement in health-promoting behaviours are recommended as the main strategy for population improvement. Health determinants and elements in psychological, personal, economic, social, and environmental aspects that reflect health situations of individuals, can be used to explain the variations in the status of health-promoting behaviours. These factors may influence how well an individual can live his life. Health behaviours of population can be affected by culture, national health policy, social norms, advertisements, mass media, and physical and social settings. In addition to the population health strategies proposed in Ottawa's Charter, family doctors who have the trust and access to the patients, can be engaged in a prominent role in promotion of health and prevention of diseases.

Variables should be taken into account in order to address behavioural risk factors in the promotion of population health, including diet, physical exercise, spiritual development, health responsibility, stress management, and interpersonal relationships. The promotion of healthy behaviours and their support are related to disease prevention. For instance, encouraging healthy behaviours can help people develop good eating and cooking habits because health is significantly influenced by nutrition. A healthier diet is linked to stronger immunity, longer life expectancy, safer pregnancies and births, and lower risk of non-communicable diseases like diabetes, hypertension, and coronary heart diseases. Appropriate food purchase and preparation allows people to have healthy diet. Hence, it can reduce their risk of having diseases which are related to poor eating habits (Spring et al., 2013). Behavioural changes of other lifestyle habits are also important for improvement of population health. For example, a reduction in tobacco use can be useful to reduce smoking-related diseases in both smokers and non-smokers, such as cancer, stroke, lung diseases, and chronic obstructive pulmonary disease (COPD) (Higgins, 2020).

Social Impacts in the Community

Social conditions affect people's health, happiness, and quality of life significantly in the community. Social determinants of health (SDOH) refer to the circumstances in the environments where a person is born, stays, studies, plays, works, and ages. In practice, SDOH can be translated into five categories of domains, i.e. access and quality of healthcare services, stability of the economy, social and community perspective, neighbourhood and environment, and access and quality of education. On the other hand, SDOH can cause negative impacts on a broad-spectrum of health, operational, and risk and outcomes of life quality if they are not addressed. Examples of SDOH include unsafe housing and transportation, exposure to polluted air and water, inaccessible nutritious foods and physical activity opportunities, unemployment, low income, low education level, discrimination, violence, racism, etc. (Islam, 2019). SDOH also contributes to the widespread health inequities and disparities. For instance, people are less likely to be well-nourished if they cannot have access to grocery stores or nutritious components or meals. This may shorten their life and raise the risk of contracting diseases. Simply encouraging healthy living choices would not be enough to eradicate the health inequities. Instead, public health organisations and stakeholders in sectors like education, transportation, and housing must work together to improve the conditions living for the population (Agarwal & Brydges, 2018; Andermann, 2016; Council on Community Pediatrics, 2016; Shen et al., 2021).

Keys to Primary Health Care in the Community

The adoption of PHC as a key strategy has been one of the most valuable and effective principles to improve health in all nations. The goal of PHC is to look into healthier populations residing in healthier neighbourhoods. The WHO has supported PHC as a crucial part of health systems since the 1978 Declaration of Alma-Ata. In 1994, the publication of Starfield's landmark article was followed by research from Canada, Europe, the United States, and other countries with various income levels (Starfield, 1994). It has been established that PHC-centred health systems will have higher patient satisfaction, fewer unnecessary hospital admissions, reduced health costs, and better population health. They also have greater socioeconomic justice. Additionally, these systems have greater screening and follow-up rates for serious conditions and are better in addressing the requirements of individuals with multimorbidity (Behzadifar et al., 2017). As a means to facilitate people, families, and communities to have access to essential health care, PHC needs appropriate development and financing in the health sector as well as in the economic and social sections. The main objective of PHC is to achieve a degree of physical, psychological, and social well-being that enables individuals to engage fairly with their surroundings. PHC is, in reality, the foundation of health systems everywhere (Jonsson & Sigurdsson, 2020).

PHC works in the communities and pursues to deal with the entire health problems of every resident. PHC that covers the promotion of health, prevention of diseases, maintenance of health, education, and rehabilitation, should become a necessary and affordable form of health services to everyone in the community, irrespective of the background of individuals. PHC aims to improve equity in the health sector, lower the expenditure of the public, expand access to health care, address status of health deficits, and, above all, engage and empower individuals in health promotion and care delivery. In 2008, the importance of PHC was reiterated by the WHO in its Health Report, "Primary health care, now more than ever". However, a significant portion of financial resources is spent on secondary health care, whereas PHC has been estimated to significantly lower the global burden of disease by up to 70% at a far lower cost (Behzadifar et al., 2017). In addition, PHC contributes to the realisation of UHC, which was strongly advocated in the 2015 Sustainable Development Goals by United Nations (Jha et al., 2016). UHC aims to offer financial risk protection by providing care without regard to the ability to pay and to ensure that everyone has access to both the essential, high-quality medical services as well as safe, affordable medications and vaccinations. Van Weel and Kidd (2018) have emphasised the significance of performance indicators in health system reform, particularly on the importance of PHC in the implementation of UHC.

Effective Promotion of Primary Health Care in the World

Nonetheless, PHC has been referred to as a "black box" for policymakers by the World Bank, the Bill and Melinda Gates Foundation, and WHO. It is complex, enigmatic, and challenging to understand PHC, which is poorly recognised by many healthcare policymakers and funders, making it challenging to measure its contributions to the health systems. PHC is worth promoting in the world as it is a valuable and effective way to enhance population health in all communities and countries. The healthcare sector can better appreciate the benefits of effective and efficient primary health care from international comparisons of performance in population health in connection to health spending and various aspects of healthcare procedures and structures. According to the WHO 2008 Health Report, the healthcare system can consider attempting four steps to promote PHC in the community. First and the foremost, the healthcare system should implement universal health coverage, where needs of the population are the priority, over financial capability. Secondly, the systems ought to be people-oriented. Therefore, health care will be responsive to the changes in social and local situations and needs. Thirdly, the system should incorporate public health with primary care. Last but not least, it should increase the reliability and capability of the governments through negotiation-based leadership (World Health Organization, 2008).

The government of every country is the key to promoting PHC. Policies and regulations about PHC should be considered to enhance PHC promotion in the community. For instance, National Health Policy was built upon preventive and promotive care in India and the National Rural Health Mission has upgraded 8,250 primary healthcare facilities and 2,313 facilities for first referral in 2017. This regulation focus on school health by making health education a requirement for graduation, encouraging good hygiene habits, and serving as a hub for basic health care. Additionally, the policy encouraged yoga and healthy living practices from AYUSH (India's indigenous medical system) in the classrooms, at work, and in the community. There was a rise in population-wide and healthcare provider health promotion practices as a result of the policy pushes. Ultimately, to make sure that primary healthcare professionals are incorporating and using the health promotion practice successfully, a thorough assessment is desirable (Pati et al., 2017).

China has tried to re-establish its PHC following the Health Care Reform in 2009. Over the last decade, China has built an extensive primary healthcare infrastructure composed of village clinics, township centres, and community health centres in the urban areas with over 400,000 trained general practitioners (GPs). It has also established a national essential medicines system and committed itself to improving PHC and public health services providing a range of primary care services for common ailments, chronic diseases, and preventive care such as vaccinations. It has shown that, during the outbreak of COVID-19, Chinese GPs played a significant role in gatekeeping and clinical responses in a pandemic, and changed their clinical practice to support and educate the community (Tse et al., 2020). Nonetheless, they are perceived as poorly equipped and of low quality by the general public because the culture of over-investigation driven by financial incentives of the health system has led to a belief that good care should be high tech and aggressive treatment (Mash et al., 2015). Governance of primary care is another problem with fragmented medical insurance coverage by different state bodies resulted in differing levels of coverage and access to health care by different insurance schemes. To address these issues, standardised validated tools such as the Primary Care Assessment Tool to regularly monitor primary care activities, integration of person-centred thinking into primary care and teaching GPs an integrated comprehensive approach, will be needed (Chen et al., 2020; Shi et al., 2020).

Moreover, other parties in the communities are significant stakeholders to the promotion of PHC. It is suggested that non-governmental organisations should be engaged to introduce primary health care to the general public. For example, knowledge, perception, and awareness in the population about disease risk factors can be increased through health talks, workshops, booth games, etc. Besides, these organisations can encourage preventive behaviour to the public by community programmes, such as cancer screenings and vaccinations. They can also guide the public towards appropriate primary healthcare resources in health promotion and education. The resulting and enhanced social support has been seen to help people meet their physical and emotional requirements as well as buffer the effects of stressful events related to the quality of life.

References

Agarwal, G., & Brydges, M. (2018). Effects of a community health promotion program on social factors in a vulnerable older adult population residing in social housing. *BMC Geriatrics, 18*, Article 95. https://doi.org/10.1186/s12877-018-0764-9

Agency for Healthcare Research and Quality. (n.d.). Primary care workforce facts and stats. https://www.ahrq.gov/research/findings/factsheets/primary/pcworkforce/index.html

Andermann, A. (2016). Taking action on the social determinants of health in clinical practice: A framework for health professionals. *Canadian Medical Assocaition Journal, 188*(17–18), E474–E483. https://doi.org/10.1503/cmaj.160177

Behzadifar, M., Mirghaed, M. T., & Aryankhesal, A. (2017). Primary health care: An important approach for health sector, missed in Iran's health system evolution plan. *Iranian Journal of Public Health, 46*(9), 1307–1308. https://ijph.tums.ac.ir/index.php/ijph/article/view/11013/5699

Chen, A., Feng, S., Zhang, L., & Shi, L. (2020). Comparison of patients' perceived quality of primary care between urban and rural community health centers in Guangdong, China. *International Journal of Environmental Research and Public Health, 17*(13), Article 4898. https://doi.org/10.3390/ijerph17134898

Council on Community Pediatrics. (2016). Poverty and child health in the United States. *Pediatrics, 137*(4), Article e20160339. https://doi.org/10.1542/peds.2016-0339

DeVoe, J. E., Bazemore, A. W., Cottrell, E. K., Likumahuwa-Ackman, S., Grandmont, J., Spach, N., & Gold, R. (2016). Perspectives in primary care: A conceptual framework and path for integrating social determinants of health into primary care practice. *Annals of Family Medicine, 14*(2), 104–108. https://doi.org/10.1370/afm.1903

Freeman, T., Baum, F., Javanparast, S., Labonté, R., Lawless, A., & Barton, E. (2021). The contribution of group work to the goals of comprehensive primary health care. *Health Promotion Journal of Australia, 32*(1), 126–136. https://doi.org/10.1002/hpja.323

Gonzalez, A. M. G., Lopez, R. G., Muniz, M. A., Ledo, M. J. V., Lugo, N. D. L. C. S., & Santiesteban, M. V. (2018). Economic considerations on Cuban public health and its relationship with universal health/Consideraciones economicas sobre la salud publica cubana y su relacion con la salud universal/Consideracoes economicas sobre a saude publica cubana e sua relacao com a saude universal. *Revista Panamericana de Salud Publica, 42*(1), NA-NA.

Hanson, K., Brikci, N., Erlangga, D., Alebachew, A., De Allegri, M., Balabanova, D., & Wurie, H. (2022). The lancet global health commission on financing primary health care: Putting people at the centre. *The Lancet Global Health, 10*(5), e715–e772. https://doi.org/10.1016/S2214-109X(22)00005-5

Hassan, O. (2022, March 7). *Access to primary health care in Pakistan*. Memon Medical Institute Hospital. https://mmi.edu.pk/blog/access-to-primary-health-care-in-pakistan/

Higgins, S. T. (2020). Behavior change, health, and health disparities 2020: Some current challenges in tobacco control and regulatory science. *Preventive Medicine, 140*, Article 106287. https://doi.org/10.1016/j.ypmed.2020.106287

Islam, M. M. (2019). Social determinants of health and related inequalities: Confusion and implications. *Frontiers in Public Health, 7*, Article 11. https://doi.org/10.3389/fpubh.2019.00011

Jha, A., Godlee, F., & Abbasi, K. (2016). Delivering on the promise of universal health coverage. *BMJ, 353*, Article i2216. https://doi.org/10.1136/bmj.i2216

Jongen, C., McCalman, J., Campbell, S., & Fagan, R. (2019). Working well: Strategies to strengthen the workforce of the Indigenous primary healthcare sector. *BMC Health Services Research, 19*(1), 1–12.

Jonsson, J. S., & Sigurdsson, E. L. (2020). The power of primary health care. *Scandinavian Journal of Primary Health Care, 38*(4), 361–362. https://doi.org/10.1080/02813432.2020.1841507

Katz, A., Chateau, D., Enns, J. E., Valdivia, J., Taylor, C., Walld, R., & McCulloch, S. (2018). Association of the social determinants of health with quality of primary care. *Annals of Family Medicine, 16*(3), 217–224. https://doi.org/10.1370/afm.2236

Larson, E. H., Andrilla, C. H. A., & Garberson, L. A. (2020). Supply and distribution of the primary care workforce in rural America: 2019. *Policy brief, 167*.

Leong, S. L., Teoh, S. L., Fun, W. H., & Lee, S. W. H. (2021). Task shifting in primary care to tackle healthcare worker shortages: An umbrella review. *European Journal of General Practice, 27*(1), 198–210.

Leslie, M., Khayatzadeh-Mahani, A., Birdsell, J., Forest, P. G., Henderson, R., Gray, R. P., Schraeder, K., Seidel, J., Zwicker, J., & Green, L. A. (2020). An implementation history of primary health care transformation: Alberta's primary care networks and the people, time and culture of change. *BMC Family Practice, 21*(1), 1–20.

Li, B., & Chen, J. (2022). Barriers to community-based primary health care delivery in urban China: A Systematic Mapping Review. *International Journal of Environmental Research and Public Health, 19*(19), 12701.

Li, X., Krumholz, H. M., Yip, W., Cheng, K. K., De Maeseneer, J., Meng, Q., Mossialos, E., Li, C., Lu, J., Su, M., Zhang, Q., Xu, D. R., Li, L., Normand, S. T., Peto, R., Li, J., Wang, Z., Yan, H., Gao, R., & Hu, S. (2020). Quality of primary health care in China: Challenges and recommendations. *Lancet (london, England), 395*(10239), 1802–1812. https://doi.org/10.1016/S0140-6736(20)30122-7

Mash, R., Almeida, M., Wong, W. C. W., Kumar, R., & Von Pressentin, K. (2015). The roles and training of primary care doctors: China, India, Brazil and South Africa. *Human Resources for Health, 13*, Article 93. https://doi.org/10.1186/s12960-015-0090-7

Mash, R., Howe, A., Olayemi, O., Makwero, M., Ray, S., Zerihun, M., Gyuse, A., & Goodyear-Smith, F. (2018). Reflections on family medicine and primary healthcare in sub-Saharan Africa. *BMJ Global Health, 3*(Suppl 3), e000662.

Muhammed, K. A., Umeh, K. N., Nasir, S. M., & Suleiman, I. H. (2013). Understanding the barriers to the utilization of primary health care in a low-income setting: implications for health policy and planning. *Journal of public health in Africa, 4*(2).

Organisation for Economic Co-operation and Development. (n.d.). *Primary care.* https://www.oecd.org/health/primary-care.htm

Pati, S., Chauhan, A., Mahapatra, S., & Sinha, R. (2017). Practicing health promotion in primary care–a reflective enquiry. *Journal of Preventive Medicine and Hygiene, 58*(4), E288-E293. https://doi.org/10.15167/2421-4248/jpmh2017.58.4.749

Poitras, M.-E., Vaillancourt, V. T., Canapé, A., Boudreault, A., Bacon, K., & Hatcher, S. (2022). Culturally safe interventions in primary care for the management of chronic diseases of urban Indigenous People: A scoping review. *Family Medicine and Community Health, 10*(Suppl 1), Article e001606. https://doi.org/10.1136/fmch-2022-001606

Rogers, H. L., Pablo Hernando, S., Núñez-Fernández, S., Sanchez, A., Martos, C., Moreno, M., & Grandes, G. (2021). Barriers and facilitators in the implementation of an evidence-based health promotion intervention in a primary care setting: a qualitative study. *Journal of health organization and management, ahead-of-print*(ahead-of-print), 349–367. https://doi.org/10.1108/JHOM-12-2020-0512

Shahzad, M., Upshur, R., Donnelly, P., Bharmal, A., Wei, X., Feng, P., & Brown, A. D. (2019). A population-based approach to integrated healthcare delivery: A scoping review of clinical care and public health collaboration. *BMC Public Health, 19*, Article 708. https://doi.org/10.1186/s12889-019-7002-z

Shen, W.-T., Yu, X., Zhong, S.-B., & Ge, H.-R. (2021). Population health effects of air pollution: Fresh evidence from China health and retirement longitudinal survey. *Frontiers in Public Health, 9*, Article 779552. https://doi.org/10.3389/fpubh.2021.779552

Shi, J., Jin, H., Shi, L., Chen, C., Ge, X., Lu, Y., Zhang, H., Wang, Z., & Yu, D. (2020). The quality of primary care in community health centers: Comparison among urban, suburban and rural users in Shanghai. *China. BMC Family Practice, 21*, 178. https://doi.org/10.1186/s12875-020-01250-6

Sivanandan, A., Kumar, S. G., & Krishnamoorthy, Y. (2020). Awareness and preference in utilizing primary health-care services from rural health center as first point-of-care: A community-based cross-sectional study in South India. *Journal of Education and Health Promotion, 9*, 85. https://doi.org/10.4103/jehp.jehp_593_19

Spring, B., Ockene, J. K., Gidding, S. S., Mozaffarian, D., Moore, S., Rosal, M. C., Brown, M. D., Vafiadis, D. K., Cohen, D. L., & Burke, L. E. (2013). Better population health through behavior change in adults: A call to action. *Circulation, 128*(19), 2169–2176. https://doi.org/10.1161/01.cir.0000435173.25936.e1

Starfield, B. (1994). Is primary care essential? *Lancet, 344*(8930), 1129–1133. https://doi.org/10.1016/S0140-6736(94)90634-3

Tse, D. M. S., Li, Z., Lu, Y., Li, Y., Liu, Y., & Wong, W. C .W. (2020). Fighting against COVID-19: Preparedness and implications on clinical practice in primary care in China. *BMC Family Practice, 21*, Article 271. https://doi.org/10.1186/s12875-020-01343-2

Van Weel, C., & Kidd, M. R. (2018). Why strengthening primary health care is essential to achieving universal health coverage. *Canadian Medical Assocaition Journal, 190*(15), E463–E466. https://doi.org/10.1503/cmaj.170784

Walraven, G. (2019). The 2018 Astana declaration on primary health care, is it useful? Journal of Global Health, 9(1). *Article, 010313*,. https://doi.org/10.7189/jogh.09.010313

Wan, G., Wei, X., Yin, H., Qian, Z., Wang, T., & Wang, L. (2021). The trend in primary health care preference in China: A cohort study of 12,508 residents from 2012 to 2018. *BMC Health Services Research, 21*, 1–15.

World Health Organization. (2008). *The world health report 2008 : Primary health care now more than ever*. https://apps.who.int/iris/handle/10665/43949

World Health Organization. (2019). *Declaration of Astana: Global conference on primary health care: Astana, Kazakhstan, 25 and 26 October 2018.* https://apps.who.int/iris/handle/10665/328123

World Health Organization. (2020). *Operational framework for primary health care: Transforming vision into action.* https://apps.who.int/iris/handle/10665/337641

World Health Organization. (2022). *The 1st International Conference on Health Promotion, Ottawa, 1986.* https://www.who.int/teams/health-promotion/enhanced-wellbeing/first-global-conference

World Health Organization. (2023). *Global Health Workforce Statistics Database.* World Health Organization. https://www.who.int/data/gho/data/themes/topics/health-workforce

World Population Review. (2023). *2023 world population by country* . 2023 World Population by Country. https://worldpopulationreview.com/

Wu, Y., Zhang, Z., Zhao, N., Yan, Y., Zhao, L., Song, Q., Ma, R., Li, C., Li, J, Liu, S., Bi, X., & Zhang, Z. (2022). Primary health care in China: A decade of development after the 2009 health care reform. *Health Care Science.*

Yuda, M. (2022). Healthcare utilization under a comprehensive public welfare program: Evidence from Japan. *Frontiers in Public Health, 10,* 895679. https://doi.org/10.3389/fpubh.2022.895679

Part II
Gaps and Actions in Health Improvement

Chapter 6
Cultural Shift in Healthcare and Ethnic Inequality—Professional Responsibilities

Francesca Quattri

Abstract The 13th target of the United Nation's Sustainability Development Goal 3 calls for strengthening "the capacity of all countries for early warning, risk reduction and management of national and global health risks". With the help of examples and practical solutions, this chapter explores two issues regarding this target, inclusiveness and culture, focusing on maternity care in the UK by the NHS. The latest studies on maternal care in the UK show health inequalities affecting safety in childbirth that particularly endanger ethnic minorities. Similarly, social reports display health inequalities triggered by social disparities. Safety reports, national guidelines and recommendations will be critically assessed to understand the preventable measures that should be implemented and what prevents them from being implemented. The chapter looks at some medical training material and the lack of socially inclusive tools for clinical students to practice medicine inclusively. A section discusses clinical trials, which are fundamental in public health for early warnings, effective cures and risk reduction but often lack inclusiveness. The author examines the notion of culture as a social construct and the coexistence of different, sometimes conflicting cultures in clinical settings. It is argued that culture should be nurtured with counterintuitive arguments and by questioning own and system biases. Cultural shifts that can provide respectful, sustainable and healthy working conditions to healthcare professionals to provide quality and safety of care to their patients are hard to achieve. This chapter explores some viable options for cultural shifts to happen.

Keywords Health inequalities · Maternity care · Inequality · Healthcare

---

F. Quattri (✉)
Department of Population Health Sciences, University of Leicester, Leicester, UK
e-mail: quattri.francesca@gmail.com

B. Y. F. Fong and W. C. W. Wong (eds.), *Gaps and Actions in Health Improvement from Hong Kong and Beyond*,
https://doi.org/10.1007/978-981-99-4491-0_6

Introduction

The World Health Organization defines health inequalities as "differences in health status or in the distribution of health determinants between different population groups" (World Health Organisation, 2014 Health Impact Assessment Glossary of Terms Used). The 13th target of the United Nation's Sustainability Development Goal 3 reminds us of this definition as it calls for strengthening "the capacity of all countries for early warning, risk reduction, and management of national and global health risks". It calls for early intervention at community, national and international levels to prevent health scares and put forward feasible and long-term actions to ensure inclusiveness and fairness in the distribution and access of medical and clinical resources to prevent and cure avoidable health risks and diseases around the globe. This target strives to avoid avoidable casualties and to narrow the gap between rich and poor so that everybody, as it is our fundamental human right, can access care when we need it, regardless of our social status or colour of the skin, ability or disability.

This chapter mainly focuses on health inequalities in maternity care. The right to life is a human right, and birth is a universal phenomenon. Maternity care, which represents a complex kind of care spanning different stages of care (antenatal, intrapartum, postnatal care), shall provide safe and quality care throughout these stages. The following sections focus on the stark contrast of healthcare safety in pregnancy for women of different ethnic minorities in the United Kingdom (UK). They show different inequalities in medical settings that affect patients and healthcare professionals (HCPs). Possible solutions are proposed, including responses by some latest research and responses by national guidelines and recommendations in the UK. The supported argument is that a change of culture is feasible and that it starts with guaranteeing healthcare practitioners safe working environments.

Equality—a Legal Duty

Racial equality is a moral and, most importantly, a legal duty. In the UK, the right to be dignified as a human being is protected by a body of articles in the UK Constitution. These articles are meant to protect the right to life.

Article 2 prohibits inhuman and degrading treatments, the same as Article 3, which, in healthcare, will manifest as ill-treating, negligently treating or non-adequately treating patients. Violations of Article 3 include carrying out procedures without the patient's consent, using physical abuse, racist abuse and discriminatory behaviour against that patient, failure to provide care or acts of negligence towards that client.

Article 8 protects the right to private and family life. Lack of patient consent, including the patient's decision about where, how and with whom to give birth, represents a violation of this article.

Article 9 protects the right to freedom of thought, conscience and religion, which includes religion-led decisions made in pregnancy and childbirth—discriminations based on faith and creed are therefore punishable.

Article 14 prohibits discrimination based on race, colour, language, religion and national or social background.

The UK Constitution is not the only regulator in matters of equality. The UK Equality Act 2010 legally protects people from discrimination in the workplace and the broader society. It also states that discrimination against people based on their membership in a group with protected characteristics is unlawful. These characteristics include age, disability, gender reassignment, marriage and civil partnership, pregnancy and maternity, religion and belief, sex, sexual orientation and race. Despite the presence of a solid legal framework protecting, among others, the rights of childbearing people in the UK, health and safety in maternity care in the UK is profoundly different based on ethnicity and what comes with it.

In the following section, it is argued that mothers and babies from specific communities and with certain backgrounds in the UK are more vulnerable to certain conditions, they might be disadvantaged, or they might get overlooked by the system of care, putting their health and the health of their babies in danger.

Health Inequalities in Maternity Care in the UK—an Overview

The UK population is knowingly multicultural and multi-ethnic—13% of the UK's total population identifies as being from a BAME (Black, Asian and Minority Ethnic) background (Knight et al., 2020a; Royal College of Obstetricians and Gynaecologists, n.d.). The recent and ongoing COVID-19 pandemic has severely affected entire populations, but the worse outcomes in maternity care have been registered among BAME people. At the pandemic's peak, 55% of individuals admitted to critical care in the UK for COVID-19 were from BAME communities, and these individuals were also at a higher risk of dying from the disease (Royal College of Obstetricians and Gynaecologists, 2020b).

Several research outputs have been pivotal in quantifying this silent toll on mothers and babies, particularly the UKOSS study and the MBRRACE-UK reports. The UKOSS study, conducted by Marian Knight and her team at the University of Oxford (Knight et al., 2020b), was the largest population-based cohort of pregnant people admitted to the hospital with COVID-19 to date. The study considered the outcomes of pregnant women and their babies admitted to hospitals in the UK between 1st March and 14th April 2020. At that time, 427 women were admitted to the hospital. 4.9 of every 1,000 women were admitted to give birth, and 1 in 10 received intensive care. The study revealed that a high proportion of these pregnant inpatients, 55%, were black or from ethnic minority groups and that, according to the investigation, black pregnant women are eight times more likely to get admitted to the hospital while infected with COVID-19 (3,135 maternities; 89 admitted while infected). Asian women are four times more likely to be admitted while infected (7,400 maternities; 103 admissions). Higher infection rates across BAME communities were found to be unrelated to the size of the city of origin of these birthing people. The study revealed that even after excluding women from London, the West Midlands and the North West of England, areas which include some of the most affluent cities and towns in the UK, Black and BAME mothers were the most affected. Since March 2020, the same research team has presented new interim data to the public, including at the Maternity Safety Conference in Birmingham in September 2021. On that occasion, Professor Knight explained that 30 women a day had been admitted to hospitals with COVID-19 during pregnancy in 2020 at the pandemic's peak, with one-fifth of them needing respiratory support. More than 99% of the recently admitted patients were not vaccinated (BabyLifeline, 2021).

Another investigation showing disparities in the UK population in maternity care and mortality is the MBRRACE-UK research and its rapid report findings (Knight et al., 2021a). The team published data regularly, between March and May 2020; June 2020-March 2021, besides ongoing investigations. According to the 2019 MBBRACE report, which analysed data through confidential enquiries and audits in the UK from 2015 to 2017 (Knight et al., 2019), Black women in the UK are five times more likely to die of pregnancy and while giving birth compared to their counterparts. Women of mixed ethnicities were three times more likely to die; Asian women double as much as their counterparts. The 2020 MBRRACE Rapid report confirmed that 7 out of 8 pregnant women dying due to COVID-19 were from BAME backgrounds and that the COVID-19 mortality rate across the investigated population was 6.2 per 100,000 people (Knight et al., 2020a). The latest 2021 MBBRACE report confirms that there continue to be racial disparities in maternity care, with Black, Asian and mixed ethnicity people at a significantly higher risk of dying in pregnancy than their white counterparts (Knight et al., 2021b).

The studies mentioned above have raised national attention on the disparities in maternal safety and pregnancy experiences affecting Black, Asian and ethnic minorities women in the UK, and rightly so, but two issues need to be mentioned.

An Ongoing Trend of Inequalities Despite Overall Improvements in Maternal and Infant Mortality Rates

One shall not forget that BAME communities have been at risk of complications and death in pregnancy for a long time (Ekechi, 2022), not just during the COVID-19 pandemic, and that these data might be a reflection of underlying, chronic, systemic issues that may have been and are still overlooked in maternity care for a long time.

For instance, according to a recent Lancet study by Quenby and colleagues, black women have a 43% higher chance than their white counterparts of having a miscarriage (Quenby et al., 2021). Most countries, including the UK, do not collect statistics

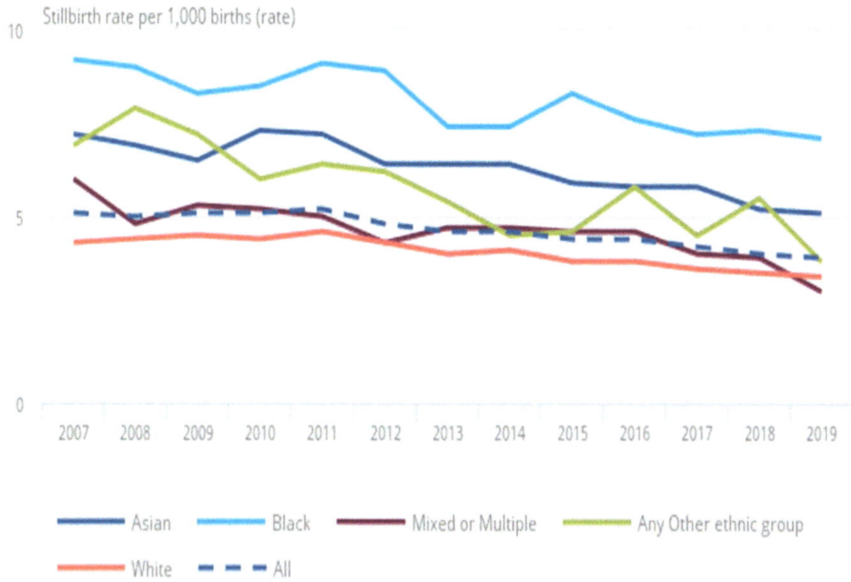

Fig. 6.1 Stillbirth rates were the highest for babies from Black ethnic group (*Source* Office for National Statistics, 2021)

on stillbirth rates, but the researchers estimate that 15% of pregnancies end in loss and that 1% of women, particularly Black women, will still experience recurrent miscarriage (Fig. 6.1). At the same time, while most go on to live a healthy life and have children, some experience traumatic loss and struggle with it. They may also experience long-term health issues, such as blood clots, heart disease and depression. The leading author of the Lancet article, Prof. Quenby, who also runs Tommy's National Centre for Miscarriage Research in the UK, stated that further research on this issue and the disparities in miscarriages are urgently needed.

A legitimate question is how the data of BAME populations compare to the overall population in the UK. Pregnancy in the UK remains very safe. Maternal death in the country has decreased significantly over the years (Fig. 6.2). From 2016–18, around 2 million pregnant people have given birth. Among them, five hundred and sixty-six died either due to direct causes (deaths up to 12 months after birth) or indirect causes, where the symptoms of a condition or a disease exacerbated during pregnancy but were unrelated to pregnancy (Knight et al., 2020c). The latest figures show a decrease of over 25% in stillbirth rates in the UK since 2010 (Department of Health and Social Care & Caulfield, 2022). This was made possible thanks to early interventions, prevention and continuity of care whenever possible. The 2021 MBBRACE UK also found that pregnancy remains very safe, with 8.8 women dying every 100,000 births (Knight et al., 2021b). As reported by Birthrights (Mohdin, 2021), the latest statistics (2021) show a slight improvement in the mortality rate of BAME people.

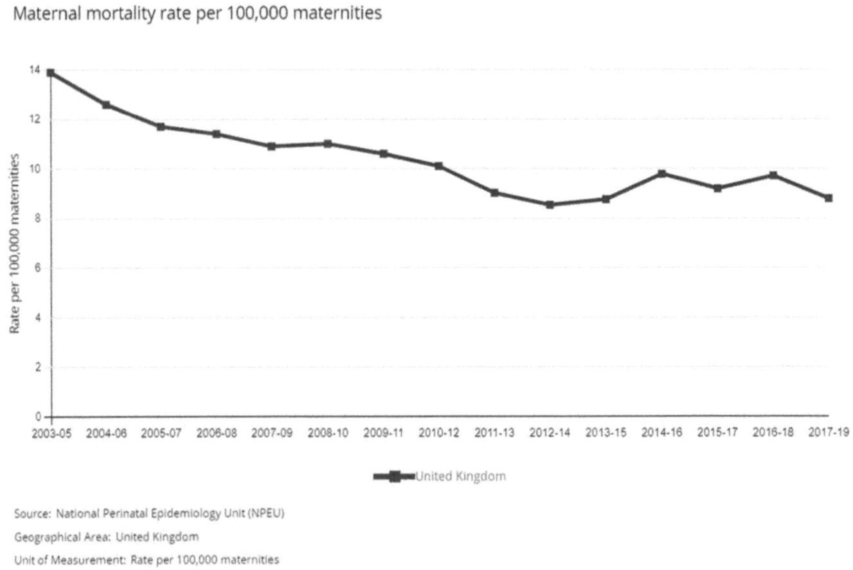

Fig. 6.2 Maternal mortality ratio (*Source* UK data for the sustainable development goals, 2021)

Notwithstanding the small steps forward, BAME communities continue to suffer. The mortality rate of black women in the UK in 2000–02 was seven times higher than the rest of the population. In 2015–17, it was still five times higher than the rest of the population (Ekechi, 2022). In 2021, it was still four times higher than their counterparts (Mohdin, 2021).

Affected Staff

It is essential to highlight that discrimination involves patients, clients *and* healthcare staff. According to recent statistics by the UK government (Fig. 6.3), staff from Other ethnic groups reported having experienced discrimination at work from peers in 97% of NHS trusts. This was the case in every region in the UK. Other than white ethnicity staff experienced abuse and discrimination almost double as much compared to their white peers. According to a recent (2020) report by the Royal College of Physicians (as reported in The Guardian on 21st October 2020), minority ethnic hospital doctors struggle to get their deserved recognition within the NHS system, climb ranks, and get promoted to consultants. According to the report, 29% of white respondents were offered a post after being shortlisted for the first time, while only 12% of BAME applicants experienced the same. An analysis of NHS salaries in England (also reported by The Guardian on 27th September 2018) has revealed that Black NHS doctors are paid on average £10,000 less than their peers and that black nurses are paid almost £3,000 less than their counterparts. This issue aggravates discourse

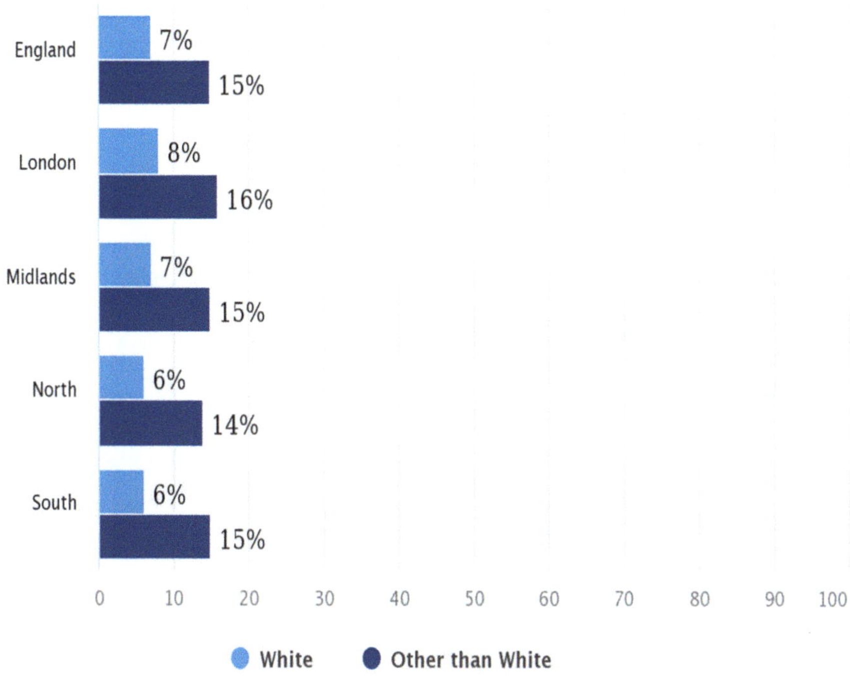

Fig. 6.3 Percentage of NHS staff experiencing discrimination at work, by ethnicity and area (*Source* NHS England, 2019a)

around NHS restoration strikes that is currently circulating in the country at the time of writing.

So far, it has been presented that the issue of racial inequalities is complex—it affects patients and healthcare staff, is rooted in history and is ongoing. Multiple factors may have led to poor or fatal outcomes for childbearing people and their babies. In the following sections, some of these triggers are explored.

Possible Triggers of Healthcare Inequalities in Maternity Care

As the MBBRACE Report 2021 highlights, there exists a "constellation" of factors that may trigger disparities in pregnancy and birth outcomes (Fig. 6.4).

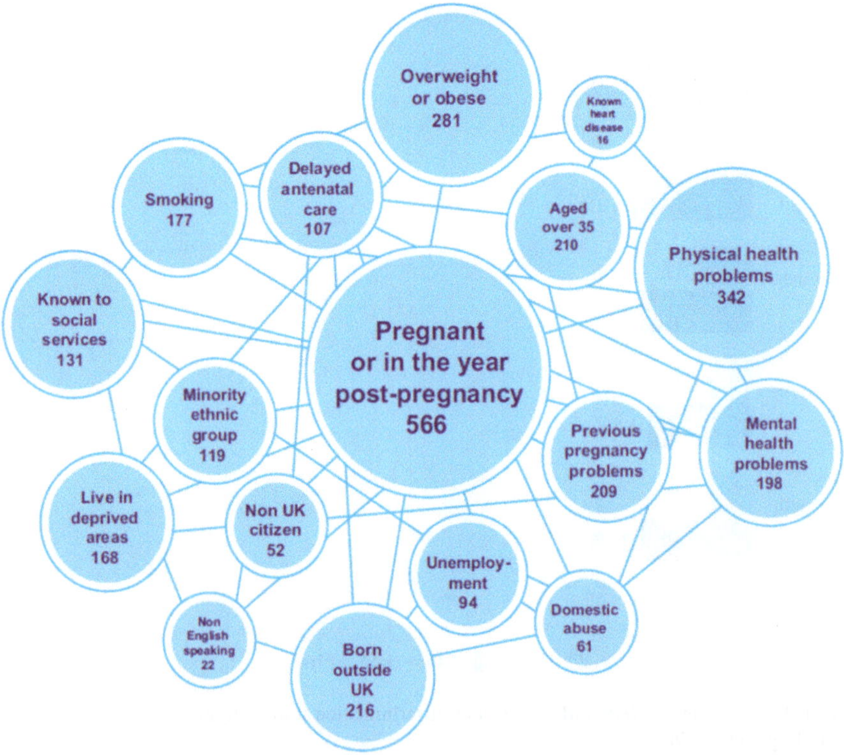

Fig. 6.4 Constellation of factors leading to maternal mortality in the UK (Knight et al., 2020c)

Socioeconomic Disparities

Social inequalities are one element worsening health inequalities. The 2020 Marmot Review, a landmark review of UK social, economic and health inequalities, has reported that health in the UK has declined for the entire population over the last decade, leaving families and children to struggle for food, income, access to education, employability and welfare. Disadvantaged social, economic and cultural factors might increase birthing people's vulnerabilities and those of their children. As stated in the 2016 *Better Births* report, a child in Tower Hamlets, UK, is more than five times more likely to be living in poverty than a child born in Wokingham and babies whose mothers live in poverty have a 57% higher risk of perinatal mortality compared to the rest of the population (The National Maternity Review, 2016). Dhawan (Dhawan, 1995) compared the birth weight of first- and second-generation Asians in the UK and found that the mean birth weight of babies of second-generation Asian women was higher than their first-generation counterparts. The paper's authors argued that this factor was due to better social integration of childbearing Asian people, including improved socioeconomic factors like stable jobs, housing, better nutrition, education and language skills.

Social Determinants of Health that are disadvantaged for some can affect birth outcomes, mothers' and babies' well-being, quality of life and even life expectancy. In pregnancy, health inequalities that are present before pregnancy reflect and influence the course of the pregnancy, the delivery and the pregnant mothers' and babies' well-being (Ockenden, 2022). According to (Knight et al., 2020c), pregnant people from disadvantaged areas in England are at a higher risk of pre-existing conditions, including a higher BMI, poor nutrition, worse mental state and hypertension when entering pregnancy than the rest of the population. These and other pre-existing conditions, which may have been triggered or exacerbated by a disadvantaged lifestyle and which may remain undiagnosed until pregnancy, may well affect pregnancy outcomes and experiences. Babies born in these situations may be premature or present with problems, affecting their later development and social integration (Clayton et al., 2022).

Societal and Cultural Factors

Societal and cultural factors can also trigger or affect inequality, including social discrimination and racial disparity. They too can affect the maternal experience and possibly lead to adverse events and adverse outcomes in pregnancy and birth. Discrimination can affect mothers and babies in multiple ways, causing stress and psychological trauma. Unfortunately, prejudice, stigma, stereotyping and racism still happen in the NHS's public healthcare system. Just recently (May 2022), the UK charity Birthrights and the law firm Leigh Day published a one-year inquiry into racial injustice and human rights in UK maternity care (Birthrights, 2022). They have reviewed over 300 testimonies of people who claimed to have suffered from gender, ethnic and racial injustice and identified some common themes in these testimonies, including lack of physical and psychological safety; being ignored as a patient, racism by caregivers, dehumanisation, lack of choice, consent and coercion, structural barriers and "anti-inclusive" culture in the healthcare workforce.

Henderson and colleagues (Henderson et al., 2013) surveyed around 24,000 BAME women aged 16 and above, in England, across 144 NHS Trusts and asked them about their service use and perceptions of care antenatally intrapartum and postnatally. They found care inequalities towards BAME populations that could be labelled as "too little too late care". Overall, they recorded poor experiences of maternity services lived and suffered by the surveyed women. According to Henderson's study, patients from ethnic minority backgrounds tended to access antenatal care later in pregnancy, and they were usually without a partner, young, multiparous and living with family members. They received fewer antenatal checks, fewer ultrasound scans and less screening compared to their white counterparts. They were also less likely to receive pain relief during labour and birth. Black African women, in particular, were more likely to deliver via c-section. The women in the survey reported staying longer in the hospital. Many breastfed but received fewer home visits from midwives compared to the rest of the patients. Although Henderson's results mentioned above go back a few years (2013), some of these findings resonate with experiences of care provision as narrated by midwives and obstetricians working for the NHS (Quattri, 2025).

Some of Henderson's findings are also similar to a previous study by (Raleigh et al., 2010) on social and ethnic inequalities in women's experiences of maternity care in England. These studies urge the need for policy and community to reform and improve childbirth experiences and outcomes for ethnic minorities as well as socially, economically and culturally disadvantaged birthing people. The physical and psychological scars resulting from a traumatic pregnancy and birthing experience can lead to long-term consequences for mothers and their babies and can gravely affect their rapport and bond. In the aftermath of an adverse event or a traumatic experience during pregnancy and during birth, a mother's self-esteem and desire to give birth again can be gravely affected, and poor and traumatic birth experiences can result in long-term healthcare physical ailments experiences.

Lack of Comprehensive Patient Data

Another factor that can seriously hinder fair and equal care to all patients is the lack of comprehensive and accessible patient data in NHS trusts and clinics. As the Ockenden team has revealed in their latest investigation of the Shrewsbury and Telford Hospital NHS Trust maternity scandals (Ockenden, 2022), there seems to be an increasing trend of harvesting and archiving incomplete data on ethnic background in maternity care across NHS trusts, big and small ones. The trust in question for the Ockenden investigation could be considered reasonably big. According to its website, which was last accessed in May 2022, the Shrewsbury and Telford Hospital NHS Trust provides hospital services "for half a million people in Shropshire". For this trust alone, the Ockenden team identified 9,276 missing ethnic background information (Ockenden, 2022), which is a substantial amount of missing data considering that about 10% of the admitted population in that hospital is BAME (Ockenden, 2022). When data are missing, hiccups occur in intervention and management strategies. For example, the Ockenden team, which was reviewing this trust's conduct and clinical leadership, could not draw any conclusion or any particular recommendation addressing ethnic and racial inequalities, as little to no evidence from minorities' experiences of care was missing from this trust.

This singular case may well reflect a trend of missing patients' information by trusts across the country, which often results in BAME women's voices, their stories, and their babies' stories likely being unknown. The lack of information on these patients and their circumstances of care also means that these patients and their families are unlikely to receive any compensation or apologies for what happened in the case of adverse events during or soon after their pregnancy. Unknowns about bad events and adverse outcomes also higher the risk of mistakes being repeated, as the clinical staff and the Clinical Commissioning Groups, the Trust Boards and the external regulatory bodies of these healthcare institutions might not be fully aware or might be oblivious of the actual extent of the damage and harm perpetrated against vulnerable patients. The saying in healthcare, "If something is not written, it does not exist", materialises in these instances. Documentation in healthcare is critical.

The Role of Clinical Leadership

The responsibility to care for patients, which includes the responsibility to collect thorough information about them and their patient histories, does not lay exclusively in the hands of the HCPs involved, but it is also the trusts' and boards' responsibility. If the best possible care is not provided to all the patients as expected, Trust Boards and clinical leadership may too be found liable for their lack of duty of care towards these patients, and liability could escalate to include clinical leaders as directly responsible if adverse events happen. Indeed, Article 2 of the UK Constitution argues that if the death of a patient was caused by systemic issues rather than by the act of negligence of a single individual, leadership, including the state, shall respond to that death.

Theoretically, corporations, healthcare organisations and clinical leaders in NHS trusts can be investigated under the Corporate Manslaughter and Corporate Homicide Act 2007 (or CM), however limitations intrinsic to this Act and the lack of a sufficient body of evidence using CM to prosecute cases make the chances for clinical leaders to be prosecuted under CM rather slim. Instead, when an adverse event happens, it is much more likely that trusts end up being investigated and prosecuted for Health and Safety violations according to the Health and Safety at Work Act (HSWA) 1974, which, although imposing hefty fines on trusts, involves far less aggravating accusations than CM (Brearey-Horne, 2013; Griffiths & Sanders, 2013; Quick, 2006; Samanta & Samanta, 2021).

Predatory Advertisement and Unfounded Evidence

The physiological predisposition for specific conditions and ailments, which has been found among some BAME members, has made these communities vulnerable to the predatory advertisement of medical products and instances of harmful overtreatment.

One example that has triggered much discontent among maternity care communities and HCPs is a NICE draft guideline on inducing labour (National Institute for Health and Care Excellence), which has been retracted. One aspect of concern in this draft was the recommendation to HCPs that induction of labour should be considered at 39 weeks for women "with a black, Asian or minority ethnic family background", regardless of whether these are nulliparous or multiparous patients or patients with high-risk or low-risk pregnancies. Several professionals and scholars have denounced the intervention as excessive, unnecessary and harmful for mothers and babies on social media (Wickham, 2021), and the UK charity Birthrights mobilised to retract the guideline.

Another example of health injustices triggered by unfounded evidence is the one reported by the latest NHS Race & Health Observatory report (Kapadia et al., 2022), raising the issue that Asian babies might be overrepresented in admissions to neonatal units for jaundice. Jaundice is a neonatal condition that can often present at birth and can be managed if identified early. Nonetheless, as pointed out by the report's authors, visual estimation of jaundice in babies is highly inaccurate, and it may be particularly unreliable in babies with skin tones other than white. Similarly, women in the same report felt poorly supported and isolated from proper care.

Already in the early 2020s and the 1990s, Anderson and colleagues (Anderson et al., 2009) and Cleeland and peers (Cleeland et al., 1997) documented the underprescription of pain medication for black patients with recurrent or metastatic cancer as a systemic issue, as there seems to exist the concerning misconception that mixed ethnicities, childbearing women and people with racial backgrounds are better at tolerating pain and they are thus more vulnerable to being prescribed the wrong medications or fewer medications. In fact, according to a relatively recent survey (Hoffman et al., 2016) with data collected from around 400 US medical students and residents, the majority believed that black people have a lower perception of pain, and therefore they would recommend them inadequate pain treatments.

The examples and cases presented so far show that healthcare inequalities can be triggered by the limitedness or absence of ethnically inclusive medical data, by clinical leadership's mismanagement, unsubstantiated evidence, and by clinical research biases, such as in the case of clinical trials.

Biased Clinical Trials and Curricula

Inequalities in healthcare happen in clinical training and research. In the following sections, examples show that the lack of comprehensive, inclusive research and clinical practice can lead to potentially biased outcomes, leading to healthcare inequalities and biased outcomes.

The scope of clinical studies and trials is to investigate the effect of a drug or treatment on the broader population. These studies are usually used to feed national and clinical guidelines, approve new drugs and start new treatments—they are important and impact patients' well-being. However, if these studies are not adequately representative of the entire population—if, for instance, only healthy individuals are recruited for these trials or if certain groups and populations get underrepresented in the trial phase—this can eventually lead to unsafe outcomes and treatments.

For instance, researchers involved in a systematic review of randomised controlled trials, RCTs, for diabetes treatment recently found that, during the patient eligibility process for RCT participation, only half of 58 selected RCTs considered the language proficiency of their participants as one eligibility criterion (Isaacs et al., 2016), which in turn may pose questions about whether the study participants understood the goal of the study and if they were adequately informed about it. According to Isaacs et al. (2016)'s research, less than a third of the considered studies recruited BAME, black Asian and ethnic minority patients, despite representing over 30% of the recruited population. Isaacs and colleagues complained in their article about the lack of standardisation in RCTs in reporting about patients' background, ethnicity, language and other sociodemographic features and the lack of standardised approaches in recruiting trial participants. In fact, while the USA legislates on the inclusion of BAME patients in medical research, other countries, including the UK, Canada and Australia, do not. However, privately funded research, including research funded by industry, does not need to apply to government regulations.

A more recent study by Rashid et al. (2021) from Keele University, UK, revealed significant disparities between BAME patients and white patients in receiving treatment for myocardial infarction caused by COVID-19, even though BAME communities have had proportionally higher levels of hospitalisation compared with white counterparts. The analysed population needed to wait longer than white patients to get treatment, suggesting delayed patient response and misuse of guidelines recommended for BAME patients affected by COVID-19 pandemic. The authors have appealed for an "urgent need" to address this social disparity with potentially fatal consequences.

Jenei and colleagues (2021) also recently conducted a systematic review of oncology trials over the last 20 years, and they found a stark underrepresentation of women in these trials. Women represented only 40% of the participants in 505 selected RCTs. These studies represent that gender and communities can and might have been underrepresented in important discoveries aiming at improving the health and well-being of society at large. Some of these disparities might as well be entrenched in history, like the historical underrepresentation of women in medicine, yet research outcomes remain uncertain without a comprehensive representation of the wider population.

Racial inequalities are also evident in clinical curricula. One example is provided by Louie and Wilkes (2018)'s investigation of the representation of race and skin tone in medical textbook imagery. The scholars analysed 4,146 images from different renewed anatomy textbooks for medical students and coded the race and skin tone of the images there. They found an overrepresentation of light skin tone, an underrepresentation of dark skin tone and a lack of diversity of skin tones across images. The problem is that these images are often used to study critical clinical cases, such as melanomas, discolourations and skin conditions. Students not actively exposed to different skin tones during their training years might be disadvantaged when detecting conditions and diseases in actual patients. This, in turn, can higher the risk of misdiagnosing, mistreating and mismanaging people of colour or BAME communities.

Possible Solutions

Responses from the Government and the NHS

There has been some progress in publicly reporting cases of healthcare inequalities, mainly thanks to the efforts of government-led and government-invited reviews and enquiries and reports by research centres, organisations and charities. In light of this latest evidence on maternal and infant mortality rates in the country, the UK government has repeatedly urged long-standing campaign groups, charities and patients' organisations to act on the matter.

The 2020 FivexMore petition asking for improved maternal mortality rates and healthcare for Black women in the UK reached 180,000 signatures. The government has recently (February 2022) established a task force, The New Maternity Disparities Taskforce, led by the current Minister for Patient Safety and Primary Care and the current Chief Midwifery Officer, which will look into some of the factors for disparities and address poor outcomes. The NHS has come forward with a long-term plan to fund more research on maternal inequalities based on race and ethnic disparities, and it has pledged that by 2024, 75% of women from BAME backgrounds will have access to continuity of care antenatally, intrapartum and postnatally, with additional midwifery time where needed (NHS England, 2019b).

Meanwhile, the latest rapid evidence review by the NHS Race & Health Observatory (Kapadia et al., 2022) has highlighted systemic racial inequalities in every stage of life and healthcare, from maternity care to mental healthcare and in all services, including primary, secondary and tertiary care in the NHS. Through their work, these teams have made a clear and overwhelming case for radical action on race and ethnic inequalities in the UK healthcare system, which are hard to ignore, and which have been picked up by the public.

Long-term plans to improve maternity care have been set up by the NHS and local organisations and charities, and several efforts have been put in place to improve inclusiveness, equity and equality. The NHS long-term plan remains committed to making England the safest place on earth to be pregnant, birth and transition into motherhood for all women from every ethnic background (NHS England, 2017, 2019b; NHS England & NHS Improvement, 2020; The National Maternity Review, 2016). In March 2022, NHS England announced an extra £127 m to be poured into maternity care for retention, recruitment and training. The much-discussed Ockenden report (Ockenden, 2022), which has metaphorically shed light on a slurry of scandals involving maternal care, starting with the investigation of the Shrewsbury and Telford NHS Hospital Trust, has set forward Local Actions for Learning (LAfL) and Immediate and Essential Actions (IEAs) to be implemented at the trust as well as across the broader maternity services in England. The team has also worked closely with NHS England, and it has been reassured multiple times, as reported in the report, that future changes within the NHS regarding reporting and monitoring adverse events will be well coordinated.

COVID-19 has taken a disproportionately higher toll on ethnic minorities, challenging leaders to act. Studies including UKOSS and MBRRACE-UK mentioned in this chapter have recommended "key mitigating actions" to contain risk and vulnerabilities antenatally, during birth and postnatally. Some of these "key mitigating actions" include the need to refer BAME patients directly to senior obstetric care at the start of their pregnancies, bypassing doulas' and midwives' care. Mental perinatal health services shall be available across the country, and vulnerable pregnant people shall receive daily obstetric reviews from competent staff (Knight et al., 2020a). Better Births, named after a National Maternity Review led by Baroness Cumberlege, has recommended that pregnant people with a Black, Asian and other minority background be promptly informed that they have a higher risk of perinatal mortality compared to the rest of the population (The National Maternity Review, 2016) and that they should therefore take particular care in treating and preventing ailments and infections. Clinicians shall also use "lower thresholds" (Dunkley-Bent, 2021) to review, consider and allow multidisciplinary escalation of BAME people as well patients presenting with co-morbidities and coexisting clinical conditions. Clinical leaders, trust managers and healthcare regulators shall carefully consider the suspension and reorganisation of maternity care services across the country, especially in communities with higher concentrations of BAME people. The Royal College of Obstetricians and Gynaecologists and the Royal College of Midwives (RCM) have repeatedly stressed the need to maintain "continuity of care" in their services and inclusiveness for all the patients (Royal College of Obstetricians and Gynaecologists, n.d., 2020). They have acknowledged that "women we care for need us more than ever", especially in light of the social isolation brought by COVID-19 (Elliott-Mainwaring, 2021) and in light of the recent scandals which have increased public mistrust against public healthcare services and facilities.

Responsibility has been called upon pregnant people as well, including women from mixed ethnic backgrounds, as the pandemic has highlighted changes in their attitudes towards obstetric and midwifery care. During the pandemic, there have been cases of pregnant women intentionally avoiding hospital visits, disengaging with maternity services and deciding to home birth despite complications—for fear of contracting the virus or maybe again due to mistrust against the public care system. These cases have sometimes led to late interventions with preventable adverse outcomes for mothers and their babies.

Education, Training and Technology

It is shocking and disconcerting to read that racial biases in pain assessment and treatment recommendations still exist in medicine to this day and that some medical students might have been trained to believe that there are biological differences between patients based on the colour of their skin, or that they might have been insufficiently trained to treat all their patients, regardless of the colour of their skin. Cultural changes, including changes in medical curricula and training, are key.

Providing medical students and HCPs with ethnically inclusive instrumentation and inclusive clinical material or ensuring that clinical studies and RCTs are representative of all different communities in society are relatively easy ways to ensure that health equality and equity are acknowledged. Advancements in technology can also help close the gap in racial disparity and inequalities. Lately, the NHS is testing a new artificial intelligence pregnancy screening tool that could slash racial disparities in baby death rates. The researchers discovered that early screening for placenta dysfunction leads to a notable decrease in perinatal mortality rates among black, Asian, and culturally diverse individuals who are expecting children. The new tool, which is still being piloted across England, is said to reduce baby deaths among BAME communities by 60% (Gregory, 2022).

Changing the Culture

As current and past reports and inquiries highlight, fixing mistakes and avoiding adverse events in clinical settings is not just a matter of better training and education at the clinical staff level but also, and sometimes most, it is a matter of transparent management and honest communication between the trust and the families involved in adverse events. It is a matter of culture—the set of values, beliefs, communication systems and different practices co-created and shaped for and in one specific workplace.

Staff is required to denounce irregularities at their places of work in the fashion of racial and ethnic inequalities, discriminatory treatments, racism or disrespect and stereotyping to their regulatory bodies, including the GMC (the General Medical Council) and the NMC (the Nursing & Midwifery Council) (Poole, 2019). Senior management and clinical leaders shall also be monitored regularly and strictly to ensure that they fulfil their duty of care towards all the patients in their trusts. Senior management and clinical leaders shall know their legal duties towards their patients well. Commissioners shall also be aware of those regulations, including the Clinical Commissioning Groups, the CCGs and the local and national system leaders. CCGs and NHS England have duties "to reduce inequalities between patients in access to health services and the outcome achieved (s.14 T; s.14Z11, s.13 T)", as well as duties to "properly and seriously" take into account health inequalities in their decision-making processes and while pondering interventions versus countervailing factors (NHS England, 2018). Relatively small changes can make a big difference too. Making sure that all the data from ethnic minorities and BAME people are appropriately reported in trusts' and clinics' data sets can also lay out a good premise in case of investigations or prosecutions.

Recommendations of inclusive healthcare made to trusts shall be followed and implemented as soon as possible. However, one shall also realistically assess whether these recommendations are feasible and easily able to penetrate the current texture or status quo of healthcare. In other words, changes without a realistic understanding of the current working conditions of the staff "on the shop floor" (i.e. those relating directly with the patients and clients) versus their management risk providing "lip service" value. We know from previous experiences that similar recommendations like those made in the latest reports have not always been followed up or implemented. For instance, if one compares the list of local actions for learning and immediate actions as recommended by the Ockenden team (Ockenden, 2020, 2022) with previous recommendations made by independent charitable organisations and public regulatory bodies (e.g. the CQC report in 2011; the Seventh and Eight Report of the Confidential Enquiries 2003–5 and 2006–8; the 2008 King's Fund report, and the 2010 Healthcare Commission Report (Brearey-Horne, 2013)), it becomes noticeable that these recommendations partially overlap with the Ockenden's and that these recommendations were also put forward in the aftermath of severe incidents endangering and ending the lives of patients, including mothers' and babies' from mixed minority groups. This shows that some lessons have yet to be learned, and some plans have yet to be implemented.

Often, when mistakes in the workplace happen, miscommunication is pointed out as the culprit for the lousy happening, while in reality, the problem might be more profound and related to culture. For instance, the disconnect that, in some cases and places of work, still exists between "the shop floor", aka the operative functioning staff in maternity care, and their management and the governing bodies might well be a cultural issue for people who do not see themselves included or reflected in the values of their work of place (Quattri, 2025). Bullying and gas-lighting as distorted cultures of power continue to thrive in healthcare settings, to the disadvantage of patients and clinical staff. As Brazier and colleagues denounce (2016), more than the fear of litigation and criminal or civil proceedings in the case of adverse events, HCPs shall probably fear the toxicity that sometimes generates and stalls in some healthcare settings, as that will prompt stress, fatigue, disillusionment and clinical mistakes, thus endangering patients' safety and denting quality of care.

As reported, in the NHS today, there are cases of gender-based, race and ethnicity-based discrimination against clinical staff by clients, patients or peers. There are wage imbalances and unfair treatments, which can also affect the overall working morale and enthusiasm in carrying on with the profession. The NHS is haemorrhaging healthcare professionals in different roles and functions, including midwives and obstetricians, who are leaving in droves due to exhaustion, disillusionment, life-changing decisions or better working and living conditions. The decimation of clinical staff due to COVID-19, the resignation and change of place of work of many, especially in the aftermath of the maternity scandals, the closure of several maternity services across the country due to financial struggles and managerial decisions, the lack of personnel which provides continuity of care as well as the challenges in keeping up with stuttering IT services at many trusts in the country are all hindering factors in the realisation of many of these recommendations aiming at better care for all. Indeed, the obstetric and midwifery teams in many hospitals in the UK are aware of this status quo and are feeling the heat of the public and internal scrutiny. However, they continue to provide high-quality care in sometimes very stressful work conditions. In these circumstances, implementing several recommendations from the top floors is highly hindered by the current state of affairs in many NHS trusts. This is not to say that by replenishing NHS staff, societal issues such as health inequalities will vanish, but they might, in some cases, be minimised, as more staff than the current figures would be available to foster one-to-one care with their patients, with the chances that more staff than currently would feel confident to denounce adverse events at work.

While recommendations and action plans can certainly prevent and contain the damage in maternity services at the moment, regulating and managing care is just one side of the interventions. The system needs to rely on a sufficient number of efficient HCPs working in their best conditions to create a really inclusive healthcare infrastructure that guarantees promptness to care and fair access to care, as mentioned in this chapter. Besides being a problem of recruitment and retainment, this may also be a matter of changing and shifting the culture in certain trusts.

Changing the culture also includes changing the social culture—redefining what we think is important and worthy, what holds potential, and defining relatively small-scale interventions to balance what is unbalanced. Fisher and colleagues have determined Julian Tudor Hart's "inverse care law", which states that people living in poverty and various forms of destitution are those who are more likely to receive the least of national healthcare. This seems to be a modern dilemma in the UK (Fisher et al., 2022). Social determinants of health inequalities are a powerful tool to assess the well-being of a nation and, consequently, of patients. Adopting appropriate intervention is key to tackling such determinants, yet as some scholars have argued, it is equally challenging.

While some interventions actively aim at tackling healthcare inequalities relative to gender, race and ethnicity, there is a dearth of evidence about practical, viable solutions to tackle social determinants of health and health inequalities in society. Bambra and colleagues have summarised recent systematic reviews on the effects of health and health inequalities of interventions. They have identified that, despite the lack of evidence in many areas of action, there exists suggestive evidence that specific categories of intervention may indeed positively impact inequalities or the health of specific disadvantaged groups. In particular, they identified housing and living environments and the work environments as two suggestive areas of improvement.

For the first, housing and living environments, renovation, updating and rehousing have been mentioned by the authors of the systemic reviews as possible solutions for both disadvantaged and frail people for them to live in healthier and safer environments (e.g. preventing falls and injury, increasing mobility, preventing diseases derived from the living conditions, such as mould or coldness). Changes mentioned for the work environment include the introduction of work schedules, shifts, team works and welfare for disadvantaged people.

Shifting culture also appeals to a more inclusive culture. Recently, the Royal College of Obstetricians and Gynaecologists has appealed for an immediate suspension of charging expectant immigrant women NHS maternity care costs, estimated to typically cost £7,000 upwards, if complex care is required (Taylor, 2022). The professionals' organisation has likewise urged the UK government to review its maternity care policies for migrants. There have been unfortunate cases of stillbirth and complications for mothers and babies among migrant women, who were reluctant to visit maternity care centres and units for fear that this would impact their immigration status or because they could not pay the medical bills. There have been complaints in some trusts that miscommunication can arise because of the unsubstantiated help in terms of translators or translating systems put in place. This, too, can endanger the quality of care and safety in care.

Finally, besides "operational" and technical changes in how healthcare is managed and organised, some HCPs argue that one's own culture change is also needed. Dr Ekechi argues that HCPs need to look introspectively at their practice, recognise their sometimes involuntary prejudices and stereotypes against certain kinds of patients and unveil the biases they might inadvertently see in their patients (Ekechi, 2022). Racism and discrimination also go the other way around, from staff to staff or from patients/clients to HCPs.

Conclusions

In this chapter, some stark inequalities in the United Kingdom, particularly concerning maternity care, have been pointed out. Ethnic inequalities in health and social care outcomes have been well documented in published research. The latest UK research on maternity mortality and infection rates shows an almost twofold difference in mortality rates of pregnant women from Asian communities than their white counterparts and an even higher difference for black pregnant people. As the latest research suggests, black women are also 40% more likely to experience miscarriage than white women. Clinical and statistical references show that UK BAME pregnant people have worse outcomes in maternity, and BAME women have reported cases of poor care and clinical staff being dismissive of their complaints. The COVID-19 pandemic has exacerbated health inequalities, with people from minority ethnic groups disproportionately affected.

To mark a difference, initiatives launched by the UK government, the NHS, charities and other organisations to contain such inequalities, efforts to improve the current status quo need to continue. Discrimination based on race and ethnicity is one of the many factors that can lead to health inequalities, but it is not the only one. This chapter has explored discrimination based on determinants of care for disadvantaged people and other factors that might also trigger health inequalities. Among them, lack of comprehensive patient data and biases in clinical education and training, where limited or poor clinical evidence, lack of critical analysis and critical thinking or the lack of comprehensive work instruments can perpetrate health inequalities. Health inequalities can also be spotted in clinical guidelines, RCTs and clinical research, and in doctor-patient relationships and HCP-HCP relationships, so one needs to consider the culture and a change thereof in places of work where inequalities exist.

Clinical staff who experience the inability to be treated equally and exercise the same rights to care, who become the subject of verbal and physical abuse and discrimination because of their race or ethnicity, are hindered in their attempt to provide the best possible care. These behaviours must be denounced and stopped, as "toxic environments" are dangerous for patients and staff. National guidelines and recommendations may provide relatively quick "fixes" and recommendations to the issues of discrimination, but the disconnection between the "shop floor" aka the personnel on the ground and the management still represents a big problem to solve. Strong bottom-up perspectives shall level out the top-down approach to care and improvement. Healthcare staff often know or shall be informed about what goes awry in their trusts, including episodes of health inequalities and unfair access to care. If they know about these episodes, they shall be able to speak freely and bring them to public attention without fear of repercussions.

References

Anderson, K. O., Green, C. R., & Payne, R. (2009). Racial and ethnic disparities in pain: Causes and consequences of unequal care. *The Journal of Pain, 10*(12), 1187–1204. https://doi.org/10.1016/j.jpain.2009.10.002

BabyLifeline. (2021). *The National Maternity Safety Conference 2021.* Retrieved September 10, 2021, from https://www.babylifeline.org.uk/conference-2021

Birthrights. (2022). *Systemic racism, not broken bodies. An inquiry into racial injustice and human rights in UK maternity care. Executive summary.* https://www.birthrights.org.uk/wp-content/uploads/2022/05/Birthrights-inquiry-systemic-racism_exec-summary_May-22-web.pdf

Brazier, M., Devaney, S., Griffiths, D., Mullock, A., & Quirk, H. (2016). Improving healthcare through the use of "medical manslaughter"? Facts, fears and the future. *Clinical Risk, 22*(5–6), 88–93. https://doi.org/10.1177/1356262217696623

Brearey-Horne, P. (2013). The Corporate Manslaughter and Corporate Homicide Act 2007 and maternal death: an opportunity to address systemic deficiencies in maternity services? In D. Griffitsh, & A. Sanders (Eds.), *Bioethics, medicine and the criminal law* (vol. 2, pp. 210–226). Cambridge University Press. https://doi.org/10.1017/CBO9781139109376.015

Clayton, C. E., Hemingway, A., Hughes, M., & Rawnson, S. (2022). The public health role of caseloading midwives in advancing health equity in childbearing women and babies living in socially deprived areas in England: The Mi-CARE Study protocol. *European Journal of Midwifery, 6*(April), Article 17. https://doi.org/10.18332/ejm/146012

Cleeland, C. S., Gonin, R., Baez, L., Loehrer, P., & Pandya, K. J. (1997). Pain and treatment of pain in minority patients with cancer. The Eastern Cooperative Oncology Group Minority Outpatient Pain Study. *Annals of Internal Medicine, 127*(9), 813–816. https://doi.org/10.7326/0003-4819-127-9-199711010-00006

Department of Health and Social Care & Caulfield, M. (2022, February 23). *New taskforce to level-up maternity care and tackle disparities* [Press release]. https://www.gov.uk/government/news/new-taskforce-to-level-up-maternity-care-and-tackle-disparities

Dhawan, S. (1995). Birth weights of infants of first generation Asian women in Britain compared with second generation Asian women. *BMJ, 311*(6997), 86–88. https://doi.org/10.1136/bmj.311.6997.86

Dunkley-Bent, J. (2021, January 13). *Midwives, maternity and COVID-19* [Keynote address]. The London Maternity and Midwifery Festival 2021, London, United Kingdom. https://www.maternityandmidwifery.co.uk/midwives-maternity-and-covid-19/

Ekechi, C. (2022, February 15). *Racial bias in women's health* [Webiner presentation]. Racial Inequalities in Maternal Healthcare - Webinars. https://www.ogpnews.com/2021/12/24-january-2022-racial-inequality-in-maternal-healthcare-webinar/83685

Elliott-Mainwaring, H. (2021, February 2). Women's needs in maternity services in a pandemic. *All4Maternity.* https://www.all4maternity.com/womens-needs-in-maternity-services-in-a-pandemic/

Fisher, R., Allen, L., Malhotra, A. M., & Alderwick, H. (2022). Tackling the inverse care law: Analysis of policies to improve general practice in deprived areas since 1990. *The Health Foundation*. https://doi.org/10.37829/HF-2022-P09

Gregory, A. (2022, February 28). NHS pilots pregnancy screening that may cut racial disparities in baby deaths. *The Guardian*. https://www.theguardian.com/lifeandstyle/2022/feb/28/nhs-pilots-pregnancy-screening-that-may-cut-racial-disparities-in-baby-deaths

Griffiths, D., & Sanders, A. (2013). The road to the dock: Prosecution decision-making in medical manslaughter cases. In D. Griffiths & A. Sanders (Eds.), *Bioethics, Medicine and the Criminal Law* (vol 2, pp. 117–158). Cambridge University Press. https://doi.org/10.1017/CBO9781139109376.010

Henderson, J., Gao, H., & Redshaw, M. (2013). Experiencing maternity care: the care received and perceptions of women from different ethnic groups. *BMC Pregnancy and Childbirth, 13*, Article 196. https://doi.org/10.1186/1471-2393-13-196

Hoffman, K., Trawalter, S., Axt, J. R., & Oliver, M. N. (2016). Racial bias in pain assessment and treatment recommendations, and false beliefs about biological differences between blacks and whites. *Proceedings of the National Academy of Sciences, 113*(16), 4296–4301. https://doi.org/10.1073/pnas.1516047113

Isaacs, T., Hunt, D., Ward, D., Rooshenas, L., & Edwards, L. (2016). The inclusion of ethnic minority patients and the role of language in telehealth trials for type 2 diabetes: A systematic review. *Journal of Medical Internet Research, 18*(9), Article e256. https://doi.org/10.2196/jmir.6374

Jenei, K., Meyers, D. E., & Prasad, V. K. (2021). The inclusion of women in global oncology drug trials over the past 20 years. *JAMA Oncology, 7*(10), 1569–1570. https://doi.org/10.1001/jamaoncol.2021.3686

Kapadia, D., Zhang, J., Salway, S., Nazroo, J., Booth, A., Villarroel-Williams, N., Becares, L., & Esmail, A. (2022). Ethnic inequalities in healthcare: A rapid evidence review. *NHS Race & Health Observatory*. https://www.nhsrho.org/wp-content/uploads/2022/02/RHO-Rapid-Review-Final-Report_v.7.pdf

Knight, M., Bunch, K., Tuffnell, D., Shakespeare, J., Kotnis, R., Kenyon, S., & Kurinczuk, J. J. (2019). Saving lives, improving mothers' care—Lessons learned to inform maternity care from the UK and Ireland confidential enquiries into maternal deaths and morbidity 2015–17. *National Perinatal Epidemiology Unit, University of Oxford*. https://www.npeu.ox.ac.uk/assets/downloads/mbrrace-uk/reports/MBRRACE-UK%20Maternal%20Report%202019%20-%20WEB%20VERSION.pdf

Knight, M., Bunch, K., Cairns, A., Cantwell, R., Cox, P., Kenyon, S., Kotnis, R., Lucas, D. N., Lucas, S., Marshall, L., Nelson-Piercy, C., Page, L., Rodger, A., Shakespeare, J., Tuffnell, D., & Kurinczuk, J. J. (2020a). Saving lives, improving mothers' care—Rapid report: Learning from SARS-CoV-2-related and associated maternal deaths in the UK. *National Perinatal Epidemiology Unit, University of Oxford*. https://www.npeu.ox.ac.uk/assets/downloads/mbrrace-uk/reports/MBRRACE-UK_Maternal_Report_2020a_v10_FINAL.pdf

Knight, M., Bunch, K., Morris, E., Simpson, N., Gale, C., O'Brien, P., Maria, Q., Peter, B., & Kurinczuk, J. J. (2020b). Characteristics and outcomes of pregnant women admitted to hospital with confirmed SARS-CoV-2 infection in UK: National population based cohort study. *The BMJ, 369*, Article m2107. https://doi.org/10.1136/bmj.m2107

Knight, M., Bunch, K., Tuffnell, D., Shakespeare, J., Kotnis, R., Kenyon, S., & Kurinczuk, J. J. (2020c). Saving lives, improving mothers' care - Lessons learned to inform maternity care from the UK and Ireland confidential enquiries into maternal deaths and morbidity 2016–18. *National Perinatal Epidemiology Unit, University of Oxford*. https://www.npeu.ox.ac.uk/assets/downloads/mbrrace-uk/reports/maternal-report-2020c/MBRRACE-UK_Maternal_Report_Dec_2020c_v10_ONLINE_VERSION_1404.pdf

Knight, M., Bunch, K., Cairns, A., Cantwell, R., Cox, P., Kenyon, S., Kotnis, R., Lucas, D. N., Lucas, S., Nelson-Piercy, C., Patel, R., Rodger, A., Shakespeare, J., Tuffnell, D., & Kurinczuk, J. J.

(2021a). Saving lives, improving mothers' care - Rapid report 2021a: Learning from SARS-CoV-2-related and associated maternal deaths in the UK. *National Perinatal Epidemiology Unit, University of Oxford*. https://www.npeu.ox.ac.uk/assets/downloads/mbrrace-uk/reports/MBRRACE-UK_Maternal_Report_June_2021a_-_FINAL_v10.pdf

Knight, M., Bunch, K., Tuffnell, D., Patel, R., Shakespeare, J., Kotnis, R., Kenyon, S., & Kurinczuk, J. J. (2021b). Saving lives, improving mothers' care - Lessons learned to inform maternity care from the UK and Ireland confidential enquiries into maternal deaths and morbidity 2017–19. *National Perinatal Epidemiology Unit, University of Oxford*. https://www.npeu.ox.ac.uk/assets/downloads/mbrrace-uk/reports/maternal-report-2021b/MBRRACE-UK_Maternal_Report_2021b_-_FINAL_-_WEB_VERSION.pdf

Louie, P., & Wilkes, R. (2018). Representations of race and skin tone in medical textbook imagery. *Social Science & Medicine, 202*, 38–42. https://doi.org/10.1016/j.socscimed.2018.02.023

Mohdin, A. (2021, November 11). Black women in the UK four times more likely to die in pregnancy and childbirth. *The Guardian*. https://www.theguardian.com/society/2021/nov/11/black-women-uk-maternal-mortality-rates

NHS England. (2017). *Implementing better births: Continuity of carer.* https://www.england.nhs.uk/wp-content/uploads/2017/12/implementing-better-births.pdf

NHS England. (2018). *Improving access for all: Reducing inequalities in access to general practice services.* https://www.england.nhs.uk/wp-content/uploads/2017/07/inequalities-resource-sep-2018.pdf

NHS England. (2019b). *The NHS Long Term Plan.* https://www.longtermplan.nhs.uk/wp-content/uploads/2019b/08/nhs-long-term-plan-version-1.2.pdf

NHS England. (2019a). *NHS staff experiencing discrimination at work.* https://www.ethnicity-facts-figures.service.gov.uk/workforce-and-business/nhs-staff-experience/nhs-staff-experiencing-discrimination-at-work/2.0

NHS England, & NHS Improvement. (2020). *Better births four years on: A review of progress.* https://www.england.nhs.uk/wp-content/uploads/2020/03/better-births-four-years-on-progress-report.pdf

Ockenden, D. (2020). *Emerging findings and recommendations from the independent review of maternity services at the Shrewsbury and Telford Hospital NHS trust.* https://assets.publishing.service.gov.uk/government/uploads/system/uploads/attachment_data/file/943011/Independent_review_of_maternity_services_at_Shrewsbury_and_Telford_Hospital_NHS_Trust.pdf

Ockenden, D. (2022). *Findings, conclusions, and essential actions from the independent review of maternity services at the Shrewsbury and Telford Hospital NHS trust.* https://assets.publishing.service.gov.uk/government/uploads/system/uploads/attachment_data/file/1064302/Final-Ockenden-Report-web-accessible.pdf

Office for National Statistics. (2021). *Births and infant mortality by ethnicity in England and Wales: 2007 to 2019.* https://www.ons.gov.uk/peoplepopulationandcommunity/healthandsocialcare/childhealth/articles/birthsandinfantmortalitybyethnicityinenglandandwales/2007to2019

Poole, N. (2019). *Clinical negligence made clear: A guide for patients and professionals.* Bath Publishing. https://bathpublishing.com/products/clinical-negligence-made-clear-a-guide-for-patients-professionals

Quattri, F. (2025). *The challenges of seeking to avoid overdiagnosis and overtreatment: Exploring defensive medicine* [Unpublished doctoral dissertation]. University of Leicester.

Quenby, S., Gallos, I. D., Dhillon-Smith, R. K., Podesek, M., Stephenson, M. D., Fisher, J., & al., e. (2021). Miscarriage matters: The epidemiological, physical, psychological, and economic costs of early pregnancy loss. *The Lancet, 397*(10285), 1658–1667. https://doi.org/10.1016/S0140-6736(21)00682-6

Quick, O. (2006). Prosecuting gross medical manslaughter: Manslaughter, discretion, and the crown prosecution service. *Journal of Law & Society, 33*(3), 421–450. https://doi.org/10.1111/j.1467-6478.2006.00365.x

RCOG. (2020a). Guidance for provision of midwife-led settings and home birth in the evolving coronavirus (COVID-19) pandemic. Royal College of Obstetricians and Gynaecologists.

RCOG. (2020b). Royal College of Obstetricians and Gynaecologists, Coronavirus infection and pregnancy, Information for pregnant women and their families [Guidance].

Raleigh, V. S., Hussey, D., & Hallt, S. K. (2010). Ethnic and social inequalities in women's experience of maternity care in England: Results of a national survey. *Journal of the Royal Society of Medicine, 103*(5), 188–198. https://doi.org/10.1258/jrsm.2010.090460

Rashid, M., Timmis, A., Kinnaird, T., Curzen, N., Zaman, A., Shoaib, A., Mohamed, M. O., de Belder, M. A., Deanfield, J., Martin, G. P., Wu, J., Gale, C. P., & Mamas, M. (2021). Racial differences in management and outcomes of acute myocardial infarction during COVID-19 pandemic. *Heart, 107*(9), 734–740. https://doi.org/10.1136/heartjnl-2020-318356

RCOG. (2020a). Guidance for provision of midwife-led settings and home birth in the evolving coronavirus (COVID-19) pandemic. UK. Royal College of Obstetricians and Gynaecologists.

Royal College of Obstetricians and Gynaecologists. (2020). *Guidance for provision of midwife-led settings and home birth in the evolving coronavirus (COVID-19) pandemic.* https://www.rcm.org.uk/media/4099/2020-05-22-guidance-for-provision-of-midwife-led-settings-and-home-birth-in-the-evolving-coronavirus-covid-19-pandemic.pdf

Royal College of Obstetricians and Gynaecologists. (n.d.). *Coronavirus (COVID-19), pregnancy and women's health.* https://www.rcog.org.uk/en/guidelines-research-services/guidelines/coronavirus-pregnancy/

Samanta, A., & Samanta, J. (2021). Death caused by negligent medical care: Reconsidering the role of gross negligence manslaughter in the aftermath of Bawa-Garba. *Medical Law International, 21*(4), 293–301. https://doi.org/10.1177/0968533221992838

Taylor, D. (2022, March 27). Stop charging migrant women for NHS maternity care, RCOG urges. *The Guardian.* https://www.theguardian.com/society/2022/mar/27/stop-charging-migrant-women-for-nhs-maternity-care-rcog-urges

The National Maternity Review. (2016). *Better births: Improving outcomes of maternity services in England - A five year forward view of maternity care.* https://www.england.nhs.uk/wpcontent/uploads/2016/02/national-maternity-review-report.pdf

UK data for the Sustainable Development Goals. (2021). *Maternal mortality rate per 100,000 maternities, and maternal mortality ratio.* https://sdgdata.gov.uk/3-1-1/

Wickham, S. (2021, June 24). *Ten reasons to question the draft NICE Guideline on inducing labour. Dr Sara Wickham.* https://www.sarawickham.com/articles-2/nice-guideline-on-inducing-labour/

Chapter 7
Filling the Gaps in Youth Health and Wellness

Helen S. M. Hsu and Fanny Y. F. Ng

Abstract The pandemic has brought health risks to young people not only physically, but also their need to adapt to new challenges in life, study and work. It is crucial for young people to return to basics, live a healthy and fulfilling life, and be positive and optimistic in attitude and action to face adversity. A report by The Hong Kong Federation of Youth Groups (HKFYG) was conducted to explore ways how young people might cope with health challenges and build resilience through understanding the concept of all-round wellness. The authors advocate the concept of the ABC of wellness, namely, building Awareness on one's health; ensuring Balance in developing physical, emotional, social, occupational, digital and environmental wellness; and building Connections from the inside out, so that young people can live a meaningful and fulfilling life.

Keywords Youth · Health · Resilience · All-round wellness

Introduction

Hong Kong has faced unprecedented challenges over the past few years. This has not been easy for the entire community, particularly for the all-round well-being of young people. No one can predict when another pandemic, collective trauma or stressor will hit. One of the most effective ways to cope, is to build strength and resilience within the community and among the young people, in order to be prepared.

There is no generally recognised definition or interpretation of "All-round Wellness". Yet, the World Health Organization (WHO) stated, as early as in 1948, that "health is a state of complete physical, mental and social well-being and not merely the absence of disease or infirmity". When this concept is applied to the young people,

H. S. M. Hsu · F. Y. F. Ng (✉)
The Hong Kong Federation of Youth Groups, Hong Kong, China
e-mail: yuefan.ng@hkfyg.org.hk

H. S. M. Hsu
e-mail: siuman.hsu@hkfyg.org.hk

B. Y. F. Fong and W. C. W. Wong (eds.), *Gaps and Actions in Health Improvement from Hong Kong and Beyond*,
https://doi.org/10.1007/978-981-99-4491-0_7

however, what concrete elements should be considered? And, as a key stakeholder in this respect, how do young people interpret such a concept?

Indeed, both comparative analyses of international data and various local studies have shown that mental health problems of Hong Kong's young people have been an area of concern for many years. According to data from the Organisation for Economic Co-operation and Development (OECD), Hong Kong students' levels of satisfaction with life and self-efficacy were lower than those in other developed economies. The level of satisfaction with life was only 52% among young people in Hong Kong, which was lower than the average level of 69% among other OECD regions (Organisation for Economic Co-operation & Development, 2019). Another study indicated that Hong Kong's young people's satisfaction towards the three areas of housing, politics and society, and the environment was lower than the pass rate of five marks (Wong, 2019). Over the past two years, under the influence of a series of social incidents and the pandemic, the city's economic environment and people's everyday lives have been seriously affected. The uncertainties under the new norm have affected the general public's social, physical and mental health. Under these circumstances, young people's situation and the pressures on them are self-evident.

A recent research has showed that adolescents with higher resilience level has a much lower socio-economic inequality in mental health, implying that resilience is the key skill that can be developed in the adolescent stages (Chung et al., 2023). Resilience building is the potential intervention for health and wellness among the youth. The gap is "how" to strengthen the resilience of young people in an effective way.

Despite the aforementioned, health issues are often not the top concern of the youth. Instead of instilling standard health knowledge into the young people, the Hong Kong Federation of Youth Groups (HKFYG) has explored ways how young people might sustain a balanced life through understanding the concept of all-round wellness. Young people here refer to people aged between 12 and 34 in both the school and community settings, who are the targeted service users of HKFYG. This chapter also shares figures and observations of the recent situation of youth. The framework of Six Dimension of Wellness is introduced, and advocated. This is to provide balanced and healthy living habits in six areas: the physical, emotional, occupational, environmental and digital at an individual level; and the building and maintaining connection of young people among peers, families and society. It is hoped that these areas will provide good reference relating to the concept of "all-round wellness", by offering up definition and composing elements, as well as the direction for potential-related service implementation, filling the recent gaps of youth health and wellness.

Basic Concepts About All-Round Wellness

Origin of the Concept of "Health"

In as early as in 1948, WHO gave a definition to "health", "as a state of complete physical, mental and social well-being and not merely the absence of disease or infirmity". Apart from being physically sound without diseases, it is equally important for people to take care of their psychological, emotional and social health. A person's health status hinges on various factors, called "Social Determinants of Health". "Health" is widely perceived to primarily come with individual factors such as a healthy diet, regular exercise and seeking medical care when feeling sick. However, health is not merely dependent on individual strength. A number of other factors, ranging from families, schools, workplaces, social life and community networks to economy and culture, bear interdependent influence on individual health. In this regard, the United States Department of Health and Human Services has proposed five social determinants of health, which affect general public (World Health Organization, 2021). These five determinants are:

1. Economic Stability
2. Education Access and Quality
3. Health Care Access and Quality
4. Neighbourhood and Built Environment
5. Social and Community Context

This extends the definition of "health" from physical health to mental, social and community levels, indicating that health not only refers to physical conditions, but also closely relates to areas such as people's psychological conditions, learning, work and surrounding environments. Since then, different academics have started to examine the composing domains of "health". With social advancements and improving quality of life, the concept of "all-round wellness" has gradually arisen. This concept of "all-round wellness" is more comprehensive than the pure promotion of health and it aims to enable each and every person to lead a more balanced life of higher quality and higher sense of satisfaction.

Broad Definitions of "All-Round Wellness"

Different bibliographic records show that there are different interpretations and definitions of the term "all-round wellness", yet most of them put emphasis on proactive attitudes and actions, as well as the values and meaning of life. The Global Wellness Institute defines "all-round wellness" as an individual's active pursuit of life, including consciously shaping his/her own life and ways of living through different kinds of activities so as to reach a healthy condition (The Global Wellness Institute, n.d.). Meanwhile, the National Wellness Institute defines "all-round wellness" as the attainment of more meaningful existence through an active process, with the ultimate goal of achieving the meaning of life (The National Wellness Institute, 1976).

Dimensions Covered in the Wellness Model

To enable the general public to better understand the concept of all-round wellness and the channels to reach this condition, academics have proposed different dimensions to evaluate individuals in this respect. Hettler (1976) proposed the Six Dimensions of Wellness Model, advocating a balanced way of life, putting forward six different dimensions by which all-round wellness is achieved only if each and every dimension is well taken care of. Along with the development of time and the progress of society, this has been extended to the Eight Dimensions of Wellness Model (Roddick, 2016; University of Northern Iowa, 2021). There is a general belief that if an individual becomes more conscious about each and every dimension in everyday life and addresses his/her own needs in every dimension and then takes related actions, he/she can achieve a holistic way of living more easily and will ultimately reach a condition of all-round wellness condition. Related concepts are elaborated in Table 7.1:

Digital Wellness Coming with Time

Given the huge popularity of advanced technology and Internet, Digital Wellness has become a key area in everyday life, gradually arousing concern over its impact on individuals' health. A significant number of overseas studies have shown that a balance in young people's everyday and social lives, between the online world and the real world, plays a decisive role in their health. Digital Wellness generally means a way of living by using digital technology in a healthy way. Otherwise, the use of technology, can affect physical, mental and psychological health (The Digital Wellness Collective, 2020). Some studies show that young people aged 11–16 are particularly interested in digital technology and that they are the most active groups on social media platforms (The Lancet Digital Health, 2020). Although digital wellness was not covered under the framework of all-round wellness in the past, the close link between the Internet and young people's everyday lives can now not be denied. Given the advancements in modern technology, digital wellness should not be neglected when considering young people's all-round wellness development. Digital Wellness Collective suggested six directions to measure the balance between life and digital technology, as shown in Table 7.2.

Table 7.1 Eight dimensions of wellness model

Psychological/ Emotional wellness	To perceive, express and adapt to one's own feeling and emotion in an appropriate way, while being able to read other people's feelings and emotions. People who are emotionally healthy can address various challenges in life more effectively and build good relationships with others
Physical wellness	Adequate physical activities, nutritious diet and enough sleep can help build physical strength for now and the future
Social wellness	To develop positive personal relationships through proactively creating social networks, so as to build positive a connection and sense of belonging with other people and society. Proactive participation in, and contributions to, organisations or groups as a member can help develop connections and improve social health
Occupational Wellness	Refers to the level of satisfaction towards selected jobs and whether a sense of achievement can be attained at work. Everyone can achieve a work-life balance and manage work stress well through doing a job which fits in with his/her values, interests and skill sets, so as to achieve occupational wellness
Financial wellness	Fully understand one's financial status and opt for suitable ways to manage one's finance. Make rational financial decisions and set short-term and long-term financial goals
Environmental wellness	Fully understand the impact of the surrounding environment on one's health and be aware of the impact of daily habits on environmental wellness and sustainable development; opt to live in a way that can support environmental wellness and sustainable development
Intellectual wellness	Stay curious about new things and be motivated to proactively acquire and share knowledge. This includes the nurturing of creativity and problem-solve capabilities, which can facilitate mental growth and help improve health
Spiritual wellness	To realise the meaning and goals in everyday lives and explore the meaning of life, with or without religion. In general, this can be achieved through participation in activities which fit in one's own values or beliefs, such as volunteer services, self-reflection, mindfulness practice, religion or getting close to nature

Source Stoewen (2017)

Theoretically, the development of appropriate attitudes and literacy relating to the use of technology products in terms of the six directions above can help people leverage technology in different domains in everyday life, while at the same time avoiding the negative impact of technology. This will ultimately enable us to enjoy the benefits brought about by technology, reaching the condition of Digital Flourishing.

Table 7.2 Six directions to measure the balance between life and digital technology

1. Physical health	Whether an individual has enough sleep, healthy eyes, sufficient rest, etc
2. Productivity	Balance with work, whether concentration is affected, whether technology is appropriately used to uplift productivity, etc
3. Digital citizenship	Privacy and network security, management of digital identity, digital literacy, etc
4. Wellbeing	Balance between online and offline lives, positive emotion, self-expression and unleashing creativity, etc
5. Relationship	Meaningful exchanges with other people, the sense of belonging and connection, etc
6. Mental health	Positive comparison, strategies to address matters that cause emotional overloads, conscious selection of content, etc

Source The digital wellnesscollective (2020)

Relationship Between All-Round Wellness and Young People

Importance of All-Round Wellness to the Young People

Factors such as individuals, families, schools and the environment all have an impact on young people's health and wellness. A study in the UK also stated that the mental and emotional health of a person at puberty had an impact on his/her personal relationships, social connectedness and productivity during adulthood (Whitney, 2021). Given the close relationship between the mental health of an adult with his/her puberty, mental health support targeting young people should be a priority concern as this can help raise the mental health level of society as a whole. After a person's mental issues develop into disorders, the intervention cost would be much higher. Taking as an example the prevention and treatment principles for general diseases, treatment for chronical physical diseases face certain limitations and the focus would only be on the control and management of related symptoms and conditions, which is not as effective as early intervention. Therefore, it is suggested that the Government allocate resources for the prevention of mental health problems targeting adolescents and intervene as early as possible in response to young people's determinants of mental health in a bid to prevent emotional distress from developing into chronic disorders.

The above shows that the all-round wellness of young people is of the utmost importance to themselves, their future and reduction in the social cost relating to mental disorders. As young people's mental health has become an area of concern, apart from intervention through treatment and rehabilitation, fundamental support should be provided to young people in more proactive ways with a comprehensive mindset in the interest of their mental health. Such support should help them maintain good physical health, strengthen self-management ability and nurture proactive and positive attitude towards life, so that young people would be equipped with sufficient basic abilities under adequate protection to face different challenges in life.

Key Factors Affecting the Young People's Health and Wellness

The study above also attempted to explore the trajectories and drivers affecting young people's emotional and mental health (Whitney, 2021). Under the study, around 5,000 young people born after the year 2000, particularly those aged 11, 14 and 17, were interviewed, to learn about the comparative impact of different social drivers on their current well-being, self-esteem, psychological health, self-values and hope. It was concluded that a series of factors, as follows, had prominent impact on young people's mental health (Whitney, 2021).

1. Interconnection between family income and young people's mental health
   People from low-income families are more likely to have a lower sense of happiness and self-esteem as well as more depressive symptoms. The current COVID-19 pandemic has accelerated prevailing social inequalities, exerting more psychological pressure on young people.
2. Positive impact of sports and physical activities on young people
   Frequent physical activities have a positive impact on young people's sense of happiness and self-esteem. It also helps curb depressive symptoms. Such a positive impact is particularly significant among male interviewees aged 14, and is observed in both male and female interviewees aged 17.
3. Negative impact attributed to overuse of social media
   The study shows that spending a lot of time on social media has a negative impact on the sense of happiness and self-esteem of female interviewees aged 14 and 17. This also has a negative impact on the health of male interviewees aged 14. Body images depicted online tend to spur negative feelings and have a negative impact on girls, while boys tend to see such online comparisons as a driving force to pursue physical fitness.
4. Obesity has a long-term impact on young people's psychological health and self-image
   The psychological health of both male and female young interviewees who are obese or overweight during childhood is relatively unfavourable. Overweight problems during childhood have a certain impact on body image and social interaction of a person during all stages of puberty.
5. Relationship with and the quality of parents and peers are of huge significance
   Bullying has a very huge and long-lasting impact on young people's psychological health, regardless of gender. Young people aged 17 and 14 who often quarrel with parents have comparatively low sense of happiness, while this exerts more psychological pressure on younger interviewees.

6. Lower academic achievement has an impact on self-esteem
   Boys aged 14 are more likely to be influenced if their academic performance is categorised as being at a relatively low level. In this respect, their scores in self-esteem are relatively low, showing the existence of the socially stigmatising effect of those labelled as having relatively bad academic performance.
7. Mothers' health conditions have an impact on young people's mental health
   The unfavourable health conditions of mothers during pregnancy lead to the reduced sense of happiness and self-esteem and increased depressive symptoms among both male and female young people. For the 17-year-old female interviewees, they are more likely to show depressive symptoms if their mothers suffer from depression disorders during their infancy.
8. Impact of neighbourhood security on girls' mental health
   Girls, regardless of their age, are of poorer health and at higher risk of suffering from depression if they think that their neighbourhood or community environment is insecure.

The findings clearly indicated that mental health of young people is interrelated with multiple factors, including their socio-economic status, parental health, physical activity level, social relationship, academic achievement and so on.

Young People's View About All-Round wellness—A Study in Hong Kong

HKFYG had conducted a comprehensive study in 2021 through questionnaires (1,099 respondents aged 12–34 who were HKFYG members), in-depth interviews (ten youth) and design thinking group for youth work practitioners, to understand the views of all-round wellness among youth and youth workers. Based on the findings, new service directions addressing young people's all-round wellness development needs could be explored while feasible suggestions to increase the effectiveness of related programmes could be given.

Young People's Interpretation of All-Round Wellness

1. The young people interviewed did not know much about all-round wellness. 64.1% of the respondents stated that they had never heard of the concept of all-round wellness. Most of them thought that this concept covered mainly physical and mental wellness.
2. 69% of the respondents agreed that a disease-free body, being psychologically healthy, the pursuit of goals, taking actions to reach the goals, living with a positive attitude and having meaning in life all make up to all-round wellness.

They saw living with a positive attitude and reaching the goals through actions as the most significant elements.

The findings showed that the concept of all-round wellness was not well-known. The corresponding youngster did not fully understand the concept. However, they generally agreed that all-round wellness should be considered as a more comprehensive concept, which is more than just physical and mental wellness and should cover the positive attitude towards living and the pursuit of life goals.

Dimensions of All-Round Wellness Emphasised and Overlooked by Young People

The study was based on the eight dimensions of all-round wellness covered in the bibliography, gathering young people's views about different dimensions and the impact of the pandemic and the social environment on them. The following is an elaboration of the dimensions that were likely to be emphasised and overlooked by young people.

1. Over 50% of the respondents would attempt to take action to improve their all-round wellness. The older the respondents were, the more attention they paid to their all-round wellness.
2. The respondents paid more attention to their emotional wellness, social life/interpersonal relationships and work-life balance, while, in general, they paid relatively less attention to their social connectedness and job satisfaction. Young people in different age groups paid more attention to different dimensions.
3. The respondents are more likely to overlook their own exercise habits, the duration and quality of their sleep and the time spent with the time spent in nature.

The findings showed that the young people paid more attention to emotional, social and occupational dimensions in all-round wellness, while physical dimensions such as eating and exercise habits as well as environmental wellness were comparatively overlooked. Spiritual and financial wellness were seldom mentioned by the respondents. Besides, many of them attempted to take actions to improve their all-round wellness, yet their efforts were relatively limited to personal levels.

Impact of the Pandemic and the Social Environment on Young People's All-Round Wellness

1. Young people encountered difficulty in adapting to the new norm, which brought them more pressure on the psychological, work or learning front.

Students needed to learn online most of the time over the past year under the pandemic, while some jobs adopted flexible working arrangements. Some of the working respondents said the pandemic had changed the traditional working mode, which brought freshmen into the workplace and students more psychological pressure, indirectly affecting their emotional wellness.

2. Social contacts were limited under the pandemic and the relationships among individuals became distant.

   The young people interviewed agreed that face-to-face interaction in everyday lives was an important way to connect with the society. Under the pandemic, many activities had to be cancelled or go online, significantly reducing interpersonal interaction. Some of the respondents said that online communication had made it more difficult to build their social circles, which had an impact on their emotional wellness.

3. Under the impact of the social environment and the pandemic, young people generally felt uneasy about the future. Some of the respondents admitted that they felt feeble facing the social issues.

   Some people believed that they were incapable of making contributions or changes to the society. This, plus the change in the social environment and the constantly fluctuating epidemic situation, resulted in the respondents feeling hesitant and uneasy about their future and prospect.

4. Although it was difficult to adapt to the new norm, this new mode had a positive impact. For example, young people could spend more time on what they wanted to do and that they were now more willing to offer help to people around them.

   To sum up, the pandemic and social environment had a certain impact on young people's emotional, social and psychological wellness. Regarding emotional wellness, the respondents found it difficult to adapt to the new norm, which put them under more psychological, work or learning pressures. Regarding social wellness, the respondents had far fewer social contacts and the connections among individuals had reduced. Although certain social contacts could be maintained online, this could not fully replace actual face-to-face contacts. Besides, under the impact of a series of social incidents, the respondents generally felt uneasy and some even felt feeble. A sense of security and hope towards the future was a key contributing factor in good health. Therefore, the society needed to face up to and address young people's uneasy feelings towards the future.

   The new norm also had its positive impact on young people's mental and social wellness. Over half of the respondents said they had more time to do what they wanted to and develop their interests over the past year. Besides, although the pandemic had obstructed face-to-face communications, the respondents became more willing to help those in need around them as they saw that many people were affected by the social environment.

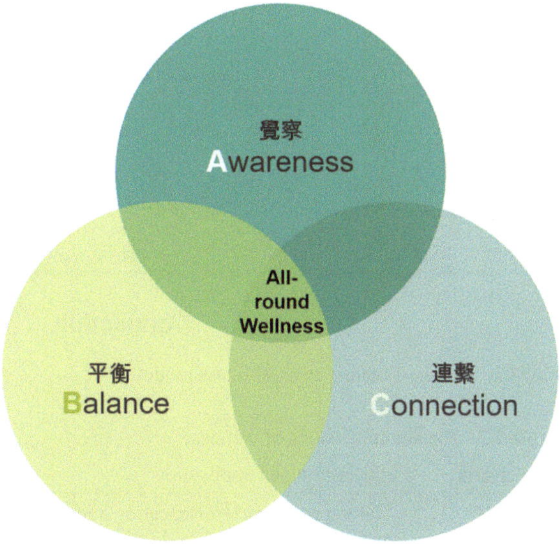

Fig. 7.1 All-round wellness

Suggestions on All-Round Wellness Development

Gaining All-Round Wellness Through "Wellness ABC"

Figure 7.1 shows that all-round wellness is an all-encompassing healthy living target that can be pursued by everyone. It has to do with "awareness", "balance" and "connection". Young people can strike a balance among different areas of life, including physical, psychological, social, occupational, digital and environment wellness through raising awareness of their own needs, while establishing good connections between themselves and the outside world, so as to live a meaningful and satisfying life.

The Six Dimensions of Wellness Model

The Six Dimensions of Wellness Model as shown in Fig. 7.2 further illustrates the balanced developments in different dimensions under all-round wellness, establishing connections between the self and the world.

Table 7.3 elaborates the definitions and application of the six dimensions of wellness:

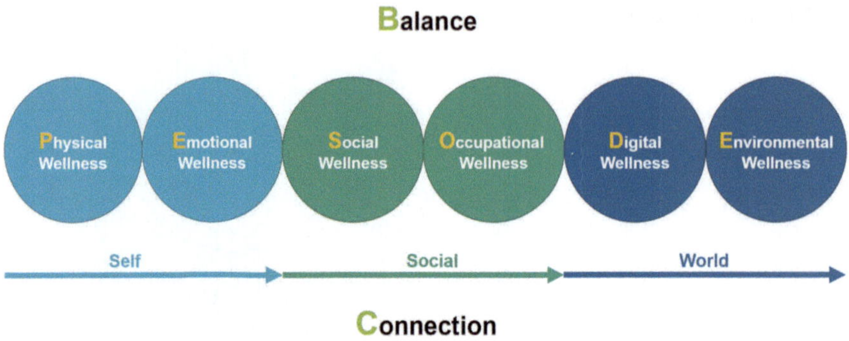

Fig. 7.2 The six dimensions of wellness model

Table 7.3 The six dimensions of wellness

Dimension	Definition and application
Physical wellness	Taking regular exercise, eating a nutritious diet and having enough sleep, etc. can help build the lifestyle and behaviours contributing to physical wellness both now and in the future
Emotional wellness	To become aware of, express and accommodate one's own feelings and emotions in appropriate ways; to understanding other people's emotions and feelings; be able to address life challenges with emotional wellness
Social wellness	To develop good interpersonal relationships through various social networks, so as to build positive connections with families, peers and the community and a sense of belonging. Proactive involvement in and contributions to organisations or groups as members can help improve social wellness
Occupational wellness	Occupational wellness is not limited to the traditional views about jobs. Instead, it covers the jobs' meaningfulness to the young people and the sense of satisfaction and achievement they can gain. To achieve occupational wellness, the young people focus on whether the jobs are in line with their values and interests, enable them to contribute their skills and allow a balance between work and rest as well as whether they can manage related pressure
Digital wellness	To consciously build the attitude towards the use of technology products and related literacy. To leverage technology in different areas of life, such as learning, work and connections with other people. To avoid the possible negative impact of technology with good attitude and literacy so as to enjoy the benefits bought about by technology
Environmental wellness	Be aware of the relationships between the environment and one's own health as well as the impact of one's own living habits on the entire environment and sustainable development. To learn to pay attention to and respect the environment through learning about the concepts of sustainable development. To understand the relationships between human beings and nature, animals and the earth. To choose to adopt a lifestyle that is environmentally friendly and supports sustainable development

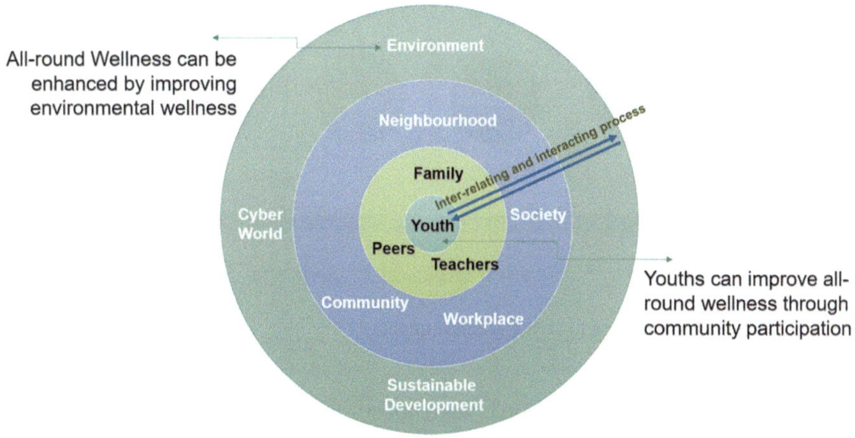

Fig. 7.3 From individual level to social level

From Individual Level to Social Level

Figure 7.3 suggests that apart from individuals' proactive efforts, the environment surrounding young people is another key determinant of their all-round wellness developments. These individual efforts and the environment are correlated. To promote the all-round wellness concept among young people, on top of individuals' all-round wellness development programmes tailor-made for the young people themselves, they should be encouraged to play a role in improving the surrounding environment. For example, they can participate in the promotion of the all-round wellness concept; improve their relationships with peers, families and teachers; take part in community improvement activities; help develop a healthier Internet culture and a more sustainable community. Improving the environment is an interactive process. Such efforts can facilitate the young people to further improve their all-round wellness, while the resulting better environment is favourable to the young people's all-round wellness developments.

Sustainable Wellness to Create Greatest Impact

All-round wellness developments are personal processes. These have to do with not only learning and experience, but also, more importantly, actions and practice, which transform related experiences into the healing process. Therefore, in order to increase the programme effectiveness, the users' pain points and barriers in their experience and practice should be considered in advance when designing any all-round wellness programmes. Figure 7.4 is a summary of the users' journey.

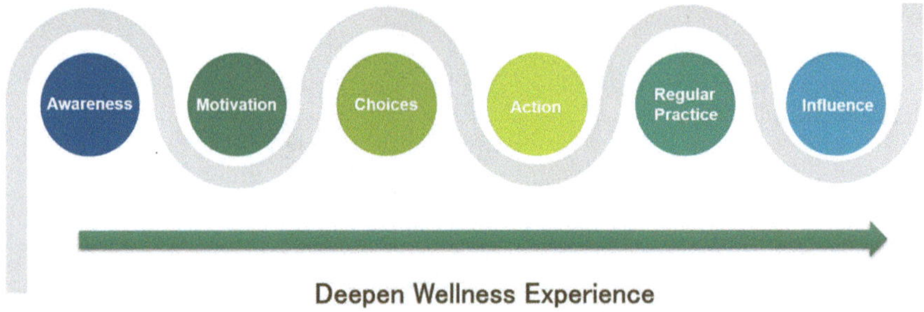

Fig. 7.4 Sustainable wellness to create greatest impact

Focusing on the areas that people were not sufficiently aware of can raise awareness of our own needs and then motivate the pursuit for all-round wellness. We may also provide the users with different options to motivate them to action. For those who have participated in all-round wellness programmes, we should think about how to further encourage the participants to apply the all-round wellness concepts to their everyday lives through the programme design. For the young people who have developed all-round wellness habits, we should encourage them to take a step further to exert their personal influence on others. In this regard, we can provide them with opportunities and platforms to share their knowledge and skills with others. This framework can help promote the all-round wellness concepts further, extending these to the young people, while at the same time increasing the quantity and effectiveness of our services.

Conclusion

With social advancements and improved quality of life, the narrow belief in the past that health and wellness is just about a disease-free body has been gradually replaced by the all-round wellness concept over the past few decades. Over the past two years, the continuous social incidents and the pandemic have had a far-reaching impact on the young people and society in Hong Kong. To both the young people and youth workers, it was a new challenge for them to accommodate themselves to various aspects including values, physical and mental health, financial conditions and employment, family harmony, interpersonal relationships, lifestyle, learning and work.

In view of the changes in the social environment in future as well as the mental health risks facing the young people under the pandemic, there is an emerging need to take immediate action in helping young people to lead a proactive life and heal themselves in the "post-pandemic era". All-round wellness practice can adopt the "consolidation of the basis and cultivation of energy" concept of Chinese medicine to produce a protective effect and help the young people face the various challenges in their lives.

Furthermore, it is important to deepen stakeholders from various sectors in the community, youth workers, and parents in the understanding of the importance of all-round wellness developments for young people. This framework aims to define all-round wellness development concepts as well as the composing elements and the directions for action in simple ways. It is hoped that under this framework of all-round wellness, each and every young person can lead a healthier life with a higher sense of satisfaction and a hopeful future in their time.

References

Chung, G.K.-K., Chan, Y.-H., Lee, T.S.-K., Chan, S.-M., Chen, J.-K., Wong, H., Chung, R.Y.-N., & Ho, E.S.-C. (2023). Socioeconomic inequality in the worsening of psychosocial wellbeing via disrupted social conditions during COVID-19 among adolescents in Hong Kong: Self-resilience matters. *Frontiers in Public Health, 11*,. https://doi.org/10.3389/fpubh.2023.1136744

Hettler, B. (1976). *Definition of wellness*. https://cdn.ymaws.com/members.nationalwellness.org/resource/resmgr/pdfs/sixdimensionsfactsheet.pdf

Organisation for Economic Co-operation and Development. (2019). *PISA 2018 results (Volume III)*. https://doi.org/10.1787/acd78851-en

Roddick, M. L. (2016, May 27). The 8 dimensions of wellness: Where do you fit in? *GoodTherapy Blog*. https://www.goodtherapy.org/blog/8-dimensions-of-wellness-where-do-you-fit-in-0527164

Stoewen, D. L. (2017). Dimensions of wellness: Change your habits, change your life. *The Canadian Veterinary Journal, 58*(8), 861–862. https://www.ncbi.nlm.nih.gov/pmc/articles/PMC5508938/

The Digital Wellness Collective. (2020). *What is digital wellness*. https://digitalwellnesscollective.com/digitalwellness

The Global Wellness Institute. (n.d.). *What is wellness?* https://globalwellnessinstitute.org/what-is-wellness/

The Lancet Digital Health. (2020). *Child and adolescent health in the digital age*. https://www.thelancet.com/journals/landig/article/PIIS2589-7500(20)30029-7/fulltext

The National Wellness Institute. (1976). *The six dimensions of wellness*. https://nationalwellness.org/resources/six-dimensions-of-wellness/

University of Northern lowa. (2021). *8 dimensions of wellness*. https://studentwellness.uni.edu/8-dimensions#physical

Whitney C. J. (2021). *Young people's mental and emotional health, Trajectories and drivers in childhood and adolescence*. https://epi.org.uk/wp-content/uploads/2021/01/EPI-PT_Young-people%E2%80%99s-wellbeing_Jan2021.pdf

Wong, S. W. D. (2019). *Young people's happiness index 2019: A comparative study between Hong Kong and Singapore* [in Chinese]. https://www.hkwecare.hk/wp-content/uploads/2019/10/%e9%9d%92%e5%b0%91%e5%b9%b4%e9%96%8b%e5%bf%83%e6%8c%87%e6%95%b82019.pdf

World Health Organization. (2021). *Social determinants of health*. https://www.who.int/health-topics/social-determinants-of-health

Chapter 8
Health Literacy in Digital World

Thomas M. C. Dao and Bean S. N. Fu

Abstract Health literacy is the cognitive and social ability of an individual to access, understand, analysis and use information for promoting and maintaining health. Individuals with a lower educational level and family income would usually have a lower health literacy and poorer access to health information yet with more chronic illnesses. Inadequate health literacy could result in suboptimal self-management skills for health problems, leading to wider health inequality and poorer health outcome in the socially disadvantaged population. In the era of digitalisation, health resources often exist in electronic forms, such as digital applications (apps) and webpages. The recent COVID-19 pandemic also drove the accelerated development of various public health measures in digital form, including the use of apps for surveillance, contact tracing, exposure notifications and provision of health advice. Thus, digital health literacy, also known as electronic health (eHealth) literacy, is an important consideration when devising public health interventions. In this chapter, ways to assess of health literacy, digital health literacy and their implications will be discussed. Various strategies to bridge the health literacy gaps and the digital divide, particularly in the low-educated and low-income population, and their ethical considerations will also be explored.

Keywords Health literacy · Digital health literacy · Digital health care · Digital divide

What is Health Literacy?

People in all age groups need health care services now and then. Even though we have no illness, we usually follow government recommendations for various health-related activities, such as vaccinations, health check and surveillance. The journey of health

T. M. C. Dao (✉) · B. S. N. Fu
Department of Family Medicine and Primary Health Care,
Kowloon West Cluster, Hospital Authority, Hong Kong, China
e-mail: thomasmcdao@hotmail.com

B. Y. F. Fong and W. C. W. Wong (eds.), *Gaps and Actions in Health Improvement from Hong Kong and Beyond*,
https://doi.org/10.1007/978-981-99-4491-0_8

care services starts from the decision of attending or not, followed by selection of service providers, making appointments, attendance of consultation and subsequent management. People have to decide, access, understand, analyse and use relevant information for promoting and maintaining health. This cognitive and social ability is known as health literacy (Ad Hoc Committee on Health Literacy for the Council on Scientific Affairs, American Medical Association, 1999). It is different from the term "Literacy" which traditionally describes general reading and numerical skills.

In 2000, Nutbeam proposed health literacy models of three different levels. The first level is the basic skills in reading and writing (functional health literacy). In patients' perspective, it refers to their ability to read disease, investigation, procedure or treatment information. The second level is the ability to derive meaning from different forms of new information and apply it in various situations (interactive health literacy). Patients are able to communicate and interact with health care providers effectively. The highest level is the critical health literacy, who analyses information critically and change policy and organisational accordingly. For instance, patients have to understand the procedure, pros and cons of an operation, so that they can decide if they will receive the surgery or not (Nutbeam, 2000).

Digital Divide

"*Digital divide*" refers to the inequality in accessing the internet or other information and communications technology devices among different social groups (Organisation for Economic Co-operation & Development, 2001). In the global COVID-19 pandemic, infectious control measures limited people's attendance to health care services. Nevertheless, this was the time of highest health care service demand. Patients with close contact, respiratory symptoms or non-specific deterioration of general condition need timely assessment by their health care providers. Due to the social distancing measures and restrictions, telecommunication has been extensively employed in health care, and it relies heavily on internet connection. It potentially exacerbates the existing digital inequality and widens the digital divide (Azzopardi-Muscat & Sorensen, 2019). The effective use of digital technology firstly depends on network coverage and hardware availability. Further, the knowledge and technological capability of an individual in using them is also important. Those living in rural areas, belonging to an older age group or having pre-existing medical conditions, including cognitive impairment, visual impairment, dexterity problems, etc., are prone to encounter difficulties in the access, knowledge and skill of digital health information.

Nowadays, most teens and adults in the developed countries possess at least one mobile device. As of April 2022, 5 billion people used the internet worldwide, which was around 63% of the global population. 4.65 billion of them were social media users. East Asia (particularly China and India) has the highest number of internet users worldwide, whereas Northern Europe has the highest global internet penetration rate (Statista Research Department, 2022). In Hong Kong, 94.4% of households have internet access. However, the access rate is only 75.2% in the families with a monthly household income below HK$10,000 (USD 1,274) (Census & Statistics Department, 2022).

The digital divide significantly impacts the competition of access to the limited health care services. It imposes barriers for individuals and families without network, particularly in understanding the choice of available services and scheduling appointments. Patients may not be able to receive timely information on health care service suspension or diversion during the pandemic. For example, many elective, non-urgent health care services were changed, or rescheduled in the beginning of COVID-19 pandemic. A significant proportion of health care workers were infected, or being close contacts of the infected. Mobile phone SMS and social media were relied heavily to announce the changes of service. Some patients, therefore, could not access health care services to manage their health problems. They became anxious on the nature and prognosis of their health problems. It might result in inappropriate use of emergency services if they could not use online resources to manage their health problems. Many health institutes now use electronic means in scheduling appointments and managing referrals to specialists and allied health services. This creates a barrier for digitally disconnected patients to access health services. Furthermore, they would be less empowered to manage their own health as they do not have access to online tools that could facilitate them to check their health record, laboratory data, medication history and so forth.

Catalysing Digital Health Care in COVID-19

The pandemic has catalysed the speedy development of eHealth services, including initial patient assessment, COVID-19 confirm cases reporting, surveillance and follow-up of many patients within a short time. By using push notifications from mobile applications (apps), the government could communicate with the public more instantly regarding important health information and relevant regulations. Many countries use digital contact tracing apps to facilitate outbreak investigations, which are traditionally done labour-intensively. The information gathered by the apps can also help predict the outbreak risk in a particular area or region using big data analytics and statistical modelling.

The suspension of routine health services during COVID-19 drove the rapid development of telemedicine. For example, the Home Online Health Consultation Systems (HOHC) used synchronous video conferencing systems or software (such as Skype or Zoom) to facilitate the communication between a health care professional in their workplace and a patient and their carer in the home. Patients must have internet access and either a computer or mobile device. It was known that some could not use the service because of internet connection issues (Almathami et al., 2020). In Hong Kong, the Hospital Authority used telemedicine to deliver care for COVID-19 patients with mild symptoms. They did not need to travel to clinics, thus reducing the risk of transmission in the community. The medications could be dispatched to their home by non-contact courier services.

Digital Health Literacy

Digital health literacy or eHealth literacy refers to people's health literacy in digital contexts and environments. It includes the skills and knowledge to search, find, understand and appraise health information on the internet. Then they can apply the knowledge to solve their health problems (Norman & Skinner, 2006b). The competency involves operational skills, navigation skills, information searching, evaluating reliability, determining relevance, adding self-generated content and protecting privacy (van der Vaart & Drossaert, 2017). Today, enhancing the general public's health literacy, even digital health literacy, has become a global goal for better health promotion, patient education and communication strategies, ultimately improving health outcomes. The World Health Organisation has put "Improving Health Literacy" under a health promotion activity (World Health Organization, n. d.).

In the scenario of this common example, a 4-year-old child has a fever of 39-degree Celsius and rashes over his tummy. The mother has to decide if she should give him some paracetamol and wait, or bring him to see a general practitioner, the emergency department or a Chinese Medicine practitioner. Apart from discussing with other family members, the mother then searches for the appropriate management on the internet and may ask experts or other parents on social media. When she decides to see a GP, she searches for any GP nearby and their operation hours, then she makes an appointment using the mobile apps. When she brings the child to see the GP, she has to scan her QR code to record her visit, demonstrating to the clinic staff that she has completed three doses of COVID vaccines. She fills in a web-based questionnaire to declare if she has any febrile illnesses or contact history. Her GP gives her electronic pamphlets for patient education of children with fever. While waiting for her drugs, she can use mobile apps to check when the drugs are available for collection. She can look up the drugs' names, dosage and side effects on the internet. She can set drug alert messages or alarms to remind the drug compliance. After the consultation, the clinic nurse may follow up on her son's condition the day after by communication apps.

The above example demonstrates how the mother with adequate digital health literacy can manage her son's illnesses with the assistance of the internet. Imagine if the mother, with neither the mobile apps in the electronic device nor internet access, or if she was illiterate, she could only make decisions herself or among the family members. She would make appointments by phone calls and receives hard copies of education material. She would communicate with health care service providers by handwritten information or direct conversation. She might access less health information, less services and less knowledge to help to increase her self-efficacy. An interesting question is, "Would the child in the first scenario have a better health outcome?".

Mörelius et al. (2021) and Donovan et al. (2020) tried to answer the above question with systematic reviews. They had a few trials using web-based portals to improve parents' health knowledge and health behaviour. Mörelius et al. found that parents were highly satisfied with the intervention and showed improvement in health literacy and disease-specific knowledge, and some changed their behaviour. Donovan et al. (2020) reviewed the studies of two apps and one website: Children's On-Call—a US advice-only app; Should I See a Doctor?—a Dutch self-triage app for any acute illness; and Strategy for Off-Site Rapid Triage (SORT) for Kids—a US self-triage website for influenza-like illness. Many parents did not find the two apps easy to use. None of the interventions demonstrated a reduced use of urgent-care services. Concerning about the improvement in health literacy after intervention, it was difficult to compare outcomes between studies because of various measuring tools (Urstad et al., 2022).

Two most frequently used tools for digital health literacy measurement are the eHealth literacy scale (eHEALS) (Norman & Skinner, 2006a) and the European Health Literacy Survey Questionnaire (HLS-EU-Q47) (Sorensen et al., 2013). The eHEALS consists of eight items that measure knowledge and trust when subjects have health related concerns. Subjects rate their perceived skills in finding, evaluating and applying electronic health information on a 5-point scale in the range from 1 (strongly disagree) to 5 (strongly agree). It is simple and easy to use by self-administration. The items are "I know how or where…" "I can tell…". The outcome is subjective, and it may not reflect the actual ability and efficacy of the subjects. The tool cannot capture the social and personal related factors which may contribute to the digital health literacy level.

In HLS-EU-Q47, there are 47 health literacy related items, covering the 12 subscales, which are based on the access, understanding, appraisal and evaluation and application of the health information in 3 domains: health care, disease prevention and health promotion. The subjects rate a 4-point scale in the range from very difficult to very easy, and the 5th item "I don't know". The questionnaire has been validated in 8 European countries. A short version of HLS-EU-Q12 contains unidimensional 12 items was developed for Norwegian population (Finbraten et al., 2018). In order to apply the short version in different populations, psychometric validation is required.

Health Problems in People with Low Health Literacy

The global health literacy level is far from satisfactory. For instance, a population survey in China found a drop of adequate health literacy level from the eastern region (33%) towards 17.6% in the western region (Li et al., 2021). The situation in Europe was highlighted in the 2011 European health literacy survey. The prevalence of low health literacy was inconsistent across Member States: Austria, Bulgaria, Germany (North Rhine-Westphalia), Greece, Ireland, the Netherlands, Poland and Spain. Overall, the health literacy among adult population was 47.6% (World Health Organization, 2018). In United Kingdom, 30% of people aged 65 and over has limited health literacy (von Wagner et al., 2007). Given that health literacy is only one of the six domains in digital health literacy, it can be estimated that the global digital health literacy should be much lower than recommended.

The factors associated with health literacy are mostly related to educational level and family income. People in poverty have less education opportunities, lower literacy and numeracy level, less time for self-study and less access to computer or internet. Yet, they tend to have more chronic illnesses, more health risk behaviour, less preventive activities and less practice of self-management. It is difficult to compare different adverse health outcomes in people with low health literacy with different illness. Mariciano et al. (2019) reviewed the association of diabetes patients' knowledge, self-care practice and glycaemic control with their health literacy level. They found diabetes knowledge is significantly associated with patients' health literacy, while the association were heterogeneous in self-care practice and glycaemic control.

The consequence of low digital health literacy is substantial. When almost everyone has at least one mobile devices, email account and social media accounts, the public are very likely to read low quality, misleading or false health information. The social media is overwhelmed with fake news. van der Linden et al. (2020) summarised the fake news in social media during COVID-19. For example, gargling with lemon or salt water and injecting oneself with bleach could cure COVID-19; the 5G cellular network worsened symptoms of COVID-19; wearing a mask actually "activated" the coronavirus. Naeem et al. (2021) found more than 1,000 fake news in the social media. Their study concluded that the COVID-19 infodemic was full of false claims, half backed conspiracy theories and pseudoscientific therapies, regarding the diagnosis, treatment, prevention, origin and spread of the virus. The fake news distorts people's risk perception, therefore changes health behaviour and people's compliance to the public health recommendation, such as the psychological resistance to vaccination.

Ethical Issues in Digital Health

Autonomy, beneficence, non-maleficence and justice are the four key ethical principles by Beauchamp and Childress in analysing biomedical issues. Very often, tension may arise in these principles in different situations. Some of the digital health interventions during COVID-19 are examined by applying the principlism (Beauchamp & Childress, 2019).

The principle of autonomy refers to the respect for self-determination of an individual and is considered a fundamental human right. In terms of medical interventions, a person should be given a choice to accept or refuse without coercion. As mentioned previously, there is widespread adoption of telecare during the pandemic. An individual should be provided adequate information regarding the process, benefits and risks of using teleconsultations before the person voluntarily chooses the service. Informed consent should be obtained by having a genuine dialogue between the user and service provider without undue influence or exaggerating the expected benefits. Incentives should be provided cautiously and appropriately. The user should also be given alternative options (e.g. retreating to routine clinical care) if he or she refuses to use telecare so that the user would not be disadvantaged or excluded from the health system.

In simple terms, principles of beneficence and non-maleficence mean "doing good" and "do no harm", respectively, with the aims of maximising the benefits and minimising the harm. There are many advantages of using digital health care, like reduction of health care costs, particularly for those living in difficult-to-reach areas, enhancement of communication between patients and health care providers, greater patient empowerment using digital health resources and provision of integrated medical records for better patient care. However, there may be potential harm if the health technology is related to the misuse of health data. Data privacy is one of the major concerns for the digitalisation of health care. Health organisations should adhere to the relevant data protection regulations and are obliged to prevent any unintended and unauthorised use of data. The data should only be used for specific purposes with the consent of the data owners.

Lastly, the principle of justice refers to equal and fair distribution of resources in health care through rationing. Each decision made needs to be transparent and accountable to gain support from the public (Brall et al., 2019). Norman Daniels and James Sabin (2002) put forward the notion of "accountability for reasonableness" to explain how a justifiable and legitimate priority-setting decision could be made. Four conditions must be satisfied upon deliberation of stakeholders: publicity, relevance, appeals and enforcement conditions (Daniels & Sabin, 2002; Nyrup, 2021).

Bridging the "Digital Divide"

The development of digital health care is inevitable in the modern era. To address the gaps in technology-driven health care for individuals with low digital health literacy, multi-sectoral collaboration involving the government, non-governmental organisations (NGOs), internet service providers, private companies, health organisations and representatives from various patient groups is essential. Before implementing digital health care, potential users should be involved in the process of designing the algorithms. Particular attention should be given to those vulnerable populations, including children and elderly, socially disadvantaged groups, people with disability, homeless people, marginalised populations and the ethnic minorities (Eyrich et al., 2021).

To bridge the digital divide and to increase the uptake of digital health care, the provision of hardware and implementation of strategies to improve digital health literacy are essential. In terms of hardware, digital infrastructure, including adequate network coverage and broadband, should be provided at an affordable price. The government and NGOs could subsidise the acquisition of mobile devices for those with financial difficulty. Free and secured network access could be provided in public places, such as libraries, community centres, hospitals and clinics, government buildings and recreational venues.

In order to improve the digital health literacy of the population, targeted strategies are needed to meet the need of different population groups. For example, the elderly may be less proficient in using mobile devices and network services. Hands-on digital skills training workshops would be beneficial for them. One must pay particular attention that while designing such workshops; the information should be delivered in simple and straightforward languages. The carers could also be empowered to provide support. Digital resources in the community should also be made known to those in need (Alkureishi et al., 2021).

On the other hand, misinformation is everywhere on the internet. Individuals with technological capability need to take extra caution to the pseudoscientific messages, especially during disasters and public health crisis like the COVID-19 pandemic. Such falsified information may mislead the general public to be sceptical towards the government policies in infection control, quarantine measures and vaccination campaigns, which in turn lead to inappropriate health-seeking behaviours and mistrust between health care professionals and patients (Chesser et al., 2016). The government should educate the general public to improve their ability to discern trustworthy or misleading sources. In the case of widespread rumours that may have an enormous impact, the government could clarify the misinformation timely to avoid inducing public anxiety and distress.

Although digitalisation of health care is unavoidable, it should be aware of the fact that some patients have limited access to the digital system because of physical disability, mental incapacity or socially disadvantage. The choice of individuals should be respected because some may prefer to use traditional communication methods. Health care organisations should provide "low-tech" communication options for users, such as telephone calls and mails, so as to avoid excluding them from the health care system. Home visits by health care workers should not be substituted entirely by virtual telecare, as examinations and some treatments could not be done without physically touching the patients.

Conclusion

Adequate digital health literacy is essential for the general public to navigate the digitalised health care system. COVID-19 pandemic has catalysed the development of a technology-driven health care model, including health education and information dissemination, doctor-patient consultations, contact tracing and outbreak containment and big data modelling for risk assessment. Although it seems promising, the government and policy-makers should avoid exacerbating the digital inequality and "digital divide". Ethical principles, particularly the principle of justice, should be carefully considered before implementing digital technologies. All should work together to improve digital health literacy for the betterment of the health of the general public.

References

Alkureishi, M. A., Choo, Z. Y., Rahman, A., Ho, K., Benning-Shorb, J., Lenti, G., Velázquez Sánchez, I., Zhu, M., Shah, S. D. & Lee, W. W. (2021). Digitally disconnected: Qualitative study of patient perspectives on the digital divide and potential solutions. *JMIR Human Factors, 8*(4), Article e33364. https://doi.org/10.2196/33364

Almathami, H. K. Y., Win, K. T., & Vlahu-Gjorgievska, E. (2020). Barriers and facilitators that influence telemedicine-based, real-time, online consultation at patients' homes: Systematic literature review. *Journal of Medical Internet Research, 22*(2), Article e16407. https://doi.org/10.2196/16407

Azzopardi-Muscat, N., & Sorensen, K. (2019). Towards an equitable digital public health era: Promoting equity through a health literacy perspective. *European Journal of Public Health, 29*(Supplement_3), 13–17. https://doi.org/10.1093/eurpub/ckz166

Beauchamp, T. L., & Childress, J. F. (2019). *Principles of biomedical ethics* (8th ed.). Oxford University Press. https://global.oup.com/ushe/product/principles-of-biomedical-ethics-9780190640873?cc=hk&lang=en&

Brall, C., Schroder-Back, P., & Maeckelberghe, E. (2019). Ethical aspects of digital health from a justice point of view. *European Journal of Public Health, 29*(Supplement_3), 18–22. https://doi.org/10.1093/eurpub/ckz167

Census and Statistics Department. (2022). *Personal computer and internet penetration.* https://www.censtatd.gov.hk/en/data/stat_report/product/C0000052/att/B11302752022XXXXB0100.pdf

Chesser, A., Burke, A., Reyes, J., & Rohrberg, T. (2016). Navigating the digital divide: A systematic review of eHealth literacy in underserved populations in the United States. *Informatics for Health and Social Care, 41*(1), 1–19. https://doi.org/10.3109/17538157.2014.948171

Committee, A. H., & on Health Literacy for the Council on Scientific Affairs, American Medical Association. (1999). Health literacy: Report of the council on scientific affairs. *JAMA, 281*(6), 552–557. https://doi.org/10.1001/jama.281.6.552

Daniels, N., & Sabin, J. E. (2002). Accountability for reasonableness. In N. Daniels, & J. E. Sabins (Eds.), *Setting limits fairly: Can we learn to share medical resources?* (pp. 43–66). Oxford University Press. https://doi.org/10.1093/acprof:oso/9780195149364.003.0004

Donovan, E., Wilcox, C. R., Patel, S., Hay, A. D., Little, P., & Willcox, M. L. (2020). Digital interventions for parents of acutely ill children and their treatment-seeking behaviour: A systematic review. *British Journal of General Practice, 70*(692), e172–e178. https://doi.org/10.3399/bjgp20X708209

Eyrich, N. W., Andino, J. J., & Fessell, D. P. (2021). Bridging the digital divide to avoid leaving the most vulnerable behind. *JAMA Surgery, 156*(8), 703–704. https://doi.org/10.1001/jamasurg.2021.1143

Finbraten, H. S., Wilde-Larsson, B., Nordstrom, G., Pettersen, K. S., Trollvik, A., & Guttersrud, O. (2018). Establishing the HLS-Q12 short version of the European Health Literacy Survey Questionnaire: latent trait analyses applying Rasch modelling and confirmatory factor analysis. *BMC Health Service Research, 18*, Article 506. https://doi.org/10.1186/s12913-018-3275-7

Li, Z., Tian, Y., Gong, Z., & Qian, L. (2021). Health literacy and regional heterogeneities in China: A population-based study. *Frontiers in Public Health, 9*, Article 603325. https://doi.org/10.3389/fpubh.2021.603325

Marciano, L., Camerini, A., & L., & Schulz, P. J. (2019). The role of health literacy in diabetes knowledge, self-care, and glycemic control: A meta-analysis. *Journal of General Internal Medicine, 34*(6), 1007–1017. https://doi.org/10.1007/s11606-019-04832-y

Mörelius, E., Robinson, S., Arabiat, D., & Whitehead, L. (2021). Digital interventions to improve health literacy among parents of children aged 0 to 12 years with a health condition: Systematic review. *Journal of Medical Internet Research, 23*(12), Article e31665. https://doi.org/10.2196/31665

Naeem, S. B., Bhatti, R., & Khan, A. (2021). An exploration of how fake news is taking over social media and putting public health at risk. *Health Information and Libraries Journal, 38*(2), 143–149. https://doi.org/10.1111/hir.12320

Norman, C. D., & Skinner, H. A. (2006a). eHEALS: The eHealth literacy scale. *Journal of Medical Internet Research, 8*(4), Article e27. https://doi.org/10.2196/jmir.8.4.e27

Norman, C. D., & Skinner, H. A. (2006b). eHealth Literacy: Essential Skills for consumer health in a networked world. *Journal of Medical Internet Research, 8*(2), Article e9. https://doi.org/10.2196/jmir.8.2.e9

Nutbeam, D. (2000). Health literacy as a public health goal: A challenge for contemporary health education and communication strategies into the 21st century. *Health Promotion International, 15*(3), 259–267. https://doi.org/10.1093/heapro/15.3.259

Nyrup, R. (2021). From general principles to procedural values: Responsible digital health meets public health ethics. *Frontiers in Digital Health, 3*, Article 690417. https://doi.org/10.3389/fdgth.2021.690417

Organisation for Economic Co-operation and Development. (2001). *Understanding the Digital Divide.* https://www.oecd.org/digital/ieconomy/1888451.pdf

Sorensen, K., Van den Broucke, S., Pelikan, J. M., Fullam, J., Doyle, G., Slonska, Z., Kondilis, B., Stoffels, V., Osborne, R.H., & Consortium, H. E. (2013). Measuring health literacy in populations: Illuminating the design and development process of the European Health Literacy Survey Questionnaire (HLS-EU-Q). *BMC Public Health, 13*, Article 948. https://doi.org/10.1186/1471-2458-13-948

Statista Research Department. (2022). *Internet usage worldwide - statistics & facts.* Retrieved from https://www.statista.com/topics/1145/internet-usage-worldwide/

Urstad, K. H., Andersen, M. H., Larsen, M. H., Borge, C. R., Helseth, S., & Wahl, A. K. (2022). Definitions and measurement of health literacy in health and medicine research: A systematic review. *BMJ Open, 12*(2), Article e056294. https://doi.org/10.1136/bmjopen-2021-056294

van der Linden, S., Roozenbeek, J., & Compton, J. (2020). Inoculating against fake news about COVID-19. *Frontiers in Psychology, 11*, Article 566790. https://doi.org/10.3389/fpsyg.2020.566790

van der Vaart, R., & Drossaert, C. (2017). Development of the digital health literacy instrument: Measuring a broad spectrum of health 1.0 and health 2.0 Skills. *Journal of Medical Internet Research, 19*(1), Article e27. https://doi.org/10.2196/jmir.6709

von Wagner, C., Knight, K., Steptoe, A., & Wardle, J. (2007). Functional health literacy and health-promoting behaviour in a national sample of British adults. *Journal of Epidemiology & Community Health, 61*(12), 1086–1090. https://doi.org/10.1136/jech.2006.053967

World Health Organization. (2018). *What is the evidence on existing policies and linked activities and their effectiveness for improving health literacy at national, regional and organizational levels in the WHO European Region?* https://apps.who.int/iris/handle/10665/326251

World Health Organization. (n. d.). *Improving health literacy.* https://www.who.int/activities/improving-health-literacy

Chapter 9
Video Conferencing-Delivered Health Intervention

Janet Lok Chun Lee and Sui Yu Yau

Abstract Videoconferencing has emerged as a form of telemedicine for delivering health interventions since the turn of the millennium. It has many advantages over other forms of telemedicine like phone calls or web-based system because of its multisensory outputs. For instance, healthcare providers and care recipients can see each other, listen and interact with each other in real time. It makes the experiences of the remote physical or psychological therapy sessions, group health education, and medical consultation more satisfying. The COVID-19 pandemic has accelerated the wide adoption of it, and there has been an upsurge of articles investigating the feasibility of videoconferencing as a form of healthcare delivery model. This chapter begins with a brief historical review of telemedicine and telehealth. Thereafter, the current evidence for the effectiveness, uniqueness, and challenges of videoconferencing-delivered health interventions is reviewed. Finally, the use of videoconferencing as an extension of space and place by traditional health institutions is discussed.

Keywords Videoconferencing · Telehealth · Tele-exercise · Tele-rehabilitation · Tele-psychiatry · Tele-palliative care

Introduction

The use of videoconferencing (VC) has emerged as a form of telemedicine for delivering health interventions since the turn of the millennium. Initially, VC was mainly used to provide remote healthcare to patients who lived in rural areas and had limited

J. L. C. Lee (✉)
Department of Rehabilitation Sciences, The Hong Kong Polytechnic University, Hong Kong, China
e-mail: lcjlee@polyu.edu.hk

S. Y. Yau
School of Nursing and Health Studies, Hong Kong Metropolitan University, Hong Kong, China
e-mail: isyyau@hkmu.edu.hk

B. Y. F. Fong and W. C. W. Wong (eds.), *Gaps and Actions in Health Improvement from Hong Kong and Beyond*,
https://doi.org/10.1007/978-981-99-4491-0_9

access to healthcare services. Before the outbreak of the coronavirus disease 2019 (COVID-19) pandemic, VC was widely used by various healthcare professionals in different disciplines. Since the pandemic, many research studies have documented the feasibility of VC-delivered health (VCH) interventions in different population sub-groups and among different healthcare professionals. These studies have found that the effectiveness of VCH interventions is similar to the effectiveness of face-to-face (F2F) health interventions for most participants (Amorese & Ryan, 2022; Berryhill et al., 2019; Steel et al., 2011). Unlike telephone-delivered or web-based systems for delivering remote healthcare, VCH interventions have unique advantages over F2F health interventions. The multisensory outputs of VC make it a more optimal communication medium than other information and communication technologies (ICTs), i.e. telephone, email, and web-based systems, which have a narrower range of sensory modalities. An increasing number of studies have shown that VCH interventions have the potential to permanently change the healthcare landscape, and instead of being a supplement or substitute for traditional F2F health interventions (Amorese & Ryan, 2022; Berryhill et al., 2019; Mallow et al., 2016; Steindal et al., 2020; Wundersitz et al., 2020). They may become an integral part of healthcare service delivery, and an extension of health services to patients' homes without the limits of physical place and space.

A Brief History of Telemedicine

VCH is a type of telemedicine, which is a term coined in the 1970s. Telemedicine has been broadly defined as the use of various types of ICTs to improve access to care and medical information with the aim of improving patient outcomes (World Health Organization, 2010). Initially, the use of ICTs in telemedicine referred to the use of videotapes and televisions to facilitate education and consultation between medical specialists and regional general practitioners in mental health disciplines (Benschoter et al., 1965). As ICTs have evolved, telemedicine now refers to the use of telephone calls or email messages for medical consultations. In recent time, telemedicine has included the use of VC technologies to improve access of healthcare for patients in rural and remote areas (Department of Health & Human Services, 2015). In general, ICTs may be divided into three main categories, namely synchronous, asynchronous, and hybrid. In the synchronous mode, real-time communication occurs for both parties. Examples of this type are VC and telephone calls. The asynchronous mode refers to 'store-and-forward' communications, which include mobile applications, email messages, online discussion forums, and web-based systems. The hybrid mode simply refers to the combination of both synchronous and asynchronous modes of communication (Rudel et al., 2011).

The terms 'telemedicine' and 'telehealth' are used interchangeably in the literature. While both terms emphasise the use of ICTs to provide remote support, 'telehealth' usually refers to broader health-related service delivery by healthcare professionals, such as allied health professionals (Rudel et al., 2011), while 'telemedicine' usually refers to clinical service delivery by physicians only (World Health Organization, 2010). In addition to the terms ‘telemedicine’ and ‘telehealth’, when describing the use of ICTs for remote care in different disciplines such as psychiatry, mental health, palliative care, rehabilitation, and exercise intervention, terms like ‘telepsychiatry’, ‘telemental health’, ‘telepalliative care’, ‘telerehabilitation’, and ‘tele-exercise’ are found in the literature.

Emergence of VC-delivered Health Interventions

As described in the previous section, when VC is used as the mode of delivery of a health intervention, it falls into the synchronous communication telehealth category and supports real-time communication between health service providers and patients or clients. It also allows two or more locations to be connected in real-time using two-way video and audio transmission (Rudel et al., 2011). The application of VC in delivering health interventions may be traced back to the 2000s in different healthcare disciplines. Studies of VC-delivered interventions for long-term chronic disease management (Banbury et al., 2018; Foucher et al., 2015), exercise intervention delivery (Wu & Keyes, 2006), long-term weight management (Ahrendt et al., 2014), and psychotherapy (Shore, 2013; Strachan et al., 2012) have been reported. These studies have explored the use of VC as a delivery mode because of its unique advantages of reaching individuals in rural areas and the lower cost of long-term management. A review revealed that patients with a wide variety of contexts and conditions (e.g. cancer, diabetes, chronic obstructive pulmonary disease, osteoporosis, and cardiovascular disease) have high levels of satisfaction with VCH interventions (Steel et al., 2011). The use of VCH interventions is especially well-adopted in the field of nursing. For instance, nurse-led clinics or interventions using VC have provided comprehensive and high-quality care for cancer patients (Kwok et al., 2022a; Reb et al., 2020), sexual assault victims (Miyamoto et al., 2021), older adults (Wong et al., 2022), and patients with prevalent chronic diseases (Whitmore et al., 2020).

The feasibility of VC as a delivery mode has been investigated, and there is both quantitative and qualitative evidence showing favourable results. There is an accumulating evidence demonstrating that patients have high levels of satisfaction with and acceptance of VCH interventions (Richardson et al., 2009). VCH interventions have become widely accepted and adopted in health disciplines that rely heavily on verbal communication or advice, such as psychotherapy, speech therapy, or dietitian-led dietary advice sessions. Conversely, it is less accepted or adopted in physical health disciplines that require a more hands-on approach (Wundersitz et al., 2020).

COVID-19 as a Turning Point for the Widespread Adoption of VC as a Delivery Mode

There had been a significant turning point in the adoption of VC during the COVID-19 pandemic, which required healthcare services to transition to remote care as a precautious measure. Telehealth became the only practical and feasible means to maintain professional connection and healthcare delivery during lock-down periods or when strict social distancing measures were in place. Since the onset of the pandemic, there have been numerous studies reporting the use of VC as an alternative for the conventional F2F healthcare services. Examples included interventional studies for individuals with mild intellectual disabilities (Oudshoorn et al., 2021), older adults (Wong et al., 2022), individuals with dementia (Greenwood-Hickman et al., 2021), youth with mental health problems (DeLuca et al., 2020), cancer patients and their caregivers (Snyder et al., 2021), adults with psychological distress (Keyan et al., 2021), individuals with Parkinson's disease (Kwok et al., 2022b), children with autism spectrum disorder (Su et al., 2021), and individuals with obesity (Calcaterra et al., 2021). Findings from these studies have demonstrated the successful transformation to the online delivery mode for most participants. The VC mode has also been positively received by most interventionists and participants.

Effectiveness of VC-delivered Health Interventions

Health Outcomes

Several review articles have shown that VCH interventions produce similar or equivalent effectiveness as F2F-delivered health interventions in health outcomes (Amorese & Ryan, 2022; Berryhill et al., 2019; Steel et al., 2011). For instance, patients with Parkinson's disease who received VCH had a similar improvement in VO_2 compared to patients who received a F2F intervention (van der Kolk et al., 2018). In the field of psychology, F2F- and VC-delivered cognitive-behavioural therapy (CBT) was found to be equally effective in reducing depressive symptoms in children. In postnatal care, VCH and F2F-delivered interventions have been shown to be equally effective, with both delivery modes resulting in a similar breastfeeding prevalence (Seguranyes et al., 2014). Research on counselling interventions for substance abusers has also shown that patients in the groups receiving a VC- or F2F-delivered intervention demonstrated a similar positive result for abstinence and with a 100% attendance when returning to less-intensive care (King et al., 2009).

Engagement

Participants' level of engagement in VCH interventions has been found to be similar to that in F2F interventions. Children with special education needs and individuals with an intellectual disability have been shown to be equally engaged in activities requiring fine and gross-motor skills during VCH and F2F interventions (Oudshoorn et al., 2021; Wynn et al., 2012). The effectiveness of VCH interventions in engaging participants is also reflected in attendance rates. For example, a VC-delivered CBT intervention for children and a VC-delivered yoga intervention for individuals with Parkinson's disease have been shown to have high attendance rates (Kwok et al., 2022b).

Empathy

While the effects and engagement ability of an intervention are essential, the establishment of a relationship between the interventionist and the participants is also important. Research has shown that VCH interventions are able to effectively convey warmth and empathy. In the field of psychiatry, while clinicians have expressed concern about the difficulty in establishing rapport and trust and showing empathy towards their clients (Wynn et al., 2012), interestingly, clients of VC-delivered psychotherapy sessions perceive therapists to be significantly more empathic and supportive during VCH interventions than F2F interventions (Sperandeo et al., 2021). A similar phenomenon was observed in VC-delivered stroke rehabilitation. It has been suggested that conveying empathy does not necessarily require physical touch or environmental proximity, because it may also be communicated through facial expression, vocal intonation, and attentive participation in an online mode (Cheshire et al., 2021).

Advantages of VC-delivered Health Interventions

VCH interventions are able to remove the barriers of distance and mobility, create unique safe spaces for patients, and cost-effectively maintain long-term management and the continuity of care.

Removing the Barriers of Distance and Mobility

It has been found that a VC-delivered exercise intervention reduces the barriers related to transportation and improves access to trained healthcare professionals for those who have geographical or mobility restrictions (Amorese & Ryan, 2022; Mois et al., 2019; Wakasa et al., 2020). Moreover, for patients with a high symptom burden, VCH interventions represent an excellent method to maintain the continuity of care by healthcare providers (Chávarri-Guerra et al., 2021).

Creating a Safe Place and Space

In the field of psychiatry, users of VC-delivered services have reported that VC-delivered care provides feelings of safety and security. They have found that the VC delivery mode reduces stigma, as care is provided in the home environment and, therefore, is more confidential and safer (Shore, 2015). Similarly, research has shown that substance abusers prefer VC-delivered counselling with mental health professionals to the F2F mode because of the increase in confidentiality (Berryhill et al., 2019). Similarly, patients receiving palliative care have reported that VC-delivered care contributes to feelings of relief, tranquillity, and security. They have also reported experiencing concentrated responsiveness from healthcare professionals and a high possibility of reaching agreement on the division of responsibilities for future health actions (Steindal et al., 2020).

Maintaining Long-term Management and Continuity of Care

VCH interventions also have greater long-term effects on weight management than F2F interventions (Ahrendt et al., 2014). Reb and colleagues (2020) found that the skills practiced during a nurse-led VCH intervention helped to ease anxiety and fears related to cancer progression in patients with advanced cancer. The severity of most symptoms, such as depression, anxiety, emotional stress, and pain severity, has been shown to decrease for cancer patients after receiving a VCH intervention (Kwok et al., 2022a; Ream et al., 2020). Most importantly, enhanced quality of life and improved self-efficacy have also been reported after VCH interventions (Chen et al., 2018; Wong et al., 2022).

Challenges of VC-delivered Health Interventions

Although VC-delivered health interventions are shown to be as effective as F2F health intervention on certain health outcomes and have its own uniqueness, health interventions delivered by VC do face some challenges. They are privacy concerns, receptiveness of service providers, and technical challenges.

Privacy Issues

As previously mentioned, some patients perceive VCH to have high confidentiality, as it is delivered at the patients' homes, where the home environment enhanced the feeling of privacy. However, some patients are worried that the remote sessions are not totally private or the sessions may be privately recorded and viewed by others (Rodda et al., 2022; Wynn et al., 2012).

Receptiveness of the Health Service Providers

Health practitioners, in general, are less receptive to VC than patients (Steel et al., 2011). There are two major reasons that affected their receptiveness. Firstly, in the field of psychiatry, psychiatric health practitioners perceive increased efforts in using VC in delivering therapy session. They perceive using higher amount of effort and energy in building rapport and demonstrating empathy to service recipients when compared to in-person sessions (Wynn et al., 2012). Secondly, perceived quality of VCH is lower. For example, in the field of integrative care, VCH that requires supervising patients' bodily movements, like VC-delivered exercise sessions, even participants used external webcams and adjustable stands; health practitioners have difficulty in viewing the participants' entire bodies, thus hindering their ability to give quality supervision or instructional adjustment to the participants (Snyder et al., 2021).

Technical Challenges

To deliver VCH, ICTs infrastructure is required. Not all health service providers have access to internet or stable internet connections. Additionally, health service providers might not have appropriate hardware or professionals with adequate knowledge to operate hardware requires for VCH. Similarly, service users may not have internet access, and device to connect to VCH (Chávarri-Guerra et al., 2021).

A Perspective Future Role of VCH Interventions in the Smart Health Era—Extending the Space and Place for Health Interventions

VCH interventions have the potential to extend the space of intervention from the clinic or hospital to the patient's home. COVID-19 has accelerated the adoption of VC in delivering health interventions and appeared to have 'permanently' changed the healthcare landscape. It has also encouraged the wider adoption of VC from lecture-based health education interventions to programmes involving exercise and physical health rehabilitation. Studies conducted during COVID-19 have provided evidence that interventions not originally planned to be delivered by VC can be successfully adjusted to be delivered by VC and achieve good adherence and engagement from participants.

It is worthwhile to highlight some potential health improvements and benefits for individuals arising from the use of VCH. VCH allows long-term lifestyle and disease management that improve a person's health in a long run. Long-term lifestyle management programmes for specific health purposes were not adequately provided to patients from health institution in the past because of the physical space limitations. The use of VC allows continuing health intervention and does not require the use of extra space from health institution. Physical fitness of a patients can be improved with the use of VCH. Research has suggested that patients are more motivated when they attend supervised VC-delivered exercise intervention in their home environment and there is a high potential in making exercise a habit (Wakasa et al., 2020). Long periods of physical rehabilitation or psychological therapy follow-up with patients will no longer take up physical space in the clinic or hospital, but can be performed in the patients' living environment. From a social health perspective, VC has the potential to help reduce the feelings of loneliness in older adults and to connect older adults in geriatric institutions with their loved ones (Naudé et al., 2021). Although individuals' technical literacy, internet access, and device ownership are challenges to the widespread adoption of VCH interventions, the benefits of VC identified above make it worthwhile to direct multilevel and multidisciplinary efforts towards addressing these challenges.

References

Ahrendt, A. D., Kattelmann, K. K., Rector, T. S., & Maddox, D. A. (2014). The effectiveness of telemedicine for weight management in the MOVE! program. *The Journal of Rural Health, 30*(1), 113–119. https://doi.org/10.1111/jrh.12049

Amorese, A. J., & Ryan, A. S. (2022). Home-based tele-exercise in musculoskeletal conditions and chronic disease: A literature review. *Frontiers in Rehabilitation Sciences, 3*, Article 811465. https://doi.org/10.3389/fresc.2022.811465

Banbury, A., Nancarrow, S., Dart, J., Gray, L., & Parkinson, L. (2018). Telehealth interventions delivering home-based support group videoconferencing: Systematic review. *Journal of Medical Internet Research, 20*(2), Article e25. https://doi.org/10.2196/jmir.8090

Benschoter, R., Eaton, M. T., & Smith, P. (1965). Use of videotape to provide individual instruction in techniques of psychotherapy. *Journal of Medical Education, 40*(12), 1159–1161. https://doi.org/10.1097/00001888-196512000-00006

Berryhill, M. B., Culmer, N., Williams, N., Halli-Tierney, A., Betancourt, A., Roberts, H., & King, M. (2019). Videoconferencing psychotherapy and depression: A systematic review. *Telemedicine and e-Health, 25*(6), 435–446. https://doi.org/10.1089/tmj.2018.0058

Calcaterra, V., Verduci, E., Vandoni, M., Rossi, V., Di Profio, E., Carnevale Pellino, V., Tranfagliam V., Pascuzzi, M. C., Borsani, B., Zuccotti, G., & Bosetti, A. (2021). Telehealth: A useful tool for the management of nutrition and exercise programs in pediatric obesity in the COVID-19 era. *Nutrients, 13*(11), Article 3689. https://doi.org/10.3390/nu13113689

Chávarri-Guerra, Y., Ramos-López, W. A., Covarrubias-Gómez, A., Sánchez-Román, S., Quiroz-Friedman, P., Alcocer-Castillejos, N., Del Pilar Milke-Garcia, M., Medina-Palma, M., Carrillo-Soto, M., Morales-Alfaro, A., Medina-Palma, M., Aguilar-Velazco, J. C., Morales-Barba, K., Razcon-Echegaray, A., Maldonado, J., & Soto-Perez-de-Celis, E. (2021). Providing supportive and palliative care using telemedicine for patients with advanced cancer during the COVID-19 pandemic in Mexico. *The Oncologist, 26*(3), e512–e515. https://doi.org/10.1002/onco.13568

Chen, Y. Y., Guan, B. S., Li, Z. K., & Li, X. Y. (2018). Effects of telehealth intervention on breast cancer patients' quality of life and psychological outcomes: A meta-analysis. *Journal of Telemedicine and Telecare, 24*(3), 157–167. https://doi.org/10.1177/1357633X16686777

Cheshire, W. P., Barrett, K. M., Eidelman, B. H., Mauricio, E. A., Huang, J. F., Freeman, W. D., Robinson, M. T., Salomon, G. R., Ball, C. T., Gamble, D. M., Melton, V. S., & Meschia, J. F. (2021). Patient perception of physician empathy in stroke telemedicine. *Journal of Telemedicine and Telecare, 27*(9), 572–581. https://doi.org/10.1177/1357633X19899237

DeLuca, J. S., Andorko, N. D., Chibani, D., Jay, S. Y., Rakhshan Rouhakhtar, P. J., Petti, E., Klaunig, M. J., Thompson, E. C., Millman, Z. B., Connors, K. M., LeeAnn Akouri-Shan, M. S. W., Fitzgerald, J., Redman, S. L., Roemer, C., Bridgwater, M. A., DeVylder, J. E., King, C. A., Pits, S. C., Reinblatt, S. P., … Schiffman, J. (2020). Telepsychotherapy with youth at clinical high risk for psychosis: Clinical issues and best practices during the COVID-19 pandemic. *Journal of Psychotherapy Integration, 30*(2), 304–331. https://psycnet.apa.org/doi/10.1037/int0000211

Department of Health and Human Services. (2015). Critical success factors: How to establish a successful telehealth service. *Victorian Government.* https://www2.health.vic.gov.au/Api/downloadmedia/%7B7BFB8453-C318-47CF-8261-3B8F27AF057E%7D

Foucher, Y., Meurette, A., Daguin, P., Bonnaud-Antignac, A., Hardouin, J.-B., Chailan, S., Neau, K., Papuchon, E., Gaboriau, S., Legendre, C., Morélon, E., Tessier, P., & Giral, M. (2015). A personalized follow-up of kidney transplant recipients using video conferencing based on a 1-year scoring system predictive of long term graft failure (TELEGRAFT study): Protocol for a randomized controlled trial. *BMC Nephrology, 16*, Article 6. https://doi.org/10.1186/1471-2369-16-6

Greenwood-Hickman, M. A., Dahlquist, J., Cooper, J., Holden, E., McClure, J. B., Mettert, K. D., Perry, S. R., & Rosenberg, D. E. (2021). "They're going to zoom it": A qualitative investigation of impacts and coping strategies during the COVID-19 pandemic among older adults. *Frontiers in Public Health, 9*, Article 679976. https://doi.org/10.3389/fpubh.2021.679976

Keyan, D., Dawson, K., Azevado, S., Yadav, S., Tran, J., & Bryant, R. A. (2021). Brief videoconferencing psychological intervention for reducing COVID-19 related distress: Study protocol for a randomized controlled trial. *BMC Public Health, 21*, Article 474. https://doi.org/10.1186/s12889-021-10529-x

King, V. L., Stoller, K. B., Kidorf, M., Kindbom, K., Hursh, S., Brady, T., & Brooner, R. K. (2009). Assessing the effectiveness of an Internet-based videoconferencing platform for delivering intensified substance abuse counseling. *Journal of Substance Abuse Treatment, 36*(3), 331–338. https://doi.org/10.1016/j.jsat.2008.06.011

Kwok, C., Degen, C., Moradi, N., & Stacey, D. (2022a). Nurse-led telehealth interventions for symptom management in patients with cancer receiving systemic or radiation therapy: A systematic review and meta-analysis. *Support Care in Cancer, 30*, 7119–7132. https://doi.org/10.1007/s00520-022-07052-z

Kwok, J. Y. Y., Lee, J. J., Choi, E. P. H., Chau, P. H., & Auyeung, M. (2022b). Stay mindfully active during the coronavirus pandemic: A feasibility study of mHealth-delivered mindfulness yoga program for people with Parkinson's disease. *BMC Complementary Medicine and Therapies, 22*, Article 37. https://doi.org/10.1186/s12906-022-03519-y

Mallow, J. A., Petitte, T., Narsavage, G., Barnes, E., Theeke, E., Mallow, B. K., & Theeke, L. A. (2016). The use of video conferencing for persons with chronic conditions: A systematic review.

E-Health Telecommunication Systems and Networks, 5(2), 39–56. https://doi.org/10.4236/etsn.2016.52005

Miyamoto, S., Thiede, E., Dorn, L., Perkins, D. F., Bittner, C., & Scanlon, D. (2021). The sexual assault forensic examination telehealth (SAFE-T) center: A comprehensive, nurse-led telehealth model to address disparities in sexual assault care. *The Journal of Rural Health, 37*(1), 91–102. https://doi.org/10.1111/jrh.12474

Mois, G., Mackin, T. E., Datta, A., Koon, L. M., Rogers, W. A., Mitzner, T. L., & Beer, J. M. (2019). Perceptions from people aging with a mobility impairment towards using tele-technology for exercise. *Proceedings of the Human Factors and Ergonomics Society Annual Meeting, 63*(1), 11–15. https://doi.org/10.1177/1071181319631040

Naudé, B., Rigaud, A.-S., & Pino, M. (2021). Video calls for older adults: A narrative review of experiments involving older adults in elderly care institutions. *Frontiers in Public Health, 9*, Article 751150. https://doi.org/10.3389/fpubh.2021.751150

Oudshoorn, C. E. M., Frielink, N., Riper, H., & Embregts, P. (2021). Experiences of therapists conducting psychological assessments and video conferencing sessions with people with mild intellectual disabilities during the COVID-19 pandemic. *International Journal of Developmental Disabilities*, 1–9. https://doi.org/10.1080/20473869.2021.1967078

Ream, E., Hughes, A. E., Cox, A., Skarparis, K., Richardson, A., Pedersen, V. H., Wiseman, T., Forbes, A., & Bryant, A. (2020). Telephone interventions for symptom management in adults with cancer. *Cochrane Database of Systematic Reviews, 6*, Article CD007568. https://doi.org/10.1002/14651858.CD007568.pub2

Reb, A. M., Borneman, T., Economou, D., Cangin, M. A., Cope, D. G., Ma, H., Ruel, N., Sharpe, L., Patel, K. S., Cristea, M., Koczywas, M., & Ferrell, B. (2020). A nurse-led intervention for fear of cancer progression in advanced cancer: A pilot feasibility study. *European Journal of Oncology Nursing, 49*, Article 101855. https://doi.org/10.1016/j.ejon.2020.101855

Richardson, L. K., Frueh, B. C., Grubaugh, A. L., Egede, L., & Elhai, J. D. (2009). Current directions in videoconferencing tele-mental health research. *Clinical Psychology: Science and Practice, 16*(3), 323–338. https://doi.org/10.1111/j.1468-2850.2009.01170.x

Rodda, S. N., Park, J. J., Wilkinson-Meyers, L., & King, D. L. (2022). The impact of COVID-19 on addiction treatment in New Zealand. *Addictive Behaviors, 127*, Article 107230. https://doi.org/10.1016/j.addbeh.2021.107230

Rudel, D., Fisk, M., & Roze, R. (2011). Definitions of terms in telehealth. *Informatica Medica Slovenica, 16*(1), 28–46. https://ims.mf.uni-lj.si/ims_archive/16-01/16a-21.pdf

Seguranyes, G., Costa, D., Fuentelsaz-Gallego, C., Beneit, J. V., Carabantes, D., Gómez-Moreno, C., Palacio-Tauste, A., Pauli Group, A., & Abella, M. (2014). Efficacy of a videoconferencing intervention compared with standard postnatal care at primary care health centres in Catalonia. *Midwifery, 30*(6), 764–771. https://doi.org/10.1016/j.midw.2013.08.004

Shore, J. (2013). Telepsychiatry: Videoconferencing in the delivery of psychiatric care. *American Journal of Psychiatry, 170*(3), 256–262. https://doi.org/10.1176/appi.ajp.2012.12081064

Shore, J. (2015). The evolution and history of telepsychiatry and its impact on psychiatric care: Current implications for psychiatrists and psychiatric organizations. *International Review of Psychiatry, 27*(6), 469–475. https://doi.org/10.3109/09540261.2015.1072086

Snyder, S., Silva, R. F., Whisenant, M. S., & Milbury, K. (2021). Videoconferenced yoga interventions for cancer patients and their caregivers during the COVID-19 pandemic: A report from a clinician's perspective. *Integrative Cancer Therapies, 20*, 1–7. https://doi.org/10.1177/15347354211019111

Sperandeo, R., Cioffi, V., Mosca, L. L., Longobardi, T., Moretto, E., Alfano, Y. M., Guerriera, C., Architravo, M., & Maldonato, N. M. (2021). Exploring the question: "Does empathy work in the same way in online and in-person therapeutic settings?" *Frontiers in Psychology, 12*, Article 671790. https://doi.org/10.3389/fpsyg.2021.671790

Steel, K., Cox, D., & Garry, H. (2011). Therapeutic videoconferencing interventions for the treatment of long-term conditions. *Journal of Telemedicine and Telecare, 17*(3), 109–117. https://doi.org/10.1258/jtt.2010.100318

Steindal, S. A., Nes, A. A. G., Godskesen, T. E., Dihle, A., Lind, S., Winger, A., & Klarare, A. (2020). Patients' experiences of telehealth in palliative home care: Scoping review. *Journal of Medical Internet Research, 22*(5), Article e16218. https://doi.org/10.2196/16218

Strachan, M., Gros, D. F., Yuen, E., Ruggiero, K. J., Foa, E. B., & Acierno, R. (2012). Home-based telehealth to deliver evidence-based psychotherapy in veterans with PTSD. *Contemporary Clinical Trials, 33*(2), 402–409. https://doi.org/10.1016/j.cct.2011.11.007

Su, W.-C., Srinivasan, S., Cleffi, C., & Bhat, A. (2021). Short report on research trends during the COVID-19 pandemic and use of telehealth interventions and remote brain research in children with autism spectrum disorder. *Autism, 25*(6), 1816–1822. https://doi.org/10.1177/136236132 11004795

van der Kolk, N. M., de Vries, N. M., Penko, A. L., van der Vlugt, M., Mulder, A. A., Post, B., Alberts, J. L., & Bloem, B. R. (2018). A remotely supervised home-based aerobic exercise programme is feasible for patients with Parkinson's disease: Results of a small randomised feasibility trial. *Journal of Neurology, Neurosurgery & Psychiatry, 89*(9), 1003–1005. https://doi.org/10.1136/jnnp-2017-315728

Wakasa, M., Odashima, T., Saito, A., Kimoto, M., Saito, I., Handa, S., Syukunobe, K., Kume, Y., & Okada, K. (2020). Telerehabilitation with tablet computers replaces face-to-face rehabilitation. *Physical & Occupational Therapy in Geriatrics, 38*(1), 85–97. https://doi.org/10.1080/02703181.2019.1660446

Whitmore, C., Bird, M., McGillion, M. H., Carter, N., Chen, R., Pierazzo, J., & Carroll, S. (2020). Impact of nurse scientist-led digital health interventions on management of chronic conditions. *Nursing Outlook, 68*(6), 745–762. https://doi.org/10.1016/j.outlook.2020.06.010

Wong, A. K. C., Bayuo, J., Wong, F. K. Y., Yuen, W. S., Lee, A. Y. L., Chang, P. K., & Lai, J. T. C. (2022). Effects of a nurse-led telehealth self-care promotion program on the quality of life of community-dwelling older adults: Systematic review and meta-analysis. *Journal of Medical Intercet Research, 24*(3), Article e31912. https://doi.org/10.2196/31912

World Health Organization. (2010). *Telemedicine: Opportunities and developments in Member states: Report on the second global survey on eHealth.* https://apps.who.int/iris/handle/10665/44497

Wu, G., & Keyes, L. M. (2006). Group tele-exercise for improving balance in elders. *Telemedicine Journal & E-Health, 12*(5), 561–570. https://doi.org/10.1089/tmj.2006.12.561

Wundersitz, C., Caelli, A., Georgy, J., Musovic, A., Manning, R., Prause, M., Robertson, J., & Taylor, N. F. (2020). Conducting community rehabilitation review sessions via videoconference: A feasibility study. *Australian Journal of Rural Health, 28*(6), 603–612. https://doi.org/10.1111/ajr.12665

Wynn, R., Bergvik, S., Pettersen, G., & Fossum, S. (2012). Clinicians' experiences with videoconferencing in psychiatry. In J. Mantas, S. K. Andersen, M. C. Mazzoleni, B. Blobel, S. Quaglini, & A. Moen (Eds.), *Quality of life through quality of information* (pp. 1218–1220). IOS Press. https://doi.org/10.3233/978-1-61499-101-4-1218

Chapter 10
Appropriate Care and Post-COVID-19 Syndrome

Leon Wai Li, Wing Tung Percy Ho, and Pui Yu Chesney Wong

Abstract Coronavirus disease 2019 (COVID-19) is caused by a new coronavirus called SARS-CoV-2 first identified in December 2019. It then became a pandemic outbreak and has been dominating activities of every country and significantly altered the form of daily life globally. In addition to its upsurge incidence rate and morbidity worldwide, the residual effects or sequelae of COVID-19 infection have been receiving more concerns including the impact on quality of life, and physical and mental health among the patients. With advancing definitions of "post-COVID-19 syndrome" by various studies, the syndrome describes an individual with a history of clinical and diagnostic SARS-CoV-2 infection with the persistence of symptoms and illness signs for more than 2–3 months which is not attributable to alternative diagnoses. The condition can be fluctuated or relapsed over time and developed into physical and mental sequelae. Despite the high incidence rate, the fatality rate is relatively low. Since there is an increasing number of patients who have recovered from COVID-19 infection but are still suffering from its complications, it is of utmost importance to identify necessary management plans and follow-up measures for the post-COVID-19 syndrome. By understanding the global situation of the post-COVID-19 syndrome, recognising the pathophysiology and clinical manifestations of the post-COVID-19 syndrome, and exploring the potential benefits gained from different post-COVID-19 management approaches, this chapter recommends a robust care plan for rehabilitation to multidisciplinary professionals in the community in the context of all for health.

Keywords COVID-19

L. W. Li (✉) · W. T. P. Ho
Hong Kong College of Community Health Practitioners, Hong Kong, China
e-mail: leonwai9413@gmail.com

P. Y. C. Wong
Department of Surgery, Queen Mary Hospital, Hong Kong, China

B. Y. F. Fong and W. C. W. Wong (eds.), *Gaps and Actions in Health Improvement from Hong Kong and Beyond*,
https://doi.org/10.1007/978-981-99-4491-0_10

The Post-COVID-19 Syndrome

With the strike of coronavirus disease 2019 (COVID-19) pandemic, the global healthcare system, healthcare resources and people's daily life had experienced an unprecedented impact. The infection of severe acute respiratory syndrome coronavirus 2 (SARS-CoV-2) can cause mild to severe symptoms, including fever, cough, fatigue, shortness of breath, sore throat, a sign of gastroenteritis, anomia, ageusia, clinical signs of pneumonia or respiratory failure (World Health Organization [WHO], 2021b). As the convalescent population has increased over the period, studies are starting to document the long-term effects of the complications and residual effects of SARS-CoV-2 infection (Michelen et al., 2021). Resources, follow-up and treatment strategies should thereby alter from focusing on primary controlling measures (e.g. treating acute COVID-19 symptoms) to developing management plans that can apply across multispecialty care in the outpatient setting to individual self-management level with the objective to reduce and alleviate the incompetence and pressure raised among people who recovered from COVID-19 (Malik et al., 2021; Vanichkachorn et al., 2021).

With varying terminology and clinical case definition mentioned in different kinds of literature regarding prolonged symptoms of COVID-19/post-COVID-19 condition, some termed the condition "post-acute COVID-19 syndrome" (Malik et al., 2021; Nalbandian et al., 2021), "chronic or post-COVID-19 syndrome" (Augustin et al., 2021; Menges et al., 2021) or "Long COVID" (Michelen et al., 2021; Sudre et al., 2021). In this chapter, the term "Post-COVID-19 syndrome" (PCS) will be used throughout the context.

To reach a uniform case definition of PCS, World Health Organization (2021a) has used the Delphi method to collect consensus data from internal and external experts, patients, clinicians, researchers, and other stakeholder groups from WHO regions, including African, American, Eastern Mediterranean, European, Southeast Asian and Western Pacific. This method is a prospective and structured communication technique that is beneficial to aggregate responses on a problem with numerous opinions and fluctuated group dynamics, especially during the pandemic period, face-to-face experts panel meetings can be hard to arrange due to infection control measures and geographical limitations (Grime & Wright, 2016). The WHO Delphi consensus determined PCS as the ongoing COVID-19 symptoms in individuals with a history of suspected or confirmed SARS-CoV-2 infection for more than 2–3 months which is not attributable to alternative diagnoses. The common symptoms of PCS can fluctuate or relapse over time, including fatigue, dyspnoea, anosmia, cognitive and psychological distress and joint and chest pain. These physical and mental sequelae can lead to a decline in quality of life as the convalescent people from COVID-19 will be hindered to be back on the normal social and occupational activities (Augustin et al., 2021; Malik et al., 2021; Vanichkachorn et al., 2021).

In this chapter, through exploring the pathophysiology and clinical manifestations of the post-COVID-19 syndrome along with medical, social and economic challenges faced by people recovering from COVID-19, an evidence-based care plan for rehabilitation by multidisciplinary professionals for the community and self-management will be recommended.

Epidemiology

Global Situation

COVID-19 is an infectious disease caused by coronavirus called SARS-CoV-2. It has caused over six million deaths worldwide since 2019. In late 2019, WHO's Country Office in People's Republic of China noticed a cluster of atypical pneumonia cases in Wuhan which were reported from the Chinese authorities. It activated Incident Management Support Team (IMST) to coordinate the emergency preparedness and response across regions and countries worldwide for public health emergency. On 30th January of 2020, the director of WHO declared a public health emergency concern and subsequently declared COVID-19 a pandemic in March of 2020 (World Health Organization, 2022a). However, the clinical presentation and tissue tropism of COVID-19 infection depend on the host species, like in human. The infection can be asymptomatic or symptomatic, and the virus is known with an extremely high mutation rates which facilitates the emergence of COVID-19 outbreaks (Sharma et al., 2021). Although the trend of new cases and mortality rate has been declining since March 2022, there are still newly diagnosed cases and new deaths found in some of the regions or countries (Table 10.1). Despite the government, non-government organisations (NGOs), researchers and pharmaceutical companies put great efforts on the prevention of COVID-19 infection and development of the COVID-19 treatment; the high transmission rate and mutation of coronavirus elude the effectiveness of the current non-pharmaceutical and pharmaceutical measures against COVID-19.

Situation in Hong Kong

The situation in Hong Kong was fluctuating and the fifth wave of the pandemic had occurred since late December of 2021. This wave was described as the worst outbreak ever in Hong Kong because it caused the collapse of healthcare system, great economic loss, high prevalence and mortality rates, despite people and government of Hong Kong had learned a lesson from SARS in 2003. As of 29 April 2022, there were 758,351 positive cases tested by PCR test and 445,496 cases tested positive by rapid antigen test (RAT) from the report of the Centre for Health Protection (CHP) report (Centre for Health Protection, 2022). There were 9,298 deaths, and the case fatality rate was higher in the older population, at 10.45% for those aged over 80 years. Among them, the death rate was higher in those who were not fully vaccinated than

Table 10.1 Newly reported and cumulative COVID-19 cases and deaths, by WHO regions, as 24 April 2022

WHO Region	New cases in last 7 days (%)	Change in new cases in last 7 days (%)	Cumulative cases (%)	New deaths in last 7 days	Change in new deaths in last 7 days	Cumulative deaths (%)
Europe	2,289,820 (50%)	−23	213,043,360 (42%)	6811 (45%)	−23	1,980,000 (32%)
Western Pacific	1,487,880 (33%)	−28	53,464,927 (11%)	2246 (15%)	−33	222,968 (4%)
Americas	550,015 (12%)	9	152,533,748 (30%)	4029 (27%)	−19	2,719,562 (44%)
South-East Asia	161,639 (4%)	−6	57,734,555 (11%)	1580 (10%)	41	783,530 (13%)
Africa	35,994 (1%)	32	8,721,105 (2%)	185 (1%)	110	171,564 (3%)
Eastern Mediterranean	22,878 (1%)	−30	21,685,928 (4%)	283 (2%)	−34	342,020 (5%)
Global	**4,548,226 (100%)**	**−21**	**507,184,387 (100%)**	**15,134 (100%)**	**−20**	**6,219,657 (100%)**

Source World Health Organization (2022c)

those who were fully vaccinated, at about 10% and 3.4%, respectively (Centre for Health Protection, 2022).

It is noteworthy the difference of daily confirmed case number with the data over the past 2 years as shown in Figs. 10.1, 10.2 and 10.3. The daily number of confirmed cases in 2022 had demonstrated a hundred times increased in the past 2 years.

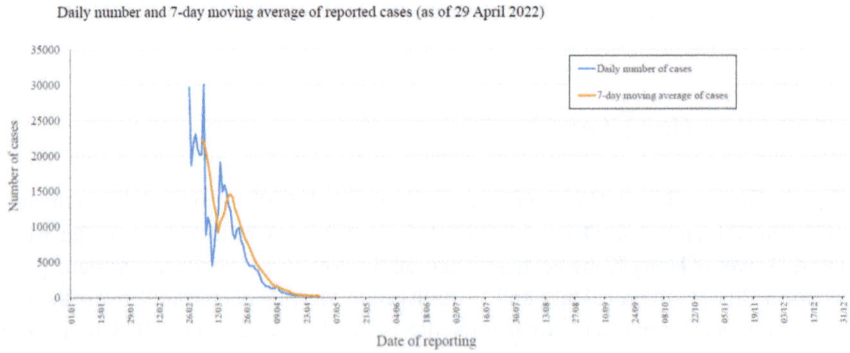

Fig. 10.1 Daily case number and 7 day moving average of cases in 2022. *Source* Centre for Health Protection (2022)

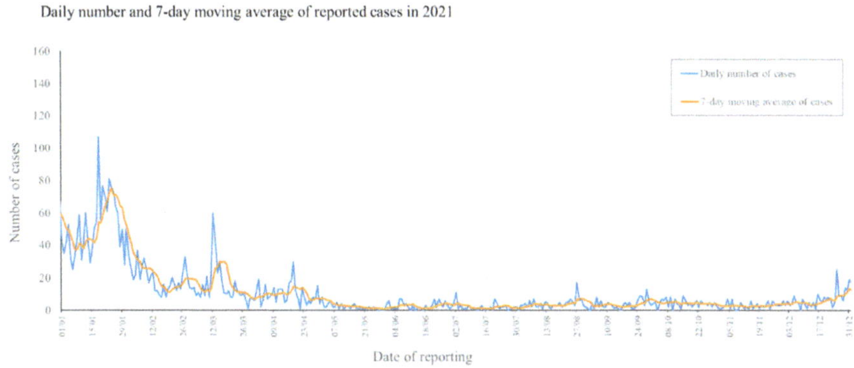

Fig. 10.2 Daily case number and 7 day moving average of cases in 2021. *Source* Centre for Health Protection (2022)

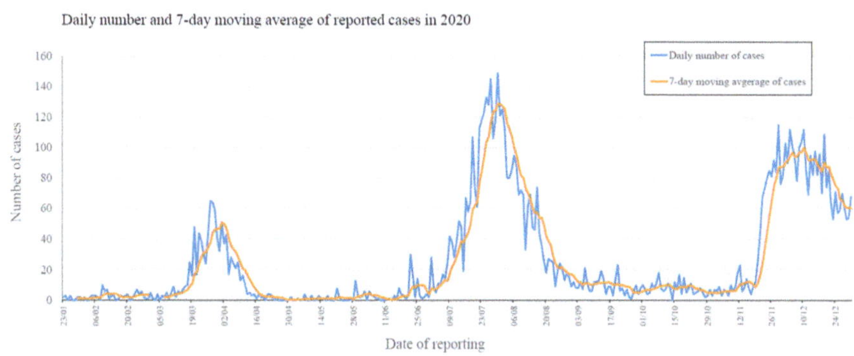

Fig. 10.3 Daily case number and 7 day moving average of cases in 2020. *Source* Centre for Health Protection (2022)

Pathophysiology

Physiological Sequalae

Fatigue, headache and anomia are the common symptoms in people with PCS, and the underlying reason could be associated with a pathogenically induced inflammatory response similar to Myalgic Encephalomyelitis/Chronic Fatigue Syndrome (ME/CFS) (Mackay, 2021). Specific pathogens that triggered the release of inflammatory mediators and stimulated the stress-integrator within the brain can overwhelm stress threshold with the continuous transmission of stress signals in humoral and neural pathways, leading to an exhausted feeling in people (Hickie et al., 2006). Based on this, Mackay (2021) and a systematic review (Polidoro et al., 2020) suggested that SARS-CoV-2 could also induce ME/CFS like symptoms due to the "cytokine-storm" that followed the infection. The over-reaction of inflammatory process can act as stressors to the neuron cluster in the hypothalamic paraventricular nucleus of the brain. Therefore, people with PCS can have clinical signs of ME/CFS, such as feeling dizziness, muscle weakness and experience occasional sleep disturbance (Bornstein et al., 2021).

Another common persisting symptom in patients with PCS is dyspnoea. Two multi-centre studies documented that the residual effect of lung damage due to severe acute illness of COVID-19 would cause a significant reduction in diffusion capacity, resulting in a higher risk of prolonged pulmonary complications (Fernández-de-las-Peñas et al., 2022; Zhao et al., 2020). These pulmonary sequelae could also relate to the inflammatory response triggered during COVID-19 infection which leads to the infusion of immune cells into alveolar space through penetration of the endothelial-epithelial barrier. The breakdown of the barrier increases the risk of subsequent bacterial infection in the area and development of pulmonary fibrosis potentially (McElvaney et al., 2020; Nalbandian et al., 2021; van Gassel et al., 2021). The over-reactive inflammatory response also caused another noticeable PCS symptom—chest pain, caused by corticosteroid use during the acute COVID-19 infection to treat immune-mediated myocarditis and additionally reduce cardiac reserve (Hatipoglu et al., 2021; Obokata et al., 2018; Puntmann et al., 2020; World Health Organization, 2021a).

Hospitalised patients have been reported to acquire gastrointestinal sequelae such as diarrhoea, gastroenteritis, loss of appetite and vomiting that can associate with a higher risk of developing PCS 3–6 months after discharge (Augustin et al., 2021; Rizvi et al., 2021). Since the intestine serves as one of the important secondary lymphoid organs in regulating immunological components, even after the recovery from the acute illness, the viral residuals can remain in the intestine and potentially alter gut microbiome and diminish commensal microorganisms that are crucial for health. The condition can eventually develop into malnutrition or significant weight loss that should receive medical support to avoid life-threatening events (Weng et al., 2021).

Neuropsychiatric Sequelae

Persisting symptoms of PCS can also lead to psychiatric symptoms and potential cognitive impairment, which can worsen patients' quality of life in association with altered socioeconomic status after COVID-19 infection (Malik et al., 2021; Menges et al., 2021). In a Chinese study, significant clinical signs of depression and anxiety troubled one-quarter of patients who recovered from acute COVID-19 infection at 6 months of follow-up, especially in patients with severe pulmonary manifestations and who required supplemental oxygen (Huang et al., 2021). Hospitalised patients with COVID-19 may particularly have a higher risk of having anxiety or depression after being discharged, as the long period of hospitalisation can arouse insecurity towards their jobs, financial costs on medical treatment etc., and the quarantine has isolated them from the outside world. All these affect patients' mental health and their perceived quality of life (Chopra et al., 2021). Combination of all physical, mental and financial stress can increase the likelihood of developing Post-traumatic stress disorder (PTSD) after recovering from COVID-19, and it can further differentiate as a predisposing risk factor to neuropathology-related deficits or cognitive impairment, such as "post-COVID brain fog" (Janiri et al., 2021; Kaseda & Levine, 2020).

Post-COVID-19 cognitive impairment, or "brain fog", is characterised by inattention, weaker memorising ability and lessened communication and executive functions (Nalbandian et al., 2021). Anatomical evidence had shown that the SARS-CoV-2 virus might invade the blood-brain and blood-cerebrospinal fluid barriers and could damage the structure of brain parenchyma, vessels and lateral orbitofrontal cortex, along with an accumulation of immune cells expressed in microglia that could eventually drive neuroinflammation and neurodegenerative conditions, resulting in cognitive-behavioural changes (Flores-Silva et al., 2021; Theoharides et al., 2021).

As the virus could infect nervous tissue by breaking the blood-brain barrier, the direct action of the virus and inflammatory reaction acting on olfactory receptors can cause anosmia (loss of smell) and ageusia (loss of taste), and these conditions can exaggerate after 6 months from COVID-19 infection (Hintschich et al., 2022). The penetration of the virus into the nasal cavity and invading the extracellular spaces of the olfactory epithelium with an accumulation of pro-inflammatory cytokine can impair the sense of smell. While SARS-CoV-2 virus also has a high tendency in occupying Angiotensin-converting enzyme 2 (ACE2) which is located in the sialic acid receptors of taste buds in the oral cavity and viral RNA primarily targets the salivary gland in upper airway that can subsequently degrade taste buds and impair salivary gland, respectively, resulting in ageusia (Lovato et al., 2020; Nalbandian et al., 2021; Neta et al., 2021; Tham et al., 2020).

Measures for Recovery and Rehabilitation

The United States

In the United States, the Mayo Clinic established a multidisciplinary COVID-19 Activity Rehabilitation Programme (CARP) in 2020. Interventions of the programme were recommended and constructed by healthcare professionals from different specialities. CARP interventions would normally be delivered to patients within at least 4 weeks of clinically confirmed SARS-CoV-2 infection and 3 main objectives were focused on prevention, diagnostics and rehabilitation throughout the programme.

The first objective of CARP is early detection and adoption of preventive measures for possible sequelae with prolonged PCS, such as pulmonary embolism, and myocardial inflammation-induced chest pain. This can be achieved through routine functional focused interviews by face-to-face visits or virtual meetings to review the pre-existing conditions in preliminary assessments, including fatigue, sleeping quality, blood pressure, signs of pulmonary embolism, dyspnoea and cognitive performance that can incorporate data from additional standard laboratory assessments, diagnostic tests and consultations towards a multidisciplinary medical care for achieving the treatment goals. The second objective is to facilitate function improvement of the body after recovery from COVID-19. Data obtained from laboratory assessments and diagnostic tests will be used for individualised physical and occupational therapies, which will be established by occupational therapists and physiotherapists to guide the patients' activities and recommend self-management skills to achieve the greatest therapeutic outcomes. Apart from physical training and self-care routines, psychosocial-based treatment is another component for the identification and removal of perceived barriers to stress management and psychological health. The third objective is to manage occupational information and control work restriction variables including the severity of persisting symptoms, perceived pain, physical and mental ability and patient's socioeconomic level, to facilitate the return to work pathway. In this part, communication between health care personnel, patients, employers and health advisors is vital to ensure the environment, health and safety policies and measures can fit the individuals' needs and increase flexibility in the job tasks (Haigh & Gandhi, 2021; Vanichkachorn et al., 2021).

The Centers for Disease Control and Prevention (2021) also established the "How Right Now campaign" to strengthen and promote emotional well-being and resiliency to populations that are adversely affected by COVID-19, in coping with related stress, anxiety, grief and loss. The campaign had partnered with local, regional and national organisations to incorporate knowledge, resources and expertise to manage post-COVID-19 conditions challenges. For example, the National Opinion Research Center (NORC) at the University of Chicago (n.d.) developed a mental health resources hub that can help people, who are bothered by the prolonged post-COVID-19 psychiatric symptoms, to access specific information that target individual needs. The multi-organisational efforts had provided great support to promote evidence-based approaches along with NORC's nationally-representative survey panel called "AmeriSpeak". The materials and resources can generalise culturally responsive and feasible content to the target audiences.

United Kingdom

In the UK, the National Institute for Health and Care Excellence (NICE) and the Royal College of General Practitioners (RCGP) had collaboratively published national guidance for managing the long-term effects of COVID-19 called the "Scottish Intercollegiate Guidelines Network" (SIGN) in 2020. The recommendations can be applied by general practitioners, primary care providers, social workers and other healthcare professionals in specialist secondary care services, including occupational therapists, cardiologists, psychiatrists, etc. The guideline also provided evidence-based guidance to the family members, carers, policymakers and support organisations to provide services and take care of people suffering from long-term symptoms of acute COVID-19.

People who have PCS will experience fluctuating symptoms and increase in anxiety due to prolonged periods of recovery. Therefore, healthcare professionals are recommended to provide accurate information about self-management tips in accessible ways and share decision making to discuss and agree with the patients on whether a further assessment is needed and be alert to individuals' health needs to urgent referrals through person-centred assessment, especially to children, the elderly and people with disability (Wallström & Ekman, 2018). The National Health Service has also established a website named "Your COVID Recovery" which provides practical knowledge and supporting information to the patients' family members, friends or relatives when facing physical and psychological challenges. If patients or carers need further medical advice, they can seek health information through a specific portal called the "Improving Access to Psychological Therapies (IAPT)" service (National Health Service, 2021).

China

The National Health Commission of the People's Republic of China (2020a) has established the Protocol on Prevention and Control of COVID-19 to ensure the adoption of evidence-based, accurate and standardised practice across all regions in the country. With the principle of "early detection, early reporting, early isolation and early treatment", the emphasis on multi-sectoral joint prevention and control efforts is shown in surveillance measures, epidemiological investigation, infection control, information sharing, risk communication and treatment. For management after discharge and follow-up treatment, patients will be recommended to have self-isolation for additional health monitoring. All provinces are encouraged to give support to the patients, while intensive research has been conducted to examine the effects of using Traditional Chinese medicine together with western medicine in helping the patients to recover from COVID-19 (Liu et al., 2022a; National Health Commission of the People's Republic of China, 2020b).

Interdisciplinary Care and Management

Post-hospital Discharge Care

Studies have shown that one in four people may develop PCS after SARS-CoV-2 infection and require further medical follow-up, especially among people with advanced age and long-term comorbidities such as cardiovascular diseases and diabetes, having a higher risk of re-hospitalisation (Bowles et al., 2021; Menges et al., 2021). Therefore, the capability of post-hospital discharge care and interdisciplinary management in COVID-19 clinics, including rehabilitation services, telehealth, social and financial support should be guaranteed for long-term access by PCS patients to improve quality of life and alleviate the challenges posed to healthcare providers and public health practitioners (Malik et al., 2021; The Lancet, 2020). To provide integrated care to patients recovering from COVID-19, and due to limited resources, prioritisation should be given to people at high risk for PCS (Melman et al., 2021). Therefore, the identification process is crucial in the design of treatment plan according to different physiological and neuropsychiatric sequelae with various clinical manifestations (Table 10.2).

Management of Physiological Symptoms

As fatigue, muscular weakness, dyspnoea and chest pain are the most commonly reported symptoms, preliminary assessments can identify these symptoms as indicators to provide further medical follow-up. To continuously monitor patients with persistent dyspnoea, home pulse oximetry devices can help the patients and family to check the arterial oxygenation level easily and seek medical help immediately if warning signs of hypoxemia are indicated (Luks & Swenson, 2020; The Government of the Hong Kong Special Administrative Region, 2022b). In addition, 4–12 weeks after hospital discharge, for people recovering from severe acute COVID-19 and still experiencing such pulmonary sequelae, the 6 min Walk Test (6MWTs) can be used along with a high-resolution computed tomography of the chest. These techniques are useful in identifying the needs for the provision of supplemental oxygen due to hypoxemia or breathing support during sleeping caused by persistent diffusion impairment and the possibility of pulmonary fibrosis (Huang et al., 2021; National Institute for Health and Care Excellence & Royal College of General Practitioners, 2020). In a Chinese and UK study, it had demonstrated the effectiveness of early follow-up assessments (e.g. chest X-ray, ultrasonography) prior to applying the medical treatment plan in treating patients with inflammatory lung disease from COVID-19 infection and at 4–6 weeks of hospital discharge (George et al., 2020; Huang et al., 2021).

Table 10.2 Treatment plans for physiological and neuropsychiatric complications

	Physiological sequalae	Neuropsychiatric sequelae
Screening Tools/ Methods	– 6 min Walk Test (6MWTs) – High-resolution computed tomography (HRCT) in chest	– EQ-VAS scale – ED-5Q-5L Questionnaires – 21-item Depression, Anxiety and Stress Scale (DASS-21) – Magnetic resonance imaging (MRI) and – Magnetic resonance angiography (MRA)
Specialists involved	– Physiotherapist – Pharmacist – Primary care physicians – Cardiologist – Neurologist – Nutritionists – Psychologist – Occupational therapists	
Treatment plans	Post Hospital Discharge periods: 1 – 3 month(s): Standard medical consultation and specialist's referral if necessary + Chest X-ray + Administration of corticosteroids if needed 3 – 6 months: Psychological assessment and consultation + Physical training + Administration of probiotics/synbiotics ≥ 6 months: Psychological assessment and consultation + Olfactory training protocol + Dietary intake of Omega-3, Zinc sulfate and Vitamin A + Follow-up consultation in primary care setting regularly	

Improving other physical functions, such as respiratory and limb muscle strength, are also crucial to alleviate the sense of fatigue and muscle weakness through physiotherapy interventions (Medrinal et al., 2021; Thomas et al., 2020). Nevertheless, as there is a possibility of having immune-mediated myocarditis in patients, physical activities should only be carried out after an asymptomatic period of at least 7 days and at best in 3–6 months post-discharge, through the adoption of a phrasal approach from low to moderate level of exercises after completed examinations like walk test, cardiac magnetic resonance imaging or endomyocardial biopsy if necessary (Salman et al., 2021).

In addition, a previous study had reported a positive correlation between low levels of gut microbiota and poorer lung function in post-acute COVID-19 patients. Hence, the management of gastrointestinal symptoms is also an important element in PCS management (Chen et al., 2021). The loss of beneficial bacteria such as Bifidobacteria, Roseburia and Faecalibacteria had been demonstrated to have potentially adverse effects on the immunomodulatory functions and deterioration of persistent symptoms of PCS at 3–6 months' recovery (Liu et al., 2022b; Tian et al., 2021). Nutritional interventions to modulate gut microbiota had been documented to promote displacement of potentially pathogenic bacteria and rebalance of the microbial commensal. Administration of probiotics including Lactobacilli and Bifidobacterium can enhance anti-inflammatory effects to relieve the ME/CFS like symptoms and promote vaccine immune efficacy against SARS-CoV-2, respectively, while boosting immuno-regulatory effects in enteric infections, mucosal inflammation and respiratory functions, with enhanced local and systemic immune responses. Additional supply of prebiotics in dietary products including carbohydrates, cellulose, xylans, resistant starch and inulin can be administrated. Moreover, to foster the generation of the intestinal barrier by microbial metabolites, such as short-chain fatty acids (SCFAs) and Tryptophan, the administration of probiotics and prebiotics combinations (namely synbiotics) can serve an effective role in maintaining the mucosal barrier and promoting recovery in respiratory tract infections (Gagliardi et al., 2018; Tian et al., 2021; Zhao et al., 2022).

Care for Neuropsychiatric Complications

Neurological complications include headaches, loss of taste and smell and cognitive impairment. Standard screening tools are required for conditions such as hemiparesis, (with a score of 4/5 on the Medical Research Council's scale (MRC scale), central face palsy, diminished deep tendon reflexes and extensor plantar reflex. Quality of life (QoL) is measured by instruments like EQ-VAS scale and ED-5Q-5L Questionnaires. The presence and severity of depression, anxiety and stress symptoms are assessed by using the 21-item Depression, Anxiety and Stress Scale (DASS-21) to evaluate the needs for specialist referral, while imaging evaluation are performed by magnetic resonance imaging (MRI) and magnetic resonance angiography (MRA) (Malik et al., 2021; Vacaras et al., 2021).

To promote neuroregeneration and improve cognitive function, the application of caffeine as an olfactory rehabilitation strategy and oral corticosteroids (e.g. fluticasone and triamcinolone) has been studied to facilitate the regain of olfactory function and increase the transmission of neurotransmitters such as dopamine, norepinephrine and glutamate that are responsible for cognitive function (Altundag et al., 2020; Neta et al., 2021). The use of corticosteroids can also provide an additional anti-inflammatory effect, especially for patients who require mechanical ventilation during acute COVID-19 infection. Clinical Olfactory Working Group also recommends the combination of olfactory training with medical treatment as a therapeutic alternative by offering a set of 36 weeks' training protocol with 3 different sets of smell sensory training with a series of olfactory stimuli to trigger regeneration of olfactory receptor neurons (Addison et al., 2021; Altundag et al., 2020). Two systematic review studies also identified the use of Omega-3 supplements could potentially promote neuroregeneration and regulate the inflammatory response of epithelial cells in the airway damaged by viral infection (Fadiyah et al., 2022; Hopkins et al., 2020).

In addition to neuropsychiatric monitoring, rehabilitation medicine and dietary interventions, the consideration of early rehabilitation with patient education, enrolment in clinical research studies and active engagement with patient advocacy and support groups are essential in the prevention of the progression of the prolonged COVID-19 symptoms of PCS that affect mental health. It also encourages the high-risk patients to seek the correct and appropriate health services in primary and community care, multidisciplinary rehabilitation services and specialist services (National Institute for Health and Care Excellence & Royal College of General Practitioners, 2020; The Government of the Hong Kong Special Administrative Region, 2022a).

Self-management Tips

As the period of PCS has not been defined yet, people should have information and support for self-management. As recommended by the National guidance for managing the long-term effects of COVID-19 published by National Institute for Health and Care Excellence and Royal College of General Practitioners (2020), a "tiered approach" can be adopted by the patients with achievable goals set in their individualised rehabilitation plan to self-manage the symptoms with community supports, including social care, patient advocacy groups, online information hub, telehealth, etc. Hence, information sharing is vital for people to ensure the continuity of care, and patients should have a baseline measurement (e.g., resting oxygen saturation, heart rate) and ongoing assessments to monitor the progress of their rehabilitation plan. In addition, as advised by World Health Organization (2020), there are sets of activities and supporting guidance for adults, who have acute COVID-19 before and have been discharged from the hospitals, to relieve the continuous COVID-19 related illness and have better directions in facing the prolonged symptoms that affect their daily lives as shown below.

Breathing Control

When people are feeling breathlessness, they can find a relaxed posture by sitting or lean-standing by a desk or chair, or with back support with a wall, and putting their hands by their sides and having their feet about a foot away from the wall and slightly apart. Afterwards, they can put one hand on the chest and the other on the stomach and slowly close their eyes to concentrate on the pace of breathing. It will be better to maintain the breathing pattern by breathing through the nose and out through the mouth.

Optimal Exercises

People are suggested to seek professional guidance and advice before returning to physical activities. Studies have indicated that after recovery from different levels of COVID-19 infection, any exercises or sports activities should be carried out at least 1–2 weeks later for the asymptomatic people. Those who have had mild to severe infection are recommended to wait for more than 3 weeks–6 months. Resumption of exercises or physical activities should start with an easily achievable target by setting up a pre-illness baseline for designing an individual's training plan, such as a 500 m walk without breathlessness, and flexibility/stretching. These light-intensity activities are suggested to gradually increase at 10–15 minutes per day at the same exertion level that an individual can tolerate (Phelan et al., 2020; Salman et al., 2021; Vasiliadis & Boka, 2021).

Before moving on to more challenging movement activities, except for seeking professional advice, an individual can also use The Borg Rating of Perceived Exertion (RPE) scale to self-assess their capability in making progress to the next phase. In this scale, the exertion rating was based on a 6–20 rating scale which can provide an estimation of the actual heart rate during physical activity (Centers for Disease Control & Prevention, 2022). In general, if an individual's Borg Scale fell between 12 and 14 and can perform physical activity at a moderate level of intensity, activities can include exercising on a treadmill, resistance exercise with light weights and side-steps. If the individuals can be capable of gradually increasing the training loads without feeling abnormal breathlessness, abnormal heart rate and excessive fatigue after an hour or the day after performing the physical activities, they can normally resume their pre-illness baseline level of activity (Salman et al., 2021). More importantly, to facilitate the return to a normal level of physical activities, World Health Organization (2020) has suggested performing cool-down exercises with different sets of muscle stretches for approximately 5 min and each set should hold for 15–20 s.

Cognitive, Mental and Emotional Training

As some people may experience memory loss, attention problem and mental problems, the support given by family or other close relatives is very important to recognise the psychiatric problems and their difficulties in dealing with the post-COVID-19 life. In addition, an individual can actively join some patient advocacy groups to seek peer support and be able to receive updated treatment information (Kruse et al., 2022). Some brain exercises can also be carried out through games, memory exercises, puzzles and reading (Adcock et al., 2020). People can make good use of mobile phone applications to set notifications of any scheduled activities and break the activities down into manageable scales to avoid overwhelmed and frustrated feelings. Regular and optimal exercises also need to play alongside cognitive training activities, which have been proved to stimulate neurogenesis, improve learning and mental performance, enhance brain health and plasticity and can provide beneficial effects on mental health including lessening depression and anxiety (Chang et al., 2019; Cotman, 2002; Savikangas et al., 2021).

Conclusion

There should be more clinical studies and active research to identify the resources that are required to meet the needs of patients with the post-COVID-19 syndrome and provide more data to develop a knowledge base and clinical guidelines on taking care of multi-organ sequelae with a multidisciplinary approach, especially the impact on neurological and mental health which can be harder to identify by the patients than physical health problems, hence delaying the time from seeking appropriate medical help. Therefore, continuous support is needed for comprehensive care for patients with PCS after discharge. Resource allocation in healthcare service planning and prioritisation of follow-up care is essential to ensure efficient utilisation of limited healthcare resources and reach the people with imminent needs for long-term care after COVID-19 infection.

More advanced treatment methods for improving the mental and physical health of patients are also required to facilitate health improvement during rehabilitation. For example, the promotion of neuromodulation therapy combining training with concurrent transcranial direct current stimulation (tDCS) through brain stimulation-assisted cognitive training in patients with post-COVID-19 cognitive impairment (Thams et al., 2022) and exploring the introduction of Traditional Chinese Medicine into treatment plan which has been advocated by some communities and the WHO (Ng et al., 2022; World Health Organization, 2022b).

Vaccination had also been reported for its potentially beneficial effect on the persistent COVID-19 symptoms by taking reference to the persistence of adverse symptoms following viral infection in the previous epidemics, including Ebola, Chikungunya and the Middle East respiratory syndrome (Strain et al., 2022). The study conducted by Strain et al. (2022) had shown that 57.9% of the subjects who had got vaccinated reported improvements in the symptoms, while a larger improvement in the symptom severity scores were observed in those receiving mRNA vaccines. Another study also demonstrated similar research results. Ayoubkhani et al. (2022) studied the associations between COVID-19 vaccination and persistent COVID-19 symptoms in adults with SARS-CoV-2 infection before vaccination. Their result had shown that the impact and period of persistent COVID-19 symptoms were seen to decrease in vaccinated subjects while the improvement was more significant in those with second dose vaccination. Further research should also be conducted to study the longitudinal effect between the health condition and the status of vaccination within the population recovering from mild to severe COVID-19, with the goal to help all the patients recovering from COVID-19 to get rid of PCS exuberantly and get back to healthy life instantaneously.

References

Adcock, M., Fankhauser, M., Post, J., Lutz, K., Zizlsperger, L., Luft, A. R., Guimarães, V., Schättin, A., & de Bruin, E. D. (2020). Effects of an in-home multicomponent exergame training on physical functions, cognition, and brain volume of older adults: A randomized controlled trial. *Frontiers in Medicine, 6*, Article 321. https://doi.org/10.3389/fmed.2019.00321

Addison, A. B., Wong, B., Ahmed, T., Macchi, A., Konstantinidis, I., Huart, C., Frasnelli, J., Fjaeldstad, A. W., Ramakrishnan, V. R., Rombaux, P., Whitcroft, K. L., Holbrook, E. H., Poletti, S. C., Hsieh, J. W., Landis, B. N., Boardman, J., Welge-Lüssen, A., Maru, D., Hummel, T., & Philpott, C. M. (2021). Clinical Olfactory Working Group consensus statement on the treatment of postinfectious olfactory dysfunction. *Journal of Allergy and Clinical Immunology, 147*(5), 1704–1719. https://doi.org/10.1016/j.jaci.2020.12.641

Altundag, A., Saatci, O., Sanli, D. E. T., Duz, O. A., Sanli, A. N., Olmuscelik, O., Temirbekov, D., Kandemirli, S. G., & Karaaltin, A. B. (2020). The temporal course of COVID-19 anosmia and relation to other clinical symptoms. *European Archives of Oto-Rhino-Laryngology, 278*(6), 1891–1897. https://doi.org/10.1007/s00405-020-06496-5

Augustin, M., Schommers, P., Stecher, M., Dewald, F., Gieselmann, L., Gruell, H., Horn, C., Vanshylla, K., Cristanziano, V. D., Osebold, L., Roventa, M., Riaz, T., Tschernoster, N., Altmueller, J., Rose, L., Salomon, S., Priesner, V., Luers, J. C., Albus, C., . . . Lehmann, C. (2021). Post-COVID syndrome in non-hospitalised patients with COVID-19: A longitudinal prospective cohort study. *The Lancet Regional Health—Europe, 6*, Article 100122. https://doi.org/10.1016/j.lanepe.2021.100122

Ayoubkhani, D., Bermingham, C., Pouwels, K. B., Glickman, M., Nafilyan, V., Zaccardi, F., Khunti, K., Alwan, N. A., & Walker, A. S. (2022). Trajectory of long COVID symptoms after COVID-19 vaccination: Community based cohort study. *BMJ, 377*, Article e069676. https://doi.org/10.1136/bmj-2021-069676

Bornstein, S. R., Voit-Bak, K., Donate, T., Rodionov, R. N., Gainetdinov, R. R., Tselmin, S., Kanczkowski, W., Müller, G. M., Achleitner, M., Wang, J., Licinio, J., Bauer, M., Young, A. H., Thuret, S., Bechmann, N., & Straube, R. (2021). Chronic post-COVID-19 syndrome and chronic fatigue syndrome: Is there a role for extracorporeal apheresis? *Molecular Psychiatry, 27*, 34–37. https://doi.org/10.1038/s41380-021-01148-4

Bowles, K. H., McDonald, M., Barrón, Y., Kennedy, E., O'Connor, M., & Mikkelsen, M. (2021). Surviving COVID-19 after hospital discharge: Symptom, functional, and adverse outcomes of home health recipients. *Annals of Internal Medicine, 174*(3), 316–325. https://doi.org/10.7326/m20-5206

Centers for Disease Control and Prevention. (2021, April 16). *Partners*. Retrieved December 17, 2021, from https://www.cdc.gov/howrightnow/partners/index.html

Centers for Disease Control and Prevention. (2022, April 27). *Perceived exertion (Borg Rating of Perceived Exertion Scale)*. Retrieved 31 May 2022, from https://www.cdc.gov/physicalactivity/basics/measuring/exertion.htm

Centre for Health Protection. (2022, April 29). *Latest situation of COVID-19 (as of 29 April 2022)*. https://www.chp.gov.hk/files/pdf/local_situation_covid19_en_20220429.pdf

Chang, P. S., Knobf, T., Oh, B., & Funk, M. (2019). Physical and psychological health outcomes of Qigong exercise in older adults: A systematic review and meta-analysis. *The American Journal of Chinese Medicine, 47*(2), 301–322. https://doi.org/10.1142/s0192415x19500149

Chen, Y., Gu, S., Chen, Y., Lu, H., Shi, D., Guo, J., Wu, W. R., Yang, Y., Li, Y., Xu, K. J., Ding, C., Luo, R., Huang, C., Yu, L., Xu, M., Yi, P., Liu, J., Tao, J. J., Zhang, H., … Li, L. (2021). Six-month follow-up of gut microbiota richness in patients with COVID-19. *Gut, 71*(1), 222–225. https://doi.org/10.1136/gutjnl-2021-324090

Chopra, V., Flanders, S. A., O'Malley, M., Malani, A. N., & Prescott, H. C. (2021). Sixty-day outcomes among patients hospitalized with COVID-19. *Annals of Internal Medicine, 174*(4), 576–578. https://doi.org/10.7326/m20-5661

Cotman, C. (2002). Exercise: A behavioral intervention to enhance brain health and plasticity. *Trends in Neurosciences, 25*(6), 295–301. https://doi.org/10.1016/s0166-2236(02)02143-4

Fadiyah, N. N., Megawati, G., & Luftimas, D. E. (2022). Potential of omega 3 supplementation for Coronavirus disease 2019 (COVID-19): A scoping review. *International Journal of General Medicine, 15*, 3915–3922. https://doi.org/10.2147/ijgm.s357460

Fernández-de-las-Peñas, C., Palacios-Ceña, D., Gómez-Mayordomo, V., Palacios-Ceña, M., Rodríguez-Jiménez, J., de-la-Llave-Rincón, A. I., Velasco-Arribas, M., Fuensalida-Novo, S., Ambite-Quesada, S., Guijarro, C., Cuadrado, M. L., Florencio, L. L., Arias-Navalón, J. A., Ortega-Santiago, R., Elvira-Martínez, C. M., Molina-Trigueros, L. J., Torres-Macho, J., Sebastián-Viana, T., Canto-Diez, M. G., … Arendt-Nielsen, L. (2022). Fatigue and dyspnoea as main persistent post-COVID-19 symptoms in previously hospitalized patients: Related functional limitations and disability. *Respiration, 101*(2), 132–141. https://doi.org/10.1159/000518854

Flores-Silva, F. D., García-Grimshaw, M., Valdés-Ferrer, S. I., Vigueras-Hernández, A. P., Domínguez-Moreno, R., Tristán-Samaniego, D. P., Michel-Chávez, A., González-Duarte, A., Vega-Boada, F. A., Reyes-Melo, I., Jiménez-Ruiz, A., Chávez-Martínez, O. A., Rebolledo-García, D., Marché-Fernández, O. A., Sánchez-Torres, S., García-Ramos, G., Cantú-Brito, C., & Chiquete, E. (2021). Neurologic manifestations in hospitalized patients with COVID-19 in Mexico City. *PLoS One, 16*(4), Article e0247433. https://doi.org/10.1371/journal.pone.0247433

Gagliardi, A., Totino, V., Cacciotti, F., Iebba, V., Neroni, B., Bonfiglio, G., Trancassini, M., Passariello, C., Pantanella, F., & Schippa, S. (2018). Rebuilding the gut microbiota ecosystem. *International Journal of Environmental Research and Public Health, 15*(8), Article 1679. https://doi.org/10.3390/ijerph15081679

George, P. M., Barratt, S. L., Condliffe, R., Desai, S. R., Devaraj, A., Forrest, I., Gibbons, M. A., Hart, N., Jenkins, R. G., McAuley, D. F., Patel, B. V., Thwaite, E., & Spencer, L. G. (2020). Respiratory follow-up of patients with COVID-19 pneumonia. *Thorax, 75*(11), 1009–1016. https://doi.org/10.1136/thoraxjnl-2020-215314

Grime, M. M., & Wright, G. (2016). Delphi method. *Wiley StatsRef: Statistics Reference Online*, 1–6. https://doi.org/10.1002/9781118445112.stat07879

Haigh, K. Z., & Gandhi, M. (2021). COVID-19 mitigation with appropriate safety measures in an essential workplace: Lessons for opening work settings in the United States during COVID-19. *Open Forum Infectious Diseases, 8*(4), Article ofab086. https://doi.org/10.1093/ofid/ofab086

Hatipoglu, S., Lyon, A. R., & Pennell, D. J. (2021). CMR unveiling the cause of post COVID-19 infection chest pain. *The International Journal of Cardiovascular Imaging, 37*, 2025–2026. https://doi.org/10.1007/s10554-021-02161-y

Hickie, I., Davenport, T., Wakefield, D., Vollmer-Conna, U., Cameron, B., Vernon, S. D., Reeves, W. C., & Lloyd, A. (2006). Post-infective and chronic fatigue syndromes precipitated by viral and non-viral pathogens: Prospective cohort study. *BMJ, 333*(7568), 575. https://doi.org/10.1136/bmj.38933.585764.ae

Hintschich, C. A., Fischer, R., Hummel, T., Wenzel, J. J., Bohr, C., & Vielsmeier, V. (2022). Persisting olfactory dysfunction in post-COVID-19 is associated with gustatory impairment: Results from chemosensitive testing eight months after the acute infection. *PLoS One, 17*(3), Article e0265686. https://doi.org/10.1371/journal.pone.0265686

Hopkins, C., Alanin, M., Philpott, C., Harries, P., Whitcroft, K., Qureishi, A., Anari, S., Ramakrishnan, Y., Sama, A., Davies, E., Stew, B., Gane, S., Carrie, S., Hathorn, I., Bhalla, R., Kelly, C., Hill, N., Boak, D., & Nirmal Kumar, B. (2020). Management of new onset loss of sense of smell during the COVID-19 pandemic—BRS consensus guidelines. *Clinical Otolaryngology, 46*(1), 16–22. https://doi.org/10.1111/coa.13636

Huang, C., Huang, L., Wang, Y., Li, X., Ren, L., Gu, X., Kang, L., Guo, L., Liu, M., Zhou, X., Luo, J., Huang, Z., Tu, S., Zhao, Y., Chen, L., Xu, D., Li, Y., Li, C., Peng, L., … Cao, B. (2021). 6-month consequences of COVID-19 in patients discharged from hospital: A cohort study. *The Lancet, 397*(10270), 220–232. https://doi.org/10.1016/s0140-6736(20)32656-8

Janiri, D., Carfì, A., Kotzalidis, G. D., Bernabei, R., Landi, F., & Sani, G. (2021). Posttraumatic stress disorder in patients after severe COVID-19 infection. *JAMA Psychiatry, 78*(5), 567–569. https://doi.org/10.1001/jamapsychiatry.2021.0109

Kaseda, E. T., & Levine, A. J. (2020). Post-traumatic stress disorder: A differential diagnostic consideration for COVID-19 survivors. *The Clinical Neuropsychologist, 34*(7–8), 1498–1514. https://doi.org/10.1080/13854046.2020.1811894

Kruse, M. H., Durstine, A., & Evans, D. P. (2022). Effect of COVID-19 on patient access to health services for noncommunicable diseases in Latin America: A perspective from patient advocacy organizations. *International Journal for Equity in Health, 21*, Article 45. https://doi.org/10.1186/s12939-022-01648-x

Liu, J., Dong, F., & Robinson, N. (2022a). State-of-the-art evidence of traditional Chinese medicine for treating coronavirus disease 2019. *Journal of Traditional Chinese Medical Sciences, 9*(1), 2–6. https://doi.org/10.1016/j.jtcms.2022.01.005

Liu, Q., Mak, J. W. Y., Su, Q., Yeoh, Y. K., Lui, G. C. Y., Ng, S. S. S., Zhang, F., Li, A. Y. L., Lu, W., Hui, D. S. C., Chan, P. K., Chan, F. K. L., & Ng, S. C. (2022b). Gut microbiota dynamics in a prospective cohort of patients with post-acute COVID-19 syndrome. *Gut, 71*(3), 544–552. https://doi.org/10.1136/gutjnl-2021-325989

Lovato, A., de Filippis, C., & Marioni, G. (2020). Upper airway symptoms in coronavirus disease 2019 (COVID-19). *American Journal of Otolaryngology, 41*(3), Article 102474. https://doi.org/10.1016/j.amjoto.2020.102474

Luks, A. M., & Swenson, E. R. (2020). Pulse oximetry for monitoring patients with COVID-19 at home. Potential pitfalls and practical guidance. *Annals of the American Thoracic Society, 17*(9), 1040–1046. https://doi.org/10.1513/annalsats.202005-418fr

Mackay, A. (2021). A paradigm for post-Covid-19 fatigue syndrome analogous to ME/CFS. *Frontiers in Neurology, 12*, Article 701419. https://doi.org/10.3389/fneur.2021.701419

Malik, P., Patel, K., Pinto, C., Jaiswal, R., Tirupathi, R., Pillai, S., & Patel, U. (2021). Post-acute COVID-19 syndrome (PCS) and health-related quality of life (HRQoL)—A systematic review and meta-analysis. *Journal of Medical Virology, 94*(1), 253–262. https://doi.org/10.1002/jmv.27309

McElvaney, O. J., McEvoy, N. L., McElvaney, O. F., Carroll, T. P., Murphy, M. P., Dunlea, D. M., Ní Choileáin, O., Clarke, J., O'Connor, E., Hogan, G., Ryan, D., Sulaiman, I., Gunaratnam, C., Branagan, P., O'Brien, M. E., Morgan, R. K., Costello, R. W., Hurley, K., Walsh, S., … McElvaney, N. G. (2020). Characterization of the inflammatory response to severe COVID-19 illness. *American Journal of Respiratory and Critical Care Medicine, 202*(6), 812–821. https://doi.org/10.1164/rccm.202005-1583oc

Medrinal, C., Prieur, G., Bonnevie, T., Gravier, F. E., Mayard, D., Desmalles, E., Smondack, P., Lamia, B., Combret, Y., & Fossat, G. (2021). Muscle weakness, functional capacities and recovery for COVID-19 ICU survivors. *BMC Anesthesiology, 21*, Article 64. https://doi.org/10.1186/s12871-021-01274-0

Melman, G., Parlikad, A., & Cameron, E. (2021). Balancing scarce hospital resources during the COVID-19 pandemic using discrete-event simulation. *Health Care Management Science, 24*(2), 356–374. https://doi.org/10.1007/s10729-021-09548-2

Menges, D., Ballouz, T., Anagnostopoulos, A., Aschmann, H. E., Domenghino, A., Fehr, J. S., & Puhan, M. A. (2021). Burden of post-COVID-19 syndrome and implications for healthcare service planning: A population-based cohort study. *PLOS One, 16*(7), Article e0254523. https://doi.org/10.1371/journal.pone.0254523

Michelen, M., Manoharan, L., Elkheir, N., Cheng, V., Dagens, A., Hastie, C., O'Hara, M., Suett, J., Dahmash, D., Bugaeva, P., Rigby, I., Munblit, D., Harriss, E., Burls, A., Foote, C., Scott, J., Carson, G., Olliaro, P., Sigfrid, L., & Stavropoulou, C. (2021). Characterising long COVID: A living systematic review. *BMJ Global Health, 6*(9), Article e005427. https://doi.org/10.1136/bmjgh-2021-005427

Nalbandian, A., Sehgal, K., Gupta, A., Madhavan, M. V., McGroder, C., Stevens, J. S., Cook, J. R., Nordvig, A. S., Shalev, D., Sehrawat, T. S., Ahluwalia, N., Bikdeli, B., Dietz, D., Der-Nigoghossian, C., Liyanage-Don, N., Rosner, G. F., Bernstein, E. J., Mohan, S., Beckley, A. A., … Wan, E. Y. (2021). Post-acute COVID-19 syndrome. *Nature Medicine, 27*(4), 601–615. https://doi.org/10.1038/s41591-021-01283-z

National Health Commission of the People's Republic of China. (2020a, March 7). *Protocol on prevention and control of COVID-19* (6 ed.). http://en.nhc.gov.cn/2020a-03/29/c_78468.htm

National Health Commission of the People's Republic of China. (2020b, September 7). *Diagnosis and treatment protocol for COVID-19 patients* (Tentative 8th ed.). http://en.nhc.gov.cn/2020-09/07/c_81565.htm

National Health Service. (2021). *Your COVID recovery*. Retrieved November 24, 2021, from https://www.yourcovidrecovery.nhs.uk/

National Institute for Health and Care Excellence, & Royal College of General Practitioners. (2020, December). *Managing the long-term effects of COVID-19*. SIGN. Retrieved November 24, 2021, from https://www.sign.ac.uk/our-guidelines/managing-the-long-term-effects-of-covid-19/

National Opinion Research Center at the University of Chicago. (n.d.). *COVID-19 mental health communications*. Retrieved December 17, 2021, from https://www.norc.org/Research/Projects/Pages/covid-19-mental-health-communications.aspx

Neta, F. I., Fernandes, A. C. L., Vale, A. J. M., Pinheiro, F. I., Cobucci, R. N., Azevedo, E. P. D., & Guzen, F. P. (2021). Pathophysiology and possible treatments for olfactory-gustatory disorders in patients affected by COVID-19. *Current Research in Pharmacology and Drug Discovery, 2*, Article 100035. https://doi.org/10.1016/j.crphar.2021.100035

Ng, T. K. C., Lo, M. F., Fong, B. Y. F., & Yee, H. H. L. (2022). Predictors of the intention to use traditional Chinese medicine (TCM) using extended theory of planned behavior: A cross-sectional study among TCM users in Hong Kong. *BMC Complementary Medicine and Therapies, 22*, Article 113. https://doi.org/10.1186/s12906-022-03598-x

Obokata, M., Reddy, Y. N., Melenovsky, V., Kane, G. C., Olson, T. P., Jarolim, P., & Borlaug, B. A. (2018). Myocardial injury and cardiac reserve in patients with heart failure and preserved ejection fraction. *Journal of the American College of Cardiology, 72*(1), 29–40. https://doi.org/10.1016/j.jacc.2018.04.039

Phelan, D., Kim, J. H., & Chung, E. H. (2020). A game plan for the resumption of sport and exercise after Coronavirus disease 2019 (COVID-19) infection. *JAMA Cardiology, 5*(10), 1085–1086. https://doi.org/10.1001/jamacardio.2020.2136

Polidoro, R. B., Hagan, R. S., de Santis Santiago, R., & Schmidt, N. W. (2020). Overview: Systemic inflammatory response derived from lung injury caused by SARS-CoV-2 infection explains severe outcomes in COVID-19. *Frontiers in Immunology, 11*, Article 1626. https://doi.org/10.3389/fimmu.2020.01626

Puntmann, V. O., Carerj, M. L., Wieters, I., Fahim, M., Arendt, C., Hoffmann, J., Shchendrygina, A., Escher, F., Vasa-Nicotera, M., Zeiher, A. M., Vehreschild, M., & Nagel, E. (2020). Outcomes of cardiovascular magnetic resonance imaging in patients recently recovered from Coronavirus disease 2019 (COVID-19). *JAMA Cardiology, 5*(11), 1265–1273. https://doi.org/10.1001/jamacardio.2020.3557

Rizvi, A., Patel, Z., Liu, Y., Satapathy, S. K., Sultan, K., & Trindade, A. J. (2021). Gastrointestinal Sequelae 3 and 6 months after hospitalization for Coronavirus disease 2019. *Clinical Gastroenterology and Hepatology, 19*(11), 2438–2440. https://doi.org/10.1016/j.cgh.2021.06.046

Salman, D., Vishnubala, D., le Feuvre, P., Beaney, T., Korgaonkar, J., Majeed, A., & McGregor, A. H. (2021). Returning to physical activity after COVID-19. *BMJ, 372*, Article m4721. https://doi.org/10.1136/bmj.m4721

Savikangas, T., Törmäkangas, T., Tirkkonen, A., Alen, M., Fielding, R. A., Kivipelto, M., Rantalainen, T., Stigsdotter Neely, A., & Sipilä, S. (2021). The effects of a physical and cognitive training intervention vs. physical training alone on older adults' physical activity: A randomized controlled trial with extended follow-up during COVID-19. *PLoS One, 16*(10), Article e0258559. https://doi.org/10.1371/journal.pone.0258559

Sharma, A., Ahmad Farouk, I., & Lal, S. K. (2021). COVID-19: A review on the novel coronavirus disease evolution, transmission, detection, control and prevention. *Viruses, 13*(2), Article 202. https://doi.org/10.3390/v13020202

Strain, W. D., Sherwood, O., Banerjee, A., van der Togt, V., Hishmeh, L., & Rossman, J. (2022). The impact of COVID vaccination on symptoms of long COVID: An international survey of people with lived experience of long COVID. *Vaccines, 10*(5), Article 652. https://doi.org/10.3390/vaccines10050652

Sudre, C. H., Murray, B., Varsavsky, T., Graham, M. S., Penfold, R. S., Bowyer, R. C., Pujol, J. C., Klaser, K., Antonelli, M., Canas, L. S., Molteni, E., Modat, M., Jorge Cardoso, M., May, A., Ganesh, S., Davies, R., Nguyen, L. H., Drew, D. A., Astley, C. M., … Steves, C. J. (2021). Attributes and predictors of long COVID. *Nature Medicine, 27*(4), 626–631. https://doi.org/10.1038/s41591-021-01292-y

Tham, A. C., Thein, T. L., Lee, C. S., Tan, G. S. E., Manauis, C. M., Siow, J. K., Leo, Y. S., & Lim, M. Y. (2020). Olfactory taste disorder as a presenting symptom of COVID-19: A large single-center Singapore study. *European Archives of Oto-Rhino-Laryngology, 278*(6), 1853–1862. https://doi.org/10.1007/s00405-020-06455-0

Thams, F., Antonenko, D., Fleischmann, R., Meinzer, M., Grittner, U., Schmidt, S., Brakemeier, E. L., Steinmetz, A., & Flöel, A. (2022). Neuromodulation through brain stimulation-assisted cognitive training in patients with post-COVID-19 cognitive impairment (Neuromod-COV): Study protocol for a PROBE phase IIb trial. *BMJ Open, 12*(4), Article e055038. https://doi.org/10.1136/bmjopen-2021-055038

The Government of the Hong Kong Special Administrative Region. (2022a, March 9). *Hospital authority enhances support for COVID-19 patients in community* [Press release]. https://www.info.gov.hk/gia/general/202203/09/P2022030800381.htm

The Government of the Hong Kong Special Administrative Region. (2022b, March 12). *Using a pulse oximeter at home for persons tested positive for COVID-19*. Retrieved April 29, 2022, from https://www.coronavirus.gov.hk/pdf/po_covid_EN.pdf

The Lancet. (2020). Facing up to long COVID. *The Lancet, 396*(10266), 1861. https://doi.org/10.1016/s0140-6736(20)32662-3

Theoharides, T. C., Cholevas, C., Polyzoidis, K., & Politis, A. (2021). Long-COVID syndrome-associated brain fog and chemofog: Luteolin to the rescue. *BioFactors, 47*(2), 232–241. https://doi.org/10.1002/biof.1726

Thomas, P., Baldwin, C., Bissett, B., Boden, I., Gosselink, R., Granger, C. L., Hodgson, C., Jones, A. Y., Kho, M. E., Moses, R., Ntoumenopoulos, G., Parry, S. M., Patman, S., & van der Lee, L. (2020). Physiotherapy management for COVID-19 in the acute hospital setting: Clinical practice recommendations. *Journal of Physiotherapy, 66*(2), 73–82. https://doi.org/10.1016/j.jphys.2020.03.011

Tian, Y., Sun, K. Y., Meng, T. Q., Ye, Z., Guo, S. M., Li, Z. M., Xiong, C. L., Yin, Y., Li, H. G., & Zhou, L. Q. (2021). Gut microbiota may not be fully restored in recovered COVID-19 patients after 3-month recovery. *Frontiers in Nutrition, 8*, Article 638825. https://doi.org/10.3389/fnut.2021.638825

Vacaras, V., Frunze, S., & Cordos, A. M. (2021). Neurological complications in COVID-19—A diagnostic challenge. *Journal of Medicine and Life, 14*(2), 216–224. https://doi.org/10.25122/jml-2021-0045

van Gassel, R. J. J., Bels, J. L. M., Raafs, A., van Bussel, B. C. T., van de Poll, M. C. G., Simons, S. O., van der Meer, L. W. L., Gietema, H. A., Posthuma, R., & van Santen, S. (2021). High prevalence of pulmonary sequelae at 3 months after hospital discharge in mechanically ventilated survivors of COVID-19. *American Journal of Respiratory and Critical Care Medicine, 203*(3), 371–374. https://doi.org/10.1164/rccm.202010-3823le

Vanichkachorn, G., Newcomb, R., Cowl, C. T., Murad, M. H., Breeher, L., Miller, S., Trenary, M., Neveau, D., & Higgins, S. (2021). Post–COVID-19 syndrome (Long haul syndrome): Description of a multidisciplinary clinic at mayo clinic and characteristics of the initial patient cohort. *Mayo Clinic Proceedings, 96*(7), 1782–1791. https://doi.org/10.1016/j.mayocp.2021.04.024

Vasiliadis, A. V., & Boka, V. (2021). Safe return to exercise after COVID-19 infection. *Sultan Qaboos University Medical Journal, 21*(3), 373–377. https://doi.org/10.18295/squmj.8.2021.124

Wallström, S., & Ekman, I. (2018). Person-centred care in clinical assessment. *European Journal of Cardiovascular Nursing, 17*(7), 576–579. https://doi.org/10.1177/1474515118758139

Weng, J., Li, Y., Li, J., Shen, L., Zhu, L., Liang, Y., Lin, X., Jiao, N., Cheng, S., Huang, Y., Zou, Y., Yan, G., Zhu, R., & Lan, P. (2021). Gastrointestinal sequelae 90 days after discharge for COVID-19. *The Lancet Gastroenterology & Hepatology, 6*(5), 344–346. https://doi.org/10.1016/s2468-1253(21)00076-5

World Health Organization. (2020, June 25). *Support for rehabilitation: Self-management after COVID-19 related illness.* https://www.who.int/publications/m/item/support-for-rehabilitation-self-management-after-covid-19-related-illness

World Health Organization. (2021a, October 6). *A clinical case definition of post COVID-19 condition by a Delphi consensus.* https://www.who.int/publications/i/item/WHO-2019-nCoV-Post_COVID-19_condition-Clinical_case_definition-2021.1

World Health Organization. (2021b, November 23). *Living guidance for clinical management of COVID-19.* https://www.who.int/publications/i/item/WHO-2019-nCoV-clinical-2021-2

World Health Organization. (2022a). *Timeline: WHO's COVID-19 response.* Retrieved May 1, 2022, from https://www.who.int/emergencies/diseases/novel-coronavirus-2019/interactive-timeline

World Health Organization. (2022b, March 31). *WHO expert meeting on evaluation of traditional Chinese medicine in the treatment of COVID-19.* https://www.who.int/publications/m/item/who-expert-meeting-on-evaluation-of-traditional-chinese-medicine-in-the-treatment-of-covid-19

World Health Organization. (2022c, April 27). *Weekly epidemiological update on COVID-19—27 April 2022.* https://www.who.int/docs/default-source/coronaviruse/situation-reports/2022c0427_weekly_epi_update_89.pdf?sfvrsn=e948ab5a_3&download=true

Zhao, S., Feng, P., Meng, W., Jin, W., Li, X., & Li, X. (2022). Modulated gut microbiota for potential COVID-19 prevention and treatment. *Frontiers in Medicine, 9*, Article 811176. https://doi.org/10.3389/fmed.2022.811176

Zhao, Y. M., Shang, Y. M., Song, W. B., Li, Q. Q., Xie, H., Xu, Q. F., Jia, J. L., Li, L. M., Mao, H. L., Zhou, X. M., Luo, H., Gao, Y. F., & Xu, A. G. (2020). Follow-up study of the pulmonary function and related physiological characteristics of COVID-19 survivors three months after recovery. *EClinicalMedicine, 25*, Article 100463. https://doi.org/10.1016/j.eclinm.2020.100463

Chapter 11
Lifestyle Risk Factor Patterns and Development Trends in Hong Kong

Wendy F. M. Chan and Cynthia S. C. Yip

Abstract Lifestyle behaviours are important risk factors for non-communicable diseases. This study had identified lifestyle risk factor patterns and their development trends in Hong Kong. Over the past decades, the Hong Kong government has taken a multi-pronged approach to promoting healthy lifestyles. According to the Hong Kong Behavioural Risk Factor Surveys conducted between 2004 and 2016, most Hong Kong adults were living with multiple lifestyle risk factors. Although the average alcohol intake among males persistently and significantly decreased and the prevalence of smoking among both males and females also decreased, the average alcohol intake among females persistently and significantly increased and the prevalence of drinking among both males and females was rapidly growing in more recent years. Although changes in the average time spent doing physical activities were non-significant, the prevalence of doing sufficient physical activity among both males and females persistently expanded. The constant population shift toward a lifestyle of eating insufficient fruit and vegetables and drinking alcohol among both males and females was observed. Despite more recent investigations indicated decreased alcohol consumption, other lifestyle factors have remained to be health concerns. Strategic intervention policy changes targeting a balance of multiple lifestyle factors among different lifestyle groups instead of a single particular risk factor are urgently needed to reverse the unhealthy population lifestyle trends.

Keywords Alcohol intake · Tobacco use · Fruit and vegetable · Physical activity · Lifestyle risk factors · Time-trend analysis

W. F. M. Chan
HKCC, The Hong Kong Polytechnic University, Hong Kong, China
e-mail: wendy.fm.chan@cpce-polyu.edu.hk

C. S. C. Yip (✉)
Hong Kong Chu Hai College of Higher Education, Hong Kong, China
e-mail: ycynthia@connect.hku.hk

B. Y. F. Fong and W. C. W. Wong (eds.), *Gaps and Actions in Health Improvement from Hong Kong and Beyond*,
https://doi.org/10.1007/978-981-99-4491-0_11

Introduction

Non-communicable diseases (NCDs), also known as chronic diseases, are the leading causes of death, particularly in developed economies. Global Comparative Risk Assessments identified that use of alcohol and tobacco, unhealthy diet, and physical inactivity were major contributors to the burden of NCDs and mortality (Feigin et al., 2016; Forouzanfar et al., 2016; Gakidou et al., 2017; Lim et al., 2012; Lock et al., 2005). The recent global burden of diseases comparative assessment report (Gakidou et al., 2017) shows that smoking had contributed to 6,321 thousand deaths, alcohol use contributed to 2,814.6 thousand of deaths, a diet low in fruit contributed to 2,361 thousand deaths, a diet low in vegetables contributed to 1,520 thousand deaths, and insufficient physical activity contributed to 1,373 thousand deaths. Based on Hong Kong's first population-based food consumption survey conducted in 2005–2007, and the best identified relative risk from systematic reviews (Yip et al., 2018, 2019a), Yip and Fielding (2017) estimated that by reducing Hong Kong adults' meat intake to 60 g per capita per day and replacing the intake energy with fruit and vegetable, it could prevent 2,519 to 7,012 premature deaths in males and 53 to 1,342 in females.

Substance Use

Obesity is a worldwide epidemic. It occurs in both developing countries as well as in more developed nations. It is one of the major chronic risk factors for atherosclerosis, hypertension, Type II diabetes, and cancer (Matsuda & Shimomura, 2013). Alcohol is not an essential nutrient, but it provides high calories of 7 kcal/g. It does not require any digestion and could be absorb rapidly from gastrointestinal (GI) tract by diffusion. It is one of the most efficiently absorbed energy sources which lead to "beer belly" or apple shape in the upper body. Although historically alcohol consumption has been taken as a buffer against the effects of stress and especially during economic crises, a recent meta-analysis shows the pre-to-post-stressor affect was non-significant (Masaoka et al., 2016), while post-stressor negative affect was significantly lower (Bresin, 2019). Another multivariate meta-analysis suggests coping-related drinking is a strong mediator for the association between post-traumatic stress disorder and harmful alcohol use (Luciano et al., 2022). A systematic review indicates that use of alcohol is associated with alcohol poisoning, foetal alcohol spectrum disorders, infectious diseases, diabetes, neuropsychiatric disorders, cardiovascular diseases (CVD), GI diseases, and injuries (Rehm et al., 2017). *Tobacco smoking releases more than 5000 chemicals such as tar, nicotine, carbon monoxide, and many of them are poisonous and up to 70 cause cancer* (Cancer Research UK, 2021). Systematic reviews and meta-analyses show that tobacco use is associated with all-cause and lung cancer mortality (Kong, 2014), prostate cancer (De Nunzio et al., 2015), bladder cancer (Masaoka et al., 2016), pancreas cancer (Matsuo et al.,

2011), oesophageal cancer (Oze et al., 2011), and diabetes (Pan et al., 2015). *Both alcoholic and tobacco use are on the International Agency for Research on Cancer classification Group 1, carcinogenic to humans.*

Dietary Nutrition and Concerns

Cereals and grains, fruit, and starchy vegetables are the most common food sources for complex carbohydrates. Carbohydrates, proteins, and lipids are essential nutrients for human health and belong to energy-yielding nutrients. Carbohydrates are the preferential source of energy especially for cells in the nervous system. Proteins are for producing vital body constituent, body growth, rebuilding and repairing, forming peptide hormones and enzymes, and contributing to production of antibodies in immune function as well as forming glucose during starvation. Carbohydrates and protein provide 4 kcal/g. Though lipids are important for production of steroid types of hormones and bile acids, participate in cell structure, they provide the highest amount of energy of 9 kcal/g. The Dietary Guidelines for Americans recommend taking 45–65% of the total calories from dietary carbohydrates intakes (U.S. Department of Agriculture and U.S. Department of Health and Human Services, 2020), while the World Health Organization (WHO) and the Food and Agricultural Organization of the United Nations recommended 55–75% of the total calories (Department of Health, 2021a).

Fruits and vegetables are rich in vitamins and dietary fibre. Vitamins are essential nutrients needed in small amounts as they cannot be synthesised in the human body with the exceptions of Vitamin B3 (niacin), B7 (Biotin), D, and K. They participate in energy-yielding processes or function as part of enzymes or coenzymes (Percival, 2011). They also have specific roles in immunity. Vitamin B6 in banana and potato takes a role in antibody production. Folate and Vitamins C and E are antioxidants which slow down the formation of free radical during the daily metabolisms and facilitate DNA repairing. Vitamin C is rich in citrus fruits whereas Vitamin E is usually found in sunflower seeds and wheat germ. Phytochemicals such as anthocyanins and lycopene are anti-carcinogens. Anthocyanins can be found in blueberries and raspberries. Lycopene is available in orange fruits and vegetables e.g., tomatoes, watermelons, and papayas, while carotenoids in cruciferous vegetables e.g., broccolis and cauliflowers.

Dietary fibre is made up of polysaccharides which cannot be digested by human digestive system. Dietary fibre can be classified according to its solubility and fermentable in the large intestine and thus affecting their roles. Soluble, viscous, more fermentable fibres such as pectin are found in oats, fruits, and green peas. Their beneficial effects on lowering blood cholesterol are via enhanced enterohepatic circulation, slow glucose absorption, slow transit of food through upper GI tract, and holding moisture in stools and increased satiety. A cross-sectional study of 1,068 adults with a mean age of 67 conducted by Ibarrola-Juardo et al. (2012) reports that dietary intake of phylloquinone in leafy green vegetables was associated with a lower prevalence of type II diabetes. Increased phylloquinone intake with a median of 5.5 years shown that a 51% reduction in the risk of diabetes onset in the elderly at high cardiovascular risk (Ibarrola-Jurado et al., 2012). Meats are rich sources of protein, energy, amino acids, vitamins, iron, calcium, zinc, selenium, and various micronutrients, which are important to human wellbeing. Systematic reviews show low fruit and vegetable intakes were associated with 22 risk-disease pairs (Yip et al., 2019a), and high meat intakes were associated with 37 risk-disease pairs (Yip et al., 2018), mainly cardiovascular diseases, cancers, and diabetes.

Physical Activity

Regular physical exercises help regulating cardiorespiratory and cardiovascular fitness, improve glycaemia and insulin response, and bring a variety of positive effects on the human body (Di Liegro et al., 2019). Physical activity is recommended as a non-pharmacologic therapy for different pathological affections and general health status maintenance. Systematic reviews and meta-analyses indicate that physical inactivity increase the risk of all-cause mortalities (Ku et al., 2018); CVD and cancer mortalities and incidences, and diabetes incidence (Biswas et al., 2015); colon, endometrial, and lung cancer (Schmid & Leitzmann, 2014); and breast cancer (Zhou et al., 2015).

Health Promotion

Over the past decade, the Department of Health, Hong Kong has taken a multi-pronged approach to reduce each of the risk factors: reduce the harmful use of alcohol as well as physical inactivity and promote smoking cessation and healthy diet. It recommends non-drinkers not to start drinking with the intent of improving health, and drinkers should limit alcohol intake to minimise alcohol-related harms (Department of Health, 2022a). It also opposes smoking and prohibits tobacco advertising and smoking in most public places. It encourages the public to follow the principles of the Healthy Eating Food Pyramid; include a variety of foods providing appropriate calories and nutrients in the diet; and decrease fat, salt, and sugar intakes (Department of Health, 2022b). It recommends eating at least two servings of fruit and three servings of vegetables per day. To improve cardiorespiratory and muscular fitness, bone health, and reduce the risk of NCDs and depression, the government urges adults aged 18–64 to follow the WHO recommendation and do at least 150 min of moderate-intensity aerobic physical activity throughout the week (converted to on average 21.43 min/day), or at least 75 min of vigorous-intensity aerobic physical throughout the week (converted to on average 10.71 min/day), or an equivalent combination of moderate- and vigorous-intensity activity (Department of Health, 2022c; World Health Organization, 2020).

Dynamic Lifestyle Trends 2004–2016

The study has identified lifestyle risk factor patterns and their development trends in Hong Kong. The Centre for Health Protection, a professional arm of the Department of Health, Hong Kong seeks to prevent communicable and NCDs. The Centre continues to strengthen the surveillance and promotion of healthy living. The Department commissioned the Social Sciences Research Centre of the University of Hong Kong to conduct Behavioural Risk Factor Surveys. The Behavioural Risk Factor Surveillance System is set up by the Surveillance and Epidemiology Branch, Centre for Health Protection of the Department of Health. It collects information of health-related Behaviours among the Hong Kong non-institutionalised adult population aged 18–64 through periodic telephone surveys. The vision of such initiative is to monitor the prevalence of and detect any changes in major Behavioural risks of the target population, and provide up-to-date information to facilitate planning and management of public health programmes. The surveys were conducted through Computer Assisted Telephone Interview (CATI). Random samples (excluding foreign domestic helpers) of Cantonese, Putonghua or English-speaking residents aged 18–64 years were drawn from the 2007 Hong Kong residential telephone directory (English version). The survey asked participants the number of days/week they ate fruit and vegetables, and the average intake/eating day. Participants were also asked to estimate their average number of cigarettes and units of drink/day. International Physical Activity Questionnaire (short form) was adopted to assess respondents' level of physical activity. Informed consent, data collection, and questionnaires details could be found in the corresponding main reports (Centre for Health Protection, 2021). Based on an investigation of the Behavioural Risk Factor Survey data collected between 2004 and 2016, the lifestyle trends among Hong Kong adult males and females were dynamic.

Alcohol Intake

The average alcohol intakes among Hong Kong adults were 1.20 and 1.29 units of 10 g ethanol/day/person for males and females, respectively, in 2016, compared to 1.63 and 0.47 unit/day/person respectively in 2004 (Fig. 11.1). While the average alcohol intake among males was gradually decreasing, the average intake among females was rapidly increasing. The decreases in the average intake among males were persistently and statistically significant since 2012 when compared to 2004. The increases in the average intake among females were also persistently and statistically significant since 2014 (Table 11.1). On the other hand, the prevalence of drinking among females increased rapidly from 28.1% in 2004 to 66.7% in 2016 (Fig. 11.2). Although male non-drinkers ate significantly more fruit and vegetables, they spent significantly more time sitting when compared with drinkers. Female non-drinkers ate significantly more fruit and spent significantly less time sitting (Table 11.2).

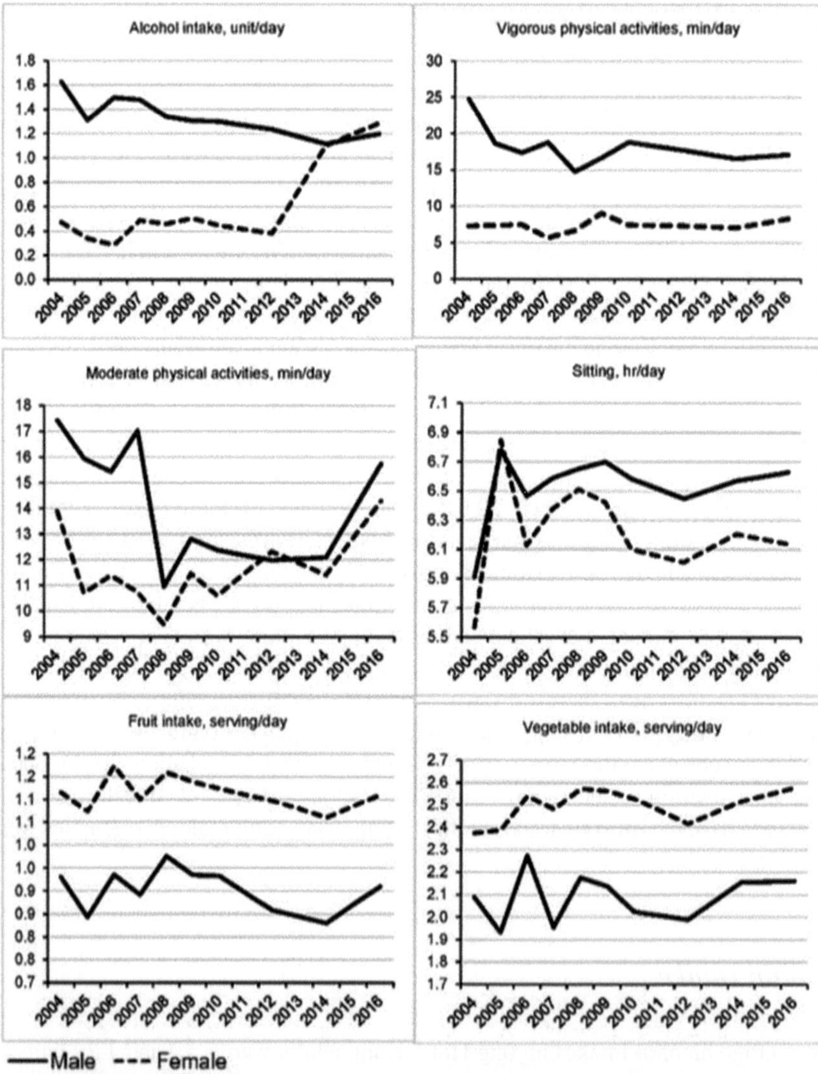

Fruit and vegetable intake mean: seven day average/day. One serving of fruit is equivalent to one medium-sized apple or orange. One medium sized banana, or 2 kiwi fruits or plums, or half a rice bowl of small fruits like grapes or strawberries. One serving of vegetables is equivalent to half a rice bowl of cooked vegetables or a rice bowl (250-300ml) of uncooked vegetables

Fig. 11.1 Hong Kong adult population age-standardised mean alcohol intake, physical activity, fruit, and vegetable intake by sex by year, 2004–2016

Table 11.1 Multiple comparison of population age-standardised means alcohol intake, physical activities, and fruit and vegetable intakes 2004 against 2012, 2014 and 2016 by sex

			Male				Female			
Dependent Variable	Independent variable			p-value	95% CI		Mean (I-J)	p-value	95% CI	
	Mean (I)	Mean (J)	Mean (I-J)		Lower	Upper			Lower	Upper
Alcohol intake, unit/day	2004	2012	0.39*	0.02	0.04	0.75	0.09	0.69	−0.06	0.24
		2014	0.51*	0.00	0.23	0.80	−0.63*	0.00	−0.80	−0.45
		2016	0.43*	0.00	0.14	0.72	−0.81*	0.00	−0.99	−0.64
Vigorous physical activities min/day	2004	2012	7.06	0.34	−2.36	16.48	−0.04	1.00	−3.77	3.69
		2014	8.22	0.08	−0.46	16.90	0.22	1.00	−3.22	3.67
		2016	7.65	0.14	−1.00	16.30	−1.03	0.99	−4.45	2.38
Moderate physical activities, min/day	2004	2012	5.45	0.18	−0.96	11.87	1.59	0.99	−3.62	6.80
		2014	5.34	0.15	−0.80	11.48	2.48	0.77	−2.02	6.98
		2016	1.69	1.00	−4.63	8.00	−0.40	1.00	−4.97	4.16
Walking, min/day	2004	2012	2.41	1.00	−10.35	15.18	5.09	0.96	−7.55	17.73
		2014	−1.52	1.00	−12.60	9.55	1.29	1.00	−9.77	12.35
		2016	−1.61	1.00	−12.47	9.24	−0.38	1.00	−11.43	10.66
Sitting, min/day	2005	2012	19.94	0.51	−9.77	49.65	45.00*	0.00	20.34	79.65
		2014	12.61	0.89	−13.81	39.03	38.48*	0.00	11.79	65.18
		2016	9.09	0.99	−17.63	35.82	42.50*	0.00	15.92	69.08
Fruit intake, serving/day	2004	2012	0.07	0.70	−0.05	0.20	0.02	1.00	−0.09	0.13
		2014	0.10*	0.03	0.01	0.19	0.06	0.62	−0.03	0.14
		2016	0.02	1.00	−0.08	0.12	0.00	1.00	−0.09	0.10

(continued)

Table 11.1 (continued)

Dependent Variable	Independent variable		Male				Female			
	Mean (I)	Mean (J)	Mean (I-J)	p-value	95% CI Lower	95% CI Upper	Mean (I-J)	p-value	95% CI Lower	95% CI Upper
Vegetable intake, serving/day	2004	2012	0.10	0.88	−0.11	0.31	−0.04	1.00	−0.24	0.15
		2014	−0.07	0.98	−0.25	0.12	−0.14	0.21	−0.32	0.03
		2016	−0.07	0.97	−0.26	0.12	−0.20*	0.01	−0.38	−0.03

All Games-Howell Post Hoc Tests. *The mean difference is significant at the 0.05 level. One unit of alcohol is equivalent to 10 g ethanol. One serving of fruit is equivalent to one medium-sized apple or orange. One medium sized banana, or 2 kiwi fruits or plums, or half a rice bowl of small fruits like grapes or strawberries. One serving of vegetables is equivalent to half a rice bowl of cooked vegetables or a rice bowl (250 ml) of uncooked vegetables

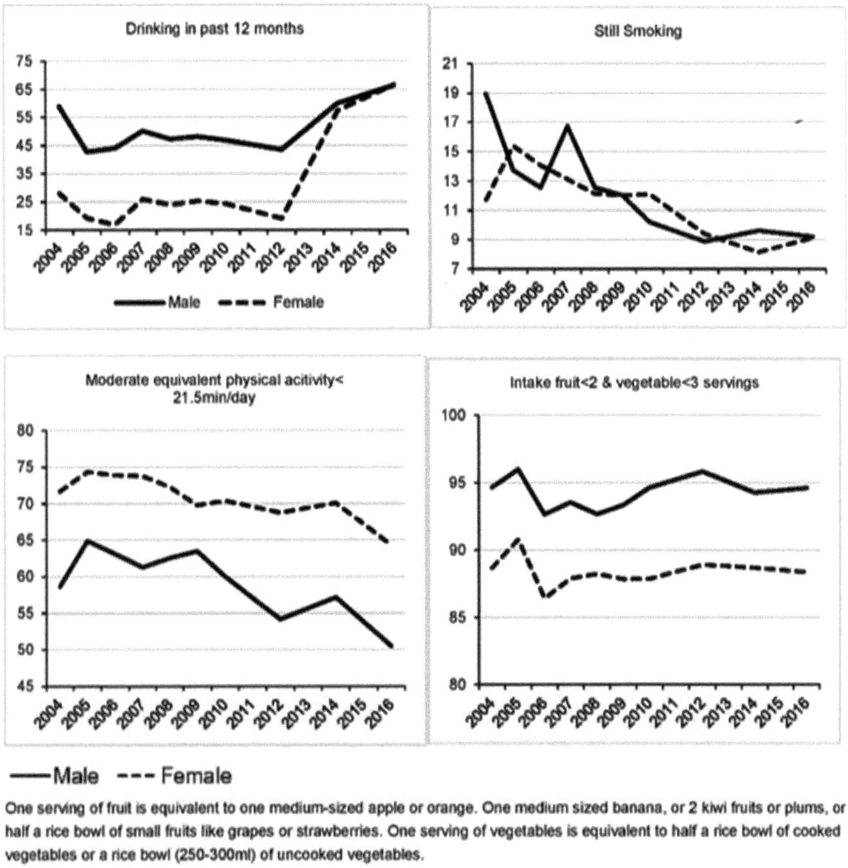

Fig. 11.2 Age-standardised percentages of Hong Kong adult population drinking, smoking and did not meet the physical activity, fruit and vegetable intake recommendations by sex by year, 2004–2016

Tobacco Use

The prevalence of smoking among both males and females decreased rapidly, from 19.0% and 11.7% in 2004 to 9.2% and 9.1% in 2016, respectively (Fig. 11.2). Male smokers drank significantly more alcohol but spent less time sitting when compared with non-smokers. Female smokers drank significantly less alcohol (Table 11.2).

Table 11.2 Multiple comparison of age-standardised mean differences by lifestyle factors by sex, 2004–2016, statistically significant at 95% confidence level

				Mean (I-J)	p-value	95% CI	
Dependent Variable	Test	Mean (I)	Mean (J)			Lower	Upper
Male							
Sitting, min/day	*	Not drinking	1 < Intake/day ≤ 2 units	30.73	0.00	15.48	45.97
Fruit intake, serving/day	#	Not drinking	Intake/day > 5 units	0.16	0.00	0.07	0.25
			2 < Intake/day ≤ 5 units	0.09	0.00	0.03	0.16
Vegetable intake, serving/day	*	Not drinking	2 < Intake/day ≤ 5 units	0.15	0.014	−0.277	−0.020
Alcohol intake, unit/day	*	Yes, and still smoking	Yes, but not now	0.39	0.00	0.16	0.62
			Never	0.25	0.01	0.06	0.43
Sitting, min/day	*	Yes, and still smoking	Yes, but not now	−25.06	0.02	−47.17	−2.94
			Never	−20.53	0.00	−35.61	−5.45
Sitting, min/day	*	Activity ≥ 21.5 min/day	0 < Activity < 21.5 min/day	−52.59	0.00	−63.91	−41.26
			Activity = 0	−28.80	0.00	−40.31	−17.29
Fruit intake, serving/day	*	Activity ≥ 21.5 min/day	0 < Activity < 21.5 min/day	0.14	0.00	0.10	0.18
			Activity = 0	0.18	0.00	0.14	0.22
Vegetable intake, serving/day	*	Activity ≥ 21.5 min/day	0 < Activity < 21.5 min/day	0.18	0.00	0.10	0.26
			Activity = 0	0.26	0.00	0.18	0.33
Alcohol intake, unit/day	*	Fruit intake ≥ 2 servings	Intake < 1 serving	−0.36	0.00	−0.49	−0.23
Activities, min/day	*	Fruit intake ≥ 2 servings	1 ≤ Intake < 2 servings	19.97	0.00	10.98	28.95
			Intake < 1 serving	20.93	0.00	12.34	29.51

(continued)

Table 11.2 (continued)

				Mean (I-J)	p-value	95% CI	
Dependent Variable	Test	Mean (I)	Mean (J)			Lower	Upper
Sitting, min/day	*	Fruit intake ≥ 2 servings	1 ≤ Intake < 2 servings	−19.23	0.01	−33.79	−4.66
			Intake < 1 serving	−35.81	0.00	−49.45	−22.17
Vegetable intake, serving/day	*	Fruit intake ≥ 2 servings	1 ≤ Intake < 2 servings	0.45	0.00	0.33	0.56
			Intake < 1 serving	0.81	0.00	0.70	0.92
Alcohol intake, unit/day	*	Vegetable intake ≥ 3 servings	2 ≤ Intake < 3 servings	0.18	0.01	0.03	0.33
Activities, min/day	*	Vegetable intake ≥ 3 servings	1 ≤ Intake < 2 servings	8.29	0.03	0.47	16.12
			Intake < 1 serving	9.57	0.04	0.30	18.83
Sitting, min/day	#	Vegetable intake ≥ 3 servings	1 ≤ Intake < 2 servings	−17.66	0.01	−32.73	−2.59
Fruit intake, serving/day	*	Vegetable intake ≥ 3 servings	2 ≤ Intake < 3 servings	0.22	0.00	0.16	0.27
			1 ≤ Intake < 2 servings	0.42	0.00	0.37	0.48
			Intake < 1	0.54	0.00	0.48	0.60
Female							
Sitting, min/day	*	Not drinking	1 < Intake ≤ 2 units	−24.00	0.00	−40.35	−7.66
			0 < Intake ≤ 1 unit	−16.53	0.01	−30.64	−2.42
Fruit intake, serving/day	#	Not drinking	Intake > 5 units	0.17	0.02	0.02	0.31
			1 < Intake ≤ 2 units	0.11	0.00	0.05	0.17
Alcohol intake, unit/day	*	Yes, and still smoking	Never	−0.10	0.02	−0.19	−0.01

(continued)

Table 11.2 (continued)

				Mean (I-J)	p-value	95% CI	
Dependent Variable	Test	Mean (I)	Mean (J)			Lower	Upper
Sitting, min/day	*	Activity ≥ 21.5 min/day	0 < Activity < 21.5 min /day	−55.68	0.00	−66.63	−44.72
			Activity = 0	−51.22	0.00	−61.58	−40.86
Fruit intake, serving/day	*	Activity ≥ 21.5 min/day	0 < Activity < 21.5 min /day	0.18	0.00	0.14	0.23
			Activity = 0	0.22	0.00	0.18	0.26
Vegetable intake, serving/day	*	Activity ≥ 21.5 min/day	0 < Activity < 21.5 min /day	0.26	0.00	0.18	0.34
			Activity = 0	0.36	0.00	0.29	0.44
Alcohol intake, unit/day	*	Activity ≥ 21.5 min/day	Activity = 0	0.15	0.00	0.07	0.23
Sitting, min/day	*	Fruit intake ≥ 2 servings	1 ≤ Intake < 2 servings	−25.48	0.00	−36.65	−14.32
			Intake < 1 serving	−74.94	0.00	−86.05	−63.82
Alcohol intake, unit/day	*	Fruit intake ≥ 2 servings	1 ≤ Intake < 2 servings	−0.09	0.01	−0.17	−0.02
			Intake < 1 serving	−0.19	0.00	−0.27	−0.12
Activities, min/day	*	Fruit intake ≥ 2 servings	1 ≤ Intake < 2 serving	10.71	0.00	6.78	14.65
			Intake < 1 serving	15.52	0.00	11.64	19.40
Vegetable intake, serving/day	*	Fruit intake ≥ 2 servings	1 ≤ Intake < 2 servings	0.49	0.00	0.41	0.58
			Intake < 1 serving	0.86	0.00	0.78	0.94
Activities, min/day	*	Vegetable intake ≥ 3 servings	2 ≤ Intake < 3 servings	6.17	0.00	2.65	9.68
			1 ≤ Intake < 2 servings	10.33	0.00	6.15	14.51
			Intake < 1 serving	12.34	0.00	7.16	17.51

(continued)

Table 11.2 (continued)

Dependent Variable	Test	Mean (I)	Mean (J)	Mean (I-J)	p-value	95% CI Lower	95% CI Upper
Sitting, min/day	*	Vegetable intake ≥ 3 servings	1 ≤ Intake < 2 servings	−28.10	0.00	−42.29	−13.91
			Intake < 1 serving	−26.07	0.01	−47.48	−4.65
Fruit intake, serving/day	*	Vegetable intake ≥ 3 servings	2 ≤ Intake < 3 servings	0.25	0.00	0.20	0.29
			1 ≤ Intake < 2 servings	0.46	0.00	0.42	0.51
			Intake < 1 serving	0.57	0.00	0.50	0.65

*Games-Howell post hoc test
#Tukey HSD post hoc test
One unit of alcohol is equivalent to 10 g ethanol
One serving of fruit is equivalent to one medium-sized apple or orange. One medium sized banana, or 2 kiwi fruits or plums, or half a rice bowl of small fruits like grapes or strawberries
One serving of vegetables is equivalent to half a rice bowl of cooked vegetables or a rice bowl of uncooked vegetables
A rice bowl is equivalent to 250 ml
Activity refers to moderate equivalent physical activities

Physical Activities

Changes in the average time spent doing vigorous and moderate physical activities, and walking among both males and females remained non-significant when compared against in 2004. The average time spent doing vigorous physical activities mostly ranged between 17 and 18 min/day/person among males and 7–8 min/day/person among females (Fig. 11.1, Table 11.1). Changes in the average time spent on sitting also remained non-significant except among females in 2006, when it was significantly decreased by 43.16 min/day/person, and then remained non-significant thereafter when compared against 2004. On the other hand, the prevalence of insufficient physical activity (spent less than 21.5 min/day on doing moderate equivalent physical activities) decreased from 58.6% and 71.7% in 2004 to 50.5% and 64.3% in 2016 among males and females respectively. Both males and females who did sufficient physical activities spent significantly less time sitting and ate more fruits and vegetables (Table 11.2).

Fruit and Vegetable Intakes

Most Hong Kong adults ate less fruits and vegetables than recommended. No persistent significant changes in the average fruit and vegetable intakes were observed. An in-depth analysis of age and sex-specific fruit intakes trend and patterns can be found in Yip et al. (2019b). The average fruit intake between 2004 and 2016 ranged 0.83–0.94 serving/day/person for males and 1.06–1.17 serving/day/person for females (Fig. 11.1, Table 11.2). The average vegetable intake between 2004 and 2016 ranged 1.96–2.18 serving/day/person for males and 2.37–2.58 serving/day person for females. Prevalence of insufficient fruit intake (eating less than 2 servings of fruit/day) also remained stable, ranged 93–96% for males and 86–91% for females (Fig. 11.2). Males and females who ate sufficient fruit ate significantly more vegetables, drank significantly less alcohol, and spent significantly more time on doing moderate equivalent activities, while males also spent significantly less time sitting. However, males who ate sufficient vegetables (more than 3 servings of vegetables/day) also drank remarkably more alcohol.

Lifestyle Patterns

Despite the rapid lifestyle shifts between 2010 and 2014 (Fig. 11.3), lifestyles P6 and P8 remained dominant among males. The prevalence of lifestyle P5 among males was expanding. It gradually replaced P6 as the second most dominant lifestyle in 2016. Among those males who ate sufficient fruit and vegetable, there were gradual shifts from lifestyle P1, lifestyle P2, and lifestyle P4 toward lifestyle P3. Among females, lifestyles P5 and P6 remained to be the dominant lifestyles, but gradual shifting from lifestyle P2 and P6 toward the other lifestyles observed.

Mixing Health Promotion Outcomes

A high proportion of Hong Kong adults consume alcohol, spend substantial time sitting, doing insufficient physical activities, and not eating enough fruit and vegetables. Most males and females are living with multiple lifestyle risk factors. Despite a series of large-scale dietary/health promotion campaigns, fruit and vegetable intakes remain stable and below the recommended levels. On the other hand, the average alcohol intake among males has persistently and significantly decreased. The prevalence of smoking among both males and females has also persistently decreased. This may reflect success in smoking cessation promotions and tobacco control policies but not necessarily in reducing alcohol intake policies and promotion. The average alcohol intake among females persistently and significantly escalated and the prevalence of drinking among both males and females has also expanded rapidly in more recent years. Although the changes in the average time spent doing physical activities were non-significant, the prevalence of doing sufficient physical activity among both males and females persistently increased. This may probably associate with the shift from a five-and-a-half-working-day/week to a five-working-day/week. As a result, more and more people may probably spend the extra free day on doing physical activities, such as joining the weekend hiking and sport activity groups, and consequently more social activities (including physical activities), which may probably eventually lead to more social drinking.

More Recent Lifestyle Trends

Hong Kong had gone through a period of social unrest in 2019–2020, then entered the burden of COVID-19. People's nobilities and social interactions have been restricted. This brings significant impacts to Hong Kong people's lifestyles. Many people have become physically and socially inactive. Alcohol consumption among the aged 15 years or above decreased in recent years from around 2.8 L per capita per year in 2018 to around 2.5 L in 2019 and 2020 (Department of Health, 2021b); the decreases in social drinking caused by the COVID-19 might make a contribution to the decrease. The prevalence of daily cigarette smokers among the aged 15 years in the recent decade, 2010–2021, has gradually decreased from 19.9% to 16.7% in males but fluctuated between 2.7% and 3.2% in females (Tobacco & Alcohol Control Office, 2022b). According to the Health Behaviour Survey 2018/2019 (Centre for Health Protection, 2020), the prevalence of smokers, whether daily or less, often decreases with age. The prevalence of smokers in 2018/2019 was 23.3% for men and 4.1%

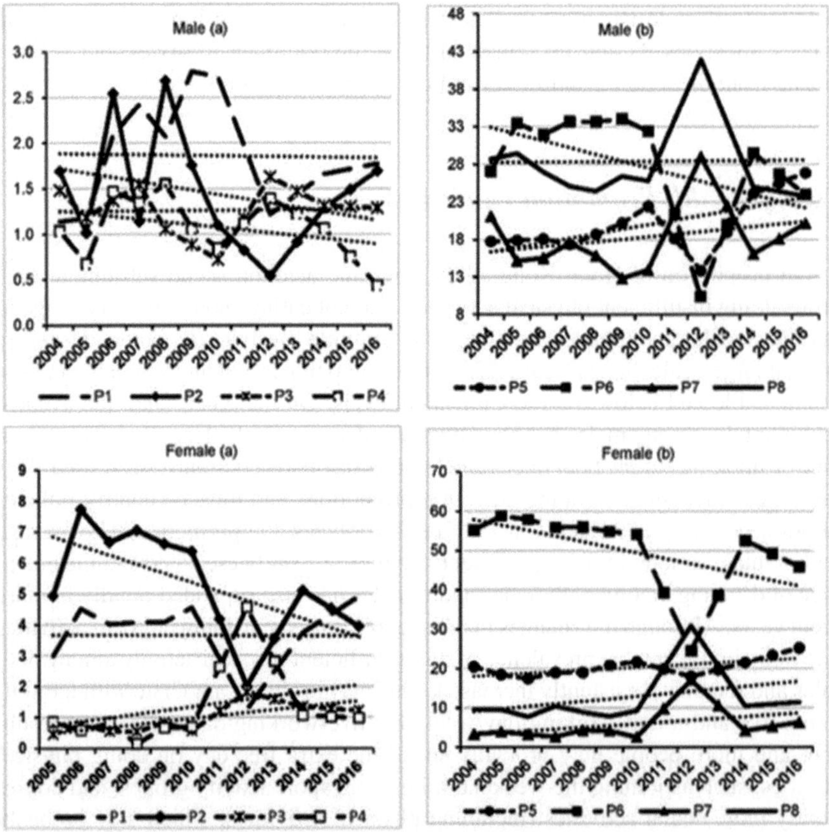

P1. Adults on average eating at least 2 servings of fruit and 3 serving of vegetables, and not smoking, and not drinking, and doing at least 21.5min/day moderate equivalent physical activities.

P2. Adults on average eating at least 2 servings of fruit and 3 serving of vegetables, and not smoking, and not drinking, and doing less than 21.5min/day moderate equivalent physical activities.

P3. Adults on average eating at least 2 servings of fruit and 3 serving of vegetables, and smoking or drinking, and doing at least 21.5min/day moderate equivalent physical activities.

P4. Adults on average eating at least 2 servings of fruit and 3 serving of vegetables, and smoking or drinking, and doing less than 21.5min/day moderate equivalent physical activities.

P5. Adults on average eating less than 2 servings of fruit or less than 3 serving of vegetables, and not smoking, and not drinking, and doing at least 21.5min/day moderate equivalent physical activities.

P6. Adults on average eating less than 2 servings of fruit or less than 3 serving of vegetables, and not smoking, and not drinking, and doing less than 21.5min/day moderate equivalent physical activities.

P7. Adults on average eating less than 2 servings of fruit or less than 3 serving of vegetables, and smoking or drinking, and doing at least 21.5min/day moderate equivalent physical activities.

P8. Adults on average eating less than 2 servings of fruit or less than 3 serving of vegetables, and smoking or drinking, and doing less than 21.5min/day moderate equivalent physical activities.

Fig. 11.3 Age-standardised percentages of Hong Kong adult population among eight different lifestyle patterns by sex and by year, 2004–2016

for women. For adults aged 18 and above, just as what the Health Behaviour Survey 2018/2019 suggests, 15.2% of males and 8.3% of females were doing insufficient physical activity—especially among those aged 85 years.

Comparing the second territory-wide food consumption survey conducted in 2018–2020 to the first population-based food consumption survey conducted in 2005–07, vegetable intake among aged 18 years or above remained relatively stable, with 191.08 g per capita per day in 2005–2007 compared to 202.65 g per capita per day in 2018–2020, while fruit consumption decreased from 146.81 g per capita per day to 120.31 g per capita per day. Red meat intakes also increased from 74.23 g per capita per day to 85.06 g per capita per day which was much higher than the recommended 60 g per capita per day or less (National Health & Medical Research Council, 2011; Yip & Fielding, 2017). This suggests Hong Kong adult's dietary habit has become unhealthier; and that reducing Hong Kong adults' meat intake to the recommended level and replacing the intake energy with fruit and vegetable could prevent even more premature deaths than what has been suggested in Yip and Fielding (2017).

Electronic cigarettes are incrementally popular in Hong Kong in recent years. Although they do not contain tobacco, it is an electronic nicotine delivery system. The e-liquid typically composes of propylene glycol, glycerin, flavourings, and other additives. The School of Public Health of the University of Hong Kong conducted School-based Survey on Smoking in 2016–2017. The findings show that within Primary 4–6 students; 2,340 (1.4%) had ever used e-cigarettes and the number of ever, and current e-cigarette users among Secondary 1–6 students were 29,380 (8.7%), and 2,770 (0.8%), respectively (Tobacco & Alcohol Control Office, 2022a). Among those primary school students who had ever used both e-cigarettes and conventional cigarettes, nearly 70% tried e-cigarettes first. Consequently, Smoking (Public Health) (Amendment) Ordinance 2021 has been enforced. Alternative smoking products were banned completely in Hong Kong from April 30, 2022. E-smokers have to either return to traditional smoking or quitting the habit completely.

Conclusions and Recommendations for Future Health Promotion

Despite more recent investigations have indicated decreased alcohol consumption, the rapidly growing prevalence of alcohol intake and other lifestyle factors have remained to be a huge public health concern. Changes in the prevalence of lifestyle risk factors have induced persistent shifts of lifestyle patterns among Hong Kong adults. More investigation is needed to identify the major determinants of increasing prevalence of alcohol intake. Strategic intervention policy changes targeting a balance of multiple lifestyle factors among different lifestyle groups instead of a single particular risk factor are urgently needed to reverse the unhealthy population lifestyle trends. As Yip et al. (2019b) have suggested, better strategies and more efforts are needed to facilitate a persistent rise in fruit and vegetable intakes among the population. Given that a diverse combination of multiple lifestyle risk factors co-existed, and the possibility that strategies successfully making behavioural change with respect to a particular risk factor may induce behavioural changes toward other risk factors. For example, quitting smoking may lead to starting or increasing drinking; increasing physical activities may increase drinking; or increase social physical activities may increase social drinking. Therefore, instead of targeting a single particular risk factor, future health intervention strategies should simultaneously target multiple risk factors in different lifestyle patterns for continuing health improvement among the population.

Acknowledgements Thanks go to Department of Health of the Hong Kong SAR Government for providing the Behavioural Risk Factor Survey data.

References

Biswas, A., Oh, P. I., Faulkner, G. E., Bajaj, R. R., Silver, M. A., Mitchell, M. S., & Alter, D. A. (2015). Sedentary time and its association with risk for disease incidence, mortality, and hospitalization in adults: A systematic review and meta-analysis. *Annals of Internal Medicine, 162*(2), 123–132. https://doi.org/10.7326/m14-1651

Bresin, K. (2019). A meta-analytic review of laboratory studies testing the alcohol stress response dampening hypothesis. *Psychology of Addictive Behaviors, 33*(7), 581–594. https://doi.org/10.1037/adb0000516

Cancer Research UK. (2021, March 25). *What's in a cigarette?* Retrieved June 14, 2022, from https://www.cancerresearchuk.org/about-cancer/causes-of-cancer/smoking-and-cancer/whats-in-a-cigarette-0

Centre for Health Protection. (2020). *Report of Health Behaviour Survey 2018/19*. Department of Health. https://www.chp.gov.hk/files/pdf/report_of_health_behaviour_survey_2018_en.pdf

Centre for Health Protection. (2021). *Behavioural risk factor survey (BRFS)*. Department of Health. https://www.chp.gov.hk/en/resources/29/327.html

De Nunzio, C., Andriole, G. L., Thompson, I. M., Jr., & Freedland, S. J. (2015). Smoking and prostate cancer: A systematic review. *European Urology Focus, 1*(1), 28–38. https://doi.org/10.1016/j.euf.2014.10.002

Department of Health. (2021a). *Carbohydrates*. Retrieved June 10, 2022, from https://www.change4health.gov.hk/en/healthy_diet/facts/calories_nutrients/carbohydrates/index.html

Department of Health. (2021b). *Estimated alcohol consumption per capita in Hong Kong*. Retrieved June 9, 2022, from https://www.change4health.gov.hk/en/alcohol_aware/figures/alcohol_consumption/index.html#:~:text=Between%202004%20and%202020%2C%20the,between%202.46%20and%202.87%20litres

Department of Health. (2022a). *Alcohol and health*. https://www.change4health.gov.hk/en/alcohol_aware/index.html

Department of Health. (2022b). *Healthy diet*. https://www.change4health.gov.hk/en/healthy_diet/index.html

Department of Health. (2022c). *Physical activity*. https://www.change4health.gov.hk/en/physical_activity/index.html

Di Liegro, C. M., Schiera, G., Proia, P., & Di Liegro, I. (2019). Physical activity and brain health. *Genes, 10*(9), Article 720. https://doi.org/10.3390/genes10090720

Feigin, V. L., Roth, G. A., Naghavi, M., Parmar, P., Krishnamurthi, R., Chugh, S., Mensah, G. A., Norrving, B., Shiue, I., Ng, M., Estep, K., Cercy, K., Murray, C. J. L., & Forouzanfar, M. H. (2016). Global burden of stroke and risk factors in 188 countries, during 1990–2013: A systematic analysis for the Global Burden of Disease Study 2013. *The Lancet Neurology, 15*(9), 913–924. https://doi.org/10.1016/S1474-4422(16)30073-4

Forouzanfar, M. H., Afshin, A., Alexander, L. T., Anderson, H. R., Bhutta, Z. A., Biryukov, S., Brauer, M., Cercy, K., Charlson, F. J., Cohen, A. J., Dandona, L., Carrero, J. J., Estep, K., Ferrari, A. J., Frostad, J. J., Fullman, N., Gething, P. W., Godwin, W. W., Griswold, M., ... Zuhlke, L. J. (2016). Global, regional, and national comparative risk assessment of 79 behavioural, environmental and occupational, and metabolic risks or clusters of risks, 1990-2015: A systematic analysis for the Global Burden of Disease Study 2015. *The Lancet, 388*(10053), 1659–1724. https://doi.org/10.1016/S0140-6736(16)31679-8

Gakidou, E., Afshin, A., Abajobir, A. A., Abate, K. H., Abbafati, C., Abbas, K. M., Abd-Allah, F., Abdulle, A. M., Abera, S. F., Aboyans, V., Abu-Raddad, L. J., Abu-Rmeileh, N. M., Abyu, G. Y., Adedeji, I. A., Adetokunboh, O., Afarideh, M., Agrawal, A., Agrawal, S., Kiadaliri, A. A., ... Murray, C. J. L. (2017). Global, regional, and national comparative risk assessment of 84 behavioural, environmental and occupational, and metabolic risks or clusters of risks, 1990-2016: A systematic analysis for the Global Burden of Disease Study 2016. *The Lancet, 390*(10100), 1345–1422. https://doi.org/10.1016/S0140-6736(17)32366-8

Ibarrola-Jurado, N., Salas-Salvado, J., Martinez-Gonzalez, M. A., & Bullo, M. (2012). Dietary phylloquinone intake and risk of type 2 diabetes in elderly subjects at high risk of cardiovascular disease. *The American Journal of Clinical Nutrition, 96*(5), 1113–1118. https://doi.org/10.3945/ajcn.111.033498

Kong, L. (2014). *A systematic review of cohort studies on the association of smoking with all-cause and lung cancer mortality in China* (Postgraduate thesis, University of Hong Kong). The HKU Scholars Hub. http://hdl.handle.net/10722/206969

Ku, P. W., Steptoe, A., Liao, Y., Hsueh, M.-C., & Chen, L.-J. (2018). A cut-off of daily sedentary time and all-cause mortality in adults: A meta-regression analysis involving more than 1 million participants. *BMC Medicine, 16*, Article 74. https://doi.org/10.1186/s12916-018-1062-2

Lim, S. S., Vos, T., Flaxman, A. D., Danaei, G., Shibuya, K., Adair-Rohani, H., Amann, M., Anderson, H. R., Andrews, K. G., Aryee, M., Atkinson, C., Bacchus, L., Bahalim, A., Balakrishnan, K., Balmes, J., Barker-Collo, S., Baxter, A., Bell, M., Blore, J., ... Kok, C. (2012). A comparative risk assessment of burden of disease and injury attributable to 67 risk factors and risk factor clusters in 21 regions, 1990–2010: A systematic analysis for the Global Burden of Disease Study 2010. *The Lancet, 380*(9859), 2224–2260. https://doi.org/10.1016/S0140-6736(12)61766-8

Lock, K., Pomerleau, J., Causer, L., Altmann, D. R., & McKee, M. (2005). The global burden of disease attributable to low consumption of fruit and vegetables: Implications for the global strategy on diet. *Bulletin of the World Health Organization, 83*(2), 100–108. https://apps.who.int/iris/handle/10665/269344

Luciano, M. T., Acuff, S. F., Olin, C. C., Lewin, R. K., Strickland, J. C., McDevitt-Murphy, M. E., & Murphy, J. G. (2022). Posttraumatic stress disorder, drinking to cope, and harmful alcohol use: A multivariate meta-analysis of the self-medication hypothesis. *Journal of Psychopathology and Clinical Science, 131*(5), 447–456. https://doi.org/10.1037/abn0000764

Masaoka, H., Matsuo, K., Ito, H., Wakai, K., Nagata, C., Nakayama, T., Sadakane, A., Tanaka, K., Tamakoshi, A., Sugawara, Y., Mizoue, T., Sawada, N., Inoue, M., Tsugane, S., & Sasazuki, S. (2016). Cigarette smoking and bladder cancer risk: An evaluation based on a systematic review of epidemiologic evidence in the Japanese population. *Japanese Journal of Clinical Oncology, 46*(3), 273–283. https://doi.org/10.1093/jjco/hyv188

Matsuda, M., & Shimomura, I. (2013). Increased oxidative stress in obesity: Implications for metabolic syndrome, diabetes, hypertension, dyslipidemia, atherosclerosis, and cancer. *Obesity Research & Clinical Practice, 7*(5), e330–e341. https://doi.org/10.1016/j.orcp.2013.05.004

Matsuo, K., Ito, H., Wakai, K., Nagata, C., Mizoue, T., Tanaka, K., Tsuji, I., Tamakoshi, A., Sasazuki, S., Inoue, M., & Tsugane, S. (2011). Cigarette smoking and pancreas cancer risk: An evaluation based on a systematic review of epidemiologic evidence in the Japanese population. *Japanese Journal of Clinical Oncology, 41*(11), 1292–1302. https://doi.org/10.1093/jjco/hyr141

National Health and Medical Research Council. (2011). *A modelling system to inform the revision of the Australian guide to healthy eating.* Department of Health and Ageing, Australian Government. https://www.eatforhealth.gov.au/sites/default/files/files/public_consultation/n55a_dietary_guidelines_food_modelling_111216.pdf

Oze, I., Matsuo, K., Ito, H., Wakai, K., Nagata, C., Mizoue, T., Tanaka, K., Tsuji, I., Tamakoshi, S., Sasazuki, S., Innoue, M., & Tsugane, S. (2011). Cigarette smoking and esophageal cancer risk: An evaluation based on a systematic review of epidemiologic evidence among the Japanese population. *Japanese Journal of Clinical Oncology, 42*(1), 63–73. https://doi.org/10.1093/jjco/hyr170

Pan, A., Wang, Y., Talaei, M., Hu, F. B., & Wu, T. (2015). Relation of active, passive, and quitting smoking with incident type 2 diabetes: A systematic review and meta-analysis. *The Lancet Diabetes & Endocrinology, 3*(12), 958–967. https://doi.org/10.1016/S2213-8587(15)00316-2

Percival, S. S. (2011). Nutrition and immunity: Balancing diet and immune function. *Nutrition Today, 46*(1), 12–17. https://doi.org/10.1097/NT.0b013e3182076fc8

Rehm, J., Gmel, G. E., Sr., Gmel, G., Hasan, O. S., Imtiaz, S., Popova, S., Probst, C., Roerecke, M., Room, R., Samokhvalov, A. V., Shield, K. D., & Shuper, P. A. (2017). The relationship between different dimensions of alcohol use and the burden of disease—An update. *Addiction, 112*(6), 968–1001. https://doi.org/10.1111/add.13757

Schmid, D., & Leitzmann, M. F. (2014). Television viewing and time spent sedentary in relation to cancer risk: A meta-analysis. *JNCI: Journal of the National Cancer Institute, 106*(7), Article dju098. https://doi.org/10.1093/jnci/dju098

Tobacco and Alcohol Control Office. (2022a). *Electronic cigarette (e-cigarette).* Department of Health. Retrieved June 14, 2022, from https://www.taco.gov.hk/t/english/infostation/infostation_ec.html

Tobacco and Alcohol Control Office. (2022b). *Pattern of smoking in Hong Kong.* Department of Health. Retrieved June 9, 2022, from https://www.taco.gov.hk/t/english/infostation/infostation_sta_01.html#a3

U.S. Department of Agriculture and U.S. Department of Health and Human Services. (2020). *Dietary guidelines for Americans 2020–2025.* https://www.dietaryguidelines.gov/sites/default/files/2020-12/Dietary_Guidelines_for_Americans_2020-2025.pdf

World Health Organization. (2020, November 26). *Physical activity.* Retrieved May 6, 2021, from https://www.who.int/news-room/fact-sheets/detail/physical-activity

Yip, C. S. C., Chan, W., & Fielding, R. (2019a). The associations of fruit and vegetable intakes with burden of diseases: A systematic review of meta-analyses. *Journal of the Academy of Nutrition and Dietetics, 119*(3), 464–481. https://doi.org/10.1016/j.jand.2018.11.007

Yip, C. S. C., Yip, Y. C., & Chan, W. (2019b). Time-trend analysis of fruit and vegetable intake in Hong Kong, 2004–2016. *Public Health, 177*, 102–111. https://doi.org/10.1016/j.puhe.2019.08.012

Yip, C. S. C., & Fielding, R. (2017). Health and greenhouse gas emission implications of reducing meat intakes in Hong Kong. *International Journal of Nutrition and Food Engineering, 11*(2), 72–81. https://doi.org/10.5281/zenodo.1339754

Yip, C. S. C., Lam, W., & Fielding, R. (2018). A summary of meat intakes and health burdens. *European Journal of Clinical Nutrition, 72*, 18–29. https://doi.org/10.1038/ejcn.2017.117

Zhou, Y., Zhao, H., & Peng, C. (2015). Association of sedentary behavior with the risk of breast cancer in women: Update meta-analysis of observational studies. *Annals of Epidemiology, 25*(9), 687–697. https://doi.org/10.1016/j.annepidem.2015.05.007

Chapter 12
Physical Activity and Health Improvement: Can More Be Achieved?

Holy Lai Man Chu

Abstract Health is essential to people of all ages and is related to good quality of sleep and nutrition in our daily lives. At the same time, regular physical activity is also one of the important elements to promote and improve health. According to the report of the World Health Organization in 2020, physical activity cannot only reduce the incidence and mortality of diseases, but also have a positive impact on mental health, intellectual development, work, and quality of life. Unfortunately, one quarter of people in the world cannot reach the amount of physical activity recommended by the WHO. There is also a major gap in terms of provision of sports facilities and, more importantly, behaviour of people in the community. To achieve All for Health, the quantity and quality of physical activity must be an in-depth discussion topic, and it is necessary to reflect on the status quo and formulate improvement plans. Three aspects will be discussed in this chapter, namely Physical Education, Sports Facilities, and the International Sports Events. All efforts and resources invested in these aspects can increase participation rate in physical activity by all populations, ultimately improving public health.

Keywords Physical activity · Health · Physical education · Sports facilities · International sports events

Introduction

Physical and mental health is essential to everyone, and they affect each other. There is no doubt that good quality of sleep and nutrition in our daily lives has always been considered an important part of maintaining health. At the same time, we should pay more attention to physical activity (PA), which is absolutely a significant factor related to our health.

H. L. M. Chu (✉)
T.W.G.Hs. Yow Kam Yuen College, Hong Kong, China
e-mail: holychulm@gmail.com

B. Y. F. Fong and W. C. W. Wong (eds.), *Gaps and Actions in Health Improvement from Hong Kong and Beyond*,
https://doi.org/10.1007/978-981-99-4491-0_12

The World Health Organization (WHO) is a public health agency of the United Nations, responsible for promoting universal health by formulating international health standards and developing guidelines for countries. According to WHO (2006), health is considered to be good physical, mental, and social conditions without illness. Regular PA is one of the important elements to promote and improve health. PA is defined as all movement involving skeletal muscles that consume energy and can appear in any of different types in our daily time, such as walking, swimming, running, cycling, etc. (World Health Organization, 2020a). PA can be divided into usual activity and exercise according to intensity (Ainsworth et al., 2000). Light-intensity activities are regarded as usual activities, such as housework, shopping, or daily tasks in life. Most of the moderate- or vigorous-intensity exercises, which are planned, structured, and repetitive to occur, results in increase in heart rate, breathing depth and frequency, and sweating, thereby improving certain components of physical fitness (Caspersen et al., 1985). In this chapter, PA, presented below, is interpreted as all types of moderate- or vigorous-intensity activities that provide health benefits. American College of Sports Medicine (ACSM) is a huge membership organisation that combines exercise science and sports medicine to improve physical fitness. To measure health fitness produced by PA, American College of Sports Medicine (2018) published ACSM's Health-Related Physical Fitness Manual, which introduces five health-related components of physical fitness, namely muscular strength, muscular endurance, flexibility, cardiovascular fitness, and body composition and develops appropriate fitness assessment testing on these five components. This basic concept mentioned above can be used as an indicator for the public to formulate different PAs to improve certain health-related components of physical fitness.

PA is beneficial to health fitness in all age groups of people, especially for the children (Júdice et al., 2017), improving components of physical fitness by attending PA has a positive influence in intelligence and academic achievement (Gil-Espinosa et al., 2020), learning, and memory (Raine et al., 2013). Regular PA leads to lower chances of depression and reduces the level of anxiety and stress among all age groups (Harvey et al., 2010; Tajik et al., 2017; Teixeira et al., 2013). In addition, there is a lot of evidence showing PA can reduce the risk of many types of cancer (Carpenter et al., 1999; Parada et al., 2020; Patel et al., 2003; Slattery et al., 1997) and non-communicable diseases (Geidl et al., 2020). PA is also recommended for people with non-communicable diseases (Geidl et al., 2020), chronic condition or disability, and for all pregnant and postpartum women without contraindication (World Health Organization, 2020a). At a time when all people around the world are facing the predicament due to COVID-19, there is ample evidence that PA can improve health before and after COVID-19 infection and reduce the severity of this disease (Sallis, 2020). Denay (2020) emphasised the significance of prioritising PA highly in our lives in order to immediately improve our overall well-being during the COVID-19 pandemic as the government issued various restrictions in order to maintain social distancing and thus to prevent infection. During the stay-at-home situation, there is a higher risk of mental health problems and physical illnesses. Regular PA is an important strategy to maintain the function of the immune system and it enhances immune system to produce antibodies against the virus that causes COVID-19 (Radom-Aizik,

2020), especially for the elderly, because the effect of vaccination is weaker with age (Edwards et al., 2020).

When many people were suffering from COVID-19, WHO (2020b) launched new guidelines and recommendations for the global population in different ages. It recommends all adults to perform at least 150 min PA per week; children and adolescents are advised to engage in PA at least 1 hour a day and 3 days a week. These activities should involve all major muscle groups to strengthen muscle and cardiovascular health (World Health Organization, 2020a, 2020b). Unfortunately, 1 in 4 adults and more than 80% of adolescents in the world are insufficiently physically active. In high-income countries, the level of physical inactivity is increasing (World Health Organization, 2021). According to a report published by the Non-communicable Disease Branch of the Centre for Health Protection of Department of Health (2020), 16.8% of adults in Hong Kong do not have enough PA. In order to improve levels of PA among all age groups, it is necessary to review the gaps and actions taken by various agencies in promoting PA to the public to improve health. The P-P-P Model (Policy-Physical Activities-Public Health Model; Fig. 12.1) illustrates the extension of the policy power amplifies participation of PA from three aspects, namely Physical Education (PE), Sports Facilities (SFs), and the International Sports Events (ISEs), thereby amplifying the diffusion of community public health.

Influence of Physical Education

Physical Literacy

To realise All for Health, PE is one of the aspects that need to be considered. Physical literacy and perception of PA constructed by PE contribute to the formation of individual PA habits. In this section, the influence of PE on physical literacy and perception, as well as strategies to increase the likelihood of participating in PA, will be discussed.

Whitehead (2013) introduced physical literacy by explaining the philosophical rationale behind the concept and proposed that physical literacy should be applied to the learning field of whole-person development, which is a popular teaching method for cultivating positive value in recent years. Physical literacy refers to the motivation, confidence, physical competence, knowledge, and understanding of its value and accountability for lifelong participation in PA (Whitehead, 2019). Physical literacy is the outcome of PE (Whitehead, 2013, 2019) and inspires people to embrace the intrinsic value of PE, which benefits our health and well-being and increases the motivation to participate in PA for life. Therefore, the promotion of physical literacy should be the most important part in any PE curriculum in both primary and secondary education. In school, when students learn the skills in structural PE, their physical literacy improves and they feel more comfortable and confident with doing all of these skills. They are more likely to be physically active for the rest of their lives.

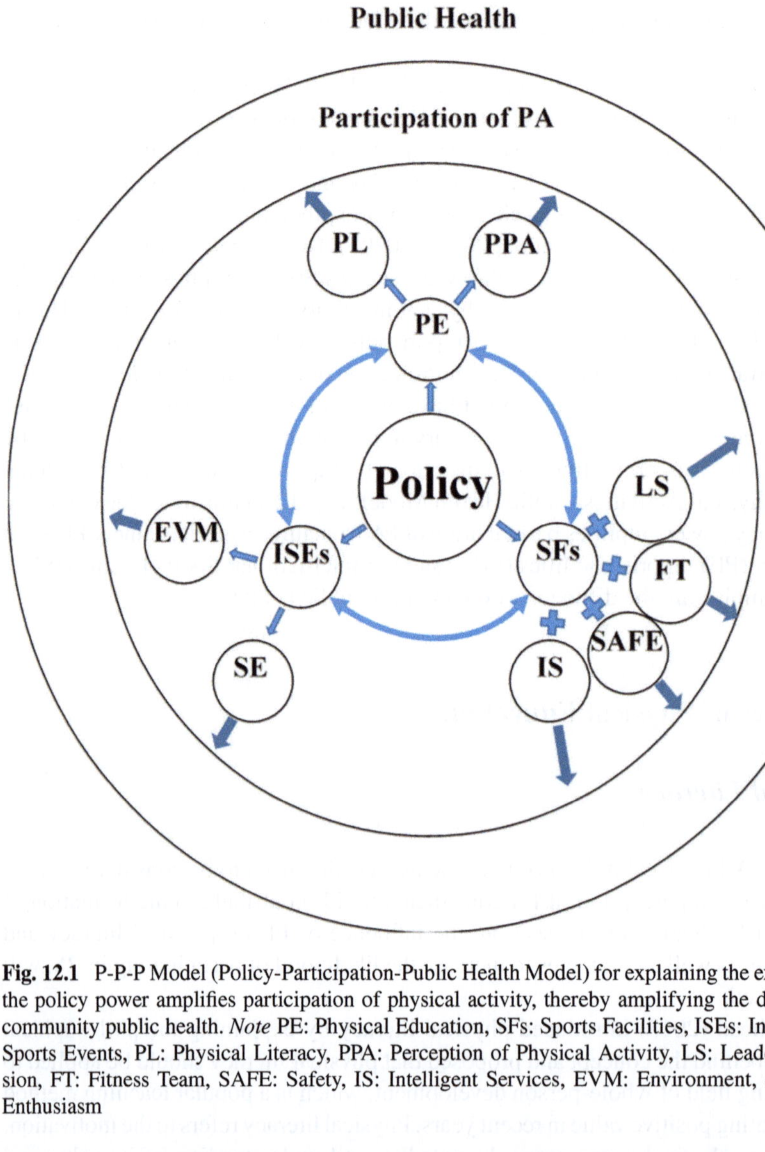

Fig. 12.1 P-P-P Model (Policy-Participation-Public Health Model) for explaining the extension of the policy power amplifies participation of physical activity, thereby amplifying the diffusion of community public health. *Note* PE: Physical Education, SFs: Sports Facilities, ISEs: International Sports Events, PL: Physical Literacy, PPA: Perception of Physical Activity, LS: Leader supervision, FT: Fitness Team, SAFE: Safety, IS: Intelligent Services, EVM: Environment, SE: Sports Enthusiasm

Therefore, physical literacy should be built early. In order to develop physical literacy in children, PE plays a vital role and is therefore an aspect that deserves attention.

Perception of Physical Activity

Perception and experience of PA is one of critical factors influencing the intention of future participation. Hardman et al. (2013) noted that the perception of PA is a kind of competitive games for those who are talented in sports, obstructing most of the general students who show up their clumsy movements during PE lesson. In school, poor and traditional PE teaching methods make students feel that PE is boring and valueless, resulting in low motivation of students towards PE (Hardman et al., 2013). Besides, women are reluctant to participate in PE because women are perceived to have more barriers than men in terms of PE goods issues, religious and cultural orientation, and parental discouragement (Hardman et al., 2013). A number of statistics show that the percentage of women with insufficient PA is higher than that of men, with a difference of 8% (Guthold et al., 2018; Huang et al., 2019). It shows consistency in perceptions and participation rate of PA across genders. Collectively, PE produces all the above-mentioned bad perceptions and experiences, which become obstacles to the motivation of participating in PA. The optimisation of PE such as curriculum content, teacher quality, and gender equality is necessary.

Review and Optimisation of Physical Education

PE is understood as an area of the school curriculum related to human movement, physical fitness, and wellness (International Council of Sport Science & Physical Education, 2010). United Nations Educational, Scientific and Cultural Organization (2013) declared "noting that physical education in school and in all other educational institutions is the most effective means of providing all children and youth with the skills, attitudes, values, knowledge and understanding for lifelong participation in society" (2013, p. 3). McLennan and Thompson (2015) noted, "physical education, as the only curriculum subject whose focus combines the body and physical competence with values-based learning and communication, provides a learning gateway to grow the skills required for success in the 21st Century" (2015, p. 6). In Hong Kong, the Education Bureau (n.d.) clearly identifies the position of PE as "education through physical activity" that aims to help students develop skills for different PAs and social communities, positive values, and attitudes for both lifelong and life-wide learning. Through PE, not only physical literacy and perception, but also comprehensive skills, are developed, which can reduce the likelihood of cursed psychological problems.

Due to the importance of PE, it is essential to review and optimise current PE. In the final report of the World-wide Survey of School Physical Education, there was a gap between policies and actual implementation of PE in schools around the world (Hardman et al., 2013). The findings showed that 29% of countries worldwide did not actually implement PE by law. Despite the rest 71% of countries officially commit to school PE through legislation, actual implementation is far from the official policy requirements (Hardman et al., 2013). The Hardman report (2013) also described the Policy to Practice Infrastructure Template of School Physical Education Basic Needs Model that listed seven elements, namely finance, qualified teachers, timetable allocation, support personnel, community partnerships, facilities and equipment and teaching resources, and national/regional governmental PE strategies. In Hong Kong, fortunately PE is a compulsory subject with all the basic needs presented in the School Physical Education Basic Needs Model. Hardman et al. (2013) also raised some concerns about insufficient quantity (time allocation) and quality (themes, content, relevance, and monitoring) of PE curriculum, as well as inadequate PE resources (Teachers, facilities, and equipment) in some countries. Reviews on specific items and plans should be conducted for improvement in PE afterwards.

The allocation time of PE is one of the direct and objective dimensions to measure the sufficiency of PE in schools. Globally, primary and secondary schools have an average allocation of 103 min (range of 25–220 min) and 100 min (range of 25–240 min) in PE each week, and the amount of allocation time shows a decreasing trend between 2000 and 2013 (Hardman et al., 2013). According to the Physical Education Key Learning Area Curriculum Guide (Primary 1-Secondary 6) issued by Curriculum Development Council (2017) of the Education Bureau in Hong Kong, schools are required to implement structured PE lessons from primary 1 to secondary 3 by accounting for 5–8% of the total lesson time (estimated to average about 100 min per week) and at least 5% of the total lesson time in senior secondary, to ensure that students can achieve whole-person development. The findings of Huang et al. (2019) showed that only 77% of 400 primary schools had 70 to 120 min of PE allocation time per week. The time allocation for PE in most schools in Hong Kong is at the global average level, but much lower than some regions with more than 200 minutes.

Guthold et al. (2018) conducted a worldwide survey investigating trends in insufficient PA from 2001 to 2016, and it was found that Latin America and Caribbean had the highest overall percentage of insufficient PA (39.1%) and Oceania had the lowest (16.3%). Hardman et al. (2013) also found a wide disparity between the indication of lower status in PE teachers in Latin America and Caribbean (47%) and Oceania (11%), and they noted, "Globally, and, with the exception of Oceania, regionally, data suggest that in actual practice PE is considered to have lower status than other subjects" (2013, p. 28). Comparing the results of Hardman et al. (2013) and those of Guthold et al. (2018), there is a correlation between insufficient PA and the status of PE subject and PE teachers. This is a sign of prioritising and scaling up the population level of PE to prevent an upward trend in insufficient PA. In addition, Oceania has a 100% gender equality rate of opportunity in three categories, namely amount, quality, and content (Hardman et al., 2013). More is needed to support gender equality.

PE plays an important role in developing individuals' physical literacy and perception of PA and should receive more attention and improvement to cultivate the habit. Once a PA habit is established, it automatically drives a healthy life.

Physical Activity Habits

Primary care is important for long-term benefits to society and future generations (Fong & Law, 2020), providing health education and promotion of healthy behaviours. Forming the PA habit depends on the persistence of PA behaviour. Fogg (2020) introduced Fogg's Behaviour Model advocating that behaviour is a combination of motivation, ability, and prompt, where motivation and ability compensate each other, and PA behaviour may not occur if one of them is deficient or without prompt. Fogg (2020) mentioned five ability factors, namely time, money, physical effort, mental effort, and routine. High Intensity Interval Training (HIIT) is a high-intensity exercise performed in a short period of time and is recommended for people who do not have time. For those who think money is a barrier to participating in PA, there are tons of workouts to play for free. Physical effort, mental effort, and routine will be difficult for most people. Fogg (2020) proposed that tiny behaviour helps people address ability factors and repeat the behaviour, then cultivate a habit. Once the behaviour has been done, reward such as positive feeling can both motivate behaviour and reinforce a habit, and over time, such habit generates a cycle formed by three elements, namely prompt, behaviour, and reward. It hence becomes self-sufficient, through which people develop a stable PA habit (Duhigg, 2013; Fogg, 2020).

Influence of Sports Facilities and Policies

Review of Provision of Sports Facilities

In order to improve public health in the community, increasing the participation rate of PA is an important way for the government to focus on and allocate resources. Numerous studies have shown that there is a positive relationship between the level of sports participation rate and level of provision of SFs. There are a number of criteria to assess the provision of SFs, namely quantity, quality, accessibility (time consumed and vehicles provided to venue locations), and availability (opening hours and permission to use) (North Northamptonshire Council, 2020). Better SFs lead to stronger intentions towards sports participation (Prins et al., 2010), and higher participation rates (Eime et al., 2017), especially in medium-sized cities (Hallmann et al., 2011). The higher participation rate of sports is also driven by the closer the distance to the SFs (Deelen et al., 2016; Sallis et al., 1990; Steinmayr et al., 2011; Zasimova, 2020), and easier access to SFs (Lee et al., 2016), because residents feel more convenient and time-saving to exercise. Therefore, quantity, quality, combined with accessibility, and availability should be the criteria of concern in the review of the current supply of SFs. The location of SFs and transportation facilities are related to the environmental design and construction of the communities, and these factors should be considered by the government to provide better sports services and opportunities to residents. Furthermore, Albaladejo et al. (2019) pointed out that the availability of SFs in two southern European cities was associated with a reduced risk of overweight in the child population, and hence, a public health strategy as well.

Owing to the differences in population structure, socio-economic development, geographical environment, community planning, and resident needs, there should not be one uniform provision guidelines for SF to implement in the world. Governments in different regions should formulate sports policies based on the analysis of the above factors, past data, and the estimation of future demands. The Hong Kong Planning Standards and Guidelines for Recreation Facilities and Open Space were approved in 1981 to provide appropriate SFs to meet the local needs and to achieve the mental and physical health of individuals and the community (Planning Department, 2022). There was a set of standards for SFs based on a range of population thresholds applied in this planning work. In the 2021 announcement, only the swimming pool category met the population standard, and the remaining three namely sports centre, football pitch, sports ground were all short of 4.6 to 12.9 units (The Government of the Hong Kong Special Administrative Region, 2021). In Hong Kong, one indicator is having one swimming pool per 287,000 people, and there was a surplus of 16.2 pools (The Government of the Hong Kong Special Administrative Region, 2021). This ratio is a far cry from that in the London Borough of Harrow, where 215,350 population share 8 pools (Genesis Strategic Management Consultants, 2009). Therefore, the number of SFs provision cannot be used as the sole criterion for reflecting the current supply and demand. In Hong Kong, the Social Surveys Section of the Census and Statistics Department collected data on public perceptions towards the provision of SFs in 2011 and the result showed that 34% of persons used SFs in the vicinity of home and over 70% of persons aged 12 and over were very satisfied or satisfied with both quality and location of SFs provided by the government (Social Surveys Section, 2011).

A decade later, there were voices from a lot of athletics and users about the insufficient and poor maintenance of SFs and equipment. This problem is prevalent in most regions of the world, with 57% of the regions having insufficient facility and equipment, while low-income countries in Africa, Latin America and the Middle East have a higher percentage of below-average quality of facility and equipment (Hardman et al., 2013). The SFs and equipment should be considered the scope of resources investment. Hardman et al. (2013) stated that provision of SFs and equipment was one of the factors that caused the difference between the policy requirements and actual conditions. Therefore, the provision of SFs is a vital aspect of analysing the implementation of government sports policies.

Review of Sports Policies and Schemes

In Hong Kong, the Culture, Sports, and Tourism Bureau is responsible for promoting sports development, while the Recreation and Sport Branch implements sports policies to achieve the three major goals of sports development, namely promoting sports in the community, supporting elite sports development, and promoting major ISEs (Culture, Sports and Tourism Bureau, n.d.). The Leisure and Cultural Services Department (LCSD) has organised a wide range of programmes in response to the three goals, including the "Healthy Exercise for All Campaign" and "Sport for All Day" launched in 2000 and 2009 respectively. The "Five-Year Plan for Sports and Recreation Facilities" formulated by the Hong Kong government has been implemented since 2017, and it helps to meet the demand of citizens to increase the sports participation rate. The "Five-year Development Programme for Team Sports" has been launched since 2018, providing monthly financial support and additional yearly funding to eight team sports, based on performance. In 2000, the "Five-year District Sports Programmes Funding Scheme" was launched with an allocation of 100 million Hong Kong Dollars to organise PA in 18 districts. The "School Sports Programme", "Student Athlete Support Scheme", and "Opening up School Facilities for Promotion of Sports Development Scheme" and other programmes are all designed to provide more opportunities for young people to participate in PA. Furthermore, 70 activities and sports training programmes are being organised for different types of disabled people, and "Elite Vote Support System for Disability Sports" supports athletes with disabilities.

The policies cover different groups of population with large budgets, but is there sufficient and appropriate allocation of resources to expand the efficacy of PA in the community? The number of participants in PAs organised by the LCSD in three years reached 7.4 million (Legislative Council Panel on Home Affairs, 2019), but the number of participants per day did not exceed 7000, and it means that the government can only provide public broadcasting services for one-thousandth of the public. Besides, in most schools in Hong Kong, the effectiveness of sports promotion programmes depends on the school's emphasis on sports development. Under the influence of traditional thinking, parents and teachers agree that academic works are more important, and tutorial classes replace students' rights to do sports, thus hindering the implementation of sports policies in schools. This conventional view is a big problem. One reason behind it has to do with the poor career development of athletes who are not able to get enough money to support their full-time athlete life and most of them are so poor that they need to work part-time jobs to make a living. Therefore, there is a need for a deep rethinking of the policies on funding and support for athletes, so as to improve their prospects and treatment.

Effectiveness of Resource Utilisation

In order to improve the utilisation of SFs and the effectiveness of sports policies, possible alternative implementation policies in other regions can be the references. The State Council of the People's Republic of China (2021) issued the National Fitness Plan (2021–2025) to promote PA among all people in the country, mainly focusing on improving primary health care. In order to achieve the goal of increasing by 1.3% and reaching 38.5% of the population participating regularly in PA by 2025, not only eight main missions but also four guaranty action plans have been proposed, namely reinforcing leader supervision, expanding fitness team, strengthening safety, and providing intelligent services (The State Council of the People's Republic of China, 2021), which are indispensable to ensure those missions can finally be accomplished. This comprehensive short-term plan makes full use of high-level big data technology such as "Sports Bank" and "Cloud Database" to render PA and fitness as part of a new fashionable way of life for people. Sihai Park in Nanshan District of Shenzhen city develops smart 5G technology to help people feel more convenient and more interested in participating in PA in life (Aisyah, 2021). To improve public health through PA, there should be a set of comprehensive action plans, combining hardware and software supports from various government departments and different stakeholders in the society. It is time to collaborate to build a culture of PA and health in the local community to achieve All for Health.

Influence of International Sports Events

International Sports Events

In addition to optimising PE and improving sports facilities, developing international sports events (ISEs) should not be neglected to increase the quality and quantity of PA to expand the effectiveness of All for Health. ISEs, commonly known as sport mega-events, are sporting events with four-large elements, large costs, large number of visitors, large media coverage, and large impact on local environment and residence (Müller, 2015). Examples include Olympic Games, FIFA World Cup, National Basketball Association, IAAF World Championships, Wimbledon Tennis, the UEFA Champions League, the Asian Games and many more.

With ISEs held in different cities for athletes from all over the world, there is often controversy over the cities to host the events in terms of resource delivery, when public money should be prioritised on housing, medical services, and education. Though hosting ISEs can raise happiness with a positive short-term "feel good" effect (Kavetsos & Szymanski, 2010), one should remark the long-term benefits which are also outcomes of ISEs. There are many studies investigating the outcomes of ISEs in terms of impact, legacy, and leveraging on host cities. The impact refers to immediate changes, legacy refers to long-term impact after the event (Preuss, 2019), and leveraging refers to the strategy to achieve the goal of the event (Chalip, 2006). Nair's (2021) research suggested that hosting ISEs had positive effects on the economy, employment, social cohesion, quality of life, and the environment. All of these dimensions are related to the mental wellness of the community, and therefore, hosting ISEs in a consummate way indirectly captures the benefits to public health.

The impact of participation in ISEs on civic sports participation is also an issue worth exploring. According to Teare and Taks (2021), most findings indicated that hosting ISEs had no effect on sports participation. However, appropriate use of the potential demonstration effect of ISEs can increase the frequency of sports participation and re-engage lost participants (Weed et al., 2015). In the promotion of health through increased public sports participation, there are many ways to achieve the goal besides participating in ISEs. In spite of heated debate among those with different perspectives on ISEs, it is time to consider the value of ISEs, both for hosting and participation, particularly the impact of past ISEs on environmental change and sports enthusiasm.

Impact on Environmental Change

The living environment is directly related to public health. With the development of society, environmental pollution is becoming more and more serious. Air pollution in China has always been a concern, and in order to improve the air quality for the Beijing 2008 Olympic Games, Campaigns of Air Quality Research in Beijing and Surrounding Regions; an international collaborative project, is responsible for formulating strategies to solve the air problem. Air pollution was controlled during the Olympic Games (Zhu et al., 2009), and this success led the government to implement follow-up actions to combat air pollution and sparked a slew of investigations into the issue. A few years later, there were reductions in air pollution and deaths from cardio-cerebrovascular and respiratory diseases in China (He et al., 2016). People avoid participation in outdoor PA due to poor air quality (Neidell, 2009), and strategies to address air pollution are the indirect ways to promote health by encouraging outdoor PA. This is a positive impact of the strict control of air quality for the Beijing Olympic Games by the Chinese government, and it continues to directly and indirectly affect people's health.

Water pollution is another issue addressed by the Olympic Games. In Tokyo, the host city of the 2020 Olympic Games, test event was cancelled due to high levels of bacteria in the water. Residents suffered from this water pollution for a long time, until the Tokyo government launched a long-term benefit project, spending 120 million yen to create a comfortable environment and improve water quality for the Tokyo Olympic Games (Bloomberg, 2021). Preparations for the Rio 2016 Olympic Games had also raised public concerns about water pollution. The state of Rio de Janeiro committed to upgrade the sewage system and finally the water pollution was improved (Watts & Vidal, 2016). The ISEs have exposed the hosting city's environmental problems, urging government policymakers to implement solutions that improve the health of residents.

Impact of Sports Enthusiasm

Winning an Olympic gold medal by Hong Kong's foil fencer Cheung Ka Long in 2021 was a great moment, and it has derived many positive impacts since then, in terms of public attention to sports, increasing resources for sports development, improving SFs for athletes, and raising participation rate in specific sports. Wen Wei Po (2021) reported that the outstanding performance of Hong Kong athletes at the Tokyo Olympics has set off a wave of sports in the city, with the number of students in training classes for fencing, karate, and even skateboarding soaring. The public has been rewarded cognitively and emotionally with extensive media coverage. They acquired sports knowledge, stimulated enthusiasm for sports, increased their recognition of the value of sports, and deepened their focus on specific types of sports, especially the sports that Hong Kong athletes participate in, such as fencing, swimming, table tennis, and so on. With the superb performance of Hong Kong athletes, a number of representatives were invited to participate in interviews to give opinions and suggestions on the development of sports. Their voices were heeded by government policymakers and positive responses were anticipated.

Great performance at ISEs is the fertiliser and driver that increase sports participation rates. How could hosting ISEs not produce this kind of chemical reaction? Admittedly, the costs of building Olympic venues and subsequent maintenance and repairs were high (Yakabuski, 2016), and often left dedicated sports infrastructure of little use after the Olympics (Baade & Matheson, 2016; NBC New York, 2022). The venues built for the Olympic Games in Sydney in 2000 (Zaccardi, 2017), Athens in 2004 (Govan, 2011), Rio de Janeiro in 2016 (Davis, 2017), and PyeongChang in 2018 (Kim, 2017) were unused and eventually demolished, due to the lack of planning and utilisation of aftercare activities. On the contrary, the Chinese government has taken a different approach, using most of the venues in the Beijing 2008 Summer Olympics for the Beijing 2022 Winter Olympics, and for sports competitions, athletic training, etc. (Prigeon, 2022). The Beijing Organising Committee (2019) proposed The Legacy Plan of the Olympic and Paralympic Winter Games Beijing 2022, which aimed to carry forward and utilise the Olympic legacy to strengthen "Healthy China".

Government policymakers are keen to pay more attention to the importance of sports policy implementation and the provision of SFs, and how they are affecting the rate of public participation in PA. The merits of ISEs in promoting sport and the positive impact on public health are worthy of widespread recognition by everyone in the community.

Interaction Between ISEs and Government Policies

ISEs interact with government policies, which involve sports development, physical education, environment, facilities, transportation, and many other aspects. Chalip et al. (2017) recommend that clear plans must be developed and managed before, during, and after the ISEs to achieve desired goals. The plans should cover sport-related and non-sport-related matters, with stakeholders including government policymakers, urban planners, sports organisations, media companies, commercial corporations, and all residences.

De Bosscher and her research team (De Bosscher et al., 2007) proposed the Sports Policy Factors Leading to International Sporting Success (SPLISS), which introduced the nine pillars of sports policy factors influencing international success, namely financial support, policy development, sport participation, talent identification, athletic and post career support, training facilities, coach development, national and international competition, scientific research, and sport medicine support. The nine pillars have a strong positive correlation with international sports success (De Bosscher et al., 2015). The Korea Sports Promotion Foundation was established to operate the Seoul 1988 Olympics (International Olympic Committee, 2020) to make their citizens unite and maintain a healthy life through sports. For the past few decades, South Korea has been at the top of every summer Olympics, partly because the development strategy of South Korean Competitive Sports has comprehensively covered all key factors for the success of competitive sports under the SPLISS Model (Chen et al., 2018). The Hong Kong government can use this as a mirror to formulate comprehensive and long-term policies to improve sports performance and thus develop the health of the citizens.

Concluding Remarks

In order to achieve All for Health through improving PA, the current situation about PA and health improvement in different regions of the world have been reviewed from three aspects. The first aspect is PE, which is considered a factor at the individual level that affects people's physical literacy and perception of PA. The government should optimise PE by formulating implementable policies, including providing adequate resources and allocation time, and improving the status of PE subject and PE teachers, so as to cultivate individual physical literacy and a good perception of PA from an early age. The second aspect is the SFs, which is considered a factor at the social level, providing exercise opportunities for the residents. The government can attract citizens to participate in PA by providing sufficient SFs, in conjunction with reinforcing leader supervision, expanding fitness team, strengthening safety, and providing intelligent services, so as to attract citizens to participate in PA. The last aspect is the ISEs, which is considered to be a factor that has attracted worldwide attention at the national level. Governments should capitalise on the positive impacts of hosting or participating ISEs, such as improving the living environment and sustaining civic sports enthusiasm, thereby improving public health. All efforts and resources invested in these aspects can increase participation rate in PA by all in the populations, ultimately improving public health for all. At the same time, they all depend on the government's policies, their implementation, and resource allocation. Therefore, in the days to come, governments should pay more attention to sports development and actively promote the physical and mental health of the public.

References

Ainsworth, B. E., Haskell, W. L., Whitt, M. C., Irwin, M. L., Swartz, A. M., Strath, S. J., O'Brien, W. L., Bassett, D. R., Schmitz, K. H., Emplaincourt, P. O., Jacobs, D. R., & Leon, A. S. (2000). Compendium of physical activities: An update of activity codes and MET intensities. *Medicine and Science in Sports and Exercise, 32*(9), S498–S504. https://doi.org/10.1097/00005768-200009001-00009

Aisyah, K. (2021, May 12). *5G technology helps China's parks to get smarter.* OpenGov Asia. https://opengovasia.com/5g-technology-helps-chinas-parks-to-get-smarter/

Albaladejo, R., Villanueva, R., Astasio, P., Ortega, P., Santos, J., & Regidor, E. (2019). Sports facilities, socio-economic context and overweight among the childhood population in two southern European cities: A cross sectional study. *BMC Pediatrics, 19*, Article 307. https://doi.org/10.1186/s12887-019-1694-1

American College of Sports Medicine. (2018). *ACSM's health-related physical fitness assessment manual.* Lippincott Williams & Wilkins. https://www.acsm.org/education-resources/books/ACSMs-Fitness-Assessment-Manual

Baade, R. A., & Matheson, V. A. (2016). Going for the gold: The economics of the Olympics. *Journal of Economic Perspectives, 30*(2), 201–218. https://doi.org/10.1257/jep.30.2.201

Beijing Organising Committee. (2019). *The legacy plan of the Olympic and Paralympic Winter Games Beijing 2022.* https://library.olympics.com/Default/doc/SYRACUSE/184888/the-legacy-plan-of-the-olympic-and-paralympic-winter-games-beijing-2022-beijing-organising-committee?_lg=en-GB

Bloomberg. (2021, July 14). Tokyo Olympics: Water at the triathlon swimming venue stinks of sewage despite clean-up efforts. *South China Morning Post.* https://www.scmp.com/news/asia/east-asia/article/3141017/tokyo-olympic-two-weeks-triathlon-water-swimming-venue-stinks

Carpenter, C. L., Ross, R. K., Paganini-Hill, A., & Bernstein, L. (1999). Lifetime exercise activity and breast cancer risk among post-menopausal women. *British Journal of Cancer, 80*(11), 1852–1858. https://doi.org/10.1038/sj.bjc.6690610

Caspersen, C. J., Powell, K. E., & Christenson, G. M. (1985). Physical activity, exercise, and physical fitness: Definitions and distinctions for health-related research. *Public Health Reports, 100*(2), 126–131. https://www.ncbi.nlm.nih.gov/pmc/articles/PMC1424733/

Chalip, L. (2006). Towards social leverage of sport events. *Journal of Sport & Tourism, 11*(2), 109–127. https://doi.org/10.1080/14775080601155126

Chalip, L., Green, B. C., Taks, M., & Misener, L. (2017). Creating sport participation from sport events: Making it happen. *International Journal of Sport Policy and Politics, 9*(2), 257–276. https://doi.org/10.1080/19406940.2016.1257496

Chen, Y. W., Kim, S., Huang, Y. C., & Tan, T. C. (2018). An investigation of South Korea's strategies for elite sport development from the perspective of the SPLISS model. *Physical Education Journal, 51*(3), 387–410. https://doi.org/10.3966/102472972018095103009

Culture, Sports and Tourism Bureau. (n.d.). *Sports policy.* https://www.cstb.gov.hk/en/policies/sports-and-recreation/sports-policy.html

Curriculum Development Council. (2017). *Physical education key learning area curriculum guide (Primary 1-secondary 6).* https://www.edb.gov.hk/attachment/en/curriculum-development/kla/pe/curriculum-doc/PEKLACG_e.pdf

Davis, S. (2017, July 18). *Rio's $700 million athletes village was turned into luxury condos but is now reportedly 'shuttered' and 93% vacant.* Business Insider. https://www.businessinsider.com/rio-olympics-athletes-village-mostly-vacant-2017-7

De Bosscher, V., De Knop, P., & Van Bottenburg, M. (2007). *Sports policy factors leading to international sporting success.* VUBPress.

De Bosscher, V., Shibli, S., Westerbeek, H., & Van Bottenburg, M. (2015). *Successful elite sport policies: An international comparison of the sports policy factors leading to international sporting success (SPLISS 2.0) in 15 nations.* Meyer & Meyer Sport. https://ussa-my.com/assets/SPLISS_report.pdf

Deelen, I., Ettema, D., & Dijst, M. (2016). Too busy or too far away? The importance of subjective constraints and spatial factors for sports frequency. *Managing Sport and Leisure, 21*(4), 239–264. https://doi.org/10.1080/23750472.2016.1255563
Denay, K. (2020, April 20). *A clinician's thoughts about self care and physical activity during COVID*. Exercise is Medicine. https://www.exerciseismedicine.org/a-clinicians-thoughts-about-self-care-and-physi/
Duhigg, C. (2013). *The power of habit: Why we do what we do and how to change*. Random House. https://www.penguinrandomhouse.com/books/202855/the-power-of-habit-by-charles-duhigg/
Education Bureau. (n.d.). *Physical education*. https://www.edb.gov.hk/en/curriculum-development/kla/physical-education/index.html
Edwards, K., Kellar, G., Marquez, D. X., & Schlicht, J. (2020, November 6). *Physical activity, COVID-19 and older adults*. Exercise is Medicine. https://www.exerciseismedicine.org/physical-activity-covid-19-and-older-adults/
Eime, R. M., Harvey, J., Charity, M. J., Casey, M., Westerbeek, H., & Payne, W. R. (2017). The relationship of sport participation to provision of sports facilities and socioeconomic status: A geographical analysis. *Australian and New Zealand Journal of Public Health, 41*(3), 248–255. https://doi.org/10.1111/1753-6405.12647
Fogg, B. J. (2020). *Tiny habits: Why starting small makes lasting change easy*. Penguin Random House. https://www.penguin.co.uk/books/438937/tiny-habits-by-bj-fogg/9780753553244
Fong, B. Y. F., & Law, V. (2020). Renewal of primary care. In *Primary care revisited: Interdisciplinary perspectives for a new era* (pp. 3–21). Springer. https://doi.org/10.1007/978-981-15-2521-6_1
Geidl, W., Abu-Omar, K., Weege, M., Messing, S., & Pfeifer, K. (2020). German recommendations for physical activity and physical activity promotion in adults with noncommunicable diseases. *International Journal of Behavioral Nutrition and Physical Activity, 17*, Article 12. https://doi.org/10.1186/s12966-020-0919-x
Genesis Strategic Management Consultants. (2009). *London borough of Harrow—Provision for swimming report*. https://www.harrow.gov.uk/downloads/file/26948/harrow-fpm-pools-jan-2009.pdf
Gil-Espinosa, F. J., Chillón, P., Fernández-García, J. C., & Cadenas-Sanchez, C. (2020). Association of physical fitness with intelligence and academic achievement in adolescents. *International Journal of Environmental Research and Public Health, 17*(12), Article 4362. https://doi.org/10.3390/ijerph17124362
Govan, F. (2011, June 23). Greece's Olympic dream has turned into a nightmare for village residents. *The Telegraph*. https://www.telegraph.co.uk/finance/financialcrisis/8595360/Greeces-Olympic-dream-has-turned-into-a-nightmare-for-Village-residents.html
Guthold, R., Stevens, G. A., Riley, L. M., & Bull, F. C. (2018). Worldwide trends in insufficient physical activity from 2001 to 2016: A pooled analysis of 358 population-based surveys with 1.9 million participants. *The Lancet Global Health, 6*(10), e1077–e1086. https://doi.org/10.1016/S2214-109X(18)30357-7
Hallmann, K., Wicker, P., Breuer, C., & Schüttoff, U. (2011). Interdependency of sport supply and sport demand in German metropolitan and medium-sized municipalities–findings from multi-level analyses. *European Journal for Sport and Society, 8*(1–2), 65–84. https://doi.org/10.1080/16138171.2011.11687870
Hardman, K., Murphy, C., Routen, A., & Tones, S. (2013). *World-wide survey of school physical education*. United Nations Educational, Scientific and Cultural Organization. https://en.unesco.org/inclusivepolicylab/system/files/teams/document/2017/8/World-wide%20survey%20on%20PE_0_0_0_0_0.pdf
Harvey, S. B., Hotopf, M., Øverland, S., & Mykletun, A. (2010). Physical activity and common mental disorders. *The British Journal of Psychiatry, 197*(5), 357–364. https://doi.org/10.1192/bjp.bp.109.075176

He, G., Fan, M., & Zhou, M. (2016). The effect of air pollution on mortality in China: Evidence from the 2008 Beijing Olympic Games. *Journal of Environmental Economics and Management, 79*, 18–39. https://doi.org/10.1016/j.jeem.2016.04.004

Huang, W. Y., Wong, S. H., Sit, C. H., Wong, M. C., Sum, R. K., Wong, S. W., & Jane, J. Y. (2019). Results from the Hong Kong's 2018 report card on physical activity for children and youth. *Journal of Exercise Science & Fitness, 17*(1), 14–19. https://doi.org/10.1016/j.jesf.2018.10.003

International Council of Sport Science and Physical Education. (2010). *International position statement on physical education.* https://www.icsspe.org/sites/default/files/International%20Position%20Statement%20on%20Physical%20Education.pdf

International Olympic Committee. (2020, June 17). *The Korea sports promotion foundation.* https://olympics.com/ioc/legacy/seoul-1988/the-korea-sports-promotion-foundation

Júdice, P. B., Silva, A. M., Berria, J., Petroski, E. L., Ekelund, U., & Sardinha, L. B. (2017). Sedentary patterns, physical activity and health-related physical fitness in youth: A cross-sectional study. *International Journal of Behavioral Nutrition and Physical Activity, 14*, Article 25. https://doi.org/10.1186/s12966-017-0481-3

Kavetsos, G., & Szymanski, S. (2010). National well-being and international sports events. *Journal of Economic Psychology, 31*(2), 158–171. https://doi.org/10.1016/j.joep.2009.11.005

Kim, T. H. (2017, December 14). *As Olympics near, South Korea agonizes over post-games costs.* Associated Press News. https://apnews.com/article/asia-pacific-business-sports-hockey-ap-top-news-04f9e1c5275e405581bfb21086309a6a

Lee, S. A., Ju, Y. J., Lee, J. E., Hyun, I. S., Nam, J. Y., Han, K. T., & Park, E. C. (2016). The relationship between sports facility accessibility and physical activity among Korean adults. *BMC Public Health, 16*, Article 893. https://doi.org/10.1186/s12889-016-3574-z

Legislative Council Panel on Home Affairs. (2019, May 27). *Promotion of sports development in Hong Kong.* https://www.legco.gov.hk/yr18-19/english/panels/ha/papers/ha20190527cb2-1500-5-e.pdf

McLennan, N., & Thompson, J. (2015). *Quality physical education (QPE): Guidelines for policy makers.* United Nations Educational, Scientific and Cultural Organization. https://en.unesco.org/inclusivepolicylab/sites/default/files/learning/document/2017/1/231101E.pdf

Müller, M. (2015). What makes an event a mega-event? Definitions and sizes. *Leisure Studies, 34*(6), 627–642. https://doi.org/10.1080/02614367.2014.993333

Nair, G. K. (2021). Hosting major international sports events in a country: A socioeconomic impact. *Emerging Markets Journal, 11*(1), 13–20. https://doi.org/10.5195/emaj.2021.207

NBC New York. (2022, January 28). *Images show abandoned Olympic venues around the world.* https://www.nbcnewyork.com/news/sports/beijing-winter-olympics/images-show-abandoned-olympic-venues-around-the-world/3171745/

Neidell, M. (2009). Information, avoidance behavior, and health the effect of ozone on asthma hospitalizations. *Journal of Human Resources, 44*(2), 450–478. https://doi.org/10.3368/jhr.44.2.450

Non-communicable Disease Branch of Centre for Health Protection of Department of Health. (2020). *Report of health behaviour survey 2018/19.* https://www.chp.gov.hk/files/pdf/report_of_health_behaviour_survey_2018_en.pdf

North Northamptonshire Council. (2020). *Sports facilities audit & needs assessment.* https://www.kettering.gov.uk/downloads/file/19369/sports_facilities_audit_and_needs_assessment_june_2020

Parada, H., McDonald, E., Bellettiere, J., Evenson, K. R., LaMonte, M. J., & LaCroix, A. Z. (2020). Associations of accelerometer-measured physical activity and physical activity-related cancer incidence in older women: Results from the WHI OPACH study. *British Journal of Cancer, 122*(9), 1409–1416. https://doi.org/10.1038/s41416-020-0753-6

Patel, A. V., Calle, E. E., Bernstein, L., Wu, A. H., & Thun, M. J. (2003). Recreational physical activity and risk of postmenopausal breast cancer in a large cohort of US women. *Cancer Causes & Control, 14*(6), 519–529. https://doi.org/10.1023/a:1024895613663

Planning Department. (2022). *Hong Kong planning standards and guidelines: Chapter 4 recreation, open space and greening*. https://www.pland.gov.hk/pland_en/tech_doc/hkpsg/full/pdf/ch4.pdf

Preuss, H. (2019). Event legacy framework and measurement. *International Journal of Sport Policy and Politics, 11*(1), 103–118. https://doi.org/10.1080/19406940.2018.1490336

Prigeon, J. (2022, February 15). *How will Beijing use their Olympic venues after the 2022 winter games?* NBC New York. https://www.nbcnewyork.com/news/national-international/how-will-beijing-use-their-olympic-venues-after-the-2022-winter-games/3554707/

Prins, R. G., van Empelen, P., Te Velde, S. J., Timperio, A., van Lenthe, F. J., Tak, N. I., Crawford, D., Brug, J., & Oenema, A. (2010). Availability of sports facilities as moderator of the intention–sports participation relationship among adolescents. *Health Education Research, 25*(3), 489–497. https://doi.org/10.1093/her/cyq024

Radom-Aizik, S. (2020, April 14). *COVID-19, exercise, children and their developing immune system*. Exercise is Medicine. https://www.exerciseismedicine.org/covid-19-exercise-children-and-their-developing-1/

Raine, L. B., Lee, H. K., Saliba, B. J., Chaddock-Heyman, L., Hillman, C. H., & Kramer, A. F. (2013). The influence of childhood aerobic fitness on learning and memory. *PLOS One, 8*(9), Article e72666. https://doi.org/10.1371/journal.pone.0072666

Sallis, J. F. (2020, April 3). *A call to action: Physical activity and COVID-19*. Exercise is Medicine. https://www.exerciseismedicine.org/a-call-to-action-physical-activity-and-covid-191/

Sallis, J. F., Hovell, M. F., Hofstetter, C. R., Elder, J. P., Hackley, M., Caspersen, C. J., & Powell, K. E. (1990). Distance between homes and exercise facilities related to frequency of exercise among San Diego residents. *Public Health Reports, 105*(2), 179–185. https://pubmed.ncbi.nlm.nih.gov/2108465/

Slattery, M. L., Potter, J., Caan, B., Edwards, S., Coates, A., Ma, K. N., & Berry, T. D. (1997). Energy balance and colon cancer—Beyond physical activity. *Cancer Research, 57*(1), 75–80. https://pubmed.ncbi.nlm.nih.gov/8988044/

Social Surveys Section. (2011, March). *Thematic household survey report No. 47*. Census and Statistics Department. https://www.statistics.gov.hk/pub/B11302472011XXXXB0100.pdf

Steinmayr, A., Felfe, C., & Lechner, M. (2011). The closer the sportier? Children's sports activity and their distance to sports facilities. *European Review of Aging and Physical Activity, 8*(2), 67–82. https://doi.org/10.1007/s11556-011-0090-0

Tajik, E., Abd Latiff, L., Adznam, S. N., Awang, H., Siew, C. Y., & Bakar, A. A. (2017). A study on level of physical activity, depression, anxiety and stress symptoms among adolescents. *The Journal of Sports Medicine and Physical Fitness, 57*(10), 1382–1387. https://doi.org/10.23736/S0022-4707.16.06658-5

Teare, G., & Taks, M. (2021). Sport events for sport participation: A scoping review. *Frontiers in Sports and Active Living, 3*, Article 655579. https://doi.org/10.3389/fspor.2021.655579

Teixeira, C. M., Vasconcelos-Raposo, J., Fernandes, H. M., & Brustad, R. J. (2013). Physical activity, depression and anxiety among the elderly. *Social Indicators Research, 113*(1), 307–318. https://doi.org/10.1007/s11205-012-0094-9

The Government of the Hong Kong Special Administrative Region. (2021, September 1). *LCQ18: Recreation and sports facilities* [Press Releases]. https://www.info.gov.hk/gia/general/202109/01/P2021090100421.htm

The State Council of the People's Republic of China. (2021, August 3). *Notice of the State Council on printing and distributing the national fitness plan (2021–2025)* [in Chinese]. http://www.gov.cn/zhengce/content/2021-08/03/content_5629218.htm

United Nations Educational, Scientific and Cultural Organization. (2013). *Declaration of Berlin*. https://unesdoc.unesco.org/ark:/48223/pf0000221114

Watts, J., & Vidal, J. (2016, August 3). What's in the water? Pollution fears taint Rio's picturesque bay ahead of Olympics. *The Guardian*. https://www.theguardian.com/sport/2016/aug/03/pollution-fears-taint-rio-bay-olympic-games

Weed, M., Coren, E., Fiore, J., Wellard, I., Chatziefstathiou, D., Mansfield, L., & Dowse, S. (2015). The Olympic games and raising sport participation: A systematic review of evidence and an interrogation of policy for a demonstration effect. *European Sport Management Quarterly, 15*, 195–226. https://doi.org/10.1080/16184742.2014.998695

Wen Wei Po. (2021, August 10). *The whole city continues sports fever, sports policies must be improved* [in Chinese]. https://www.wenweipo.com/a/202108/10/AP6111bde2e4b08d3407d3466c.html

Whitehead, M. (2013). Definition of physical literacy and clarification of related issues. *Journal of the International Council of Sport Science and Physical Education's Bulletin, 65*, 29–34. https://www.icsspe.org/sites/default/files/bulletin65_0.pdf

Whitehead, M. (2019). *Physical literacy across the world*. Routledge. https://doi.org/10.4324/9780203702697

World Health Organization. (2006). *Constitution of the World Health Organization*. https://cdn.who.int/media/docs/default-source/documents/publications/basic-documents-constitution-of-who179f0d3d-a613-4760-8801-811dfce250af.pdf?sfvrsn=e8fb384f_1&download=true

World Health Organization. (2020a, November, 26). *What is physical activity?* https://www.who.int/news-room/fact-sheets/detail/physical-activity

World Health Organization. (2020b). *WHO guidelines on physical activity and sedentary behaviour: Web annex: Evidence profiles*. https://apps.who.int/iris/handle/10665/336657

World Health Organization. (2021, October 14). *WHO calls for better and fairer opportunities for physical activity to improve health*. https://www.who.int/news/item/14-10-2021-who-calls-for-better-and-fairer-opportunities-for-physical-activity-to-improve-mental-and-physical-health

Yakabuski, K. (2016, August 8). Summer Olympics: 40 years on, Quebeckers are still footing the bill. *The Globe and Mail*. https://www.theglobeandmail.com/opinion/summer-olympics-40-years-on-quebeckers-are-still-footing-the-bill/article31295801/

Zaccardi, N. (2017, November 27). *Sydney Olympic stadium to be torn down*. NBC Sports. https://olympics.nbcsports.com/2017/11/27/sydney-olympic-stadium-demolition/

Zasimova, L. (2020). Sports facilities' location and participation in sports among working adults. *European Sport Management Quarterly*, 1–21. https://doi.org/10.1080/16184742.2020.1828968

Zhu, T., Li, X., Hu, M., Tang, X., & Team, C. (2009). Air pollution characteristics before, during, and after the Beijing Olympics. *Epidemiology, 20*(6), S250. https://doi.org/10.1097/01.ede.0000362836.37333.86

Chapter 13
Sustainable Green Environment and Health Improvement

Wang-Kin Chiu and Alan K. T. Leung

Abstract Advance of chemical technology has led to improvement in various aspects of life such as enhancement of process efficiency, synthesis of functional materials and development of new drug compounds. However, with the rapid technological advance and extensive chemical applications in daily life, there have been growing environmental concerns due to increasing chemical pollution. Numerous studies have also reported on the adverse effects of chemical pollution to human health. In view of the deteriorating environmental quality and adverse impact on public health, actions requiring the concerted efforts across education, policy, research, and industrial practice have been called upon to mitigate pollution and contamination for the prevention of associated diseases and health improvement. Under the Sustainable Development Goal (SDG) 3 which focuses on promotion of good health and well-being, one of the important targets put forward is to have substantial reduction on the number of deaths and illnesses resulted from hazardous chemicals and environmental pollution by the year of 2030. In recent years, issues related to environmental sustainability have been a major research agenda. Meanwhile, the concepts and practice of green and sustainable chemistry have gained considerable attention due to their promising potential for chemical innovations and advancement to contribute to the achievement of the SDGs and their targets. In this chapter, the hazardous effects of chemical pollution will be reviewed. Research investigations addressing the important issues of green chemistry and sustainable environment will be summarised. Implications for health promotion and disease prevention will also be discussed.

Keywords Sustainable environment · Sustainable education · Green chemistry · Green environment · Pollution

W.-K. Chiu (✉)
Division of Science, Engineering and Health Studies, College of Professional and Continuing Education, The Hong Kong Polytechnic University, Hong Kong, China
e-mail: oscar.chiu@cpce-polyu.edu.hk

A. K. T. Leung
School of Professional Education and Executive Development, The Hong Kong Polytechnic University, Hong Kong, China

B. Y. F. Fong and W. C. W. Wong (eds.), *Gaps and Actions in Health Improvement from Hong Kong and Beyond*,
https://doi.org/10.1007/978-981-99-4491-0_13

Background

In recent decades, there has been rapid advancement in chemical science and technology, leading to significant improvements in quality of life contributed by various aspects such as enhanced efficiency of industrial processes, synthetic discoveries of functional materials and development of new drugs. Meanwhile, concerns have also been growing tremendously, particularly towards the sustainability of environment with increasing levels of pollutions. The environmental quality is seriously affected by chemical pollution, with various studies having reported the association of health problems due to chemical contaminants in the environment, which is not just limited to air, but also includes water and food consumed in daily life (Chiu & Fong, 2022; Simoni et al., 2015). Therefore, the deteriorating environmental quality represents a major threat to public health, which is of particular concern in consideration of the growing worldwide ageing population due to increasing global life expectancy and declining fertility rate (Fong et al., 2021).

A sustainable green environment is indispensable for improving health and well-being. The importance of a green environment is also reflected by the Sustainable Development Goal (SDG) 3, which has several major targets aiming at a significant reduction on the number of deaths and illnesses resulted from exposure to hazardous chemicals and environmental pollution, as well as focusing on promoting good health and well-being. Green chemistry is an emerging science discipline that focuses on the innovation of chemical products and implementation of chemical processes for reducing and preventing the use and production of harmful or hazardous substances (Beach et al., 2009). Targeting at the ultimate goal of moving the society towards a sustainable future, green chemistry advocates innovations in the design and utilisation of materials and energy such that increased performance is achieved without compromising human health and the environment. Integrating the concepts of sustainability into scientific innovations, the principles of green chemistry have been pivotal to the business sector and the environment. The elements of economy, society and environment must be considered when moving towards sustainability while trade-offs are inevitable when achieving different goals with regard to the three elements. In the long term, it should be ensured that the goals of environment, society and economy are working in a concerted and synergistic way, with the applications of the Twelve Principles of Green Chemistry having demonstrated the promising prospect as an essential tool contributing to sustainability, as well as achieving the desired synergism by focusing the work at the most fundamental levels, i.e. from the molecular perspectives (Manley et al., 2008).

With the advancement in green chemistry for the reduction on the use of hazardous chemicals, its implementation in the design of chemical products and processes is imperative to the environment and public health of the continually growing global population, as well as seeking solutions to various global challenges including climate change, energy resources, toxins in the environment and sustainable agriculture (Horváth & Anastas, 2007; Kirchhoff, 2005). Given the promising values in contributing to the achievement of SDGs, there has been a surging rise of research studies investigating the applications of green chemistry towards a sustainable environment. However, mere advancement in scientific knowledge and technologies is not sufficient. It is noteworthy that health promotion and education are equally important. How to educate the emerging scientific concepts while nurturing global citizenships are important issues behind (Chiu et al., 2022; Mahaffy et al., 2019a). In this chapter, fundamental aspects related to chemical pollution and the relationship between implementation of green chemistry and a sustainable environment will be described. The advancement in research investigations of green chemistry and education, as well as the important implications behind, will be further discussed.

Chemical Pollution

Synthetic chemicals are essential to everyday life, but they are often unintentionally released, affecting the environmental quality. These chemical pollutions are a global phenomenon that affects the health of people all over the world, especially for regions with dense population or high traffic volumes. For example, in the case of Hong Kong, emissions from vehicles are a major source of chemical pollutions. Many people prefer to use diesel cars because less fuel would be consumed, resulting in a lower expense (Carwow Staff, 2022). However, diesel vehicles release more air pollutants, resulting in poorer air quality. In addition, the number of private cars in Hong Kong increases every year. According to official statistics, the number of private cars has escalated from about 470,000 in 2011 to about 630,000 in 2019 (Statista Research Department, 2022). All these have led to serious concern, as exemplified by the case of Hong Kong, where the street canyon effect due to the densely packed tall buildings has aggravated roadside pollution in the major urban areas (Rakowska et al., 2014; Wong et al., 2019). In recent decades, the associated environmental health hazards due to exposure to traffic-related chemical pollutants have been extensively investigated and there have also been various studies reporting the strategies for the mitigation of roadside air pollution and improvement of urban ventilation (Huang et al., 2021; Lo & Ngan, 2017; Lv et al., 2021). It is noteworthy that vehicular emissions just represent one of the major sources of chemical pollutants in the environment. Industrial processes, and many other types of human activities with excessive use of hazardous chemicals, are leading to rising levels of chemical pollution and posing serious threats to the environment and public health (Chiu & Fong, 2022).

Situations in Developing Countries

The most common chemical pollutants do not readily degrade in nature and exposure to these chemical contaminants can lead to adverse health effects. However, most of daily products are made up of chemicals and they are used widely. With extensive applications of chemicals, it was reported that since 2017, there had been a significant increase in chemical pollution, with over 10,000,000 tons of chemical pollutants (Eurostat Statistics Explained, 2021). Many of these pollutants originated from the extensive use of registered chemicals which led to serious environmental pollution, especially in developing countries where the populations are in particular vulnerable to chemical attack and toxic pollutants resulting from various industrial processes (Özkara et al., 2016).

However, when comparing the amount of waste produced in developed countries with that in developing countries, it is found that developed countries produce more waste than developing countries. For example, the average amount of waste produced per person per day in Japan is about 1.1 kg. In contrast, the average amount of waste produced per person in the Philippines is only about 0.7 kg per day (Ali & Sion, 2014). This shows that developing countries do not necessarily produce more waste, but rather developed countries can possibly produce more solid waste, including electronics and plastics (Browning et al., 2021; Nnorom & Osibanjo, 2008).

Nevertheless, some developed countries dispose of waste by simply dumping their own waste in developing countries. They are only responsible for paying the corresponding bills and dispose of large amounts of waste. It has been reported that the Philippines has received more than 4,000 tonnes of plastic waste in 2017 from Korea (Green Peace, 2018). The situation was getting worse, with the Philippines having received more than 11,000 tonnes of plastic waste from South Korea between January and September 2018. This was an increase of more than double when compared to that of previous year (Green Peace, 2018). The situation is alarming considering the worldwide increasing generation of solid waste and in particular for less developed countries where ineffective waste management systems are presenting serious challenges (Bundhoo, 2018).

Furthermore, there are capacity constraints in developing countries to effectively manage the proper use of chemicals (Wang et al., 2020). For example, vehicles and power stations may not be up to standard and release large amounts of toxic gases into the environment. Meanwhile, in some cases, because of the lack of a well-developed legal system, these countries face huge challenges in regulating the air quality and protecting the environment effectively (UN Environment Programme, n.d.).

Another prevailing issue is the environmental risks arising from the extensive applications of agrochemicals. Agricultural pollution has caused growing global concern due to its alarming level, especially in developing countries, where frequent agricultural activities represent major sources of chemical contaminants in the environment (Chen et al., 2017; Yang et al., 2018).

In agriculture, large quantities of pesticides and fertilisers are used to ensure an efficient production process and to reduce pests and diseases. It has been reported that from a global perspective, the loss due to pre-harvest pests accounted for an average of 35% of potential crop yield (Oerke, 2006). Therefore, use of agricultural pesticides in developing countries is very common and the importance of these chemicals is undeniable considering the continuing challenges from pests to agricultural producers (Özkara et al., 2016). However, the environmental risks associated with the use of agrochemicals and their impact on human health are also emerging key problems. Many pesticides do not degrade easily or completely, and their residues can be found in various types of foods and beverages such as fruits, vegetables, water and wine (Chourasiya et al., 2015; Nicolopoulou-Stamati et al., 2016). While the use of pesticides has made significant contributions to increased food availability in the recent decades, chemical pollution from agricultural activities has adversely impacted the environment and human health (Tang et al., 2021).

Chemical Threats to Human Health

Most of the health problems caused by chemical pollution are caused by air pollutants. More than one-third of people with heart disease and more than 40% of people who suffer from a stroke can be prevented by reducing their exposure to chemicals such as air pollutants (Prüss-Ustün et al., 2016). Air pollution can also affect the embryos of pregnant women, resulting in the risk of low birth weight, premature birth and death (Leonardi-Bee et al., 2011). In addition, air pollution can also lead to the development of respiratory diseases. According to World Health Organization (2016), more than 30% of lower respiratory tract infections are caused by air pollution and second-hand smoke. For children, respiratory infections are a major cause of death. The cause of asthma is also related to the air quality, and when air pollution level is high, it can worsen asthma. This can also lead to the development of asthma in outdoor workers when they are exposed to the polluted environment (Choudhary & Tarlo, 2014).

Polluted atmospheres commonly contain volatile organic compounds (VOCs) which refer to a wide variety of hydrocarbon compounds. Some of them, such as 1,3-butadiene, formaldehyde and benzene, are known to be toxic and the presence of these chemicals in the air presents a serious threat to human health (World Health Organization, 2000). The major exposure pathway to VOCs occurs through inhalation. Either short-term or long-term exposure can lead to adverse impact on human health. Short-term exposure to high level of VOCs can result in irritations to eyes, nose, throat and lungs. It may also cause damage to the kidney, liver and central nervous system. On the other hand, at a low concentration, long-term exposure to VOCs can cause weakened pulmonary functions, asthma, cardiovascular disease and cancers (Mo et al., 2021; Soni et al., 2018). Vehicles, solvent use and paint consumption represent significant emission sources of VOCs. The fine chemical and pharmaceutical industries are also examples of the major source sectors contributing to the release of VOCs, due to the fact that large quantities of solvents are required in different reaction stages of producing complex molecules, such as during the synthesis, extraction and purification of healthcare products and drugs.

Besides air pollution, water pollution is also an important factor that affects people's health. Factories often discharge toxic chemicals and release them directly into rivers, polluting the drinking water of residents. This problem is not common in cities, where tap water is treated before it is available to the public (Jabeen et al., 2011). However, people living in rural areas may not have facilities to treat their wastewater, and the hygiene condition in rural areas is worse than those in urban cities, so they often drink wastewater containing nitrogen compounds released from factories (Jabeen et al., 2011). The consumption of contaminated water can also have negative effects on pregnant women, resulting in babies being born underweight and affecting their health (Currie et al., 2013). Factories can also release heavy metals to contaminate water sources. Aquatic animals have the chance to absorb large amounts of heavy metals, which can lead to health problems such as hair loss or kidney failure when people consume aquatic animals from the contaminated aquatic environment (Ahmed et al., 2016). Notably, although cities and industries have been considered widely as major sources of pollution, recent studies and assessments have identified agricultural activities as one of the leading causes of water pollution due to release of huge quantities of contaminants such as agrochemicals, nutrients and drug residues (Evans et al., 2019; Sharpley et al., 2015).

Chemical Contamination of the Food Chain

Chemical contamination of the food chain affects pregnant women and their breast milk, resulting in the chance of the infant absorbing contaminated breast milk and lowering the infant's immunity (Naidu et al., 2021; van den Berg et al., 2017). At the same time, pregnant women are exposed to various foods with added chemicals, and according to studies, over 10,000 chemicals are used to process food (Trasande et al., 2018). Therefore, pregnant women have a high chance of consuming foods that are chemically treated or processed nowadays. In developing countries which do not have established regulations and laws in relation to chemically processed food, large amounts of preservatives are used to increase the storage time of food while pesticides are also widely applied to increase crop production (Awata et al., 2017).

Under these circumstances, the soil, water, and local organisms and crops are adversely affected (Tang et al., 2021). The infiltration of pesticides into the nearby pond results in an increase in phytoplankton in the pond, which blocks sunlight from penetrating to the plants in water. Plants at the bottom of the pond are important to aquatic life as they can absorb sunlight and carry out photosynthesis to supply oxygen to the pond organisms (Tang et al., 2021). Furthermore, when the phytoplankton continues to grow and expand due to exposure to more sunlight, the pH of the aquatic environment may rise to a level that is not suitable for aquatic life. Ultimately, this disrupts the original ecology of the pond, killing most of the aquatic organisms and disrupting the pond's food chain.

In the case of soil, through which most food is grown, the reduction in available arable land represents a decline in food production. In developing countries, in particular, the loss of land due to chemical pollution has led to problems in the country's food supply (Naidu et al., 2021). According to Cameron et al. (2015), more than one-third of the earth's land is now uncultivable due to chemical contamination. This impacts not only the food supply for humans but also the lives of local animals. The reduction in agricultural land means less food for animals and affects the quality of food (Naidu et al., 2021). If animals are exposed to contaminated crops, there is a risk that their health may be seriously affected, which would lead to death. The decline in herbivore populations influences ecosystem development, reducing the chances of survival for carnivores and disrupting local food chains.

When water and land continue to be polluted, local biodiversity is disturbed. It has been suggested that chemical pollution has led to the loss of over 40% of invertebrates which help to pollinate crops, and their reduction indirectly upsets biodiversity (Beketov et al., 2013; Goulson, 2013). In addition, nitrogen pollution also affects ecosystems in different places. It has been suggested that close to one-quarter of the terrestrial natural environment in the USA has suffered loss of species due to nitrogen pollution (Southon et al., 2013). In addition, Diaz and Rosenberg (2008) noted that human activities had produced too many chemicals to the oceans, resulting in the contamination of a large number of marine areas and marine ecosystems, which thus leads to the disappearance of some marine flora and fauna. The loss of native organisms has the potential to increase the number of invasive species, disrupting the local ecosystem and indirectly impacting the food chain for humans and animals.

Advance in Green Chemistry for Sustainable Environment and Health

The severity of worldwide pollution is one of the major factors leading to the surge of extensive investigations in recent years for the development and applications of green chemistry. This is in accordance with the SDGs and is responding to the environmental health risks from the heavy pollution levels across the globe (Chen et al., 2020). The twelve principles of green chemistry, postulated by Anastas and Warner (1998), are still widely applied nowadays in green chemistry research studies which focus on the basis of entire life cycles of chemicals, minimisation of the use of hazardous chemicals and toxic solvents in chemical processes, as well as preventing the generation of harmful residues from these industrial processes (de Marco et al., 2019). The concepts of green chemistry have been applied in various studies in relation to different industries, such as the pharmaceutical sector and fine chemical synthesis. It has been reported that the raw materials for preparing active pharmaceutical ingredients can be up to 85% solvent by mass (Sheldon, 2005). In addition, for many different drug manufacturing processes, when going through the early development stage to the final commercial processing stage, the demand for the use of solvents remains high (Roschangar et al., 2017). Notably, according to the review study by Clark et al. in 2015, it was estimated that the annual industrial production of organic solvents has almost reached the level of 20 million metric tons. Due to rapid urbanisation and industrialisation, tremendous amounts of VOCs are being emitted to the atmosphere from these sources every day and the effects are of particular concern in densely built environment where the pollutants are easily trapped (Mo et al., 2016; Ramírez et al., 2012). Moreover, due to extensive use of organic solvents in various chemical reactions and industrial processes, VOCs also pose adverse effects on the health of occupational painters and industrial workers (Mo et al., 2021).

The consumption of organic solvents is a dilemma. On the one hand, excessive use of non-renewable and toxic solvents is considered as a remarkable example of unsustainable practices, leading to profound environmental impact and adverse effects on human health (Clarke et al., 2018). On the other hand, solvents are indispensable components in many chemical processes. Critical roles and effects of solvents, particularly in organic reactions, have been well established (Reichardt & Welton, 2011). Therefore, in recent years, sustainable solvents have received growing interests as one of the emerging topics in green chemistry from both the chemical industry and the research community. Due to the increasing public awareness of the impact of VOCs on pollution, efforts have been directed towards the development and applications of more sustainable solvent alternatives and, in the meantime, more industrial processes are being scrutinised for solvent consumption (Clarke et al., 2018; Savelski et al., 2017).

Efforts to address these important issues have also been put on environmental directives and legislation. For example, the Clean Air Act Amendments of 1990 is a market-based environmental policy in search of efficient and economic control strategies for VOCs (Moretti & Mukhopadhyay, 1993). Other prominent examples include the European Union Solvents Emission Directive 1999/13/EC (Council of the European Union, 1999) and Registration, Evaluation, Authorisation and Restriction of Chemicals, which aim to achieve reduced solvent emissions as well as effective regulation on the use of potentially harmful or environmentally damaging chemicals (Kerton & Marriott, 2013).

Despite various measures being put forward, the use of solvents in chemical industry is inevitable. Many chemical processes are still dependent on various harmful and toxic solvents, with some developing countries having increased the consumption of harmful solvents such as dichloromethane, due to lower cost and higher availability (Clarke et al., 2018; Leedham Elvidge et al., 2015). Therefore, the development of sustainable chemicals requires serious consideration on the importance of economic factors, which is also largely related to user accessibility and market viability (Welton, 2015). Overall, the development of such processes is challenged with the complexity of interconnected components, and therefore, multi-disciplinary efforts are greatly demanded.

Future Directions and Implications

Education for a Sustainable Environment

In addition to scientific advancement, what remains as one of the core components in contributing to a sustainable environment is human behaviours. Health promotion and education play a crucial role in raising public awareness towards the impact of using harmful chemicals on the environment. They are considered as essential components of achieving a green environment for sustainable health. The importance of nurturing global citizenship has also led to growing research studies regarding the promotion of sustainable environment in the context of education. One of the important agenda in educational research is about the incorporation of systems thinking in the teaching of science subjects. Embedment of systems thinking in education is important for equipping the young generation the skills to meet the SDGs (Hurst, 2020). This is of particular importance to green chemistry education in which realising the interconnections between the chemical system and many other systems would influence people's choices of consumptions and perceptions towards green products and processes.

Moreover, a mindset of systems thinking is also imperative for professionals to engage in the innovation and development of green technologies with a holistic perspective, as well as supporting inter-disciplinary collaborations for a sustainable future (Zuin et al., 2021). In view of the promising prospects of systems thinking in contribution to sustainable environment, there have been a growing number of studies in recent years reporting the incorporation of systems thinking in education for a green environment and the possibility of supporting relevant education with advance technology and artificial intelligence (Chiu, 2021; Hurst, 2020). Recently, Miller et al. (2019) have reported a game-based learning approach for systems thinking. In their study, the activity "Green Machine" was designed as a competitive strategy card game to facilitate a systems thinking approach for learning material recycling processes and green chemistry in agreement with the SDGs. In addition to card games as educational resources, system-oriented concept map extension (SOCME) diagrams have also been devised as important resources (Aubrecht et al., 2019). The SOCME diagrams served as visualisation tools for facilitating the realisation of the complexity and interconnections between the chemical system and other systems. For example, two SOCME diagrams related to Haber process were developed for the use in general chemistry courses (Mahaffy et al., 2019b). Recently, the design of a SOCME diagram concerning the chemicals released from degradation of plastics was reported in a collaborative study across disciplines of health and chemical sciences (Chiu et al., 2022). In the study, the importance of a sustainable environment for healthy ageing was also discussed. It is further suggested that more educational resources should be developed for incorporation of systems thinking in education for a sustainable environment.

In order to have genuine utilisation and recognition of green products, promoting green chemistry to the public for health purposes are essential. This will increase public awareness of green chemistry, and when people know that green chemistry can help alleviate health and environmental problems, they will be more willing to practise green chemistry. To achieve all these, the American Chemical Society (ACS) has incorporated the Green Chemistry Institute (GCI) as part of the ACS (American Chemistry Society, n.d.). Exploration of community-level education and lifelong learning for a green environment is necessary, and effective implementation can be drawn from the experience of related programmes conducted in different regions. For example, indirectly implemented in a mandatory school curriculum, the GCI organised a one-week summer course on green chemistry to enable more students to learn about green chemistry and sustainable energy (American Chemical Society, n.d.). During the course, students were able to listen to lectures by professors and scientists working on green chemistry and sustainable energy, and participated in discussion sessions to learn more about application of green chemistry in specific areas such as apparel chemistry, thus allowing students to become the next generation of professionals in promoting green chemistry (American Chemical Society, n.d.). The ACS has established research in green oxidation and materials at the University of Hong Kong and has created a PhD degree in green chemistry (American Chemical Society, n.d.). Furthermore, the ACS has published a number of books focusing on green chemistry, for example, to understand how green chemistry can be applied to other disciplines, or to provide basic information on green chemistry to a wider audience (American Chemical Society, n.d.). Looking ahead, more collaborations between health and chemical science can enhance the integration of health knowledge and the promotion in education of the young generation for a sustainable environment (Aubrecht et al., 2019; Chiu et al., 2022).

Green Chemistry in Relation to Sustainable Health and Environment

In accordance with the SDGs, green chemistry aims at reducing the use of toxic compounds to encourage good health and well-being of individuals. Applying the concepts of green chemistry in synthetic research, the method of synthesis of nylon has been transformed. Previously, nylon was mainly synthesised using carcinogenic benzene to produce adipic acid (Umesh, 2022), a key intermediate in the manufacturing of nylon. Later, scientists created genetically-altered bacteria that acts as catalysts in glucose to synthesise adipic acid in a different way, reducing the risk of cancer from workers making nylon (Umesh, 2022). In addition, scientists have investigated different methods of producing hydrazine. Previously, hydrazine was manufactured through the Raschig process, but this method utilises dangerous chemicals such as ammonia and sodium hypochlorite, which produces sodium chloride as a by-product (Agency for Toxic Substances & Disease Registry, 1997). However, green chemistry research has shed light on the ability to improve such production method by replacing the previous method with a peroxide process. The only by-product of this method is water, and it reduces the use of more hazardous chemicals and human exposure to toxic compounds. In the future, more research studies incorporating the principles of green chemistry are expected for making synthesis and production processes greener, especially those processes originally employing the use of toxic and harmful chemicals.

Green chemistry is not only concerned with chemical synthesis or industrial pollution, but it should also be applied in daily life. In 1845, Jean-Baptiste Jolly discovered that paraffin could remove stains from clothes. Therefore, he created a dry-cleaning system to remove stains from clothes that could not be washed in water (EcoClean, n.d.). However, the use of petroleum solvents for cleaning caused fires and explosions, and oil was in short supply. Finally, scientists used green chemistry, replacing petroleum solvents with chlorinated solvents, which reduced the human harm caused by explosions and reduced oil consumption (EcoClean, n.d.). Being one of the most investigated topics nowadays, more studies to promote and facilitate the applications of green chemistry in daily life will be of importance to human health and the environment (Nasrollahzadeh et al., 2019; Saini, 2018).

Environmental pollution reduces the habitat of organisms and leads to the disappearance of certain species from the ecosystem. The species that disappear most quickly are larger species with slower survival cycles (Hutchings et al., 2012). Conversely, smaller species with shorter life cycles have increased in abundance due to a reduction in predators (Keesing & Young, 2014). However, the species with shorter life cycles are more likely to transmit zoonotic pathogens (Plourde et al., 2017). When a virus outbreak occurs, the chances for animals or humans becoming ill are greatly increased. Green chemistry can solve the problem of habitat loss due to environmental pollution. Green chemistry research can investigate to degrade toxic pesticides, turn them into environmentally friendly products and recycle environmentally damaging pesticides (United States Environmental Protection Agency, n.d.). In addition, green chemistry reduces global warming and reduces the chance of species disappearing, thereby increasing biodiversity and reducing the chance of species spreading viruses (United States Environmental Protection Agency, n.d.).

Green chemistry protects the environment and biodiversity, and indirectly leads to more resources for biomedical scientists to develop new treatments for diseases. Take breast cancer as an example. In 2020, it was estimated that more than 2,000,000 women worldwide suffered from breast cancer, and nearly 700,000 of them died of the disease, indicating the high mortality rate of breast cancer and its impact on women's health (World Cancer Research Fund International, n.d.). However, Duffy et al. (2020) found that bee venom can inhibit the growth of breast cancer. In addition, bee venom may also have the potential to treat lung and stomach cancers, opening new treatment options for cancer. In addition to reducing the adverse effects of drug use, honeybee venom could also trim down the cost of cancer treatment and benefit people especially in less developed countries (Duffy et al., 2020).

Green chemistry can maintain biodiversity and increase the number of bees' reproduction. Furthermore, there are many resources in the world that scientists have yet to explore. A recent study by RL Morlighem et al. (2018) has reported integrative analyses on marine enzymes, which have a high potential for applications in green synthesis of organic compounds, as well as in pharmaceutical and industrial biotechnology. Investigations of green chemistry strategies for drug synthesis will contribute to the achievement of sustainable health and environment, with recent studies showing the promising prospects in addressing the health research gap. A study by Yap et al. (2020) has demonstrated a sustainable biomimetic scheme to produce cyclic disulphide-rich peptides which are a group of specific chemicals finding versatile applications in drug design but formerly inaccessible through large-scale chemical synthesis, thereby leading to reduced environmental burden in the drug synthesis.

Conclusion

Extensive applications of hazardous chemicals have led to rising levels of chemical pollution with growing concern over the associated environmental health risks. Further development and implementation of green chemistry, as well as more research investigations of applying green chemistry principles in various sectors such as the pharmaceutical and fine chemical industries, would be expected to play critical roles in achieving sustainable environment and health, as in accordance with various targets set in SDGs. With increasing levels of pollutions over the world and the prevalence of associated diseases in different population groups, a clean environment is becoming more significant in the promotion of good health and well-being for all at all ages. Continued investigations of green and sustainable chemistry will further pave the way for achieving a sustainable green environment due to its versatile prospects in the improvement of health for all age groups. This can be accomplished by various contributions such as reducing the use and production of hazardous substances, designing synthetic processes with ambient conditions and enhanced energy efficiency, as well as developing inherently safer chemistry for preventing accidents. As we human would be the one to design the operation of industrial processes as well as to make decisions on the use of chemicals, public awareness on the importance of environmental sustainability and the chemical impact on different systems should be well enhanced. After all, it should be noted that efforts from multi-disciplinary professionals are equally important in both advancing the scientific innovations and education for a sustainable future.

References

Agency for Toxic Substances and Disease Registry. (1997). *Toxicological profile for hydrazines.* https://www.atsdr.cdc.gov/toxprofiles/tp100.pdf

Ahmed, T., Scholz, M., Al-Faraj, F., & Niaz, W. (2016). Water-related impacts of climate change on agriculture and subsequently on public health: A review for generalists with particular reference to Pakistan. *International Journal of Environmental Research and Public Health, 13*(11), Article 1051. https://doi.org/10.3390/ijerph13111051

Ali, N. E., & Sion, H. C. (2014). Solid waste management in Asian countries: A review of solid waste minimisation (3'r) towards low carbon. *IOP Conference Series: Earth Environment Science, 18*, 012152. https://iopscience.iop.org/article/10.1088/1755-1315/18/1/012152/pdf

American Chemical Society. (n.d.). *Green chemistry history.* https://www.acs.org/content/acs/en/greenchemistry/what-is-green-chemistry/history-of-green-chemistry.html

Anastas, P. T., & Warner, J. C. (1998). *Green chemistry: Theory and practice*. Oxford University Press. https://global.oup.com/ushe/product/green-chemistry-9780198506980?cc=hk&lang=en&

Aubrecht, K. B., Dori, Y. J., Holme, T. A., Lavi, R., Matlin, S. A., Orgill, M., & Skaza-Acosta, H. (2019). Graphical tools for conceptualizing systems thinking in chemistry education. *Journal of Chemical Education, 96*(12), 2888–2900. https://doi.org/10.1021/acs.jchemed.9b00314

Awata, H., Linder, S., Mitchell, L. E., & Delclos, G. L. (2017). Association of dietary intake and biomarker levels of arsenic, cadmium, lead, and mercury among Asian populations in the United States: NHANES 2011–2012. *Environmental Health Perspectives, 125*(3), 314–323. https://doi.org/10.1289/EHP28

Beach, E. S., Cui, Z., & Anastas, P. T. (2009). Green chemistry: A design framework for sustainability. *Energy & Environmental Science, 2*(10), 1038–1049. https://doi.org/10.1039/B904997P

Beketov, M. A., Kefford, B. J., Schäfer, R. B., & Liess, M. (2013). Pesticides reduce regional biodiversity of stream invertebrates. *Proceedings of the National Academy of Sciences, 110*(27), 11039–11043. https://doi.org/10.1073/pnas.1305618110

Browning, S., Beymer-Farris, B., & Seay, J. R. (2021). Addressing the challenges associated with plastic waste disposal and management in developing countries. *Current Opinion in Chemical Engineering, 32*, 100682. https://doi.org/10.1016/j.coche.2021.100682

Bundhoo, Z. M. (2018). Solid waste management in least developed countries: Current status and challenges faced. *Journal of Material Cycles and Waste Management, 20*, 1867–1877. https://doi.org/10.1007/s10163-018-0728-3

Cameron, D., Osborne, C., Horton, P., & Sinclair, M. (2015). A sustainable model for intensive agriculture. *Grantham Centre for Sustainable Futures, 2*.

Carwow Staff. (2022, August 26). Petrol vs diesel cars: Should I buy a diesel car? *Carwow*. https://www.carwow.co.uk/guides/choosing/petrol-diesel-878#gref

Chen, T. L., Kim, H., Pan, S. Y., Tseng, P. C., Lin, Y. P., & Chiang, P. C. (2020). Implementation of green chemistry principles in circular economy system towards sustainable development goals: Challenges and perspectives. *Science of the Total Environment, 716*, Article 136998. https://doi.org/10.1016/j.scitotenv.2020.136998

Chen, Y. H., Wen, X. W., Wang, B., & Nie, P. Y. (2017). Agricultural pollution and regulation: How to subsidize agriculture? *Journal of Cleaner Production, 164*, 258–264. https://doi.org/10.1016/j.jclepro.2017.06.216

Chiu, W. K. (2021). Pedagogy of emerging technologies in chemical education during the era of digitalization and artificial intelligence: A systematic review. *Education Sciences, 11*(11), Article 709. https://doi.org/10.3390/educsci11110709

Chiu, W. K., & Fong, B. Y. F (2022). Chemical pollution and healthy ageing: The prominent need for a cleaner environment. In B. Y. F. Fong & V. T. S. Law (Eds.), *Ageing with dignity in Asia—Holistic and humanistic care*. Springer.

Chiu, W. K., Fong, B. Y., & Ho, W. Y. (2022). The importance of environmental sustainability for healthy ageing and the incorporation of systems thinking in education for a sustainable environment. *Asia Pacific Journal of Health Management, 17*(1), 84–89. https://doi.org/10.24083/apjhm.v17i1.1589

Choudhary, H., & Tarlo, S. M. (2014). Airway effects of traffic-related air pollution on outdoor workers. *Current Opinion in Allergy and Clinical Immunology, 14*(2), 106–112. https://doi.org/10.1097/aci.0000000000000038

Chourasiya, S., Khillare, P. S., & Jyethi, D. S. (2015). Health risk assessment of organochlorine pesticide exposure through dietary intake of vegetables grown in the Periurban sites of Delhi, India. *Environmental Science and Pollution Research, 22*(8), 5793–5806. https://doi.org/10.1007/s11356-014-3791-x

Clark, J. H., Farmer, T. J., Hunt, A. J., & Sherwood, J. (2015). Opportunities for bio-based solvents created as petrochemical and fuel products transition towards renewable resources. *International Journal of Molecular Sciences, 16*(8), 17101–17159. https://doi.org/10.3390/ijms160817101

Clarke, C. J., Tu, W. C., Levers, O., Brohl, A., & Hallett, J. P. (2018). Green and sustainable solvents in chemical processes. *Chemical Reviews, 118*(2), 747–800. https://doi.org/10.1021/acs.chemrev.7b00571

Council of the European Union. (1999). *Council Directive 1999/13/EC of 11 March 1999 on the limitation of emissions of volatile organic compounds due to the use of organic solvents in certain activities and installations.* https://eur-lex.europa.eu/legal-content/EN/TXT/PDF/?uri=CELEX:31999L0013

Currie, J., Graff Zivin, J., Meckel, K., Neidell, M., & Schlenker, W. (2013). Something in the water: Contaminated drinking water and infant health. *Canadian Journal of Economics, 46*(3), 791–810. https://doi.org/10.1111/caje.12039

de Marco, B. A., Rechelo, B. S., Tótoli, E. G., Kogawa, A. C., & Salgado, H. R. N. (2019). Evolution of green chemistry and its multidimensional impacts: A review. *Saudi Pharmaceutical Journal, 27*(1), 1–8. https://doi.org/10.1016/j.jsps.2018.07.011

Diaz, R. J., & Rosenberg, R. (2008). Spreading dead zones and consequences for marine ecosystems. *Science, 321*(5891), 926–929. https://doi.org/10.1126/science.1156401

Duffy, C., Sorolla, A., Wang, E., Golden, E., Woodward, E., Davern, K., Ho, D., Johnstone, E., Pfleger, K., Redfern, A., Iyer, K. S., Baer, B., & Blancafort, P. (2020). Honeybee venom and melittin suppress growth factor receptor activation in HER2-enriched and triple-negative breast cancer. *NPJ Precision Oncology, 4,* Article 24. https://doi.org/10.1038/s41698-020-00129-0

EcoClean. (n.d.). *History of dry cleaning.* https://ecocleanaustin.com/wet-cleaning/history-of-dry-cleaning/

Eurostat Statistics Explained. (2021). *Chemicals production and consumption statistics.* https://ec.europa.eu/eurostat/statistics-explained/index.php?title=Chemicals_production_and_consumption_statistics#Total_production_of_chemicals

Evans, A. E., Mateo-Sagasta, J., Qadir, M., Boelee, E., & Ippolito, A. (2019). Agricultural water pollution: Key knowledge gaps and research needs. *Current Opinion in Environmental Sustainability, 36*, 20–27. https://doi.org/10.1016/j.cosust.2018.10.003

Fong, B. Y., Chiu, W. K., Chan, W. F., & Lam, T. Y. (2021). A review study of a green diet and healthy ageing. *International Journal of Environmental Research and Public Health, 18*(15), Article 8024. https://doi.org/10.3390/ijerph18158024

Goulson, D. (2013). An overview of the environmental risks posed by neonicotinoid insecticides. *Journal of Applied Ecology, 50*(4), 977–987. https://doi.org/10.1111/1365-2664.12111

Green Peace. (2018). *South Korea needs to be reminded that Philippines is not a waste dump, won't solve its 'waste problem'.* https://www.greenpeace.org/philippines/press/1262/south-korea-needs-to-be-reminded-that-philippines-is-not-a-waste-dump-wont-solve-its-waste-problem/

Horváth, I. T., & Anastas, P. T. (2007). Innovations and green chemistry. *Chemical Reviews, 107*(6), 2169–2173. https://doi.org/10.1021/cr078380v

Huang, Y., Lei, C., Liu, C. H., Perez, P., Forehead, H., Kong, S., & Zhou, J. L. (2021). A review of strategies for mitigating roadside air pollution in urban street canyons. *Environmental Pollution, 280,* Article 116971. https://doi.org/10.1016/j.envpol.2021.116971

Hurst, G. A. (2020). Systems thinking approaches for international green chemistry education. *Current Opinion in Green and Sustainable Chemistry, 21,* 93–97. https://doi.org/10.1016/j.cogsc.2020.02.004

Hutchings, J. A., Myers, R. A., García, V. B., Lucifora, L. O., & Kuparinen, A. (2012). Life-history correlates of extinction risk and recovery potential. *Ecological Applications, 22*(4), 1061–1067. https://doi.org/10.1890/11-1313.1

Jabeen, S., Mahmood, Q., Tariq, S., Nawab, B., & Elahi, N. (2011). Health impact caused by poor water and sanitation in district Abbottabad. *Journal of Ayub Medical College Abbottabad, 23*(1), 47–50. https://www.ayubmed.edu.pk/JAMC/23-1/Sadia.pdf

Keesing, F., & Young, T. P. (2014). Cascading consequences of the loss of large mammals in an African savanna. *BioScience, 64*(6), 487–495. https://doi.org/10.1093/biosci/biu059

Kerton, F. M., & Marriott, R. (2013). Green solvents legislation and certification. In F. Kerton & R. Marriott (Eds.), *Alternative solvents for Green Chemistry* (pp. 31–50). Royal Society of Chemistry. https://doi.org/10.1039/9781849736824-00031

Kirchhoff, M. M. (2005). Promoting sustainability through green chemistry. *Resources, Conservation and Recycling, 44*(3), 237–243. https://doi.org/10.1016/j.resconrec.2005.01.003

Leedham Elvidge, E. C., Oram, D. E., Laube, J. C., Baker, A. K., Montzka, S. A., Humphrey, S., O'Sullivan, D., & Brenninkmeijer, C. A. M. (2015). Increasing concentrations of dichloromethane, CH 2 Cl 2, inferred from CARIBIC air samples collected 1998–2012. *Atmospheric Chemistry and Physics, 15*(4), 1939–1958. https://doi.org/10.5194/acp-15-1939-2015

Leonardi-Bee, J., Britton, J., & Venn, A. (2011). Secondhand smoke and adverse fetal outcomes in nonsmoking pregnant women: A meta-analysis. *Pediatrics, 127*(4), 734–741. https://doi.org/10.1542/peds.2010-3041

Lo, K. W., & Ngan, K. (2017). Characterizing ventilation and exposure in street canyons using Lagrangian particles. *Journal of Applied Meteorology and Climatology, 56*(5), 1177–1194. https://doi.org/10.1175/JAMC-D-16-0168.1

Lv, W., Wu, Y., & Zang, J. (2021). A review on the dispersion and distribution characteristics of pollutants in street canyons and improvement measures. *Energies, 14*(19), Article 6155. https://doi.org/10.3390/en14196155

Mahaffy, P. G., Matlin, S. A., Holme, T. A., & MacKellar, J. (2019a). Systems thinking for education about the molecular basis of sustainability. *Nature Sustainability, 2*(5), 362–370. https://doi.org/10.1038/s41893-019-0285-3

Mahaffy, P. G., Matlin, S. A., Whalen, J. M., & Holme, T. A. (2019b). Integrating the molecular basis of sustainability into general chemistry through systems thinking. *Journal of Chemical Education, 96*(12), 2730–2741. https://doi.org/10.1021/acs.jchemed.9b00390

Manley, J. B., Anastas, P. T., & Cue, B. W., Jr. (2008). Frontiers in green chemistry: Meeting the grand challenges for sustainability in R&D and manufacturing. *Journal of Cleaner Production, 16*(6), 743–750. https://doi.org/10.1016/j.jclepro.2007.02.025

Miller, J. L., Wentzel, M. T., Clark, J. H., & Hurst, G. A. (2019). Green machine: A card game introducing students to systems thinking in green chemistry by strategizing the creation of a recycling plant. *Journal of Chemical Education, 96*(12), 3006–3013. https://doi.org/10.1021/acs.jchemed.9b00278

Mo, Z., Shao, M., & Lu, S. (2016). Compilation of a source profile database for hydrocarbon and OVOC emissions in China. *Atmospheric Environment, 143*, 209–217. https://doi.org/10.1016/j.atmosenv.2016.08.025

Mo, Z., Lu, S., & Shao, M. (2021). Volatile organic compound (VOC) emissions and health risk assessment in paint and coatings industry in the Yangtze River Delta, China. *Environmental Pollution, 269*, Article 115740. https://doi.org/10.1016/j.envpol.2020.115740

Moretti, E. C., & Mukhopadhyay, N. (1993). VOC control: Current practices and future trends. *Chemical Engineering Progress (United States), 89*(7).

Naidu, R., Biswas, B., Willett, I. R., Cribb, J., Singh, B. K., Nathanail, C. P., Coulon, F., Semple, K. T., Jones, K. C., Barclay, A., & Aitken, R. J. (2021). Chemical pollution: A growing peril and potential catastrophic risk to humanity. *Environment International, 156*, Article 106616. https://doi.org/10.1016/j.envint.2021.106616

Nasrollahzadeh, M., Sajadi, S. M., Sajjadi, M., & Issaabadi, Z. (2019). Applications of nanotechnology in daily life. *Interface Science and Technology, 28*, 113–143. https://doi.org/10.1016/B978-0-12-813586-0.00004-3

Nicolopoulou-Stamati, P., Maipas, S., Kotampasi, C., Stamatis, P., & Hens, L. (2016). Chemical pesticides and human health: The urgent need for a new concept in agriculture. *Frontiers in Public Health, 4*, Article 148. https://doi.org/10.3389/fpubh.2016.00148

Nnorom, I. C., & Osibanjo, O. (2008). Overview of electronic waste (e-waste) management practices and legislations, and their poor applications in the developing countries. *Resources, Conservation and Recycling, 52*(6), 843–858. https://doi.org/10.1016/j.resconrec.2008.01.004

Oerke, E. C. (2006). Crop losses to pests. *The Journal of Agricultural Science, 144*(1), 31–43. https://doi.org/10.1017/S0021859605005708

Özkara, A., Akyıl, D., & Konuk, M. (2016). Pesticides, environmental pollution, and health. In M. L. Larramendy & S. Soloneski (Eds.), *Environmental health risk—Hazardous factors to living species*. IntechOpen. https://doi.org/10.5772/63094

Plourde, B. T., Burgess, T. L., Eskew, E. A., Roth, T. M., Stephenson, N., & Foley, J. E. (2017). Are disease reservoirs special? Taxonomic and life history characteristics. *PLoS ONE, 12*(7), Article e0180716. https://doi.org/10.1371/journal.pone.0180716

Prüss-Ustün, A., Wolf J., Corvalán, C., Bos, R., & Neira, M (2016). Preventing disease through healthy environments: A global assessment of the environmental burden of disease. *World Health Organization*. https://apps.who.int/iris/rest/bitstreams/908623/retrieve

Rakowska, A., Wong, K. C., Townsend, T., Chan, K. L., Westerdahl, D., Ng, S., Močnik, G., Drinovec, L., & Ning, Z. (2014). Impact of traffic volume and composition on the air quality and pedestrian exposure in urban street canyon. *Atmospheric Environment, 98*, 260–270. https://doi.org/10.1016/j.atmosenv.2014.08.073

Ramírez, N., Cuadras, A., Rovira, E., Borrull, F., & Marcé, R. M. (2012). Chronic risk assessment of exposure to volatile organic compounds in the atmosphere near the largest Mediterranean industrial site. *Environment International, 39*(1), 200–209. https://doi.org/10.1016/j.envint.2011.11.002

Reichardt, C., & Welton, T. (2011). Solvents and solvent effects in organic chemistry. *Wiley*. https://doi.org/10.1002/9783527632220

RL Morlighem, J. É., Huang, C., Liao, Q., Braga Gomes, P., Daniel Pérez, C., De Brandão Prieto-da-Silva, Á., Ming-Yuen Lee, S., & Radis-Baptista, G. (2018). The holo-transcriptome of the zoantharian Protopalythoa variabilis (Cnidaria: Anthozoa): A plentiful source of enzymes for potential application in green chemistry, industrial and pharmaceutical biotechnology. *Marine Drugs, 16*(6), Article 207. https://doi.org/10.3390/md16060207

Roschangar, F., Colberg, J., Dunn, P. J., Gallou, F., Hayler, J. D., Koenig, S. G., Koenig, S. G., Kopach, M. E., Leahy, D. K., Mergelsberg, I., Tucker, J. L., Sheldon, R. A., & Senanayake, C. H. (2017). A deeper shade of green: Inspiring sustainable drug manufacturing. *Green Chemistry, 19*(1), 281–285. https://doi.org/10.1039/C6GC02901A

Saini, R. D. (2018). Green chemistry in daily life. *International Journal for Research in Applied Science & Engineering Technology, 6*(11), 70–73. https://doi.org/10.22214/ijraset.2018.2012

Savelski, M. J., Slater, C. S., Tozzi, P. V., & Wisniewski, C. M. (2017). On the simulation, economic analysis, and life cycle assessment of batch-mode organic solvent recovery alternatives for the pharmaceutical industry. *Clean Technologies and Environmental Policy, 19*(10), 2467–2477. https://doi.org/10.1007/s10098-017-1444-8

Sharpley, A. N., Bergström, L., Aronsson, H., Bechmann, M., Bolster, C. H., Börling, K., Börling, K., Djodjic, F., Jarvie, H. P., Schoumans, O. F., Stamm, C., Tonderski, K. S., Ulén, B., Uusitalo, R., & Withers, P. J. (2015). Future agriculture with minimized phosphorus losses to waters: Research needs and direction. *Ambio, 44*(2), 163–179. https://doi.org/10.1007/s13280-014-0612-x

Sheldon, R. A. (2005). Green solvents for sustainable organic synthesis: State of the art. *Green Chemistry, 7*(5), 267–278. https://doi.org/10.1039/B418069K

Simoni, M., Baldacci, S., Maio, S., Cerrai, S., Sarno, G., & Viegi, G. (2015). Adverse effects of outdoor pollution in the elderly. *Journal of Thoracic Disease, 7*(1), 34. https://doi.org/10.3978/j.issn.2072-1439.2014.12.10

Soni, V., Singh, P., Shree, V., & Goel, V. (2018). Effects of VOCs on human health. In N. Sharma, A. Agarwal, P. Eastwood, T. Gupta, & A. Singh (Eds.), *Air pollution and control* (pp. 119–142). Springer. https://doi.org/10.1007/978-981-10-7185-0_8

Southon, G. E., Field, C., Caporn, S. J., Britton, A. J., & Power, S. A. (2013). Nitrogen deposition reduces plant diversity and alters ecosystem functioning: Field-scale evidence from a nationwide survey of UK heathlands. *PLoS ONE, 8*(4), Article e59031. https://doi.org/10.1371/journal.pone.0059031

Statista Research Department. (2022). *Number of private cars registered in Hong Kong from 2011 to 2019*. https://www.statista.com/statistics/674231/hong-kong-registration-of-private-cars/
Tang, F. H. M., Lenzen, M., McBratney, A., & Maggi, F. (2021). Risk of pesticide pollution at the global scale. *Nature Geoscience, 14*(4), 206–210. https://doi.org/10.1038/s41561-021-00712-5
Trasande, L., Shaffer, R. M., Sathyanarayana, S., Lowry, J. A., Ahdoot, S., Baum, C. R., Bernstein, A. S., Bole, A., Campbell, C. C., Landrigan, P. J., Pacheco, S. E., Spanier, A. J., & Woolf, A. D. (2018). Food additives and child health. *Pediatrics, 142*(2), Article e20181410. https://doi.org/10.1542/peds.2018-1410
Umesh, K. (2022, July 19). Green chemistry. *EMBIBE*. https://www.embibe.com/exams/green-chemistry/
UN Environment Programme. (n.d.). *Air pollution hurts the poorest most*. https://www.unep.org/news-and-stories/story/air-pollution-hurts-poorest-most
United States Environmental Protection Agency. (n.d.). *Benefits of green chemistry*. https://www.epa.gov/greenchemistry/benefits-green-chemistry
van den Berg, M., Kypke, K., Kotz, A., Tritscher, A., Lee, S. Y., Magulova, K., Fiedler, H., & Malisch, R. (2017). WHO/UNEP global surveys of PCDDs, PCDFs, PCBs and DDTs in human milk and benefit–risk evaluation of breastfeeding. *Archives of Toxicology, 91*(1), 83–96. https://doi.org/10.1007/s00204-016-1802-z
Wang, Z., Walker, G. W., Muir, D. C. G., & Nagatani-Yoshida, K. (2020). Toward a Global Understanding of Chemical Pollution: A First Comprehensive Analysis of National and Regional Chemical Inventories. *Environmental Science & Technology, 54*(5), 2575–2584. https://doi.org/10.1021/acs.est.9b06379
Welton, T. (2015). Solvents and sustainable chemistry. *Proceedings of the Royal Society A: Mathematical, Physical and Engineering Sciences, 471*(2183), Article 20150502. https://doi.org/10.1098/rspa.2015.0502
Wong, P. P., Lai, P. C., Allen, R., Cheng, W., Lee, M., Tsui, A., Tang, R., Thach, T.-Q., Tian, L., Brauer, M., & Barratt, B. (2019). Vertical monitoring of traffic-related air pollution (TRAP) in urban street canyons of Hong Kong. *Science of the Total Environment, 670*, 696–703. https://doi.org/10.1016/j.scitotenv.2019.03.224
World Cancer Research Fund International. (n.d.). *Breast cancer statistics*. https://www.wcrf.org/cancer-trends/breast-cancer-statistics/
World Health Organization. (2000). *Air quality guidelines for Europe* (2nd ed.). https://apps.who.int/iris/handle/10665/107335
World Health Organization. (2016). *The public health impact of chemicals: Knowns and unknowns*. https://apps.who.int/iris/handle/10665/206553
Yang, Q., Li, Z., Lu, X., Duan, Q., Huang, L., & Bi, J. (2018). A review of soil heavy metal pollution from industrial and agricultural regions in China: Pollution and risk assessment. *Science of the Total Environment, 642*, 690–700. https://doi.org/10.1016/j.scitotenv.2018.06.068
Yap, K., Du, J., Looi, F. Y., Tang, S. R., de Veer, S. J., Bony, A. R., Rehm, F. B. H., Xie, J., Chan, L. Y., Wang, C. K., Adams, D. J., Lua, L. H. L., Durek, T., & Craik, D. J. (2020). An environmentally sustainable biomimetic production of cyclic disulfide-rich peptides. *Green Chemistry, 22*(15), 5002–5016. https://doi.org/10.1039/D0GC01366H
Zuin, V. G., Eilks, I., Elschami, M., & Kümmerer, K. (2021). Education in green chemistry and in sustainable chemistry: Perspectives towards sustainability. *Green Chemistry, 23*(4), 1594–1608. https://doi.org/10.1039/D0GC03313H

Chapter 14
Exploring Socio-Cultural Influences on Active Transportation Behaviour for Health Improvement

Sui Yu Yau

Abstract Socio-cultural factors refer to the group-level attributes of the life cycle circumstances such as modelling, social support, social climate, and culture. The social environment is considered an important contributor to active transport behaviour for health improvement by a number of researchers. An individual's interaction with various social environments impacts health-related behaviour such as physical activity participation. In turn, participating in physical activity contributes to the social well-being of individuals. Research studies on health behaviour often concentrate on investigating the individual characteristics of health-related behaviour or lifestyle that form certain health behaviours. As a result, interventional studies focused on changes in health behaviour have often yield unsatisfactory results due to neglecting to include the influence of the broader social contexts that shape behaviour. Although it is known that certain behaviours could lead to disease development, how the behaviours appear, and are maintained and modified remains unclear. Thus, there is a growing concern to study the role of social context in shaping health behaviour for health improvement.

Keywords Active transportation · Physical activity · Health behaviour · Socio-cultural influences

Introduction

Socio-cultural factors refer to the group-level attributes of the life cycle circumstances (Alfonzo, 2005) such as modelling, social support, social climate, crime, and culture (Sallis et al., 2006). The social environment is considered an important contributor to physical activity participation by a number of researchers (Hu et al., 2021; Lisboa et al., 2021; Van Luchene & Delens, 2021). An individual's interaction

S. Y. Yau (✉)
School of Nursing and Health Studies, Hong Kong Metropolitan University, Hong Kong, China
e-mail: isyyau@hkmu.edu.hk

B. Y. F. Fong and W. C. W. Wong (eds.), *Gaps and Actions in Health Improvement from Hong Kong and Beyond*,
https://doi.org/10.1007/978-981-99-4491-0_14

with various social environments impacts health-related behaviour such as physical activity participation (Hu et al., 2021). In turn, participating in physical activity contributes to the social well-being of individuals (World Health Organization, 2018). Research studies on health behaviour often concentrate on investigating the individual characteristics of health-related behaviour or lifestyle that form certain health behaviours (Fiorilli et al., 2022; Glass & McAtee, 2006). As a result, interventional studies focused on changes in health behaviour have often yielded unsatisfactory results due to neglecting to include the influence of the broader social contexts that shape behaviour (Glass & McAtee, 2006; McKinlay & Marceau, 2000). Although it is known that certain behaviours could lead to disease development, how the behaviours appear, and are maintained and modified remains unclear (Glass & McAtee, 2006). Thus, there is a growing concern to study the role of social context in shaping health behaviour. This chapter focuses on the complexity of the socio-cultural influences on active transport by walking (ATW) behaviours for health improvement.

Socio-Cultural Factors Influencing Active Transport Behaviours

Social environment is "the sum total of social and cultural conditions, circumstances, and human interactions that encompass human beings" (Kirst-Ashman, 2000, p. 5). It includes the social relationships and the culture that an individual interacts with (Barnett & Casper, 2001). For instance, all of the individuals, friends, families, groups, organisations, communities, and system are involved in the social environment (Kirst-Ashman, 2000). In addition, the power relations, race, social inequalities, cultural processes, art, religion, and beliefs constitute the components of a social environment (Barnett & Casper, 2001).

Health behaviour is determined by multiple variables, with the social context of an individual being one of the variables that can impact on health behaviour (Bandura, 1986; Hu et al., 2021; Lisboa et al., 2021; Van Luchene & Delens, 2021). Social influences are known to be multidimensional constructs (Mourali et al., 2005) and the differences in social context are associated with different health behaviours (Nettle, 2010).

The social environment including having friends or knowing neighbours living within walking distance of the neighbourhood promotes walking amongst adolescents or children (Johansson & Hartig, 2011; Rybråten et al., 2019). King and colleagues (2002) highlighted conceptual approaches to physical activity and categorised the socio-cultural environment to include a micro-environment of the immediate local environment within an individual's home or workplace, including such items as the operant conditions, social learning, and social cognitive influences.

Within the socio-ecological framework, cultural, and social factors across time entwine with intrapersonal factors to form our behaviours, that if rehearsed become habits. The behaviours or habits we adopt, contribute to the formation of cultural and social norms that in turn impact the behaviours of those proximal to us, and contribute to broader cultural influences more distally.

This chapter reports the socio-cultural factors influencing active transportation behaviour for a group of thirteen young adults who grew up at a metropolitan city, Hong Kong, as part of a large scale study (Yau & O'Connor, 2021). The influences by peers as supportive resources and family practice were supported as facilitators and barriers for ATW. Data from this study added support to the notion of the power of interpersonal, social, and cultural structures, over time, to impact health behaviour.

Peers as Supportive Resources

Peers played an important role in establishing social norms and encouraging social connectedness through ATW and were consequently highlighted by the participants as key resources or assets for ATW. This aspect of social and cultural behaviour as a key resource for ATW is worth considering in the Hong Kong context, particularly in contrast to other Westernised cities where transport is often researched, planned for, and promoted as an individualised behaviour. How the peers within a social group perceived walking for ATW and adopted it as practice was influential in directing the behaviours of group members. Choosing the travel mode for a destination, for example, was mentioned as a social process by all thirteen participants. This is exemplified by Lau who stated:

> We [Lau and her friends] will decide what kind of travel mode we want to choose when we are going to a place. Usually, we will go there together by the same travel mode. We never go to a place by different travel mode… it's because it seems we can experience better relationships with each other by travelling together. (Lau)

Similarly, Ho described her active transport with friends as a social practice when she stated:

> Here are my friends who always walk with me after study. We gather together after lessons… and then walk … it's our practice. (Ho)

Once a norm for group travel was established, it appeared to regulate individual behaviours. For instance, So described an established behavioural pattern for her and her friends to meet at the railway station every morning where they would travel to the University by walking for about 30 min. Without her friends, So indicated it would be highly unlikely she would engage in ATW, but rather utilise other motorised modes of transport such as a minibus instead. Similarly, Fung expressed: "I like to walk with them [the friends] after study… and I am eager to walk… otherwise…" (Fung). Fung suggested that without the social group, he would lack the motivation to walk.

This sense of social connectedness mediated individual motives and decisions towards ATW. Leung mentioned how mode of travel varied according to the influence of the social group:

> I will not go to Mong Kok by walking alone. However, when I am with my friends, we will walk there, because my friends usually go to Mong Kok by walking… (Leung)

Yau pointed out that his own choice of travel mode was highly influenced by peer choice. Leung shared similar views, whilst Hung indicated:

> I could chat with my friends if I walk with them. I am happier as someone is accompanying me. We could discuss what was happening in the day… I don't get bored. Thus, I will follow whatever travel mode my friends choose…If they [the friends] are going to Monk Kok by walking after school, I will walk with them. If they are not willing to walk, I will wait for their decisions on the mode of travel. If they want to go there by minibus, I will follow them as well. (Hung)

Ng also emphasised that it was "important to have friends to accompany me during active transport. I enjoy the time spent walking with them" (Ng). She elaborated that being accompanied by friends was a major factor motivating her to walk. So, shared that, she "…loved walking with friends…" (So) as she could chat during walking.

Cheung even pointed out travelling together was a shared experience within the social group that was highly valued and considered as an integral part of daily life:

> I want to have a shared experience with my friends during the journey… we know what's happening while we walk and we know what we encounter during the journey… (Cheung)

In contrast to joining with peers and the resultant connectedness, not wanting to show disconnectedness was also a factor in compelling participation. Ten participants noted that not joining the social group during any mode of travel could potentially affect peer relationships and to do so could be considered rude. Law highlighted this potential for feeling socially isolated if he didn't undertake travel with the social group when he noted, "if not joining with them… it seems that I am [an outlier]… I would feel a bit strange… and detached from the social group" (Law). Just as active transport could serve to be social glue, four participants demonstrated how it could be used to get distance from unwanted friends as noted by Kwan:

> I won't walk with people that I don't like. For example, if I need to leave at the same time as an unwanted friend… if I know that he or she is leaving by walking, then, I will be leaving by another mode. I want to minimise the contact with that unwanted friend. I feel better if I don't need to travel with him or her. (Kwan)

Unpacking the social group's role in mediating ATW required an exploration of the role of decision-makers within the collective. Nine of the participants nominated that their peers played an important and influential role in initiating their transport mode decisions. Within social groups, there would be some who adopted the dominant practice of the group (followers) and others who would set the agenda for travel (leaders). Four participants, Ho, Cheung, Yau, and Tsui, indicated that they frequently tried to persuade their friends to engage in ATW. These four participants expressed that they enjoyed active transport and would initiate opportunities to walk with their peers. For example, "I always invite them [the friends] to join me walking… and they always listen to and follow me" (Ho). Ho went on to elaborate that on the day of the interview, despite her friends feeling tired and unwilling to go home by walking, Ho persuaded them to walk with her. Like Ho, Cheung indicated that she persuaded her friends to walk with her and she did so by making advocacy arguments for walking as active transport.

It appeared social leadership within a social group was a driver for initiating active transport behaviours of those in the peer group. These four participants were self-described advocates for active transport and clearly articulated their roles in initiating others behaviour. In the context of Chinese culture, males are often considered to hold superior decision-making positions to women. This culture appeared to impact active transport behaviour for one of the participants in particular within this study. Ho, whilst clearly articulating her ability to advocate for active travel behaviour amongst her peers, felt subordinate to her boyfriend and his choice of travel mode. Ho indicated that she was "obliged to follow my boyfriend's decision" (Ho) in relation to travel mode. She further highlighted that her boyfriend was her advocate for all of her personal affairs and she pointed out that the closer their relationship, the greater his influence on her. Thus, despite her own sense of strong leadership that she felt she displayed amongst her peers, her capacity to make choices about travel mode were influenced by her boyfriend who preferred more sedentary travel behaviour.

This finding may have some broader significance given the potentially heavy influence of Chinese culture within Hong Kong. Concepts of individual behaviour choice in relation to transport mode were not isolated from historical cultural and gendered practices. Gendered practices around choice of travel played an important role in mediating active transport behaviour for at least one participant in this study where the male was the key decision-maker in the context of a culturally reproduced hierarchical relationship.

Family Practice Supports Active Transport

Of the thirteen participants in the study, ten expressed their current active transport behaviours as being built from a history of practice, heavily influenced by the modelling of behaviour from family. The role that significant others, particularly parents, played in shaping behaviour was apparent in the data. The findings for how family practices mediated active transport suggest a history of family practice is a resource that supports individuals' active transport behaviour. Cheung highlighted how the habits of his parents influenced the formation of his own active transport behaviour:

> it's influenced by my family… when I went out with my dad and mum when I was young, we walked together. Walking is habitual for them and I am influenced. (Cheung)

Fung shared the same view and highlighted in the following statement:

> I walked with my dad and mum when I was a child. They liked to walk whenever they could… I am fine walking with them… it (walking) becomes my habit as well. (Fung)

Another participant, Law whose parents also walked for transport since he was a child, highlighted:

> my parents love to walk… I think their habits really influence me… I was walking with them when I was a child, their behaviours definitely impacted on my current practice… (Law)

The adoption of the parent practice for walking is clearly not a one to one determinant of behaviour, but for these participants, parental influence was raised as a powerful influence on current practice. Ho further pointed out that "I may not be eager to walk now if my parents drove private cars when I was young…" (Ho).

For many of these participants, parental influence was identified as a powerful mediator of current practice. Through time spent walking with their parents as children, it is likely participants in this study adopted strategies for coping with barriers and established a familiarity bias together with an affinity for place as highlighted by Cheung that "I used to walk with my parents when I was young… I love to observe the environment".

In contrast to the ten participants whose parents were actively engaged in active transport, three participants noted how their own parents did not participate in active transport, yet they and their siblings did. These participants could provide no accounts of their parents supporting or promoting active transport. For instance, Ng stated that, "my parents do not like walking, they loved to travel by car" (Ng). Although Ng's parents were adopting more sedentary modes of travel through their own practices, the practices did not necessarily impact on Ng's active transport engagement. Similarly, Lau and Fung also noted that given the choice, their parents would not choose to walk on most occasions.

The parental practice was one of the socio-cultural framings that showed impact on their children's active transport participation which might form as behaviours and become habits. Although the three participants' parents were adopting more sedentary modes of travel through their own practices, the practices did not necessarily impact on the three participants' active transport engagement. It seemed that parental practices might be a positive driver on the participants' current active transport practice as indicated earlier. However, parental role modelling was not essential for active travel amongst this particular cohort as stated by socio-ecological models that multiple influences would impact on individual's health behaviour.

Conclusion

Data within the interpersonal domain supported the finding that mode of travel choice was influenced by a desire to maintain social connectedness and conversely avoid being perceived as unsociable. How individuals chose to participate in active transport for this group of young university students (or not) was highly influenced by the social context. The extent to which this social factor exists across different cross sections of the community or simply remains unique to this particular cohort is unclear. What was clear, however, was the extent to which social ties amongst this group of active commuters influenced individual adoption of active transport. It would seem that for these young adults; active transport was viewed positively when it facilitated socialisation and provided opportunities to talk. ATW was enhanced as a consequence of it being a social experience and this presented a significant source of motivation. When commuting with others, active transport was perceived as relaxing and consequently the act of walking was not viewed as a physical exercise, a chore or laborious.

Data also suggested that champions for ATW exist within the social groupings of these young Hong Kong adults and these champions might offer a strategic way to leverage other group members to engage in active transportation modes. Finally, family role modelling appeared to play some role in ATW for these young Hong Kong adults. Connecting the social spaces of young adults with active transport offers a potential line of inquiry for exploring further how active transport can be considered a supportive social experience and how this social experience can in turn support active modes of transport.

Implications for Policy Decision-Making

The findings in this study were the first known to the author that had discussed how Chinese culture has impacted individual's ATW participation. How the cultural factors have mediated ATW behaviour for the participants within Chinese society is worthy of further attention. Despite Hong Kong being a culturally mixed Western and Chinese city, the impact of traditional Chinese culture and values were evident in the data. Chinese values and beliefs, namely collectivism, hierarchical decision-making, notions of conformity, filial piety, the philosophy of Confucianism, stereotyped roles, familism, and the ideology of yin and yang, mediated engagement in ATW.

In addition, the social networks and social norms of peers and parents were important assets that impacted ATW behaviours amongst the cohort of young adults. The findings revealed that these values and beliefs associated with the social network were also likely linked to Chinese culture and guided the ATW behaviour of participants.

Several important observations have arisen in this study. First, unlike the individualistic nature of Western society, the notion of collectivism and social isolation in Chinese society appeared to influence individual behaviour within the peer group travel. Therefore, some collective control over individual travel mode was evident in this study. This was particularly noticeable when participants spoke of being socially isolated if they were unable to travel with the peer group. Second, there was evidence of hierarchical decision-making within peer groups that impacted ATW. Decision-making hierarchies were evident in the data with the notion of following a leader prominent in Chinese society. The social leaders made advocacy arguments for group ATW behaviour and appeared influential in setting the agenda for travel. Third, the notions of conformity within the cultural values of Chinese society are a potentially powerful influence on the choice of travel mode. The Chinese place great importance on an individual's identity conforming within a social group, whilst following the peers' choice of travel mode served to confirm socially acceptable behaviour without the risk of being labelled as an "outsider". Fourth, the central values and beliefs of familism and filial piety in the Confucian ideological system emphasises the centrality of the family, authoritarian and controlling parenting, and the practice of obeying parental decisions. The values and belief on how individuals are embedded within a family and the close social ties within the Chinese family critically impact on individual behaviour. The findings identified the significance of parental influence as a powerful mediator of an individual's current practice. Last, the long and rich history of gender stereotyped roles, especially males dominating decision-making in Chinese culture, carried over into decisions about ATW. This was partially explained by the familial domain of Confucianism and the ideology of yin and yang in Chinese culture that differentiates the social status for both genders. The gender stereotyping supports males as being strong masculine leaders and females as being obedient. The findings signal that males may play a pivotal role in determining ATW behaviour within a social group. These findings do not seek to confirm or deny there are gendered mediators, or any other social mediators on travel mode choice within the limited data provided. They do however signal that there should be a consideration of the culturally reinforced gender roles impacting ATW.

The findings have potentially shed some light for policy-makers on strategies helpful for facilitating ATW behaviour in Hong Kong or similar urbanised contexts. Previous studies, which have adopted direct and objectively measured methods to investigate the policy environment necessary for facilitating ATW, have focused too much on what is not working and not paying enough attention to the bidirectional influences across multiple level influences within socio-ecologies. This study contends that policy decision-making should be based on the perception and needs of individuals within these broader contexts. Thus, the implications for the policy environment, explored in the current study, are believed to provide a more appropriate policy approach to implementation focused on the unique socio-cultural environment within the Hong Kong context. Last but not least, through addressing and promoting socio-cultural impacts on ATW behaviour, it would possibly a strategy to achieve "health for all, all for health" in the community.

References

Alfonzo, M. A. (2005). To walk or not to walk? The hierarchy of walking needs. *Environment and Behavior, 37*(6), 808–836. https://doi.org/10.1177/0013916504274016

Bandura, A. (1986). *Social foundations of thought and action: A social cognitive theory*. Prentice Hall.

Barnett, E., & Casper, M. (2001). A definition of "social environment." *American Journal of Public Health, 91*(3), 465. https://doi.org/10.2105/ajph.91.3.465a

Fiorilli, G., Buonsenso, A., Centorby, M., Calcagno, G., Iuliano, E., Angiolillo, A., Ciccotelli, S., di Cagno, A., & Di Costanzo, A. (2022). Long term physical activity improves quality of life perception, healthy nutrition, and daily life management in elderly: A randomized controlled trial. *Nutritions, 14*, Article 2527. https://doi.org/10.3390/nu14122527

Glass, T. A., & McAtee, M. J. (2006). Behavioral science at the crossroads in public health: Extending horizons, envisioning the future. *Social Science & Medicine, 62*(7), 1650–1671. https://doi.org/10.1016/j.socscimed.2005.08.044

Hu, D., Zhou, S., Crowley-McHattan, Z. J., & Liu, Z. (2021). Factors that influence participation in physical activity in school-aged children and adolescents: A systematic review from the social ecological model perspective. *International Journal of Environmental Research and Public Health, 18*(6), 3147–3168. https://doi.org/10.3390/ijerph18063147

Johansson, M., & Hartig, T. (2011). Psychological benefits of walking: Moderation by company and outdoor environment. *Health and Well-Being, 3*(3), 261–280. https://doi.org/10.1111/j.1758-0854.2011.01051.x

King, A. C., Stokols, D., Talen, E., Brassington, G. S., & Killingsworth, R. (2002). Theoretical approaches to the promotion of physical activity: Forging a transdisciplinary paradigm. *American Journal of Preventive Medicine, 23*(Suppl. 2), 15–25. https://doi.org/10.1016/S0749-3797(02)00470-1

Kirst-Ashman, K. K. (2000). *Human behavior, communities, organizations and groups in the macro social environment: An empowerment approach.* Brooks/Cole.

Lisboa, T., da Silva, W. R., Silva, D. A. S., Felden, E. P. G., Pelegrini, A., Lopes, J. J. D., & Beltrame, T. S. (2021). Social support from family and friends for physical activity in adolescence: Analysis with structural equation modeling. *Reports in Public Health, 37*(1), Article e00196819. https://doi.org/10.1590/0102-311x00196819

McKinlay, J. B., & Marceau, L. D. (2000). Upstream healthy public policy: Lessons from the battle of tobacco. *International Journal of Health Services, 30*(1), 49–69. https://doi.org/10.2190/2v5h-rhbr-ftm1-kgcf

Mourali, M., Laroche, M., & Pons, F. (2005). Individualistic orientation and consumer susceptibility to interpersonal influence. *Journal of Services Marketing, 19*(3), 164–173. https://doi.org/10.1108/08876040510596849

Nettle, D. (2010). Why are there social gradients in preventative health behavior? A perspective form behavioral ecology. *PLoS ONE, 5*(10), Article e13371. https://doi.org/10.1371/journal.pone.0013371

Rybråten, S., Skår, M., & Nordh, H. (2019). The phenomenon of walking: Diverse and dynamic. *Landscape Research, 44*(1), 62–74. https://doi.org/10.1080/01426397.2017.1400527

Sallis, J. F., Cervero, R. B., Ascher, W., Henderson, K. A., Kraft, M. K., & Kerr, J. (2006). An ecological approach to creating active living communities. *Annual Review of Public Health, 27*, 297–322. https://doi.org/10.1146/annurev.publhealth.27.021405.102100

Van Luchene, P., & Delens, C. (2021). The influence of social support specific to physical activity on physical activity among college and university students: A systematic review. *Journal of Physical Activity and Health, 18*(6), 737–747. https://doi.org/10.1123/jpah.2020-0713

World Health Organization. (2018). *Global action plan on physical activity 2018–2030: More active people for a healthier world.* https://apps.who.int/iris/bitstream/handle/10665/272722/9789241514187-eng.pdf

Yau, S. Y., & O'Connor, J. (2021). Shaping built environments for community health: A qualitative exploration of active transport by walking. In B. Y. F. Fong & M. C. S. Wong (Eds.), *The Routledge handbook of public health and the community* (pp.196–211). Routledge. https://doi.org/10.4324/9781003119111-18-21

Part III
The All for Health Strategies

Chapter 15
Equity in Healthcare for Ethnic Minorities

John Lee and David Briggs

Abstract This chapter traverses published research about healthcare for ethnic minorities across the Asia Pacific countries from differing perspectives to identify contemporary practice, policy, and challenges in ensuring all for health and health for all in ethnic communities. Healthcare has now become a globalised concept and there has been concern in the Asia Pacific about equity of access to health services across the region with a focus on disparity between rich and poor, urban, and rural and of marginalised groups that include migrants, refugees, and other ethnic minorities, in situ within nation states. The diversity of approaches across Asia Pacific nations to the status and delivery of healthcare for ethnic communities is described using contemporary published research. Concepts around ethnic communities are diverse and complex but generally are said to be influenced by culture, behaviours, values, and the context in which they are described as being an ethnic minority. The impact on these groups based on disease category is also traversed. Lessons learned and implications for the future and the importance of leadership, technology, and empirical research are discussed. Consistent with the book title this chapter describes the experience of nation states across the Asia Pacific to analyse, compare, and contrast approaches in addressing 'Gaps and actions in health improvement from Hong Kong and beyond' utilising a 'health for all' perspective.

Keywords Ethnic minorities · Migrants · Refugees · Healthcare · Access and equity · Universal healthcare · Socio-economic determinants of health · Leadership · Management

---

J. Lee (✉)
United Christian Nethersole Community Health Service, Hong Kong, China
e-mail: johnlkh@connect.hku.hk

D. Briggs
University of New England, Armidale, NSW, Australia

B. Y. F. Fong and W. C. W. Wong (eds.), *Gaps and Actions in Health Improvement from Hong Kong and Beyond*,
https://doi.org/10.1007/978-981-99-4491-0_15

Introduction

This chapter responds to the challenges of the title wherein it is published, that addresses 'Gaps and Actions in Health Improvement: Health for All, All for Health' and, as such must address issues of access, fairness, and impetus for equity across communities, populations, and nation states. These themes are addressed throughout the chapter. In this case, one of the authors has professional clinical experience of ethnic minorities access to the health system of Hong Kong and the second author has worked extensively with health systems of the Asia Pacific and from those interests we take an approach that reflects an international and inter-disciplinary approach in an Asia Pacific context. This chapter traverses published research about healthcare for ethnic minority groups across Asia Pacific countries from differing perspectives to identify contemporary practice, policy, and challenges in ensuring all for health and health for all in ethnic communities.

The Geographic and Demographic Context of Ethnic Healthcare

Migration from low to middle income to highly industrialised high-income countries is known to have a detrimental impact on health, voluntary migrants achieve a positive 'health migrant effect' and the longer the duration of residence, the higher prevalence of risk factors, leading to morbidity and mortality from chronic conditions. Forced migrants can face higher risks and, for example, cardiometabolic risks are different between and within ethnic groups (Gallegos et al., 2019). Refugees are often cast in the light of being challenged about the extent of access to health and other services in the country that they have sought refuge. This is despite the nature and values of the host nation and aspirations of health professionals and health systems and governments. In fact, many health professionals are activists in asserting for the rights and freedoms of refugees to gain equivalency of access to healthcare in similar fashion to that of the majority population (Ferdowsian, 2021). Shum (2011) in an article on refugees also took the wider perspective around physical space, power relationships to space available and environment as did Wong et al. (2017), who broadened the debate by suggesting a framework based on the socio-economic determinants of health (SOECD).

Wong et al. (2017) described in an article about African asylum seekers and refugees in Hong Kong, wherein the United Nations High Commissioner for Refugees (UNHCR) suggests that 51.2 million people were forcibly displaced in 2014 and that Hong Kong, as a 'hot spot' for transit, has over 10,000 asylum seekers, refugees, and torture claimants (ASRs) in 2016; approximately 10% of these are from the African continent. Interestingly, this article describes this population utilising the Social Determinants of Health as a framework (CSDH) provided by Solar and Irwin (2010). The impact of extended periods of immigration detention has been researched in several counties where detainees experienced pervasive difficulties long after their detention ended as they struggled to rebuild their lives, with poor self-esteem, depression, and anxiety amongst other experiences (Coffey et al., 2010).

Healthcare has now become a globalised concept, exemplified by the recent focus on addressing the coronavirus disease 2019 (COVID) pandemic and the need for nations states and health professionals to develop and address preventative strategies across nation state boundaries. We need to acknowledge that someone who has been defined as a minority 'ethnic' in one nation state may have come from a majority population in another country. They may also be Indigenous or Aboriginal in their own country, but a minority in the population of the present.

During the pandemic of COVID 19, the vaccination rate amongst ethnic minorities group has also shown a hesitancy to participate from the ethnic minorities community (Chua et al., 2022), which proves the diversity of all for health amongst ethnic minorities is not implanted or executed comprehensively. A recent systematic review by Chauhan et al. (2020) suggested that patients from an ethnic minority may have experienced disparity in the quality and safety of care through a range of socio-cultural influences. However, there is also available evidence about the nature of the care of this group that will allow development of safe care interventions for the future.

Equity of Access to Healthcare

There has been concern in the Asia Pacific about equity of access to health services across the region with a focus on disparity between rich and poor, urban and rural, and of marginalised groups that include migrants and ethnic minorities. Fong (2021) provides an extensive and contemporary overview in a bioethics paper on equitable healthcare systems that clearly defines and emphasises the importance of equity and the dimensions of international approaches to equity. In that article, equity is defined as the absence of differences in health status of people that encompasses perspectives of socio-economic differences, including ethnicity, class, geographic location, and levels of education (p. 547).

In current contexts, most countries can also include refugees escaping conflict or persecution and economic poverty. These issues were addressed in a background paper by the UN Regional Thematic Working Group on Health (TWGH) to suggest remedies to overcome existing inequities. Key interests of this group included how to increase regional coordination, alignments, and coherence of services. As a result, health was defined as one of five priorities and created a Thematic Working Group on Health (TWGH). At that time and in that context government expenditure on health was described as one of the lowest in most Asia Pacific countries being below five percent of GDP. Malaysia, Sri Lanka, and Thailand were exampled as demonstrating better and more efficient health spending (Durairaj, 2007).

Countries are challenged to achieve universal access to healthcare (UHC) in the Asia Pacific because improvements in policies, strategies, and activities through greater targeted government investment accrue mostly to underserved disadvantaged countries and populations. Government and private expenditure across the region are in—equitability distributed. Out of pocket and catastrophic spending is significant and impacting on the poverty levels of some countries. Health spending is said to be low in countries where the disease burden is high. As is the case in most countries health systems, public health, and preventative services are less appropriately funded in comparison to that received by curative services. Physical access to care is also likely to be concentrated in high-income urbanised areas (Durairaj, 2007).

Fong (2021, p. 552) further addresses the earlier work of Mate and Wyatt who propose five ways to make health equity a core strategy. These authors suggest health equity is a leader-driven priority with organisation wide structures and processes that are designed to support equity, address the social determinants of health, and address all forms of discriminatory health practice and reflect practice based on partnerships with community organisations.

We now turn to address the literature of how the differing nation states of the Asia Pacific are addressing these challenges, commencing with Hong Kong and mainland China, Thailand and Cambodia, Malaysia, Australia, Singapore, Japan, Vietnam, Indonesia, and New Zealand. Given the global nature of the movement of refugees and ethnic minorities, narrative about North America and Europe is also included. Readers are encouraged to compare and contrast the differing national experiences and to identify themes relevant to your individual circumstances and contexts.

Hong Kong and Mainland China

In the last decade, the population of ethnic minority residents in Hong Kong, China, has increased by 30%, excluding those who are 'foreign domestic helpers' from Indonesia and the Philippines and who originate from South Asian, India, Pakistan, and Nepal. All these groups have poorer health literacy in Chinese and English, differing cultural perspectives and health literacy, making access to all aspects of healthcare more difficult. This demonstrates that health professionals and health systems need better understanding of the knowledge, understanding, and attitudes (KAP) of ethnic minorities who seek access to care and who require greater education in the use of information (Wong et al., 2017).

Wong and colleagues (2017) in Hong Kong describe significant demographic change with rapid population ageing and immigration. They further suggest ethnic minorities find accessing services difficult in a first-time study of Nepalese older adults. While their needs are assessed as like the local Chinese, the study showed that they also faced a 'range of structural, knowledge and attitudinal barriers' to access to long-term care, despite access entitlement and the WHO Age-Friendly Cities framework (AFC). This framework proposes collaborative interventions based on eight domains of 'economic, social, physical, personal, behavioural, and service factors. The domains include outdoor, spaces and buildings, transportation, housing, social participation, respect, social inclusion, civic participation, employment, communication and information, community support, and health services (Amoah et al., 2019, p. 3). They challenge the reader to take an SOECD approach to healthcare. It will be interesting to see how well this framework also addresses its potential for ethnic minorities in communities. Both Hong Kong and China face high demand from existing populations for healthcare with differing funding and delivery systems and with no commonality about how those differences and demand for services might be met (Kong et al., 2015).

In Mainland China, a systematic review of maternal and child health outcomes of ethnic minorities in Western China suggests that minority populations across the world often have worse health social and health outcomes, although there is variability within the groups. The reasons are complex and variable but are said to relate to elements of employment, income, education, food security, policy, and systems perspectives as well as social and cultural norms. There are 55 ethnic minority populations in China that represent a highly heterogeneous population. Despite positive policy approaches and extensive data, research has been limited and a need to improve information is emphasised. This review provided strong evidence of poorer health outcomes on maternal and child health outcomes than the general population in Western China (Huang et al., 2018).

Non-communicable diseases (NCDs) are responsible for an estimated 63% of global deaths and China is facing an increased burden of NCDs when ethnicity is seen as an important risk factor, with different outcomes for cancer, diabetes, cardiovascular and respiratory disease, compared to majority populations. Zhao and Associates (2021) provide an extensive China Multi-ethnic (CMEC) study that is community based, prospective observational study aimed at understanding NCDs prevalence and risk.

Thailand and Cambodia

In contrast, in Thailand, ethnic minority populations have poorer healthcare utilisation than Thais on the Thai-Myanmar border region because of lack of health insurance coverage, geographic and physical barriers making access difficult. Various cultural differences with language, belief, and religion also impact access. Some of these beliefs extend to 'spiritual beliefs' together with a lack of Thai language for groups such as Karen and Mon, adding to these difficulties. Hu and Podhisita (2008) detail the extensive nature of these ethnic minorities in Thailand. Civil conflict in Myanmar has seen the displacement of ethnic minority groups into Thailand where an estimated 3.7 million migrants are estimated to be living, with the largest number from Myanmar. While presenting challenges in managing these types of populations, particularly in managing infectious diseases, Thailand and Cambodia have managed well, in registering migrants to provide access to health insurance and using a one stop shop model to achieve both registration and health insurance conjointly. The use of migrant's navigators to and through health systems is also suggested (Murray et al.,

2016). An inter-ethnic, cross-sectional study amongst Thai older adults and retired Japanese residents in Chang Mai into differences in body composition concluded that ethnicity had a clinically important effect on body composition. The potential differences existed between the two groups and 'the sarcopenia prevention strategies should take ethnicity into account' (Yoda et al., 2021, p. 6).

Malaysia

In an article describing healthcare delivery in Malaysia, Thomas et al. (2011) describe a changing context in Malaysia towards greater equitable financing, a greater focus on wellness services in a context of public, private provision, traditional, complimentary, and western medicine. Constituting for about 5% of the Malaysian population, a million people are described as 'immigrant workers', potentially harbouring communicable diseases that require specific attention to this ethnic minority. The authors also describe the Asia Pacific as the most varied region in the world that includes the country with the largest population and varying paces of transition from communicable diseases to a widening burden of chronic diseases. They also suggest that 'various countries and the WHO are taking control of progress through primary health care (PHC)' (Thomas et al., 2011, p. 95).

Thomas et al. (2011, p. 95) describe how a large proportion of the population is transitioning through economic transition, where deaths from chronic disease are beginning to predominate. While PHC is variable across nations, accessibility of basic care and equity is improving. In Malaysia, they cite increases in diabetes, hypertension, and for women malnutrition and high morbidity in the less developed countries. Their article (Thomas et al., 2011, p. 95) identifies that 'the populations most in need are Aborigines, the poor, the disadvantaged and disabled. In this article it is also suggested that multidisciplinary interventions are required to promote health financing, health care and disease prevention (Low 2008)'.

Again Chauhan et al. (2020, p. 25) in their systematic review conclude that ethnic minorities 'may experience inequity in the safety of care' have 'higher risk of safety events'. They further conclude that health systems and services must consider 'ethnic variations to understand where and how to invest resources to enhance equity in the safety of care'.

Australia

Ethnic minorities are often described in the literature by race, language, and the capacity for English language and by the country of origin. Australia is seen as the land of Aboriginal and Torres Strait Islander peoples historically but is also defined as a nation of migrants and one that is culturally diverse with a population in excess of 25 million, coming from 190 different countries, 300 different ancestral backgrounds and 30 separately identified languages spoken at home (Woodland et al., 2021). The Australian health system is described more fully elsewhere (Briggs, 2017) and is ranked 1st in terms of equity and health outcomes, 8th for access, and 3rd in overall rankings but is 9th out of 11 countries for a ranking for access to care. Australia demonstrates equity through a mix of spending caps that are 'lower for low-income earners, with incentives to seek primary care with 86% of citizens facing no 'out of pocket' expenses for primary care visits (Schneider et al., 2021, p. 11). There is a disproportionate burden of disease amongst ethnic groups within Australia and variability between groups of different country of origin and of different types of migrants such as 'family reunion' and 'refugee' (Gallegos et al., 2019).

Aboriginal and Torres Strait Islanders (ATSI) in Australia in demographic terms are a minority population of about 3.3% of the total population. There are diverse linguistic and cultural groups within the ATSI definition and geographically they are as much an urban dweller as rural, regional, and remote. In some cases, they are the majority population in rural regional and remote communities. Despite having 'equal' access to the Australian health system there is reluctance to engage based on cultural and colonial historical distrust of the agencies of government. Politically, there is strong commitment to improving morbidity, health outcomes, and lifestyle which are well below those of the general population. This is known as 'closing the gap' and includes a deliberate higher per capita expenditure by government for Indigenous people. There are also specific Aboriginal controlled medical services that are more culturally acceptable to that community, by being more holistic in physical, emotional, cultural, spiritual, and ecological well-being for individuals and community. While Aboriginal community controlled, they also provide services to the local general population. Access continues to be a problem in rural areas because of inadequate workforce and poor public transport. Considerable effort is made to increase the Aboriginal health workforce (Australian Institute of Health & Welfare, 2022).

It is notable that 23–32% direct home care and residential care workers in the general population were born outside Australia and 18% of providers, employ workers from culturally and linguistically diverse (non-English speaking countries). International students that have been absent from Australia during the COVID Pandemic are normally an important ingredient of both the casual health workforce and the general workforce, and Australia is increasingly dependent on an imported overseas workforce for its health and agricultural sectors (Australian Institute of Health & Welfare, 2021). Critically, Australia's rural, regional, and remote medical workforce continues to depend on overseas trained doctors, despite efforts to improve self-sufficiency (O'Sullivan et al., 2019).

A study into care sensitive conditions (ACSAs), also known as Avoidable Hospital Conditions (AHCs), conducted a systematic review that included some findings for the Asia Pacific region. The study suggests that 'avoidable hospital admissions (AHS) can be used as an outcome measure of accessibility and overall effectiveness of primary health care (PHC) for people with a range of characteristics including ethnic minorities and migrants' (Dalla Zuanna et al., 2017, p. 861). They make the point that migration, ethnicity, and race are complex and overlapping concepts and differ in the national contexts in which they are used, sometimes they are used synonymously, or overlap in meaning. They suggest that in countries where migration is well established such as New Zealand and Australia, they cannot be considered to be synonymous. They also cannot be homogeneous, nor can rates of utilisation of healthcare be solely ascribed to ethnicity alone, but it may be access to PHC or preferences for traditional medicine and cultural considerations.

Singapore

Singapore in a recent study into a specific condition diabetes is described as a multi-ethnic country with a Chinese majority and ethnic minority groups of Malay and Indians. The country has a regionalised predominantly public health system. In the study described by the authors as one of the largest Asian studies conducted, suggested that one inter-ethnic disparity finding was that Indians and Malays comprised the highest proportion of the highest risk group of diabetes-related complications compared with the Chinese. Both these groups have also been shown to have poorer diabetes control compared with the Chinese. The authors suggest an interplay of complex environment and socio-economic factors as well as genetic predisposition to insulin disposition in these groups, defining the need for education focussed on their cultural dietary requirements (Seng et al., 2020). Riandini and colleagues (2021) undertook a 10-year observational study of diabetes, a growing epidemic of major concern in Asia into related complications in the multi-ethnic Asian population of Singapore. The study revealed important ethnic differences in the risk of diabetes-related low limb complications (DRLEC) with higher risk for Malays.

Vietnam

Recent research in Vietnam suggests inequities in the ethnic minority populations, women's experience between that group and PHC professionals in remote and rural communities. These inequities persist despite progress generally in maternal and child health in recent decades. There are 54 officially recognised ethnic groups in Vietnam, who are more likely to be poorer than the majority population. These groups, while said to be 'treasured' as demonstrating the cultural diversity of the nation, and where, attempts to improve living standards, are seen to be at the expense of that traditional culture. Geographical, and distance, poor transport, together with low levels of investment in physical and human capital are defined as factors of concern. This study demonstrated scope for better two-way communication and interpersonal communication and patient centred approaches between health professionals and with pregnant women (McKinn et al., 2017).

Interestingly, there are increasing opportunities for Asia Pacific nations to come together to enable regional agenda setting and networking between health systems.

A recent example is a collaborative network for setting a mental health disaster network and agenda. This network has established five priorities of strengthening community engagement and integrating planning and evaluation; assessing capacity for disaster response; optimising emerging technologies in mental health; addressing mental health impacts of climate change; prioritising support for high-risk groups. The convenors of this network record that the Asia Pacific has the highest frequency of hazards and the greatest number of people affected disasters annually with a significant proportion of mental health need not being met. The network is open to all Asia Pacific nations with current participation from Australia, Japan, China, Nepal, Sri Lanka, India, and the USA (Newnham et al., 2020).

Japan

Japan who has joined the above network does so from a base where its population is regarded as homogeneous in ethnicity and where access to mental health services is low. Those that do are likely to come from China, Philippines, Korea, and Brazil. Those that do access services suffered from neurotic and stress related disorders and required family and professional interpreter support (Takubo et al., 2020). Takenaka (2009) asserts that studies in Japan pay little attention to the mobility patterns of foreign migrants as the number of foreign migrants is estimated at 1.5% of the total population meaning that there is tendency to focus on achieved status of education and skill levels rather than an ascribed status of ethnic and national status.

Indonesia

Laksono et al. (2020, p. 584) provide an article about the concept of illness amongst ethnic groups in Indonesia in a meta-ethnographic study concluding that 'the concept of illness in ethnic communities in Indonesia was different from the concept of disease in the modern medical world'. The article traverses the differences in the meaning of illness that creates a social role and behaviours of the concepts and relationships of patients, doctors, and nurses, that persist, even when they might move to other regions. In this study of the available literature, 15 different ethnicities were obtained. There are more than 1,340 ethnic groups in Indonesia with diversity in religion and local languages. The findings indicate illness is defined when individuals are unable to perform normally, 'unable to move normally', causes are ascribed to the 'supernatural or magical things' and because of the 'violation of taboos' (Laksono et al., 2020, p. 586). These metaphors define the health seeking behaviours in ethnic groups in Indonesia and the government policy recognises and regulates traditional medicine and encourages an empirical context to its conduct.

New Zealand

Women in New Zealand 'experience high breast cancer incidence and mortality rates… and it accounts for nearly 28% of cancer registrations and 16% of all cancer deaths. It is worse amongst indigenous Māori women, with a 60% higher incidence. This study intended to examine barriers to access by ethnicity. Besides Indigenous Māori, it included a composite group of people self-identifying as Samoan, Cook Island Māori, Tongan, Tokelauan, Niuean, Fijian, and some from other Pacific Islands who together, comprise 7% of the population with 74% of England, European origins and 12% Asian people. The 'non-Māori/non-Pacific women' reported fewer barriers to access with the highest amongst Pacific women, followed by Māori women. Details to barriers to access and treatment are well described and explored in the detail of the study (Ellison-Loschmann et al., 2015). In another New Zealand study into cardio-vascular disease (CVD), the burden of the disease was greatest amongst Indigenous Māori, Pacific, and Indian people. Amongst the findings, 'Māori and Pacific people had much higher prevalence of smoking, obesity, heart failure, atrial fibrillation and prior CVD'. The study called for strong political commitment and cross-sectorial action (Selak et al., 2020, p. 14).

North America and Europe

In the Northern American context, there has been recent initiatives in improving immigrant and ethnic minority healthcare using community navigators, noted by Shommu et al. (2016) in a systematic review of the use and effectiveness of community navigators in Canada and in the USA. The review suggests evidence of improved health outcomes for a range of disease groups and for the health outcomes of ethnic minority groups. In the European context, there has been a significant and growing proportion of ethnic minorities with significant inflows to most European countries. Earlier assumptions were that infectious diseases were the main concern for health services, but this has now changed to chronic disease and in higher rates than the general population. This context will require scientific and cultural training of health workers, collection of data, and culturally adapted preventative health to give greater emphasis to the health of ethnic minorities (Modesti et al., 2016).

Health Inequality Amongst Minorities

Health inequalities are obvious and a defining theme throughout the narrative of this chapter, depending on the nation states and ethnic communities traversed and within urban and rural contexts and the variety of healthcare providers. These inequalities and the diversity of approaches will be discussed further in this chapter. Taking

Hong Kong as an example, some of the Non-Governmental Organisations (NGOs) in Hong Kong have introduced services focusing on ethnic minority populations for better health outcomes. For instance, the United Christian Nethersole Community Health Service in 2007 introduced a healthcare service named the 'Ethnic Minorities Health Services' to provide primary healthcare service, from preventive to clinical, amongst minorities population in Hong Kong. This should be considered as the initiation in this text of the title to aim for 'All-for-Health'. The service was funded by The Community Chest of Hong Kong, an independent, non-profit charity (https://www.commchest.org/en). While health inequality still exists the fundamental health of the minority's communities, has been secured at least. The initiative of the United Christian Nethersole Community Health Service is described at https://www.ucn.org.hk/en/services/preventive-medicine-and-clinical-service/ethnic-minority-health/ and the detailed service provision is at https://www.ucn-emhealth.org/.

The population who received the South Asian support programme of this service has increased from 21,834 to 23,511 from the year of 2017–2018 to 2018–2019. One of the innovation highlights described in the above links is the smoking cessation service for ethnic minorities and new immigrants. That is part of the services that provide health education, prevention, and treatment measures to minorities population with tobacco abuse. The population of service receivers increased from 2017 to 2019, from 3,438 to 4,973.

In contrast to the initiative of an innovative NGO, the Hospital Authority, responsible for the public sector services provides interpreter and translation services and multi-lingual information in all public hospitals. Vandan and colleagues (2020) identified in a recent study that South Asia participants in a 'Chinese-orientated society' reported lower health system responsiveness but were positive about the care experience. These authors suggested more concerted effort from providers and policy-makers to improve systems for these groups. This contrast raises the question as to how best to provide health services to ethnic communities and are services available to the general population sufficient or should they be specific to the ethnic community? Generally, the answer might be that there is potential for public, private, and not for profit charities to play a role, and perhaps differing roles.

In the meantime, the lack of support in clinical communication amongst ethnic minorities in Hong Kong is always an issue which the stakeholders of ethnic minorities are fighting for. This also includes refugees and asylum seekers who need medical service. Although some of the NGOs in Hong Kong keep developing interpreter service in out-patients and community health services, the demand from the minorities is always greater than the actual availability of services. In contrast, proficiency in Cantonese, English, and even Mandarin is always expected and is often included in the job requirements of healthcare providers, but not even mentioning ethnic minorities languages. This latter context is reflecting the lack of understanding of the importance of both communication and effective engagement of healthcare personnel with demanding language skills in Hong Kong, result in immature primary healthcare support to a multi-diversity community.

Friel et al. (2012) address the social and environmental determinants of health inequity in the Asia Pacific and go to the centrality of NGOs in those approaches. They suggest that 'tackling health inequalities is a political imperative' (p. 897). The article goes to the broader needs of ethnic minorities to the physical living environment for healthy living, improved workplace, and social protection, reducing workers vulnerabilities, providing universal coverage, comprehensive PHC, and equitable access to medicine. These approaches need to be delivered in a way that promotes social inclusion and equity in governance and, a greater emphasis on education, amongst other things. This also implies intersectoral action and active community participation, the involvement of civil society and advocacy. These concepts emphasise 'health for all and all for health' rather than a focus on health systems and services.

The discourse in this chapter also goes to greater consideration of innovation to address the health needs of ethnic minorities as described in some nation states. As cited, Shum (2011) in an article on refugees also took the wider perspective around physical space, power relationships to space available and environment, also currently being considered as an approach in wider health service planning in Australia. Wong et al. (2017) also broadened the debate by suggesting a framework based on the socio-economic determinants of health (SOECD). Using community navigators as described by Shommu et al. (2016) in a systematic review of the use and effectiveness of community navigators in Canada and in the USA, is another example of innovation in healthcare, one that is currently being explored as an approach in primary healthcare in Australia. The potential for specific use of non-government organisations, across sectors and alongside public and private sector providers as described in Hong Kong above and occurring in Australia into commissioning similar organisations in primary healthcare as providers are notable in their innovation. These initiatives reflect a wider emphasis on health reform through innovation, technology, leadership, and across sectorial approaches as discussed below.

Health Reform Through Innovation, Technology, Cross-Sectorial Approaches, and Leadership

One approach for all to consider is to adopt a more innovative approach to service provision. Technology is quickly improving access through telehealth, miniaturised and wearable monitors, and biotechnology and digitalised data are relatively new as is the use of artificial intelligence (AI), but rapidly advancing in use. In the regional and rural context in Australia where communities both general, first nation as Aboriginal & Torres Strait Islanders, and ethnic migrant refugees there is an emphasis on developing innovative approaches that are beginning to see the insertion of navigator positions into local communities to assist individuals to gain access to healthcare and to help them 'navigate' their way through and around service providers. There is also a focus on ensuring that providers are connected through networks of practice (NOP) locally and through distributed networks of practice (DNOP) across wider regional areas (Briggs et al., 2019). This places the emphasis of health reform on how best to deliver and access services across organisational barriers and sectors, rather than attempting to change the structure of the organisations. To achieve this objective, we need well-educated and experienced health professionals, managers, and leaders we need to engage in collaborative research that allows engagement with others in the analysis of data to allow us to move forward utilising evidence based to best practice.

Leadership and management need to be empowered to engage, make sense of what they see in the complexity before them and work across boundaries to deliver or extend services. Leadership requires strategic capacity and critical skills of being flexible, being a systems thinker, being focussed, and an influencer. In the sense-making role leaders should understand the diversity of need, differences in geographic location of populations, culture of ethnic communities and populations and be able to achieve intersectoral collaboration (Briggs, 2021). This suggests the need for authentic leadership that requires self-awareness, relational transparency, balanced processing, and having an internalised moral perspective (Olley, 2021).

Discussion

The research traversed above provides the authors and readers of this text with complex context, a term of 'ethnic minorities' that is not easily defined and, in fact is a term, that has multiple meanings to us all. Ethnic minorities can in fact be Indigenous, such as in Australia where increasingly they are referred to as 'First Nations' and in New Zealand, Māori and Pacific Islands and Indonesia with extensive ethnic minority groups. Hong Kong and Mainland China have extensive ethnic minority groups as part of its domestic workforce, while it is also challenged by refugees in transit and others like Thailand and Cambodia have extensive ethnic minorities who have escaped persecution and war in surrounding countries such as Myanmar, formerly called Burma.

The lesson here is that there is not a simple definition of the term and that it has a range of meanings within and between countries. The provision of healthcare to these groups is also variable and, even where intentions are good, the health outcomes are generally not as good as that of the majority population in each country. In some cases, the variability is seen as disease specific but generally there are poorer outcomes across the chronic diseases. There is also variability of health outcomes based on predisposition for some groups. As ably demonstrated in the article from our colleagues from Indonesia culture, beliefs, and values, heavily influenced health behaviours and how healthcare behaviours need to be socially constructed to be effective (Laksono et al., 2020).

This brings us back to the question as to the value of mainstream services versus specific ethnic healthcare services and their respective effectiveness and our readers will have formed some views about that from having read this chapter. Again, a complex question with no simple answer. Most national health systems, even those with positive policies of universal access tend towards one service model that fits all circumstances. However, the evidence in the research we have presented suggests that a variety of approaches are implemented in different countries to respond to the perspective that the effectiveness of healthcare outcomes is influenced by culture, genetic disposition, the environment, health behaviours and the values, beliefs, training, and education of both health professionals and of the recipients of healthcare.

The authors that have been quoted in this chapter clearly understood the importance of empirical evidence by measuring the effectiveness of health outcomes for ethnic minorities and comparing those results with that of the majority population (Dalla Zuanna et al., 2017, p. 861). In Australia, health pathways are developed to inform clinicians, health systems, and patients of the appropriate health pathway for their specific needs. This is a reasonably simple way, using an empirical approach to measure and determine where health improvements can be identified, and solutions adopted, either individually by clinicians or by health systems. It is an opportunity to use collaborative or participatory action research (CAR/PAR) or continuous qualitative improvement methodologies to secure improved care.

Thailand has been impressive in its more systems approach to health reform by adopting innovation in the use of socio-economic determinants, district health services, millennium development goals, and then sustainable development goals to place general practice and PHC as the centrepiece of access to local health service instead of at hospitals. Collaborative research with a focus on social determinants and SDG3 is central to 'ensure healthy lives and promote well-being for all at all ages. This approach requires a platform to integrate health and social services and encourage participation of all sectors to work together to improve their local people's quality of life (Tejativaddhana et al., 2018, p. 44).

Friel and Associates (2012, pp. 897–899) provide a comprehensive review of policy approaches to address the social and environmental determinants of health inequity in Asia Pacific and propose translating a global vision into regional and local action. They propose that inequities are not inevitable and present an action framework to move forward. Briggs and Isouard (2016) suggest that the language of health reform plays an important part in how we make progress in improving, reforming, and developing both health services and health systems. They suggest that we need to ask the critical questions when considering health reform as what problem are we attempting to address (and) whose interests are being served? They traverse the multiple directions that past frameworks and declarations have influenced and affected our progress. Importantly, they emphasise the importance of localism and the principle of subsidiarity in effecting change, 'locally' where services are being delivered. Briggs (2020, p. 1) in asking where to from here, suggests:

> health development and health reform (should occur) within a framework that encompasses a wider societal context that is based on trusting relationships within a wider community and organisational settings that place valuing health above healthcare and that have a wholistic, patient centred focus.

This is the challenge that we place before those involved in delivering ethnic healthcare in their endeavours to both progress the access and quality of that care and in demonstrating improved outcomes. This chapter demonstrates the importance in ethnic healthcare that culture and our respective values are central to the success of that healthcare and to a concept of holistic care which acknowledges the close relationship between 'body, mind and soul or spirit' (Briggs, 2020, p. 1).

References

Amoah, P. A., Mok, K. H., Wen, Z., & Li, L. W. (2019). Achieving the aged city agenda: An interventional study in Hong Kong's Island district. *Journal of Asian Public Policy, 14*(3), 333–352. https://doi.org/10.1080/17516234.2019.1663981

Australian Institute of Health and Welfare. (2022). *Profile of indigenous Australians*. Retrieved May 17, 2022, from https://www.aihw.gov.au/reports/australias-health/profile-of-indigenous-australians

Australian Institute of Health and Welfare. (2021). *Welfare workforce*. Retrieved May 17, 2022, from https://www.aihw.gov.au/reports/australias-welfare/welfare-workforce

Briggs, D. S. (2017). Challenges for health systems: Australian perspectives. *Public Administration and Policy: An Asia-Pacific Journal, 20*(1), 6–17. https://www.hkpaa.org.hk/_files/ugd/e89acc_2763e81429cf4c08bbb9f13fa84b16fe.pdf

Briggs, D. S. (2020) Health development and health reform: Where to from here? *Journal of Public Health and Development, 18*(1), 67–72. https://he01.tci-thaijo.org/index.php/AIHD-MU/article/view/240600

Briggs, D. S. (2021). From procrastination to reaction! What leadership is required to SHAPE the future of healthcare? *Asia Pacific Journal of Health Management, 16*(4), 5–10. https://doi.org/10.24083/apjhm.v16i4.1321

Briggs, D. S., & Isouard, G. (2016). The language of health reform and health management: Critical issues in the management of health systems. *Asia Pacific Journal of Health Management, 11*(3), 38–44. https://doi.org/10.24083/apjhm.v11i3.153

Briggs, D. S., Nankervis, R., Baillie, J., Turner, C., Rigby, K., & Livingstone, L. (2019). Innovation to improve patient care in an Australian Primary Health Network: An insider's perspective. *Public Administration and Policy: An Asia-Pacific Journal, 22*(2), 111–114. https://doi.org/10.1108/PAP-09-2019-0017

Chauhan, A., Walton, M., Manias, E., Walpola, R. L., Seale, H., Latanik, M., Mears, S., & Harrison, R. (2020). The safety of health care for ethnic minority patients: A systematic review. *International Journal for Equity in Health, 19*, Article 118. https://doi.org/10.1186/s12939-020-01223-2

Chua, G. T., Yan, C. L., Wong, W. H., Sridhar, S., To, K. K., Lau, J., Gurung, S., Mahtani, S., Ho, R., Li, W. S., Cs Yam, J., Rosa Duque, J. S., Wong, I. C. K., Lung Lau, Y., Yat Wah Kwan, M., & Ip, P. (2022). COVID-19 vaccine acceptance and hesitancy among ethnic minorities in Hong Kong. *Human Vaccines & Immunotherapeutics, 18*(5), Article 2054261. https://doi.org/10.1080/21645515.2022.2054261

Coffey, G. J., Kaplan, I., Sampson, R. C., & Tucci, M. M. (2010). The meaning and mental health consequences of long-term immigration detention for people seeking asylum. *Social Science & Medicine, 70*(12), 2070–2079. https://doi.org/10.1016/j.socscimed.2010.02.042

Dalla Zuanna, T., Spadea, T., Milana, M., Petrelli, A., Cacciani, L., Simonato, L., & Canova, C. (2017). Avoidable hospitalization among migrants and ethnic minority groups: A systematic review. *The European Journal of Public Health, 27*(5), 861–868. https://doi.org/10.1093/eurpub/ckx113

Durairaj, V. (2007). Enhancing equity in access to health care in the Asia-Pacific region: Remediable inequities. *World Health Organization*. https://asiapacific.unfpa.org/sites/default/files/pub-pdf/enhancing%20equity%20in%20access%20to%20health%20in%20A-P%20%282007%29.pdf

Ellison-Loschmann, L., Firestone, R., Aquilina, L., McKenzie, F., Gray, M., & Jeffreys, M. (2015). Barriers to and delays in accessing breast cancer care among New Zealand women: Disparities by ethnicity. *BMC Health Services Research, 15*, Article 394.

Ferdowsian, H. R. (2021). Ecological justice and the right to health: An introduction. *Health and Human Rights, 23*(2), 1–5. https://cdn1.sph.harvard.edu/wp-content/uploads/sites/2469/2021/12/editorial_ecological-justice.pdf

Fong, B. (2021). Bioethics Equitable Healthcare Systems. *Medical Law, 40*(4), 547–558.

Friel, S., Loring, B., Aungkasuvapala, N., Baum, F., Blaiklock, A., Chiang, T. L., Loring, B., Aungkasuvapala, N., Baum, F., Blaiklock, A., Chiang, T.-L., Cho, Y., Dakulala, P., Guo, Y., Hashimoto, H., Horton, K., Jayasinghe, S., Matheson, D., Thanh Nguyen, H., … & Surjadi, C. (2012). Policy approaches to address the social and environmental determinants of health inequity in Asia-Pacific. *Asia Pacific Journal of Public Health, 24*(6), 896–914. https://doi.org/10.1177/1010539512460569

Gallegos, D., Do, H., To, Q. G., Vo, B., Goris, J., & Alraman, H. (2019). Differences in cardiometabolic risk markers among ethnic groups in Queensland, Australia. *Health & Social Care in the Community, 27*(4), e449–e458. https://doi.org/10.1111/hsc.12745

Hu, J., & Podhisita, C. (2008). Differential unitlization of health care services among ethnic groups on the Thailand-Myanmar border: A case study of Kanchanaburi Province, Thailand. *Journal of Population and Social Studies, 17*(1), 115–134.

Huang, Y., Shallcross, D., Pi, L., Tian, F., Pan, J., & Ronsmans, C. (2018). Ethnicity and maternal and child health outcomes and service coverage in western China: A systematic review and meta-analysis. *The Lancet Global Health, 6*(1), e39–e56. https://doi.org/10.1016/S2214-109X(17)30445-X

Kong, X., Yang, Y., Gao, J., Guan, J., Liu, Y., Wang, R., Xing, B., Li, Y., & Ma, W. (2015). Overview of the health care system in Hong Kong and its referential significance to mainland China. *Journal of the Chinese Medical Association, 78*(10), 569–573. https://doi.org/10.1016/j.jcma.2015.02.006

Laksono, A. D., Wul, R. D., Nantabah, Z. K., Agustina, Z. A., Aimanah, I. U., Rukmini, R., Fitrianti, Y., Fauzia Wardhani, Y., Effendi, D., Suharmiati, S., Lestari, H., ayani, Pratiw, N., & Pratiwi, N. L. (2020). The Concept of Illness among Ethnic Groups in Indonesia: A Meta-Ethnographic Study. *Systematic Reviews in Pharmacy, 11*(9), 584–591. https://doi.org/10.31838/srp.2020.9.85

McKinn, S., Duong, T. L., Foster, K., & McCaffery, K. (2017). 'I do want to ask, but I can't speak': A qualitative study of ethnic minority women's experiences of communicating with primary health care professionals in remote, rural Vietnam. *International Journal for Equity in Health, 16*, Article 190. https://doi.org/10.1186/s12939-017-0687-7

Modesti, P. A., Perticone, F., Parati, G., Agabiti Rosei, E., & Prisco, D. (2016). Chronic disease in the ethnic minority and migrant groups: Time for a paradigm shift in Europe. *Internal and Emergency Medicine, 11*(3), 295–297. https://doi.org/10.1007/s11739-016-1444-4

Murray, J. K., DiStefano, A. S., Yang, J. S., & Wood, M. M. (2016). Displacement and HIV: Factors influencing antiretroviral therapy use by ethnic Shan migrants in Northern Thailand. *Journal of the Association of Nurses in AIDS Care, 27*(5), 709–721. https://doi.org/10.1016/j.jana.2016.04.006

Newnham, E. A., Dzidic, P. L., Mergelsberg, E. L., Guragain, B., Chan, E. Y. Y., Kim, Y., Leaning, J., Kayano, R., Wright, M., Kaththiriarachchi, L., Kato, H., Osawa, T., & Gibbs, L. (2020). The Asia Pacific disaster mental health network: Setting a mental health agenda for the region. *International Journal of Environmental Research and Public Health, 17*(17), Article 6144. https://doi.org/10.3390/ijerph17176144

O'Sullivan, B., Russell, D. J., McGrail, M. R., & Scott, A. (2019). Reviewing reliance on overseas-trained doctors in rural Australia and planning for self-sufficiency: Applying 10 years' MABEL evidence. *Human Resources for Health, 17*, Article 8. https://doi.org/10.1186/s12960-018-0339-z

Olley, R. (2021). A focused literature review of power and influence leadership theories. *Asia Pacific Journal of Health Management, 16*(2), 7–15. https://doi.org/10.24083/apjhm.v16i2.807

Riandini, T., Pang, D., Toh, M. P., Tan, C. S., Liu, D. Y., Choong, A. M., Chandrasekar, S., Shyong Tai, E., Tan, K. B., & Venkataraman, K. (2021). Diabetes-related lower extremity complications in a multi-ethnic Asian population: A 10 year observational study in Singapore. *Diabetologia, 64*(7), 1538–1549.https://doi.org/10.1007/s00125-021-05441-3

Schneider, E. C., Shah, A., Doty, M. M., Tikkanen, R., Fields, K., & William, R. D. (2021). *Mirror, mirror 2021: Reflecting poorly—Health care in the U. S. compared to other high-income countries*. https://www.commonwealthfund.org/publications/fund-reports/2021/aug/mirror-mirror-2021-reflecting-poorly

Selak, V., Poppe, K., Grey, C., Mehta, S., Winter-Smith, J., Jackson, R., Wells, S., Exeter, D., Kerr, A., Riddell, T., & Harwood, M. (2020). Ethnic differences in cardiovascular risk profiles among 475,241 adults in primary care in Aotearoa, New Zealand. *The New Zealand Medical Journal (Online), 133*(1521), 14–27. https://researchspace.auckland.ac.nz/bitstream/handle/2292/53539/Ethnic%20differences.pdf?sequence=2

Seng, J. J. B., Kwan, Y. H., Lee, V. S. Y., Tan, C. S., Zainudin, S. B., Thumboo, J., & Low, L. L. (2020). Differential health care use, diabetes-related complications, and mortality among five unique classes of patients with type 2 diabetes in Singapore: A latent class analysis of 71,125 patients. *Diabetes Care, 43*(5), 1048–1056. https://doi.org/10.2337/dc19-2519

Shommu, N. S., Ahmed, S., Rumana, N., Barron, G. R., McBrien, K. A., & Turin, T. C. (2016). What is the scope of improving immigrant and ethnic minority healthcare using community navigators: A systematic scoping review. *International Journal for Equity in Health, 15*, Article 6. https://doi.org/10.1186/s12939-016-0298-8

Shum, T. (2011). Refugee protection and spaces: Seeking asylum in Hong Kong. *Oxford Monitor of Forced Migration, 1*(2), 17–20. https://repository.vtc.edu.hk/thei-fac-gen-ed-sp/59

Solar, O., & Irwin, A. (2010). A conceptual framework for action on the social determinants of health. *World Health Organization*. https://apps.who.int/iris/handle/10665/44489

Takenaka, A. (2009). How ethnic minorities experience social mobility in Japan: An ethnographic study of Peruvian Migrants. In H. Ishida & D. H. Slater (Eds.), *Social class in contemporary Japan: Structures, sorting and strategies* (pp. 239–256). Routledge.

Takubo, Y., Nemoto, T., Iwai, M., Kashima, M., Yamaguchi, E., Maruyama, A., Miura, S., Saito, H., Tsujino, N., & Mizuno, M. (2020). Demographic and clinical characteristics of foreign nationals accessing psychiatric services in Japan: A multicentre study in a metropolitan area. *BMC psychiatry, 20*, Article 569. https://doi.org/10.1186/s12888-020-02951-z

Tejativaddhana, P., Briggs, D., Singhadej, O., & Hinoguin, R. (2018). Developing primary health care in Thailand: Innovation in the use of socio-economic determinants, Sustainable Development Goals and the district health strategy. *Public Administration and Policy: An Asia-Pacific Journal, 21*(1), 36–49. https://doi.org/10.1108/PAP-06-2018-005

Thomas, S., Beh, L., & Nordin, R. B. (2011). Health care delivery in Malaysia: Changes, challenges and champions. *Journal of Public Health in Africa, 2*(2), 93–97. https://doi.org/10.4081/jphia.2011.e23

Vandan, N., Wong, J. H., Gong, W. J., Yip, P. F., & Fong, D. T. (2020). Health system responsiveness in Hong Kong: A comparison between South Asian and Chinese patients' experiences. *Public Health, 182*, 81–87. https://doi.org/10.1016/j.puhe.2020.01.019

Wong, W. C. W., Cheung, S., Miu, H. Y. H., Chen, J., Loper, K. A., & Holroyd, E. (2017). Mental health of African asylum-seekers and refugees in Hong Kong: Using the social determinants of health framework. *BMC Public Health, 17*, Article 153. https://doi.org/10.1186/s12889-016-3953-5

Woodland, L., Blignault, I., O'Callaghan, C., & Harris-Roxas, B. (2021). A framework for preferred practices in conducting culturally competent health research in a multicultural society. *Health Research Policy and Systems, 19*, 24. https://doi.org/10.1186/s12961-020-00657-y

Yoda, T., Saengrut, B., Miyamoto, K., Rattanasathien, R., Saito, T., Ishimoto, Y., Chunjai, K., Pudwan, R., Sirimuengmoon, K., & Katsuyama, H. (2021). Differences of body composition and physical strength among Japanese and Thai older adults living in Chiang Mai, Thailand: an inter-ethnic cross-sectional study. *Environmental Health and Preventive Medicine*, *26*, Article 97. https://doi.org/10.1186/s12199-021-01017-0

Zhao, X., Hong, F., Yin, J., Tang, W., Zhang, G., Liang, X., Li, J., Cui, C., Li, X., & China Multi-Ethnic Cohort (CMEC) Collaborative Group. (2021). Cohort profile: The China Multi-Ethnic cohort (CMEC) study. *International Journal of Epidemiology*, *50*(3), 721–721l. https://doi.org/10.1093/ije/dyaa185

Chapter 16
Gaps in Sexual and Reproductive Health in Young People

William Chi Wai Wong

Abstract Sexual and reproductive health (SRH) is not merely about physical health, whether one is suffering from a certain medical condition, but it is also about mental and social well-being—the exercise of human rights and respecting the rights of others. SRH is particularly essential for adolescents' overall well-being, as they are at the age of developing sexual desire and attraction. At this phase of transition from children to adults, confusion might arise regarding sexual identity and SRH needs. Special attention to the needs and the rights of the sexual minority groups, namely lesbian, gay, bisexual and transgender (LGBT) communities, as they are likely to experience stigmatisation, bullying and violence, relating to higher rates of depression and suicidal attempts. Sex education is needed to increase young people's biological knowledge of human physiology and their rights in society and, importantly, to empower them to make informed decisions regarding sexual behaviours and practice. Without the appropriate sex education and support, they could lead to serious health consequences, including sexually transmitted infections (STIs) and HIV. Unsafe sexual practices and associated unintended pregnancies also pose huge global health burden. Acknowledging and addressing the barriers to accessing contraception at macro- and micro-levels could help meet young people's need for contraception, reducing the risk of STIs and unplanned pregnancies. Health professionals should make use of their unique position and every opportunity to promote health awareness and educate adolescents over safe sex and contraception. Law and policies would further align beyond the diverse sex education curricula in different countries to promote the rights of an individual.

Keywords Sexual health · Sexuality · Sexually transmitted infection · Youth

---

W. C. W. Wong (✉)
Department of Family Medicine and Primary Care, School of Clinical Medicine, Li Ka Shing Faculty of Medicine, The University of Hong Kong, Hong Kong, China
e-mail: wongwcw@hku.hk

B. Y. F. Fong and W. C. W. Wong (eds.), *Gaps and Actions in Health Improvement from Hong Kong and Beyond*,
https://doi.org/10.1007/978-981-99-4491-0_16

Introduction

The World Health Organization (WHO) defines "young people" as individuals aged 10–24 years, in which "youth" refers to the 15–24 year age group and "adolescents" cover the age range of 10–19 years (World Health Organization, n.d.). During this transitional phase between childhood and adulthood, adolescents develop independency, establishing life skills and new relationships. On account of physical and hormonal changes in puberty, sexual feelings arise, giving them the urge to explore their sexual identity and find intimate relationships. Being the foundation of all human relationships, romantic and sexual relationships can be exciting and precarious. Sexual feelings and thoughts might be pleasurable yet confusing to the young people concerned. Therefore, learning about relationships and exploring sexual intimacy is crucial for them to develop their own sexual identity and avoid adverse risks such as unwanted pregnancy or even sexual violence.

Sexual Identity

Adolescents, at the age of developing their own identity, experience the need to realise and express their sexual orientation and gender identity. First, we have to go beyond the binary notions of gender and be aware of the idea that one's biological sex does not equate to his/her gender identity as the "genderbread" person below is illustrated (Fig. 16.1). Biological sex, as it literally means, refers to a person's physical structure of the body, including external sex organs and intrinsic sex chromosomes. Gender identity refers to one's internal belief of being male, female or of another gender. Although the majority of individuals have their gender identity aligned with their biological sex (i.e. cisgender), misalignment of them can happen naturally, particularly among children and adolescents, such as agender (no gender), bigender (two genders), pangender (non-binary multigender), transsexual (opposite of biological gender), etc. In addition, sexual orientation is about one's held sense of being attracted physically, emotionally and/or romantically to others. Lesbian, gay, bisexual and transgender (LGBT) communities are individuals whose attraction is not confined to the opposite gender in the binary system.

Compared to cisgender, rates of bullying and violence were higher among LGBT youths (Toomey & Russell, 2016). Consequently, these youths experienced more "bias-based bullying", associated with 5–6 times the odds of suicide attempts (Ybarra et al., 2015). Bullying victimisation was also associated with other significant health outcomes. Therefore, physicians as the first port of contact can play a role, as a (health policy) advocate, mentor, health educationist/promotion and even role models—to change the attitudes and behaviours that perpetuate abuse; and build connections within communities, healthcare providers and non-governmental organisations (NGOs) in order to improve quality of life for the young people. Secondary preventive activities include shelter, counselling, safety planning and protective orders, while

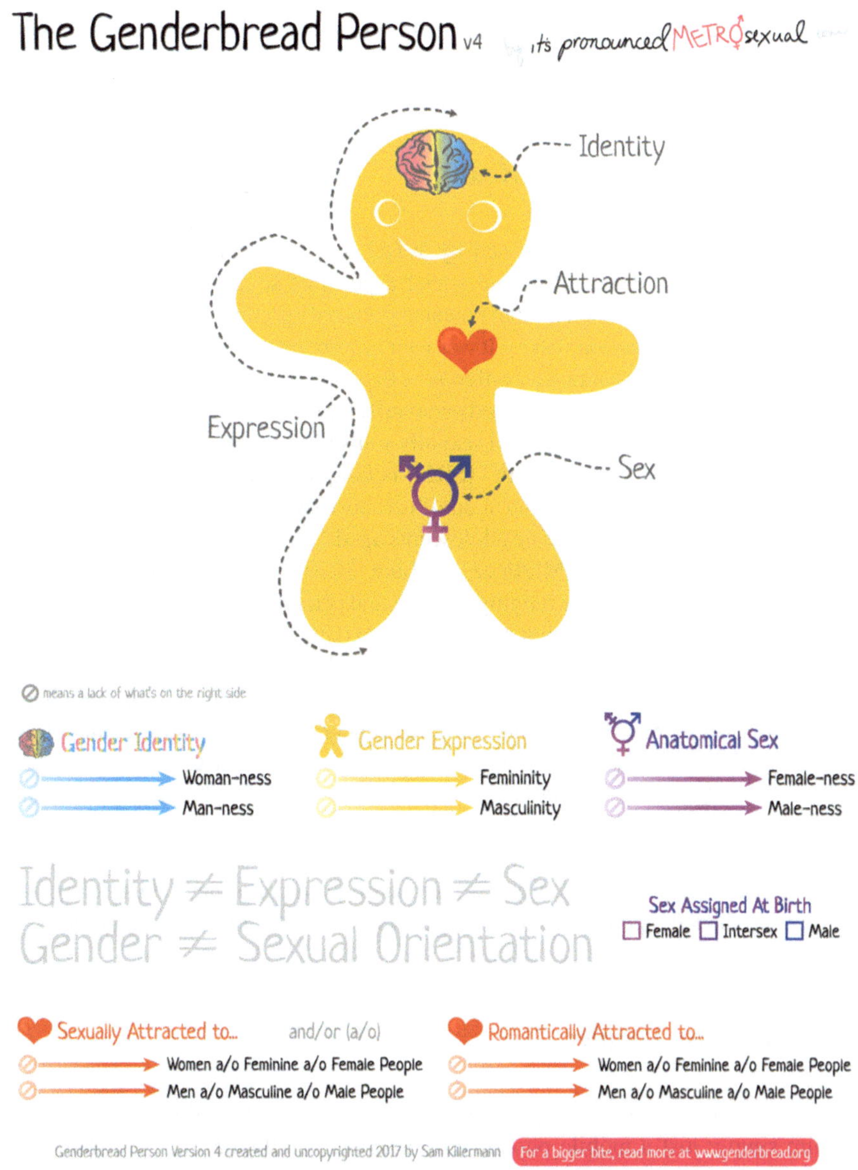

Fig. 16.1 Sexual orientation, appearance, preference and expression (gender bread man) (*Source* The Genderbread Person [2017])

tertiary prevention focuses on ongoing support to victims and ongoing accountability for abusers that can address the long-term consequences of domestic violence.

Sexual and Reproductive Health

"Sexual health" was initially defined by WHO in 1975 as "the integration of the somatic, emotional, intellectual, and social aspects of sexual well-being in ways that are positively enriching and that enhance personality, communication, and love" (World Health Organization, 1975). It was later incorporated with reproductive health in a United Nations international conference, in which the purpose of it was communicated as "the enhancement of life and personal relations, and not merely counselling and care related to reproduction and sexually transmitted diseases" (Paul, 1994).

"Sexual and reproductive health" (SRH) is ubiquitous in all human life cycles. The US Centers for Disease Control and Prevention (CDC) reported that in 2015–2017, 38–42% of female and male adolescents aged 15–19 years in the United States had had sexual intercourse (Martinez & Abma, 2020). The issues related to it are comprehensive and extensive ranging from sexual orientation and gender identity to medical conditions such as sexual dysfunction, sexually transmitted infections (STIs) and HIV, pregnancy-related issues and beyond. SRH services comprise a wide range of preventive and treatment care, including family planning, counselling, testing and treatment of STIs, breast and gynaecological cancer screening, and vaccination for human papillomavirus (HPV), antenatal, maternal and postpartum care, etc. These services are often provided in social health clinics, family planning centres and out-patient clinics in hospitals or primary care settings. SRH often involves sensitive topics encompassing personal (e.g. erectile dysfunction, extramarital sex, illegal drugs), emotional (child sexual abuse) and even political issues (abuse of power, corruption); hence, open to debates, controversy or even political manipulation.

SRH in Young People

In the digital era, we are all living in today, dating and exploring intimate relationships require simply just a mobile phone. With a world population of 7,954 million in 2022 (The United Nations Population Fund, n.d.), the number of smartphone users exceeded 6,500 million (O'Dea, 2022) and young people could meet new friends and share common interests anytime and anywhere. Nevertheless, studies have shown that the use of dating apps could be associated with higher sexual risks. An Australian survey found that boredom (59.7%), casual sex (45.1%) and casual dating (42.8%) were the top reasons for using dating apps (Garga et al., 2021). The users reported that their sexual behaviour changed after the use of those apps: increasing sexual activities (70.0%); having more sexual partners (57.1%) and sexual experimentation (42.1%). Consistently, Lehmiller and Ioerger found that the dating app users had more sexual partners compared to non-users and were also more likely to have a medical history of STIs (Lehmiller & Ioerger, 2014). Supported by Choi et al. (2016), dating app usage in Hong Kong was significantly associated with inconsistent condom usage and unprotected sex, with more than half (57.1%) of the respondents did not use a condom in their last sexual encounter. This was partly attributed to the users' cursory review of their sexual partners' STI status (Garga et al., 2021).

Sexually Transmitted Infections (STIs)

Among the 26 million new STI cases in 2018, youths accounted for nearly half of them (Centers for Disease Control & Prevention, 2021a). The most prevalent STIs were chlamydia, gonorrhoea, syphilis and trichomoniasis (World Health Organization, 2022d). Unlike Western countries like the United States and the United Kingdom, China had a higher chlamydia prevalence (2.6% for women and 2.1% for men) (Parish et al., 2003). In Hong Kong, although the overall prevalence of chlamydia was low (1.4%), it was relatively high in young women and men aged 18–26 years who were sexually active (5.8% and 4.8%, respectively) (Wong et al., 2017). STIs can lead to direct health conditions and costs of medical care to the infected individuals and society (Ryan et al., 2008). Particularly those with a "silent" nature like chlamydia. Chlamydia sequelae include pelvic inflammatory disease, chronic pelvic pain, ectopic pregnancy and infertility (Wiesenfeld, 2017).

Screening would be an effective way to detect these asymptomatic cases within the population unaware of the infection, hence, reducing the burden of disease in the economy and on the healthcare system (Wong et al., 2019). Our recent study found that the most cost-effective strategy to control chlamydia was targeted screening on the high-risk population characterised by the number of partners, with contact tracing included (Montes-Olivas et al., 2022). For STI testing and management services to be carried out effectively, barriers to screening and strategies to improve uptake rates should be identified and addressed. In a discreet choice experiment, the biggest concern among Hong Kong people was cost and the staff's attitude towards STIs (Ong et al., 2021). A systematic review of 19 previous systematic reviews included found that the use of electronic health records and self-collection in home-testing kits could facilitate testing (Wong et al., 2019). Interventions with education, advisory elements and outreach community/parent centres and homeless shelters could increase screening rates significantly (Wong et al., 2019).

To assess one's sexual history, the US CDC suggested the "Five P's approach", involving partners, practices, protection from STIs, history of STIs and pregnancy intention (Workowski et al., 2021). As it often "takes two parties to dance", healthcare providers would have to reach out to the patients' partners and address their sexual practices. For example, family physicians should be more aware of the adolescents' sexual health issues even if they are seen for other trivial matters such as sexual orientation and sexual life, in a sensitive and non-judgemental way. To control the spread of STIs in the population, particularly the asymptomatic cases, contact tracing is crucial. In Hong Kong as elsewhere, young people tend not to notify their partners of STIs due to negative emotional experiences resulting from stigma, embarrassment, lack of knowledge, fear of blame or other negative emotions from partners (Chitneni et al., 2020; Lau et al., 2021). Accurate risk assessment is crucial for the proper diagnosis, care and prevention of STIs. The other side of the coin i.e. over-diagnosis and over-treatment in Asia settings like Hong Kong is often observed as a result of the adoption of the Syndromic Approach.

The most common bacterial STIs can be treated with antibiotics while antivirals are used to control herpes and HIV so that the course of the disease can be modulated (World Health Organization, 2022d). However, antimicrobial resistance (AMR) in STIs, particularly to N. gonorrhoea, has made its management challenging. Gonorrhoea and chlamydia are currently treated with ceftriaxone and azithromycin. In China, approximately one-fifth and more than 10% of the gonorrhoea cases were resistant to azithromycin and ceftriaxone, respectively (Yin et al., 2018). Despite the "urgent" need for new antibiotics for gonorrhoea, only three new candidate drugs were under research and development in phase II and III trials (Alirol et al., 2017).

Human Papilloma Virus (HPV)

HPV is one of the most common STIs passed on by having vaginal, anal or oral sex with the infected partner with significant consequences, i.e. cervical cancer, the fourth most common cancer in women. In contrast, men can get cancers of the anus, penis, and mouth/throat caused by HPV infections. Although it is not curable once infected, vaccination is an effective means to prevent and control the spread of HPV. The vaccine is recommended for girls and boys aged 9–14 years as it can protect them best when it is administered before sexual activities started (Centers for Disease Control & Prevention, 2021b; World Health Organization, 2022c). Its effects expose complex health equity issues with approximately 600, 000 incidents in 2020, 342,000 women deceased, 90% of whom happened in low- and middle-income countries (World Health Organization, 2022c). One of the barriers to HPV vaccine uptake among youths was the lack of knowledge and the high cost of the vaccine (D'Errico et al., 2020; Singh, 2022), which can be partly improved by education (Singh, 2022). Other than voluntary vaccination, several countries including Australia, Canada, the USA, Brazil, Germany and New Zealand adopted universal vaccination programmes to protect the young populations (Prue et al., 2018). The merits of their strategy evidenced by substantial health and economic benefits point out the importance of universal HPV vaccination.

Contraceptives

Unsafe sex is the leading risk in females aged 15–49 years among the 19 risk factors for the global burden of STIs, measured by the disability-adjusted life years (DALYs) (Institute for Health Metrics & Evaluation, 2022). Though inconclusive, the authors noted based on the analysis of the 2010 DALYs' risk factors affecting the burden of disease in later life of young people that "unsafe sexual practices would probably account for a large fraction of global health burden" (World Health Organization, 2014). According to the data from 1,247 surveys for 195 regions of the world, the most common contraceptives were female sterilisation and male condom (United Nations, 2019). Unlike Europe and Northern America where oral contraceptive pills (OCP) and male condoms were the preferred form of contraception, the most commonly used contraceptive method among women in Eastern and South-Eastern Asia was the intrauterine device, while female sterilisation was the most common contraceptive in Central and Southern Asia (United Nations, 2019). However, the data stratified by region and age groups showed a different trend. Among young people in Hong Kong, the most common contraceptive method was male condoms, accounting for 89% as reported in the Youth Sexuality Survey (YSS) of the Hong Kong Family Planning Association (HKFPA) in 2022.

Barriers to accessing contraception include the lack of sexual knowledge and financial constraints, and, at policy levels, the laws in the contraceptive provision regarding age and marital status (World Health Organization, 2022b). In a patriarchal society like Oman, uneducated girls like to relinquish their decision-making power in contraception to their partners (Al Riyami et al., 2004). Women's unmet need for contraception was also associated with myths about OCP regarding body image, side effects, health risks and method of use, in Asian settings (Hamani et al., 2007). These myths have to be addressed at the macro- and micro-levels before women can choose the most suitable form of contraception for them.

Unintended Pregnancy

Complications from pregnancy and childbirth have become one of the leading causes of mortality in adolescents and youths (World Health Organization, 2022a). In the developing world, adolescent pregnancy is a serious problem, with approximately 21 million getting pregnant and 12 million childbirths at 15–19 years and more than 777,000 women giving birth before the age of 15 years (World Health Organization, 2022a, 2022b). Out of these childbirths, nearly half (47.6%) of them were unplanned and unwanted (World Health Organization, 2022b), in which half of them ended up in abortions (African Population and Health Research Center et al., 2013; Sully et al., 2018). Other than sexual abstinence and the use of contraceptives, increasing sexual knowledge among adolescents would be essential to address the current situation of SRH in youths. Many countries including the United States and China have been adopting comprehensive sex education, which teaches young people various aspects of sexuality. Ending unintended pregnancies among young people by 2030 was one of the agenda of the Sustainable Development Goals (SDGs) (The United Nations Population Fund China, 2018). With comprehensive sexuality education, SRH in youth will be improved and young people can be aware of their rights in society.

Sex Education

These worrying trends indicate the urgent need to improve current sex education programmes. According to Women UN and The United Nations Children's Fund, sex education should go beyond the biological knowledge of human physiology, reproductive system or STI prevention, and empower young people to make informed decisions, experience mutual pleasure and consensual sexual behaviours, and achieve physical, emotional, psychological, social and sexual well-being (The United Nations Population Fund, 2018). However, some countries may emphasise abstinence as the safest behaviour to avoid the risks of unwanted pregnancy and STIs (Kirby, 2008), denying young people as legitimate sexual subjects who have the right to express their sexual feelings (Allen, 2008). Taking Asian regions such as Hong Kong and Mainland China as examples, the existing practice of sex education often focuses on the knowledge of birth control, eugenics and contraception, and rarely takes into account empowerment and equity (Leung et al., 2019). Thus, theoretical-based sex education curricula that include both biomedical and sociocultural aspects of sexuality will be the way forward.

Legal and Ethical Aspects of SRH

In contemporary societies, love and sex are regulated by social rules and law under the broad umbrella of human rights and population control. Ambiguous legislative provisions could lead to stigmatisation or even criminalisation. In many countries and regions, there are regulations on the age of consent for sexual activity and marriage. This, on the other hand, could create barriers to accessing SRH services among young people, who, in turn, would not seek medical treatment for fear of prosecution, particularly in countries that criminalise consensual sexual acts among adolescents (The United Nations Population Fund East & Southern Africa Regional Office, 2017). Despite some evidence showing that same-sex marriage legislation could protect sexual minorities from suicidal attempts due to stigmatisation, it is not legalised in most places in Asia (Raifman et al., 2017). Moreover, in developing countries such as East Africa, laws and policies would be required to eliminate harmful cultural, religious and traditional practices including female genital mutilation and child marriage (The United Nations Children's Fund, n.d.).

All for Health-Ways Forward for SRH in Youth

Adolescents' sexual health and welfare should be addressed at macro- and micro-levels. Health policies should focus on SRH in youth, adopting the services to their culture and changes in habitat. Many existing information or apps on sexual health are not accurate or tailor-made to their needs. Given the popularity of the use of social media among adolescents, public health campaigns can be held online to engage large groups of young people at a relatively lower cost.

To ensure affordability and access to SRH services, they should come into different forms and be comprehensive as possible, e.g. home STI testing, online doctors and universal health coverage. At the micro-level, family physicians should be more aware of health issues in youths and take on opportunistic care and screening, as the first port of call in the healthcare system. They should also be more involved in sex education to increase public awareness of STIs and use of contraceptives, reducing stigma and discrimination against sexuality and SRH issues (Wong et al., 2006). To address these "All for Health" issues, young people should be aware and equipped with essential skills to deal with sexuality and intimate partner violence issues.

References

African Population and Health Research Center, Ipas & Guttmacher Institute. (2013). *Incidence and complications of unsafe abortion in Kenya: Key findings of a national study.* https://aphrc.org/wp-content/uploads/2019/07/Incidence-and-Complications-of-Unsafe-Abortion-in-Kenya-Key-Findings-of-a-National-Study.pdf

Al Riyami, A., Afifi, M., & Mabry, R. (2004). Women's autonomy, education and employment in Oman and their influence on contraceptive use. *Reproductive Health Matters, 12*(23). https://doi.org/10.1016/s0968-8080(04)23113-5

Alirol, E., Wi, T., Bala, M., Bazzo, M., Chen, X., Deal, C., Dillon, J.-A. R., Kularatne, R., Heim, J., van Huijsduijnen, R. H., Hook, E. W., Lahra, M. M., Lewis, D. A., Ndowa, F., Shafer, W. M., Tayler, L., Workowski, K., Unemo, M., & Balasegaram, M. (2017). Multidrug-resistant gonorrhea: A research and development roadmap to discover new medicines. *PLoS Medicine, 14*(7), Article e1002366. https://doi.org/10.1371/journal.pmed.1002366

Allen, L. (2008). They think you shouldn't be having sex anyway': Young people's suggestions for improving sexuality education content. *Sexualities, 11*(5), 573–594. https://doi.org/10.1177/1363460708089425

Centers for Disease Control and Prevention. (2021a). *Adolescents and young adults.* https://www.cdc.gov/std/life-stages-populations/adolescents-youngadults.htm

Centers for Disease Control and Prevention. (2021b). *Reasons to get HPV vaccine.* https://www.cdc.gov/hpv/parents/vaccine/six-reasons.html

Chitneni, P., Beksinska, M., Dietrich, J., Jaggernath, M., Closson, K., Smith, P., Lewis, D. A., Matthews, L. T., Smit, J., Ndung'u, T., Brockman, M., Gray, G., & Kaida, A. (2020). Partner notification and treatment outcomes among South African adolescents and young adults diagnosed with a sexually transmitted infection via laboratory-based screening. *International Journal of STD & AIDS, 31*(7), 627–636.https://doi.org/10.1177/0956462420915395

Choi, E., Wong, J., Lo, H., Wong, W., Chio, J., & Fong, D. (2016). The impacts of using smartphone dating applications on sexual risk behaviours in college students in Hong Kong. *PLoS ONE, 11*(11), Article e0165394. https://doi.org/10.1371/journal.pone.0165394

D'Errico, M. P., Tung, W.-C., Lu, M., & D'Errico, R. (2020). Barriers and recommendations associated with human papillomavirus vaccination among college students. *The Journal for Nurse Practitioners, 16*(7), 533–537. https://doi.org/10.1016/j.nurpra.2020.04.011

Garga, S., Thomas, M. T., Bhatia, A., Sullivan, A., John-Leader, F., & Pit, S. W. (2021). Motivations, dating app relationships, unintended consequences and change in sexual behaviour in dating app users at an Australian music festival. *Harm Reduction Journal, 18*, Article 49. https://doi.org/10.1186/s12954-021-00493-5

Hamani, Y., Sciaki-Tamir, Y., Deri-Hasid, R., Miller-Pogrund, T., Milwidsky, A., & Haimov-Kochman, R. (2007). Misconceptions about oral contraception pills among adolescents and physicians. *Human Reproduction, 22*(12), 3078–3083. https://doi.org/10.1093/humrep/dem259

Institute for Health Metrics and Evaluation. (2022). *Unsafe sex—Level 2 risk*. https://www.healthdata.org/results/gbd_summaries/2019/unsafe-sex-level-2-risk

Kirby, D. B. (2008). The impact of abstinence and comprehensive sex and STD/HIV education programs on adolescent sexual behavior. *Sexuality Research and Social Policy, 5*(3), 18–27. https://doi.org/10.1525/srsp.2008.5.3.18

Lau, B., Liu, L., Chan, C., Chan, C., Ong, J., Holroyd, E., & Wong, W. (2021). De-sexualizing partner notification: A Qualitative Study on Chinese young adults with chlamydia. *International Journal of Environmental Research and Public Health, 18*(8), Article 4032. https://doi.org/10.3390/ijerph18084032

Lehmiller, J., & Ioerger, M. (2014). Social networking smartphone applications and sexual health outcomes among men who have sex with men. *PLoS ONE, 9*(1), Article e86603. https://doi.org/10.1371/journal.pone.0086603

Leung, H., Shek, D., Leung, E., & Shek, E. (2019). Development of contextually-relevant sexuality education: Lessons from a comprehensive review of adolescent sexuality education across cultures. *International Journal of Environmental Research and Public Health, 16*(4), Article 621. https://doi.org/10.3390/ijerph16040621

Martinez, G. M., & Abma, J. C. (2020). *Sexual activity and contraceptive use among teenagers aged 15–19 in the United States, 2015–2017* (NCHS Data Brief No. 366). https://www.cdc.gov/nchs/products/databriefs/db366.htm

Montes-Olivas, S., Ozten, Y., Homer, M., Turner, K., Fairley, C. K., Hocking, J. S., Tse, D., van Rees, N. V., Wong, W. C. W., & Ong, J. J. (2022). Evaluating the impact and cost-effectiveness of chlamydia management strategies in Hong Kong: A modelling study. *Frontiers in Public Health, 10*, Article 932096. https://doi.org/10.3389/fpubh.2022.932096

O'Dea, S. (2022). *Number of smartphone subscriptions worldwide from 2016 to 2021, with forecasts from 2022 to 2027*. https://www.statista.com/statistics/330695/number-of-smartphone-users-worldwide/

Ong, J., Fairley, C., Hocking, J., Turner, K., Booton, R., Tse, D., & Wong, W. (2021). Preferences for chlamydia testing and management in Hong Kong: A discrete choice experiment. *Sexually Transmitted Infections, 98*, 408–413. https://doi.org/10.1136/sextrans-2021-055182

Parish, W., Laumann, E. O., Cohen, M., Zheng, H., Hoffman, I., & Wang, T. (2003). Population-based study of chlamydial infection in China: A hidden epidemic. *JAMA, 289*(10), 1265–1273. https://doi.org/10.1001/jama.289.10.1265

Paul, S. (1994). Report on the international conference on population and development. *Ageing Internation, 21*, 49–51. https://doi.org/10.1007/BF02681115

Prue, G., Baker, P., Graham, D., Nutting, C., Greenhouse, P., & Lawler, M. (2018). It is time for universal HPV vaccination. *The Lancet, 392*(10151), 913–914. https://doi.org/10.1016/S0140-6736(18)31821-X

Raifman, J., Moscoe, E., Austin, S., & McConnell, M. (2017). Difference-in-differences analysis of the association between state same-sex marriage policies and adolescent suicide attempts. *JAMA Pediatrics, 171*(4), 350–356. https://doi.org/10.1001/jamapediatrics.2016.4529

Ryan, C. A., Kamb, M., & Holmes, K. K. (2008). STI care management. In K. K. Holmes, P. F. Sparling, W. E. Stamm, P. Piot, & J. N. Wasserheit (Eds.), *Sexually transmitted diseases* (pp. 855–875). McGraw Hill.

Singh, C. (2022). Increasing knowledge of human papillomavirus among young adults. *The Journal for Nurse Practitioners, 18*(6), 618–621. https://doi.org/10.1016/j.nurpra.2022.03.006

Sully, E., Dibaba, Y., Fetters, T., Blades, N., & Bankole, A. (2018). Playing it safe: Legal and clandestine abortions among adolescents in Ethiopia. *Journal of Adolescent Health, 62*(6), 729–736. https://doi.org/10.1016/j.jadohealth.2017.12.015

Toomey, R., & Russell, S. (2016). The role of sexual orientation in school-based victimization: A meta-analysis. *Youth & Society, 48*(2), 176–201. https://doi.org/10.1177/0044118X13483778

The Genderbread Person. (2017). *Genderbread person v4.0*. https://www.genderbread.org/resource/genderbread-person-v4-0

The United Nations Children's Fund. (n.d.). *UNICEF data: Monitoring the situation of children and women*. https://data.unicef.org/

The United Nations Population Fund. (n.d.). *World population dashboard*. UNFPA. https://www.unfpa.org/data/world-population-dashboard

The United Nations Population Fund. (2018). *International technical guidance on sexuality education. An evidence-informed approach*. https://www.unfpa.org/publications/international-technical-guidance-sexuality-education

The United Nations Population Fund China. (2018). *Ending unintended pregnancies among Chinese youth by 2030*. https://china.unfpa.org/en/publications/unfpa-china-policy-brief-ending-unintended-pregnancies-among-chinese-youth-2030

The United Nations Population Fund East and Southern Africa Regional Office. (2017). *Harmonizing the legal environment for adolescent sexual and reproductive health and rights: A review of 23 countries in East and Southern Africa*. https://esaro.unfpa.org/en/publications/harmonizing-legal-environment-adolescent-sexual-and-reproductive-health-and-rights-0

United Nations. (2019). *Contraceptive use by method 2019: Data booklet*. https://www.un.org/development/desa/pd/sites/www.un.org.development.desa.pd/files/files/documents/2020/Jan/un_2019_contraceptiveusebymethod_databooklet.pdf

Wiesenfeld, H. (2017). Screening for chlamydia trachomatis infections in women. *The New England Journal of Medicine, 376*(8), 765–773. https://doi.org/10.1056/NEJMcp1412935

World Health Organization. (n.d.). *Adolescent health*. https://www.who.int/southeastasia/health-topics/adolescent-health

World Health Organization. (1975). *Education and treatment in human sexuality: The training of health professionals, report of a WHO meeting [held in Geneva from 6 to 12 February 1974]*. https://apps.who.int/iris/handle/10665/38247

World Health Organization. (2014). *DALYs and health-related behaviours*. https://apps.who.int/adolescent/second-decade/section3/page6/dalys-&-behaviours.html

World Health Organization. (2022a). *Adolescent and young adult health*. https://www.who.int/news-room/fact-sheets/detail/adolescents-health-risks-and-solutions

World Health Organization. (2022b). *Adolescent pregnancy*. https://www.who.int/news-room/fact-sheets/detail/adolescent-pregnancy

World Health Organization. (2022c). *Cervical cancer*. https://www.who.int/news-room/fact-sheets/detail/cervical-cancer

World Health Organization. (2022d). *Sexually transmitted infections (STIs)*. https://www.who.int/news-room/fact-sheets/detail/sexually-transmitted-infections-(stis)

Wong, W., Lau, S., Choi, E., Tucker, J., Fairley, C., & Saunders, J. (2019). A systematic literature review of reviews on the effectiveness of chlamydia testing. *Epidemiologic Reviews, 41*(1), 168–175. https://doi.org/10.1093/epirev/mxz007

Wong, W., Lee, A., Tsang, K., & Lynn, H. (2006). The impact of AIDS/sex education by schools or family doctors on Hong Kong Chinese adolescents. *Psychology, Health & Medicine, 11*(1), 108–116. https://doi.org/10.1080/13548500500156105

Wong, W. C., Zhao, Y., Wong, N. S., Parish, W. L., Miu, H. Y., Yang, L. G., Emch, M., Man Ho, K., Yeung Fong, F., & Tucker, J. D. (2017). Prevalence and risk factors of chlamydia infection in Hong Kong: A population-based geospatial household survey and testing. *PLoS ONE, 12*(2), Article e0172561. https://doi.org/10.1371/journal.pone.0172561

Workowski, K., Bachmann, L., Chan, P., Johnston, C., Muzny, C., Park, I., Reno, H., Zenilman, J. M., & Bolan, G. (2021). Sexually transmitted infections treatment guidelines, 2021. *Morbidity and Mortality Weekly Report Recommendations and Reports, 70*(4), 1–187. https://doi.org/10.15585/mmwr.rr7004a1

Ybarra, M., Mitchell, K., Kosciw, J., & Korchmaros, J. (2015). Understanding linkages between bullying and suicidal ideation in a national sample of LGB and heterosexual youth in the United States. *Prevention Science, 16*(3), 451–462. https://doi.org/10.1007/s11121-014-0510-2

Yin, Y., Han, Y., Dai, X., Zheng, H., Chen, S., Zhu, B., Yong, G., Zhong, N., Hu, L.-H., Cao, W.-L., Zheng, Z.-J., Wang, F., Zhi, Q., Zhu, X.-Y., & Chen, X. (2018). Susceptibility of Neisseria gonorrhoeae to azithromycin and ceftriaxone in China: A retrospective study of national surveillance data from 2013 to 2016. *PLoS Medicine, 15*(2), Article e1002499. https://doi.org/10.1371/journal.pmed.1002499

Chapter 17
Promotion of Breastfeeding as an All for Health Strategy

Candy Yuen Yee Tsoi and Yim Fan Chan

Abstract Obesity is one of the worldwide health problems and the cause of many chronic diseases, such as diabetes in adulthood. Most obesity begins from childhood. Thus, it is imperative to build a healthy foundation for the newborns. Breastfeeding has long-term health benefits for the infants, lasting into adulthood. Breastmilk is the ideal food for infants to build up the best health foundation. It is safe, clean and contains rich antibodies to protect the infant against most childhood illnesses. According to the World Health Organization, breastfed children have higher intelligence test marks and less overweight or obesity. Breastfeeding is also beneficial to the mothers, who will have lower health risks, too. The society will gain with more mothers breastfeeding infants, resulting in saving lives and health dollars, and protecting the workforce and environment. Breastfeeding builds up the best healthy life foundation for generations. Breastfeeding is all for health. Initial and sustain breastfeeding success is an all for health global strategy. Promoting and supporting breastfeeding is an all-important health strategy to promote and maintain population health in Hong Kong in 2022 and beyond. This chapter will describe the gaps of healthcare practice, clarify the discrepancy between reality and current practice in healthcare and identify the desired or optimal healthcare situation and intervention to support the all for health strategies.

Keywords Breastfeeding · Baby-friendly hospital · Lactation

C. Y. Y. Tsoi (✉)
Hong Kong College of Midwives, Hong Kong, China
e-mail: ctsoi@cihe.edu.hk

Y. F. Chan
Hong Kong College of Paediatric Nursing, Hong Kong, China
e-mail: chanyf3@ha.org.hk

B. Y. F. Fong and W. C. W. Wong (eds.), *Gaps and Actions in Health Improvement from Hong Kong and Beyond*,
https://doi.org/10.1007/978-981-99-4491-0_17

Definition of Baby-Friendly Hospital Initiative

Breastfeeding builds up the best healthy life foundation for generations. Breastfeeding is all for health. Initial and sustain breastfeeding success is an all for health global strategy. The Baby-Friendly Hospital Initiative (BFHI) is a global movement for breastfeeding success. BFHI was launched by the World Health Organization (WHO) and the United Nations Children's Fund (UNICEF) in 1991 following the Innocenti Declaration of 1990. The initiative programme was a major part of the WHO's global strategy for infant and young child feeding. It was a worldwide effort to ensure the implementation of health practices that protect, promote and support breastfeeding (World Health Organization, 2009). The BFHI programme recognises hospitals with maternity units and birthing centres that have achieved an optimal level of nursing care for breastfeeding. The initiative has a continuing improving system with measurable practices. The designation of "baby friendly hospitals or centres" is given to health facilities which implement the "Ten nursing practice to Successful Breastfeeding". In addition, follow strictly the rules and regulations of the World Health Assembly resolutions (the Code) and the International Code of Marketing of Breast-milk Substitutes, many hospitals have been designated as "baby-friendly" (World Health Organization, 2009).

The aim of the BFHI programme is to ensure every newborn receives the best nutrition, from own mother's milk, immediately at birth. The health strategy is to set up policies and guidelines that providing an environment where breastfeeding is the usual practice to increase the success. In essence, infants are being breastfed exclusively for the first six months or more. This is the key point of the programme in not only helping healthy growth and development of infant, but also reducing the levels of infant morbidity and mortality. The programme started in hospitals and has extended to the community facilities, to promote infant breastfeeding further to two years old or more. A healthcare environment encouraging breastfeeding in the whole society should be the norm in all societies, regions and countries (World Health Organization, 2009).

Benefits of Breastfeeding

Breastfeeding is the gold standard—the best, the most natural and healthy feeding to infants. The mother's milk contains optimal nutrients, growth factors, immunological and anti-inflammatory properties that benefit infant growth. The newborn can digest breastmilk easily and this prevents gas and colic. It is safe and clean and contains rich antibodies to protect the infant against most childhood illnesses. The mother makes breastmilk specifically for her own infant. Naturally, breastfeeding provides nutritional, cognitive and emotional nurturing the healthy development of infants (Lawrence & Lawrence, 2021). The first few days immediately after birth is critical for a newborn to adapt the extra-uterine life. It is also the turning point period for a mother to be a mother, starting to nurture her newborn. It is essential for health professionals to provide adequate and appropriate support to the mothers due to start breastfeeding. UNICEF and WHO have launched the Baby-Friendly Hospital Initiative programme worldwide to encourage governments and health facilities to implement the support breastfeeding policy and guidelines (World Health Organization, 2018).

Breastfeeding has long-term health gain for the infants, lasting into adulthood. After weaning, the health benefits from breastfeeding stay with the children till they grow up. Breastmilk is the ideal food for infants to build up the best and long-lasting health foundation. According to WHO, breastfed children have higher intelligence test marks and less overweight or obesity (Eidelman & Schanler, 2012). Moreover, breastfeeding not only helps mother recover from childbirth faster, but also reduces the risk of ovarian and breast cancers (Anstey et al., 2017; Babic et al., 2020) and other chronic diseases, such as diabetes, hypertension and cardiovascular diseases (Lawrence & Lawrence, 2021). Breastfeeding is also beneficial to the family and society, being convenient and economical. The mother is free to breastfeed her infant at any time and any place, building healthy future citizens for the society. Breastfeeding saves money from the purchase of infant formula milk powder, bottles and teats. It is natural and friendly to the environment too and contributing to the sustainable development in the world (Riordan & Wambach, 2014).

Successful Breastfeeding

The "Ten Steps to successful breastfeeding" (World Health Organization, 2018) are:

1. A written breastfeeding policy—routinely communicated to staff and parents, with continuous monitoring;
2. Training of staff in breastfeeding with updated knowledge to build capacity and capability;
3. To inform and discuss with all antenatal women and their families about the advantages and management of breastfeeding;
4. To support mother-newborn skin-to-skin contact immediately after birth for initiating breastfeeding;
5. To support mothers in the management of common breastfeeding difficulties and sustainability of breastfeeding for 2 years and beyond;
6. No other food or fluid except breastmilk or breastfeeding should be given to breastfed newborns unless medically indicated;
7. To keep mothers and newborns in the same room, 24 h a day, to facilitate unrestricted breastfeeding around the clock;
8. To help mothers to recognise the infants' cues for feeding and respond to them accordingly;
9. To educate and counsel mother, who are not able to breastfeed, in switching to bottle feeding with infant formulae; and

10. To coordinate and provide ongoing breastfeeding support and care in the community setting for sustainable development of breastfeeding.

Implementation of nursing procedures of "Ten Steps to Successful Breastfeeding" has been found to promote optimal clinical care for new mothers to breastfeed their newborns successfully. This, together with the compliance with the critical management procedures, and the International Code of Marketing of Breast-milk Substitutes and relevant World Health Assembly resolutions has significantly improved the breastfeeding rates (World Health Organization, 2018). A systematic review of 58 studies on maternity and newborn care demonstrated that adherence to the Ten Steps had impacts on early initiation of breastfeeding immediately after birth, exclusive breastfeeding and total duration of breastfeeding (Gavine et al., 2017).

The Choice to Mothers

Many factors are contributing breastfeeding baby by mothers. The actual success of breastfeeding initiation and breastfeeding duration rates depend on various factors at different time, different people and different environment around her. All of them may have a positive or negative impact on breastfeeding behaviour. Firstly, at the individual level, the nursing mother needs to know how breastfeeding can provide the optimum nutrition for her newborn baby. She makes the informed choice to breastfeed. The attitudes of the mother and family members, their relationship and the family environment affect the decision to initiate and keep on breastfeeding. Secondly, at the social level, it depends on if the social environment is breastfeeding-friendly or not. This will affect the sustainability of breastfeeding. Social measures, including social acceptance and consideration of family and community, occupation and workplaces, will help to facilitate the mothers and needs of individuals. The third level to be considered is the structural situation, such as applicable legislative framework, policies and supporting services for breastfeeding women. Maternal protection by the law is essential for mothers to breastfeed in public and in the workplaces. Healthcare organisations and facilities should provide women with information and education of breastfeeding. Moreover, the right attitude and skills of healthcare professionals should add to the assistance and counselling in response to mothers' needs. These three levels have important influence on the initiation and duration of breastfeeding among nursing mothers (Federal Ministry of Food & Agriculture, 2021).

Supports to Mothers

Women and families often turn to health professionals for health advice. People and parties around them play an important role in influencing the women. The families will seek information from community and social support services. Women may search and receive information from the internet, relatives, friends, colleagues, workplaces, nursery, baby-care centres, etc. The information and advice will influence the women in making the decision on breastfeeding. Breastfeeding Project team of the Australia National Aboriginal Community Controlled Health Organisation has identified the continuity and consistency of high-quality education of breastfeeding as part of the essential procedures to keep mothers in breastfeeding. The breastfeeding support should be accessible and well-coordinated by various parties in the community (National Aboriginal Community Controlled Health Organisation, 2017).

Nevertheless, failure of continuity of care within the healthcare field is not unusual. It is often arising from the following three causes:

i. Ineffective communication when different information is given by healthcare professionals and healthcare service settings. Often, the organisations or institutes are without a proper hand-over system. They pass conflicting messages. This happens when there is a lack of policy or procedure guidelines.
ii. Breakdowns in the continuity of patient education, in which women are receiving confused recommendations or treatment plans. They do not understand what they should follow, how to make the decision and how to follow the medical advice.
iii. Accountability breakdown when women are under the care of various healthcare teams in different healthcare settings. There is a question of which professional team should be accountable for the adverse outcome of care? For example, a new mother discharged from the hospital may come across various healthcare professionals in different healthcare settings. She may consult the obstetrician, paediatrician or health professionals of Maternal and Child Health Centres (MCHCs) for breastfeeding.

Without effective coordination and communication in breastfeeding programmes, nursing mothers are less likely to continue breastfeeding when they go home or back to work. Therefore, improving the continuity care in the community will increase breastfeeding care and support to mothers, resulting in greater success of the programmes (National Aboriginal Community Controlled Health Organisation, 2017).

Promotion and Gaps of Breastfeeding in Hong Kong

In 1989, global strategy in support of breastfeeding introduced the special role of maternity units in promoting breastfeeding. The guidelines of "Promoting, Protecting and Supporting Breastfeeding: The Special Role of Maternity Services" was guiding healthcare facilities with maternity care to implement the Ten practical nursing procedures to enhance the initiation and continuity of breastfeeding (Ten Steps). Following the ten steps, maternal care services helped to promote an optimal environment to support and engage mothers in breastfeeding. Hospitals with maternity services were required to complete a self-reporting questionnaire survey yearly to demonstrate the implementation of the Ten Steps, for the purpose to monitor the progress (World Health Organization, 2018). Following the Innocenti Declaration of 1990, there has been a global effort to implement practices that protect, promote and support breastfeeding (World Health Organization, 2018) in the Baby-friendly Hospital programme. The Baby-friendly Hospital Initiative Hong Kong Association (BFHIHKA) was set up by WHO and UNICEF in 1991 in Hong Kong. The main objective of BFHIHKA was to promote, support and sustain breastfeeding successfully for the mothers and babies. The association has been assisting all health facilities in Hong Kong in meeting the health strategy needs of breastfeeding.

International Baby Food Action Network Asia has developed an assessment tool, The World Breastfeeding Trends Initiative (The World Breastfeeding Trends Initiative, 2012), to assess the implementation of the WHO Global Strategy for Infant and Young Child Feeding. The assessment identifies the gaps and recommends improvement measures in infant feeding. The first assessment, performed in Hong Kong in 2008, was carried out by the Consumer Council and BFHIHKA. The other participating parties included the Hospital Authority Breastfeeding Promotion Subcommittee; the Family Health Service of the Department of Health, the School of Public Health of Li Ka Shing Faculty of Medicine at the Hong Kong University, the Department of Paediatrics and Adolescent of the Hospital Authority and the Department of Paediatrics of the Faculty of Medicine at The Chinese University of Hong.

The assessment consisted of two parts. Five indicators on infant feeding practices, forming the first part of the assessment, examined the actual results of how policy and programmes support the practices in the community.

1. Percentage of babies breastfed within one hour immediately after birth.
2. Percentage of babies from birth to six months of age exclusively breastfed in the last 24 h.
3. The average duration of the number of months of breastfeeding for babies.
4. Percentage of breastfed babies, aged less than 6 months old, receiving other foods or drink from nursing bottles.

5. Percentage of breastfed babies receiving complementary foods around 6–9 months of age.

The other ten indicators were included in the second part of the assessment. They were criteria based on the Innocenti Declaration to develop the targets of the Global Strategy.

1. National Policy, Programme and Coordination
2. Baby-Friendly Hospital Initiative (Ten Steps to Successful Breastfeeding)
3. Implementation of the International Code
4. Maternity Protection
5. Health and Nutrition Care System
6. Mother Support and Community Outreach
7. Information Support
8. Infant Feeding and HIV
9. Infant Feeding during Emergencies
10. Monitoring and Evaluation

In the year 2012, another assessment was carried out and it found some gaps in the support of breastfeeding. For the first part of the assessment, percentages of exclusive breastfeeding, receiving other foods or drinks from bottle, or complementary foods were not available. In the second part, there was "*Zero score out of ten on National Policy, Programme and Co-ordination*", indicating an absence of an infant feeding policy, a central breastfeeding committee and breastfeeding co-ordinator. Another area of 0 score was found in infant feeding during emergencies. Furthermore, a low score, one out of ten, appeared in the Baby-Friendly Hospital Initiative. In 2012, no hospital in Hong Kong had achieved the Baby-Friendly status while only a low score was achieved in the compliance of the International Code of Marketing of Breast-milk Substitutes, a voluntary Code (The World Breastfeeding Trends Initiative, 2012).

However, there were some areas of significant improvement. The discontinuation of the acceptance of free supplies of infant formula was implemented in public hospitals in 2010 in accordance with the Code. It also served as pathway for the Department of Health to prepare for a voluntary code on marketing of breastmilk substitutes to be promulgated in Hong Kong in 2012. The assessment had called hospitals with maternity units the interest to acquire the Baby-Friendly Hospital status. To monitor the local breastfeeding trends, monthly reports of breastfeeding rates are being collected from public and private hospitals with birthing units. The Breastfeeding Surveys on breastfeeding rates in the first year of life in the Hong Kong Maternal and Child Health Centres (MCHCs) are conducted regularly by the Department of Health. Most of babies born in Hong Kong are covered (Department of Health, 2021).

The COVID-19 Pandemic

In 2020, breastfeeding support services in public or private hospitals and community MCHCs were substantially scaled down during the COVID-19 pandemic. Breastfeeding support services, including antenatal breastfeeding promotion, skills education, breastfeeding assessment, counselling and coaching, were reduced because of the social distancing measures. The support had been partially resumed from June 2021. Online health education on breastfeeding had been developed. The Hospital Authority had gradually resumed antenatal classes and education workshops for breastfeeding (Department of Health, 2021). However, the infection control and precautious measures for the pandemic had complicated breastfeed and become barriers for mothers in directly breastfeeding the babies. Healthcare professionals were thus reminded and required to balance the immediate and long-term health benefits against the impact of pandemic isolation and infection control measures on the mothers and babies, the family and the community (World Health Organization, 2020).

Baby-Friendly Hospital Initiative Hong Kong

In Hong Kong, the BFHIHKA had initiated the Baby-Friendly Hospital programme and awarded health facilities as baby-friendly since 2013 (Baby-Friendly Hospital Initiative Hong Kong Association, 2022). All eight public hospitals and twelve private hospitals with birthing units were invited to participate in the yearly breastfeeding survey. Over the years, six public hospitals with maternity unit have been designated as baby-friendly hospitals. In 2021, this was translated to 50% of births being taken place in baby-friendly hospitals. The remaining two public hospitals and one private hospital were undergoing various stages of accreditation towards the reward. Three community maternal and child health centres that provided breastfeeding support to mothers in the antenatal and postnatal periods had also been designated as baby-friendly MCHCs. Another five MCHCs had started to proceed to the designation.

The Way Forward

Hong Kong has only a self-reporting breastfeeding survey by Maternal Health Care Centres and hospitals. There is still no government policy on breastfeeding, or infant and young child feeding in Hong Kong. Moreover, there is no Central Breastfeeding Committee with the authority to implement continuous monitoring of breastfeeding practice. The whole society, other than Department of Health and hospitals, should join hands together in supporting and sustaining breastfeeding.

The first step of the revised "Ten Steps" Implementation breastfeeding guideline expands not only breastfeeding training to staff, but also management procedures. The revised WHO guideline has addressed on the leadership, management and supervision to achieve the breastfeeding goals in various breastfeeding management programme with ongoing monitoring and data-management systems (World Health Organization, 2018). The HKSAR government and leaders of the society should allocate appropriate resources and consider legislations for successful breastfeeding to build a healthy community and to achieve health for all.

Specialty lactation professionals provide breastfeeding supporting services to hospitals and community. The services of lactational home visits or in Specialist Lactation Clinics should be free and easily accessible. Special lactation programmes should be implemented to assist women with medically complex pregnancies or deliveries and breastfeed their newborns. Multi-disciplinary health professional teams, including obstetricians, neonatologists, physicians, midwives, nurses, lactation consultants, physiotherapists and occupational therapists, should be involved (American College of Obstetricians & Gynecologists Committee Opinion, 2018, 2021).

Breastfeeding and breastmilk are well-known to be the best to baby's health, growth and development. In emergency, breastfeeding can ensure the survival of the baby. It is best to build up the best health foundation from newborn to adulthood. Breastfeeding is of benefit to the mothers, babies, families, society and to environment. Healthcare professionals should educate mothers about the benefits of breastfeeding. Immediate assistance should be provided after childbirth. A multisectoral approach that involves family, healthcare professionals, community and society should be strengthened to promote, support and sustain breastfeeding in the effort of all for health in the region. Breastfeeding is the best healthy life foundation for generations. Breastfeeding is all for health. Promotion of breastfeeding success is an all for health strategy worldwide. The Government and health assistance agencies should advocate for policy changes to facilitate breastfeeding. Continuous improvement lactation programmes, within hospitals and in the community should be implemented to achieve the supreme and golden breastfeeding goal, leading to health for all.

References

American College of Obstetricians and Gynecologists Committee Opinion. (2018). Optimizing support for breastfeeding as part of obstetric practice. *Obstetrics & Gynecology, 132*(4), e187–e196. https://doi.org/10.1097/aog.0000000000002890

American College of Obstetricians and Gynecologists Committee Opinion. (2021). Breastfeeding challenges. *Obstetrics & Gynecology, 137*(2), e42–e53. https://doi.org/10.1097/aog.0000000000004253

Anstey, E. H., Shoemaker, M. L., Barrera, C. M., O'Neil, M. E., Verma, A. B., & Holman, D. M. (2017). Breastfeeding and breast cancer risk reduction: Implications for black mothers. *American Journal of Preventive Medicine, 53*(3), S40–S46. https://doi.org/10.1016/j.amepre.2017.04.024

Babic, A., Sasamoto, N., Rosner, B. A., Tworoger, S. S., Jordan, S. J., Risch, H. A., Harris, H. R., Rossing, M. A., Doherty, J. A., Fortner, R. T., Chang-Claude, J., Goodman, M. T., Thompson, P. J., Moysich, K. B., Ness, R. B., Jensen, A., Schildkraut, J. M., Titus, L. J., Cramer, D. W., & Terry, K. L. (2020). Association between breastfeeding and ovarian cancer risk. *JAMA Oncology, 6*(6), e200421–e200421. https://doi.org/10.1001/jamaoncol.2020.0421

Baby Friendly Hospital Initiative Hong Kong Association. (n.d.). *Healthcare facilities.* www.babyfriendly.org.hk/en/healthcare-facilities/

Department of Health. (2021). *Breastfeeding survey 2021.* www.fhs.gov.hk/english/reports/files/BF_survey_2021.pdf

Eidelman, A. I., & Schanler, R. J. (2012). Breastfeeding and the use of human milk. *Pediatrics, 129*(3), e827–841. https://doi.org/10.1542/peds.2011-3552

Federal Ministry of Food and Agriculture. (2021). *National strategy for the promotion of breastfeeding.* https://www.bmel.de/SharedDocs/Downloads/EN/Publications/breastfeeding-strategy.pdf?__blob=publicationFile&v=2

Gavine, A., McFadden, A., Macgillivray S., & Renfrew M. J. (2017). Evidence reviews for the Ten Steps to Successful Breastfeeding initiative. *Journal of Health Visiting, 5*(8), 378–380. https://doi.org/10.12968/johv.2017.5.8.378

Lawrence, R. A., & Lawrence, R. M. (2021). *Breastfeeding: A guide for the medical professional* (9th ed.). Elsevier. https://doi.org/10.1016/C2018-0-02113-1

National Aboriginal Community Controlled Health Organisation. (2017). *Breastfeeding and continuity of care: Closing the care gap.* https://www.naccho.org/uploads/downloadable-resources/Breastfeeding-Continuity-Care.pdf

Riordan, J., & Wambach, K. (2014). *Breastfeeding and human lactation* (5th ed.). Jones and Bartlett Learning.

The World Breastfeeding Trends Initiative. (2012). *Hong Kong Special Administrative Region (HKSAR) China second assessment report 2012.* https://www.babyfriendly.org.hk/wp-content/uploads/2017/04/WBTi-HKSAR2012.pdf

World Health Organization. (2009). *Baby-friendly hospital initiative: Revised, updated and expanded for integrated care.* https://www.ncbi.nlm.nih.gov/books/NBK153471/

World Health Organization. (2018). *Implementation guidance: Protecting, promoting and supporting breastfeeding in facilities providing maternity and newborn services—The revised Baby-friendly hospital initiative.* https://www.unicef.org/media/95191/file/Baby-friendly-hospital-initiative-implementation-guidance-2018.pdf

World Health Organization. (2020). *Frequently asked questions: Breastfeeding and COVID-19 for health care workers.* https://cdn.who.int/media/docs/default-source/maternal-health/faqs-breastfeeding-and-covid-19_805d4ce8-2329-4227-9261-695afa68b32c.pdf?sfvrsn=d839e6c0_5

Chapter 18
Preventive Health Visit

Peter T. K. Lau

Abstract Screening for asymptomatic disease, through the application of laboratory tests, clinical examinations, or other procedures on apparently healthy persons, is a core element of secondary prevention and health promotion. The ultimate aim is early identification of health risks and timely implementation of effective interventions. The preventive health visit, also known variously as periodic health examination and multiple screening, is an important tool to conduct secondary prevention on a community and population level. In this chapter, the historical context and scientific basis of screening, its potential benefit, drawback, resource allocation and ethics will be discussed, with a special focus on the early diagnosis of cancer and cardio-metabolic disease, and an emphasis on the role of the primary care physician. In addition to evidence-based professional guidelines, citizen preferences should also be taken into account when considering choices for a screening programme. Other possible benefits of a preventive programme are facilitating marginalised groups to attend a healthcare service, and optimising the management of chronic disease. Moreover, recent advances in telehealth and genetic sequencing do have an impact on screening strategies. Enhancing the uptake of well-planned preventive programmes in the community will play a key part in achieving the goal of "Health for All".

Keywords Prevention · Health examination · Screening guideline · Cancer · Primary care · COVID-19

Historical Context

Preventive care is traditionally associated with the "periodic health examination" which often refers to a yearly clinical visit for screening tests. This has a long history and is said to have its origins as far back as the Industrial Revolution when workers

P. T. K. Lau (✉)
Jockey Club School of Public Health and Primary Care, The Chinese University of Hong Kong, Hong Kong, China
e-mail: plau@townhealth.com

B. Y. F. Fong and W. C. W. Wong (eds.), *Gaps and Actions in Health Improvement from Hong Kong and Beyond*,
https://doi.org/10.1007/978-981-99-4491-0_18

went for annual physicals so that the employers could maintain a healthy workforce. The American Medical Association also began to publish guidance on preventive examinations in the 1920s (Breslow, 1959; Ponka, 2014).

In the past, there has been some distinction between "periodic health examination" (conducted by the physician with an emphasis on history taking and physical examination) and "multiple screening" (a battery of screening tests performed by technicians, only individuals with abnormal test results were referred to a physician) (Breslow, 1959). While these terms traditionally represent two slightly different approaches to regular screening, in actual practice the distinction is often blurred. Moreover, terms such as "preventive health screening" and "periodic preventive health visits" are often employed to denote similar preventive healthcare activities. The author prefers the term "preventive health visit", emphasising both the preventive nature of the exercise and the preference for a visit to the healthcare provider.

While it is generally accepted that regular screening tests can catch risk factors and diseases early, the periodic health examination need not and should not be conducted on a rigid annual basis. A focused approach, with regard to the demographics and risk profile of the target population, is of much better value and utility. Whether offered as an annual physical or selective periodic preventive health examinations, screening should be a lifelong process beginning at birth (Breslow & Somers, 1977).

Annual Visit or Opportunistic Screening

Although the periodic health examination has a long history, in modern times there have been calls to abandon the comprehensive annual physical and replace it with opportunistic screening, squeezing prevention into visits for other reasons (Birtwhistle et al., 2017; Oboler et al., 2002; Ponka, 2014). However, studies have also found that a significant proportion of the populace still desired an annual physical checkup. In the United States (US) at least, the annual physical remains an important ritual for many. Although no randomised control study has proven a clear-cut morbidity and mortality benefit from the periodic health examination, strategies to incorporate preventive screening within the context of visits for another problem fared no better. It is common experience that acute care visits often leave little time for effective preventive counselling or intervention (Laine, 2002). Moreover, a regular visit to one's physician for preventive checkup when well decreases the risk of having to seek help from an unfamiliar doctor when suffering from a serious ailment. The author feels that if nothing else, the nurturing of a good client-physician relationship is sufficient justification for retaining the periodic preventive visit. Regular contact with the physician, accompanied by physical examination and well-chosen laboratory tests, helps to build up a trusting rapport and ensures that the client receives timely interventions (Laine, 2002).

The author believes that both periodic and opportunistic screening have a place in different settings. A regular primary preventive visit may be valuable in encouraging attendance of marginalised groups and optimising the management of chronic diseases (Ponka, 2014). The Royal Australian College of General Practitioners (2016) suggests systematic approaches for prevention of specifically targeted conditions including childhood immunisations, and screening for diabetes, as well as cervical, breast and colorectal cancers. Most other preventive activities in Australia would be done in opportunistic settings when the preventive activity is an add-on for patients presenting with other reasons.

Principles of Screening

A landmark publication by Wilson and Jungner (1968) more than half a century ago ushered in a new era of modern screening. The principles were adopted by the World Health Organization (WHO) and other organisations as the basis of general screening programmes. Screening was, and still is, defined as "the presumptive identification of unrecognised disease or defect by the application of tests, examinations, or other procedures". This is indeed the essence of "Secondary Prevention" in primary healthcare.

The stated principles to determine the usefulness of screening include:

1. The health problem should be an important one, with a recognisable latent or early symptomatic phase that is adequately understood.
2. The screening tests should be conveniently available and well validated, and the process should be acceptable to the screened public.
3. The treatment of the screened condition should be accessible and effective.
4. The outcome of screening should be evidence based. There should be an agreed policy on whom to treat as patients. Cost effectiveness should be considered, and the public should be educated to reach an informed decision (Royal Australian College of General Practitioners, 2016; Wilson & Junger, 1968; World Health Organization, 2020).

Current Practice

Nowadays almost all major medical and health organisations worldwide publish guidelines on screening. In one form or another, and to varying degrees, preventive health practices are incorporated into national and local healthcare systems. Most preventive strategies emphasise vaccination and developmental screening in the paediatric population. For the adult and elderly population, screening of cancers, cardiovascular diseases and diabetes, the leading causes of morbidity and mortality, becomes more important. Recommended guidelines, while broadly similar, do differ in certain areas. They also evolve over time in the light of new research findings (Fong, 2020). Illustrative examples of screening for adults, and how guidelines change over time, will be discussed in this chapter.

Scientific and Evidence Based

Not all screening measures are equally effective, and what is being offered to the public must be evidence based. Screening for the following conditions is generally considered of proven value: cervical cancer, colorectal cancer, breast cancer, diabetes and hypercholesterolemia (Eyre et al., 2004). The benefits of screening the asymptomatic population for hypertension, anaemia and kidney diseases are less clear. Targeted screening for prostate cancer (by PSA) and lung cancer (by low dose CT) may be controversial as there are arguments both for and against screening. Screening for osteoporosis and dementia should be cost-effective if targeted at the appropriate population.

Locally, the Hong Kong reference framework for preventive care of older adults includes health education on vaccination and lifestyle, together with screening of the following conditions: hypertension, diabetes, hyperlipidemia, obesity (and underweight), cervical cancer, colorectal cancer and functional impairment (Health Bureau, 2021). Breast cancer and osteoporosis are conspicuous by their absence. In the view of the author, such omission could be due to cost-effective or cost benefit considerations, or the inability of the public sector to offer these services on a population wide basis.

Changing Guidelines but Unchanged Goals

Screening guidelines evolve over time, sometimes drastically. The author vividly recalls the days when population screening for diabetes was not considered worthwhile. Now almost all major authorities recommend some form of diabetic screening for the general population. Looking at the chronology of American Cancer Society (ACS) recommendations for cancer screening in asymptomatic people, the changes are remarkable and may be confusing to the general public unless they are guided by a knowledgeable family physician. For example, monthly breast self-examination was recommended in the 1980s, but had been replaced solely by mammography by 2015. While sigmoidoscopy has always been one of colorectal cancer screening options since 1980, the latest recommendations now include, among other things, full colonoscopy, CT colonography and stool DNA testing (American Cancer Society, 2021). Although the methodology changes, the goal of screening remains the same: "to identify disease early when they are amenable to intervention, based on latest evidence on emerging screening techniques, and new study findings supporting or refuting the value of traditional tests".

Screening for Cancers and Cardiovascular Diseases: Specific Examples

Cervical Cancer

Cervical cancer is a classic example of effective prevention by detecting the cancer in its pre-malignant stage. It has been over 60 years since Dr. George Papanicolaou developed the cervical Pap smear test, and it saves many lives. Cervical cancer was once a leading cause of death among women, but the death rate dropped markedly when the Pap test became widely implemented. The Pap test is now recognised as one of the most significant advances in the fight against cancer, making cervical cancers not only curable but totally preventable. Today, even after the introduction of HPV vaccination and testing, Dr. Papanicolaou's method remains an essential component of cervical cancer prevention (Mammas & Spandidos, 2012; Vilos, 1998).

Recommendations for cervical cancer screening have evolved over the years, influenced by greater understanding of the role of high-risk human papillomavirus (HPV) in cancer causation, and the emergence of HPV testing. The current trends are towards a transition from cytology to HPV testing, an older age to begin screening, and lengthening the screening interval. In the most recent update of the ACS guideline for an average-risk individual, cervical cancer screening with HPV testing is recommended to begin at age 25 years and cease at age 65 years, with an interval every 5 years. Cytology testing alone every 3 years is an acceptable option if HPV testing is not available (Fontham et al., 2020).

In Australia, women aged 25 to 74 years are recommended to undertake a cervical HPV test every 5 years (Royal Australian College of General Practitioners, 2016). The Hong Kong guideline recommends women aged between 25 and 64 years to have cervical cytology test every 3 years after two consecutive normal annual tests. Screening may be discontinued after age 65 years if three previous consecutive tests are normal. HPV testing is not specifically mentioned (Health Bureau, 2021), perhaps due to lack of resources in the public sector.

Colorectal Cancer

Global incidence of colorectal cancer (CRC) is on the rise, but this malignancy is eminently treatable and curable if detected at an early stage and is, therefore, a good candidate for effective screening. Faecal immunochemical test (FIT) of stool is traditionally preferred due to its low cost and non-invasive nature. Colonoscopy, although much more expensive and carries certain procedural risks, can detect and remove pre-malignant colon polyps before they develop into cancer. Like the cervical smear, colonoscopy goes beyond screening and can actually prevent the onset of cancer. Using colonoscopy as CRC screening is gradually gaining wider acceptance, and not only in rich or developed countries. Two recent studies have indicated the feasibility and cost effectiveness of colonoscopy in low- or middle-income countries even when compared with FIT (Krzeczewski et al., 2021; Phisalprapa et al., 2019).

Both the American Cancer Society and the US Preventive Services Task Force (USPSTF) acknowledge colonoscopy every 10 years as one of the options for CRC screening. However, colonoscopy is not recommended by RACGP (2016) as a screening test for people at average risk of CRC. In Hong Kong, the emphasis is naturally on faecal occult blood testing every 1–2 years (Health Bureau, 2021). The government does offer heavily subsidised colonoscopy for individuals who are enrolled in its screening programme and tested positive for FIT (The Government of the Hong Kong Special Administrative Region, 2020).

Breast Cancer

Breast cancer is a leading cause of premature mortality in women. The benefits of screening are obvious. However, the risks of overdiagnosis and overtreatment cannot be underestimated, and the benefits over harm may be less clear-cut than that of cervical cancer screening. Mammography has been in use since the 1970s, and guidelines from Western countries invariably recommend mammogram screening. ACS suggests women aged 40–54 years to have regular mammography, and those 55 years or older should continue screening as long as they are in overall good health (Smith et al., 2019). Australia recommends screening mammograms every two years for asymptomatic, low-risk women aged 50–74 years (Royal Australian College of General Practitioners, 2016). The Hong Kong guideline is less enthusiastic, quoting insufficient evidence to recommend for or against population-based mammography screening (Health Bureau, 2021). In some countries such as China, mammography is either not readily accessible or not well accepted by the public due to the cost, radiation and discomfort. Moreover, it is well known that mammography has a low sensitivity in women with dense breasts. Ultrasound is not typically used as a routine screening test for breast cancer in Western countries. In China and Hong Kong, however, ultrasound is widely employed for breast cancer screening, either alone or supplemental to mammography. Studies have shown that supplemental ultrasonography could detect occult breast cancers missed by mammogram. In addition, primary ultrasonography without mammogram might have comparable performance to primary mammogram, and be utilised as primary screening tool in low-resource settings where mammography is unavailable. (Sood et al., 2019; Yang et al., 2020).

Prostate Cancer

Screening for prostate cancer is controversial and is a prime example of how conflicting expert opinions can confuse the public. Screening recommendations are controversial because the supporting evidence is equivocal. Prostate specific antigen

(PSA) screening of asymptomatic and low-risk men for prostate cancer is not generally recommended because of the lack of clear-cut survival benefits (Beck, 1999). It has even been argued that the sons of men diagnosed with prostate cancer are stigmatised in that they themselves might be at increased risk of prostate cancer, hence the burden of overdiagnosis is being passed to the next generation (Justman, 2012).

The USPSTF (2018) has concluded that there is a small net benefit of PSA-based screening for prostate cancer in some men aged 55 to 69 years, and that "the decision to undergo periodic PSA-based screening should be an individual one and should include discussion of the potential benefits and harms of screening with their clinician". The USPSTF continues to advise against PSA-based screening in men aged 70 years and older in large part because of the increased risk of harms from false-positive PSA results, biopsies, overdiagnosis, and treatment in men of advanced age. The ACS likewise recommends PSA testing for men aged 50 years and over, after an informed decision making with their healthcare provider, but places no upper age limit for screening (Smith et al., 2019). Local guideline cites the lack of convincing evidence for or against prostate cancer screening (Health Bureau, 2021). Prostate cancer is heterogeneous with a widely variable course and prognosis. New biomarkers supplementing PSA may become useful tools to reduce unnecessary biopsies, stratify low-risk from high-risk tumours and inform personalised treatment decisions. These would include biochemical markers such as percentage free PSA, prostate health index (PHI) or the 4K score, or novel genomic biomarkers (Cucchiara et al., 2018; Duffy, 2020).

Hypercholesterolemia

Elevated cholesterol, in particular LDL-Cholesterol, is an important risk factor for cardiovascular diseases such as myocardial infarction and stroke. Australian guideline suggests individuals to have blood lipids, preferably full lipid profile, assessed every five years starting at age 45 years (Royal Australian College of General Practitioners, 2016). Hong Kong guideline also recommends periodic screening for adults aged 50 to 75 years (Health Bureau, 2021). American guidelines extend the target population age to adults aged 20 years and above, albeit screened at longer intervals of 4–6 years than older adults (Grundy et al., 2019). Given that lipid profile blood test is inexpensive and readily available, the author feels that it is a valuable test that can go a long way in mitigating the future burden of cardiovascular morbidity.

Diabetes

Diabetes is often asymptomatic in its early stages and therefore may remain undetected for years without targeted screening. Early detection, coupled with timely interventions, has been shown to mitigate progression of pre-diabetes to diabetes and reduce the risk of complications of diabetes. Universal screening for all adults older than 45 years of age regardless of risk factors, and regardless of age for adults who are overweight plus at least one additional risk factors, is recommended by the American Diabetes Association (Eyre et al., 2004). Recommendations of the American Association of Clinical Endocrinology are broadly similar. The USPSTF recommendation, however, restricts screening to adults who have overweight or obesity and aged 35 to 70 years. Screening tests for pre-diabetes and type 2 diabetes include fasting plasma glucose, HbA1c, or oral glucose tolerance test (Davidson et al., 2021). Local guidelines recommend screening of diabetes mellitus for adults from age 45 years with fasting blood sugar (Health Bureau, 2021).

Expanding the Scope of Screening

Screening is not limited to physical diseases. In suitable settings, screening can and should expand to mental issues ranging from mood and substance use to pain and cognition (Sewell et al., 2020). It has also been advocated that social determinant of health should be included in preventive screening. This would include screening for domestic violence, as well as abuse of vulnerable children and adults (Krist et al., 2019).

Limitations and Potential Harm

Adverse outcome from screening is certainly unintended but also inevitable. Potential harm includes overdiagnosis, overtreatment, inaccurate test results (false positive and false negative) and diversion of precious health resources to screening measures with dubious benefits (World Health Organization, 2020).

Overdiagnosis and Overtreatment

A frequent criticism of preventive screening is the possibility of overdiagnosis, which is the incidental finding of a condition that will not lead to significant morbidity or premature mortality over the patient's lifetime. This is often seen in cases of indolent cancers, such as some forms of thyroid and prostate cancers, where the tumour can be so slow growing that the patient often dies with, not of the disease (Bell et al., 2017). People who are screened positive for relative benign conditions may receive excessive treatment that may result in excessive morbidity. Examples would include impotence from aggressive treatment of early prostate cancer, or surgical removal of benign breast lesions (World Health Organization, 2020).

False Positive and False Negative

A preliminary positive test can, and frequently does, lead to a battery of follow up investigations, causing both anxiety and expenses. It is worse if the final verdict is a false-positive screening result. Screening done wrong may even make the patient less healthy as a result. On the other hand a false negative screening can result in complacency, a false sense of security and missed warning signs of disease. The value of screening can sometimes be overestimated because of "lead time bias" (Beck, 1999). Essentially, this means when a disease is detected at an earlier stage, its prognosis and course are not altered and the end result is the same regardless of whether screening has been done. Nevertheless, even if the disease course is not altered, some people might wish to have advance knowledge of what to expect so as to properly plan their work and family life (World Health Organization, 2020).

The Unique Case of Occupational Health Check

Employee health screening, also known as industrial health examination in the past, is commonly utilised to screen potential candidates for a job or to assess the continued suitability to perform their duties. However, such health screenings do have the potential of being abused. Breslow (1959) lamented that the pre-employment checkup, which might be useful for health screening purposes, was often misused as a means to preclude certain people from employment. While the pre-employment checkup might offer an individual early awareness of health risks, when a person is denied employment because of such health issues the resulting unemployment is also detrimental to health. In Hong Kong, there is legislation against employment discrimination based on medical conditions, but protection generally is not extended to the pre-employment stage. It is essential to ensure that when employees submit themselves to such examinations, they can benefit from the screening at least as much as their employers (Wilson & Jungner, 1968).

Balancing Benefits and Harms in Health Screening

While there are both empirical and anecdotal evidence attesting to the benefits of preventive screening, both individuals and physicians are often over optimistic on the potential benefits while underestimating the harms associated with screening. Shared decision making should be undertaken, where the physician and the individual have an informed discussion on the merits and pitfalls of the screening test and reach a mutually accepted course of action (Bell et al., 2017).

Enhancing Uptake

The value of identifying and treating diseases early, particularly for chronic diseases such as diabetes and cardiovascular ailments, is well recognised. And as discussed earlier in this chapter, effective screening measures are readily available. Unfortunately, there still appears to exist an implementation gap between the burden of chronic diseases and the utilisation of effective intervention measures to mitigate the onset of diseases, or their early detection through screening. Reasons for the underutilisation of useful clinical preventive measures include lack of financial incentive in prevention, and an emphasis on "volume based" reimbursement instead of a "value-based" model where the long-term health outcomes are more important. Healthcare providers are more often than not paid to treat rather than to prevent diseases. Enhancing uptake of preventive services requires a multi-pronged approach to shift the institutional culture into recognising the benefits of prevention, and efforts to engage and educate individuals on the value of preventive care (Levine et al., 2019). Lobbying the government, employers and health insurance companies for more subsidies in preventive intervention should also prove to be useful in enhancing uptake.

Financial Constraints

People may not be motivated enough to go for preventive checkup considering the time and money involved. This can be alleviated to a certain extent if such health screenings are subsidised, either by the government or the employer (Hakro & Li, 2019). In China, it has been common practice for employers to provide annual health check to their employees. In Hong Kong, some large businesses also offer renumeration for health screening expenses. The government provides free screening to those under age 18 years, and heavily subsidised screening for elders aged 65 and above. However, most adults need to pay for preventive checkup out of their own pockets.

Users of Preventive Services: Patients or Clients?

By definition, preventive services such as screening are targeted for the healthy population without symptoms or known diseases. However, when reviewing the literature on prevention and screening the term "patients", with its connotation of ill health and suffering, is often used to denote attendees of preventive services. Even the term "healthy adult patient" has been used in some papers. There are studies to explore the issue of what to call people attending health services, and alternatives such as client, consumer, customer or even survivor (of cancer) have been proposed. It has also been found that the majority of healthcare providers and even users themselves prefer the term "patients", justifying its use with the concept of "caring" for people (Costa et al., 2019; Loudon et al., 2012). The author, however, prefers the use of "client" and does use it in his own practice. The term "client" empowers people in ways that "patient" cannot. Moreover, users of preventive health services are generally well people and they should be differentiated from those "patients" who are really ill.

Preventive Health Care During the COVID-19 Pandemic

Like almost all aspects of healthcare, preventive services were severely hampered by the pandemic. Utilisation of vaccination and periodic checkup fell sharply, as people were confined to their homes and the healthcare sector was overwhelmed in coping with COVID-19 patients (Allahqoli et al., 2022; Mularczyk-Tomczewska et al., 2022).

Although we can expect preventive services to pick up as we move out of the pandemic, lasting damage may have been done as vaccines are missed and certain major diseases like cancers and ischaemic heart diseases are diagnosed late. However, there is always a silver lining behind the dark cloud of COVID-19. Both clients and healthcare providers are forced deeper into the electronic age. Priority setting to retain the most important, evidence-based screening programmes have become acutely important (Dickinson et al., 2020). The public is more willing to embrace telehealth and other forms of remote consultation, and some of the physical barriers limiting the uptake of health services for those with mobility or access issues can be mitigated.

Moreover, demand for wellness checkup can appear unexpectedly. The author experienced a dramatic upsurge in screening tests for cardio-metabolic diseases during a government drive to encourage COVID-19 vaccination in 2021, as people wanted to make sure their body was fit for vaccination. This desire was of course not evidence based, as the vaccines are considered safe and suitable for the majority of the population. The author, however, was able to identify quite a number of hidden hypertension, hypercholesterolemia or diabetes patients during the exercise; cases that might go undetected for years if not for this sudden rush to screen. In the view of the author, this was a small but not insignificant upside amidst the grim toll of COVID-19.

Future Trends, Telehealth, Genetic Screening

Web-based or smartphone-based wellness portals or applications may be useful in enhancing awareness and provide information and advice on preventive health services based on individual health needs. With the fast-paced advances in technology into the genomic age, more and more new disease genes are being identified.

Healthcare professionals and policymakers need to assess the potential benefits and pitfalls of current or emerging genetic screening programmes (Andermann et al., 2008). A novel model of "Smart Health Communities" (SHC) has been proposed to address the issue of the evolving landscape of health care systems especially after the challenges of COVID-19. SHC relies on primary health care and embraces the use of digital health, wearable devices and electronic health records to enhance care in the community level, with a particular focus in encouraging disease prevention and overall wellbeing (Ng et al., 2021). While a smart community may be easier to realise in a smart, healthy city, the use of electronic and virtual technology may help to bridge the disparity between urban and rural localities (Lau, 2021), enabling preventive care to be delivered more equitably.

Role of the Primary Care Physician

A screening test is not intended to be diagnostic. Persons with positive or suspicious findings must be referred to their physicians for diagnosis and necessary treatment. While it is possible to offer preventive health services through employer-based programmes, direct mass marketing appeals, public health campaigns and legislation such as taxation and prohibition, primary care remains the optimal means to deliver quality preventive healthcare. As mentioned earlier in this Chapter, preventive healthcare may be delivered during one of two types of office visits, either a separate, standalone "preventive health visits or wellness visit", or visits for medical conditions. Continuous care with an established physician–patient relationship is perceived as integral to the success of preventive care delivery (Murugan et al., 2018).

For primary care to be effective, the providers should work closely with the local community to prioritise the most important services to be delivered at optimal intervals. Clinical guidelines may be imprecise or lack local relevance. Citizen involvement in guideline development may help to complement the experts' perspective with the concern of the general public (Sommer et al., 2021). Indeed preference of the general public in setting priorities for preventive health care programmes might deviate from a traditional health maximisation approach based simply on cost-effective analysis, and with emphasis on prevention more than cure (Luyten et al., 2015). Therefore, the primary care physicians, in collaboration with the community, should enlighten the public and encourage participation in preventive care. Such an interdisciplinary approach would do well in achieving the supreme goal of "health for all" (Fong & Law, 2020).

References

Allahqoli, L., Mazidimoradi, A., Salehiniya, H., & Alkatout, I. (2022). Impact of COVID-19 on cancer screening: A global perspective. *Current Opinion in Supportive and Palliative Care, 16*(3), 102–109. https://doi.org/10.1097/SPC.0000000000000602

American Cancer Society. (2021). *History of ACS recommendations for the early detection of cancer in people without symptoms.* https://www.cancer.org/health-care-professionals/american-cancer-society-prevention-early-detection-guidelines/overview/chronological-history-of-acs-recommendations.html

Andermann, A., Blancquaert, I., Beauchamp, S., & Déry, V. (2008). Revisiting Wilson and Jungner in the genomic age: A review of screening criteria over the past 40 years. *Bulletin of the World Health Organization, 86*(4), 317–319. https://doi.org/10.2471/BLT.07.050112

Beck, L. H. (1999). Periodic health examination and screening tests in adults. *Hospital Practice, 34*(12), 117–126. https://doi.org/10.3810/hp.1999.11.175

Bell, N. R., Grad, R., Dickinson, J. A., Singh, H., Moore, A. E., Kasperavicius, D., & Kretschmer, K. L. (2017). Better decision making in preventive health screening: Balancing benefits and harms. *Canadian Family Physician, 63*(7), 521–528. https://www.cfp.ca/content/63/7/521.long

Birtwhistle, R., Bell, N. R., Thombs, B. D., Grad, R., & Dickinson, J. A. (2017). Periodic preventive health visits: A more appropriate approach to delivering preventive services: From the Canadian task force on preventive health care. *Canadian Family Physician, 63*(11), 824–826. https://www.cfp.ca/content/63/11/824

Breslow, L. (1959). Periodic health examinations and multiple screening. *American Journal of Public Health and the Nation's Health, 49*(9), 1148–1156. https://ajph.aphapublications.org/doi/pdf/10.2105/AJPH.49.9.1148

Breslow, L., & Somers, A. R. (1977). The lifetime health-monitoring program: A practical approach to preventive medicine. *The New England Journal of Medicine, 296*(11), 601–608. https://doi.org/10.1056/NEJM197703172961104

Costa, D. S. J., Mercieca-Bebber, R., Tesson, S., Seidler, Z., & Lopez, A.-L. (2019). Patient, client, consumer, survivor or other alternatives? A scoping review of preferred terms for labelling individuals who access healthcare across settings. *BMJ Open, 9*(3), Article e025166. https://doi.org/10.1136/bmjopen-2018-025166

Cucchiara, V., Cooperberg, M. R., Dall'Era, M., Lin, D. W., Montorsi, F., Schalken, J. A., & Evans, C. P. (2018). Genomic markers in prostate cancer decision making. *European Urology, 73*(4), 572–582. https://doi.org/10.1016/j.eururo.2017.10.036

Davidson and M. J., Mangione, C. M., Cabana, M., Caughey, A. B., Davis, E. M., Donahue, K. E., Doubeni, C. A., Krist, A. H., Kubik, M., Li, L., Ogedegbe, G., Owens, D. K., Pbert, L., Silverstein, M., Stevermer, J., Tseng, C.-W., & Wong, J. B. , 2021 Davidson, K. W., Barry, M. J., Mangione, C. M., Cabana, M., Caughey, A. B., Davis, E. M., Donahue, K. E., Doubeni, C. A., Krist, A. H., Kubik, M., Li, L., Ogedegbe, G., Owens, D. K., Pbert, L., Silverstein, M., Stevermer, J., Tseng, C.-W., & Wong, J. B. (2021). Screening for prediabetes and type 2 diabetes: US preventive services task force recommendation statement. *JAMA, 326*(8), 736–743. https://doi.org/10.1001/jama.2021.12531

Dickinson, J. A., Thériault, G., Singh, H., Szafran, O., & Grad, R. (2020). Rethinking screening during and after COVID-19: Should things ever be the same again? *Canadian Family Physician, 66*(8), 571–575. https://www.cfp.ca/content/66/8/571.long

Duffy, M. J. (2020). Biomarkers for prostate cancer: Prostate-specific antigen and beyond. *Clinical Chemistry and Laboratory Medicine, 58*(3), 326–339. https://doi.org/10.1515/cclm-2019-0693

Eyre, H., Kahn, R., Robertson, R. M., Clark, N. G., Doyle, C., Gansler, T., Glynn, T., Hong, Y., Smith, R. A., Taubert, K., & Thun, M. J. (2004). Preventing cancer, cardiovascular disease, and diabetes: A common agenda for the American Cancer Society, the American Diabetes Association, and the American Heart Association. *CA: A Cancer Journal for Clinicians, 54*(4), 190–207. https://doi.org/10.3322/canjclin.54.4.190

Fong, B. Y. F. (2020). Use of clinical practice guidelines. *Hong Kong Medical Journal, 26*(5), 367–369. https://doi.org/10.12809/hkmj205106

Fong, B. Y. F., & Law, V. (2020). Renewal of primary care. In B. Y. F. Fong, V. T. S. Law, & A. Lee (Eds.), *Primary care revisited: Interdisciplinary perspectives for a new era* (pp. 3–21). Springer. https://doi.org/10.1007/978-981-15-2521-6_1

Fontham, Wolf, A. M. D., Church, T. R., Etzioni, R., Flowers, C. R., Herzig, A., Guerra, C. E., Oeffinger, K. C., Shih, Y. T., Walter, L. C., Kim, J. J., Andrews, K. S., DeSantis, C. E., Fedewa, S. A., Manassaram-Baptiste, D., Saslow, D., Wender, R. C., & Smith, R. A. (2020). Cervical cancer screening for individuals at average risk: 2020 guideline update from the American Cancer Society. *CA: A Cancer Journal for Clinicians, 70*(5), 321–346. https://doi.org/10.3322/caac.21628

Grundy, S. M., Stone, N. J., Bailey, A. L., Beam, C., Birtcher, K. K., Blumenthal, R. S., Braun, L. T., de Ferranti, S., Faiella-Tommasino, J., Forman, D. E., Goldberg, R., Heidenreich, P. A., Hlatky, M. A., Jones, D. W., Lloyd-Jones, D., Lopez-Pajares, N., Ndumele, C. E., Orringer, C. E. … Yeboah, J. (2019). 2018 AHA/ACC/AACVPR/AAPA/ABC/ACPM/ADA/AGS/APhA/ASPC/NLA/PCNA guideline on the management of blood cholesterol: A report of the American college of cardiology/American heart association task force on clinical practice guidelines. *Circulation, 139*(25), e1082–e1143. https://doi.org/10.1161/CIR.0000000000000625

Hakro, S., & Li, J. (2019). Workplace employees' annual physical checkup and during hire on the job to increase health-care awareness perception to prevent disease risk: A work for policy-implementable option globally. *Safety and Health at Work, 10*(2), 132–140. https://doi.org/10.1016/j.shaw.2018.08.005

Health Bureau. (2021). *Hong Kong reference framework for preventive care for older adults in primary care settings*. https://www.healthbureau.gov.hk/pho/rfs/english/reference_framework/pre_care_for_older_adults.html

Justman, S. (2012). Uninformed consent: Mass screening for prostate cancer. *Bioethics, 26*(3), 143–148. https://doi.org/10.1111/j.1467-8519.2010.01826.x

Krist, A. H., Davidson, K. W., Ngo-Metzger, Q., & Mills, J. (2019). Social determinants as a preventive service: U.S. preventive services task force methods considerations for research. *American Journal of Preventive Medicine, 57*(6), S6–S12. https://doi.org/10.1016/j.amepre.2019.07.013

Krzeczewski, B., Hassan, C., Krzeczewska, O., Wieszczy, P., Pisera, M., Ciopinska-Chaber, A., Rupinski, M., Sliwczynski, A., Pastusiak, R., Regula, J., & Kaminski, M. F. (2021). Cost-effectiveness of colonoscopy in an organized screening program. *Polish Archives of Internal Medicine, 131*(2), 128–135. https://doi.org/10.20452/pamw.15779

Laine, C. (2002). The annual physical examination: Needless ritual or necessary routine? *Annals of Internal Medicine, 136*(9), 701–703. https://doi.org/10.7326/0003-4819-136-9-200205070-00013

Lau, P. T. K. (2021). Health and urban living. In B. Y. F. Fong & M. C. S. Wong (Eds.), The Routledge handbook of public health and the community (pp. 21–35). Routledge. https://doi.org/10.4324/9781003119111-3-4

Levine, S., Malone, E., Lekiachvili, A., & Briss, P. (2019). Health care industry insights: Why the use of preventive services is still low. *Preventing Chronic Disease, 16*, Article 180625. https://doi.org/10.5888/pcd16.180625

Loudon, J., Baird, A., Haider, Z., Sein, E., Prabakar, I., & Gebbie, A. (2012). Patients, clients, users or customers: What should we call people attending sexual health services? *Journal of Family Planning and Reproductive Health Care, 38*, 19–22. https://doi.org/10.1136/jfprhc-2011-0112

Luyten, J., Kessels, R., Goos, P., & Beutels, P. (2015). Public preferences for prioritizing preventive and curative health care interventions: A discrete choice experiment. *Value in Health, 18*(2), 224–233. https://doi.org/10.1016/j.jval.2014.12.007

Mammas, I. N., & Spandidos, D. A. (2012). George N. Papanicolaou (1883–1962): Fifty years after the death of a great doctor, scientist and humanitarian. *Journal of BUON, 17*(1), 180–184. https://jbuon.com/archive/17-1-180.pdf

Mularczyk-Tomczewska, P., Żarnowski, A., Gujski, M., Sytnik-Czetwertyński, J., Pańkowski, I., Smoliński, R., & Jankowski, M. (2022). Preventive health screening during the COVID-19 pandemic: A cross-sectional survey among 102,928 internet users in Poland. *Journal of Clinical Medicine, 11*(12), Article 3423. https://doi.org/10.3390/jcm11123423

Murugan, H., Spigner, C., McKinney, C. M., & Wong, C. J. (2018). Primary care provider approaches to preventive health delivery: A qualitative study. *Primary Health Care Research & Development, 19*(5), 464–474. https://doi.org/10.1017/S1463423617000858

Ng, F., Briggs, D., & Liu, Y. (2021). Smart health communities: From sick care to health care. In B. Y. F. Fong & M. C. S. Wong (Eds.), *The Routledge handbook of public health and the community* (pp. 302–312). Routledge. https://doi.org/10.4324/9781003119111-27-31

Oboler, S. K., Prochazka, A. V., Gonzales, R., Xu, S., & Anderson, R. J. (2002). Public expectations and attitudes for annual physical examinations and testing. *Annals of Internal Medicine, 136*(9), 652–659. https://doi.org/10.7326/0003-4819-136-9-200205070-00007

Phisalprapa, P., Supakankunti, S., & Chaiyakunapruk, N. (2019). Cost-effectiveness and budget impact analyses of colorectal cancer screenings in a low- and middle-income country: Example from Thailand. *Journal of Medical Economics, 22*(12), 1351–1361. https://doi.org/10.1080/13696998.2019.1674065

Ponka, D. (2014). The periodic health examination in adults. *Canadian Medical Association Journal, 186*(16), 1245. https://doi.org/10.1503/cmaj.141125

Royal Australian College of General Practitioners. (2016). *Guidelines for preventive activities in general practice, 9th edition.* https://www.racgp.org.au/download/Documents/Guidelines/Redbook9/17048-Red-Book-9th-Edition.pdf

Sewell, R., Cottrell, E., Gutman, K., Clemons, M., Friedman, D., Kotin, E., Smith, E., Whitehouse, J., & Pratt, C. (2020). Which behavioral health screening tool should you use-and when? *The Journal of Family Practice, 69*(9), 454–460. https://doi.org/10.12788/jfp.0089

Smith, R. A., Andrews, K. S., Brooks, D., Fedewa, S. A., Manassaram-Baptiste, D., Saslow, D., & Wender, R. C. (2019). Cancer screening in the United States, 2019: A review of current American Cancer Society guidelines and current issues in cancer screening. *CA: A Cancer Journal for Clinicians, 69*(3), 184–210. https://doi.org/10.3322/caac.21557

Sommer, Titscher, V., Szelag, M., & Gartlehner, G. (2021). What are the relevant outcomes of the periodic health examination? A comparison of citizens' and experts' ratings. *Patient Preference and Adherence*, 15, 57–68. https://doi.org/10.2147/PPA.S281466

Sood, R., Rositch, A. F., Shakoor, D., Ambinder, E., Pool, K.-L., Pollack, E., Mollura, D. J., Mullen, L. A., & Harvey, S. C. (2019). Ultrasound for breast cancer detection globally: A systematic review and meta-analysis. *Journal of Global Oncology, 5*(5), 1–17. https://doi.org/10.1200/JGO.19.00127

The Government of the Hong Kong Special Administrative Region. (2020). *Eligibility of Colorectal Cancer Screening Programme updated.* https://www.info.gov.hk/gia/general/202012/30/P2020123000566.htm

US Preventive Services Task Force. (2018). Screening for prostate cancer: US preventive services task force recommendation statement. *JAMA, 319*(18), 1901–1913. https://doi.org/10.1001/jama.2018.3710

Vilos, G. A. (1998). The history of the Papanicolaou smear and the odyssey of George and Andromache Papanicolaou. *Obstetrics and Gynecology, 91*(3), 479–483. https://doi.org/10.1016/s0029-7844(97)00695-9

Wilson, J. M. G., & Jungner, G. (1968). Principles and practice of screening for disease. *World Health Organization.* https://apps.who.int/iris/handle/10665/37650

World Health Organization. (2020). *Screening programmes: A short guide. Increase effectiveness, maximize benefits and minimize harm.* https://apps.who.int/iris/handle/10665/330829

Yang, L., Wang, S., Zhang, L., Sheng, C., Song, F., Wang, P., & Huang, Y. (2020). Performance of ultrasonography screening for breast cancer: A systematic review and meta-analysis. *BMC Cancer, 20*, Article 499. https://doi.org/10.1186/s12885-020-06992-1

Chapter 19
Digital Health and Technology Adoption

Fowie S. F. Ng, Mark Brommeyer, and Zhanming Liang

Abstract The pursuit of the goal of 'All for Health' can be enabled by the adoption of 'Digital Health' and 'Technology' in all levels of care which can facilitate greater cooperation between health sectors and across different health systems. This chapter will review the development of e-health into the era of 'Digital Health' with the emphasis on technological advancement in connected patient care concerning health improvement, health protection, consumer participation as well as improvement of health service effectiveness and efficiency. Case studies from Australia and Hong Kong are used to highlight the rationale, importance, policy, and implementation issues of adopting digital technologies and innovative models of care that contribute to achieving healthcare goals in different health system contexts. Together with the advocation of 'Smart City' and 'Smart Health' by a lot of countries, government initiatives and commitments from key stakeholders are the important factors that facilitate this international movement. Similarly, a well-developed specialised digital health workforce and the competence of health services managers and health information managers in supporting the health system in transitioning into the era of 'Digital Health' are critical. A holistic approach in developing the workforce that can lead and manage digital health transformation is also discussed.

Keywords Digital health · Information and communications technology · Electronic health record · Innovation and technology · Competency development

F. S. F. Ng (✉)
Tung Wah College, Hong Kong, China
e-mail: fowieng@twc.edu.hk

M. Brommeyer
College of Business, Government and Law, Flinders University, Adelaide, SA, Australia
e-mail: mark.brommeyer@flinders.edu.au

Z. Liang
College of Public Health, Medical and Veterinary Science, James Cook University, Queensland, Australia
e-mail: zhanming.liang@jcu.edu.au

B. Y. F. Fong and W. C. W. Wong (eds.), *Gaps and Actions in Health Improvement from Hong Kong and Beyond*,
https://doi.org/10.1007/978-981-99-4491-0_19

Introduction

The failure to achieve the World Health Organization (WHO) global strategy for health for all by the year 2000 highlights the importance of removing the barriers to equity in access to services, in particular for people who are socially and economically disadvantaged and people who are living in remote areas in both developed and developing countries (Whitehead et al., 2001). It also reinforces the need to focus health system reform on strengthening primary healthcare (Zwi & Yach, 2002). With such goal in mind, in the financial constraint climate which has been worsened by COVID-19 pandemic, health systems are pressured to adopt innovative ways in providing high quality of care across different spectrums with efficiency. The most noticeable movements are the adoption of digital technologies in digitalising patient data—electronic health records (EHR) since the late 1990s; the provision of fast health services without physical contacts such as 'Telehealth', 'Telemedicine', and 'Telepharmacy', and the incorporation of 'Remote Patient Monitoring (RPM) and 'Geographic Information System' (GIS) to tackle the impact of COVID-19 (Tabacof et al., 2021). However, the success in digital health transformation and the adoption of digital health technologies does not happen without substantial planning and the implementation of strategies that enables required changes to take place. Cross learning between different healthcare contexts can certainly contribute to addressing the challenges facing the adoption of 'Digital Health' and 'Technology' into the 'New Normal' and indeed the 'Next Normal' in healthcare. Australia, a country with a population of 26 million occupying the vast 7.6 million square kilometres of land, and Hong Kong, a city with a dense population of 7.3 million people living on 1104 square kilometres of land, are chosen for such purposes.

Transitioning to Digital Health

The concept of 'Digital Health' is not new in the healthcare industry, but universal agreement on its definition or scope is lacking (Fatehi et al., 2020). In the publication by the WHO titled 'Global Strategy on Digital Health 2020–2025', it is defined as 'the field of knowledge and practice associated with the development and use of digital technologies to improve health' (World Health Organization, 2021. p. 39). The definition includes three key elements: what do we know about digital health technology, how do we use digital health technology, and the ultimate goal of digital health is to improve the health of the population. Digital health also embraces other adoption of digital technologies for health such as the Internet of things, artificial intelligence, big data, and robotics. This WHO Global Strategy on Digital Health has been adopted by the World Health Assembly in 2020 to provide the roadmap for counties to improve health outcomes with the latest development in digital health and innovation (World Health Organization, n.d.).

A number of professional institutions have played a key role in supporting the advancement of digital health transformation in healthcare. Internationally, Healthcare Information and Management Systems Society (HIMSS) (https://www.himss.org/) is the global advisor and thought leader in information and technology with more than 111,000 members with five types of membership of individual, corporate, organisational affiliate, non-profit partner and student from North America, Europe, the Middle East as well as Asia Pacific (Healthcare Information and Management Systems Society, n.d.-b). HIMSS has developed a blueprint for digital health advancement that guides healthcare providers worldwide to apply frameworks, models, and tools to build, measure and advance health system transformation. HIMSS (n.d.-a) defines digital health as 'connects and empowers people and populations to manage health and wellness, augmented by accessible and supportive provider teams working within flexible, integrated, interoperable and digitally enabled care environments that strategically leverage digital tools, technologies and services to transform care delivery' (Healthcare Information and Management Systems Society, n.d.-a). The organisation regularly conducts Certification Examination to provide qualified health professionals the status of the 'Certified Professional in Digital Health Transformation Strategy' (CPDHTS). This significantly contributes to developing healthcare executives and informatics professionals' competency in meeting the international standard in digital health transformation strategy to advance their career in digital health strategy through continuous education.

In Australia, the Australian Institute of Digital Health (AIDH) (https://digitalhealth.org.au/) is the leading professional organisation advocating Australasia's digital movement following the merger of the Health Informatics Society of Australia (HISA) and the Australasian College of Health Informatics (ACHI) in February 2020 (Australasian Institute of Digital Health, n.d.). A white paper published by AIDH outlined the rationale to promote and incorporate digital health for delivering the future of health (Rowlands, 2020). This digital health era represents a paradigm shift but not just a new term or jargon for 'e-Health'. It is seen as a distinct and important evolution in the delivery of health services that has been through four distinct stages with the first wave starting in the 1950s when Information Technology (IT) and telecommunications were implemented in the health sector. It was followed by the proliferation of computing networks with increasing bandwidth to facilitate the expansion of Information and Communications Technology (ICT) in the second wave of 'Health ICT' in the mid-1960s. 'E-Health' represents the third wave corresponding to the period of the 2000s with the use of enterprise-wide shared health records at individual, regional, and national levels.

The focus of e-health is to connect the healthcare delivery system through information technology, digitisation of images with increased quantity of health data, mobile technologies, social media, and so on to quest for healthcare interoperability. It coincided with the three domains of the conceptual model for e-Health proposed by Professor Tim Shaw and colleagues (2017) in Australia (Shaw et al., 2017). They revealed three prominent but overlapping domains including 'health in our hands', 'interacting for health', and 'data enabling health'. This practice-based model of e-Health tried to solve the lack of consistency in defining the term by supporting

Table 19.1 7 Major shifts of the digital health era

Major Shifts	Descriptions
Citizen and consumer centricity	Citizens choose where and how they store their data, who they share it with and expect service models to fit their life flows
New entrants	Big tech disruption with non-healthcare companies becoming health data companies
Industry convergence	The boundaries of health service delivery overlapping with other sectors/industries
Role convergence	Boundaries of clinical professional practice diverge and meld
Origin of data	Vast amounts of new health and health-relevant data captured outside of traditional clinical care settings
Analytics and algorithms	New analytical capabilities drive new models of care
Broader than health	Dissolving the arbitrary boundaries place between health, aged care, mental health, social services and disability sectors

Source Rowlands (2020, p. 17)

healthcare professionals in applying e-Health to different clinical and management situations in their professional or discipline contexts. The fourth wave of 'Digital Health' in the 2020s has witnessed an exponential growth of Internet of Things (IoT) or Internet of Medical Things (IoMT). The proliferation of the use of health apps, wearables, the ubiquitous use of technology, data analytics, algorithms, artificial intelligence (AI), machine learning, robotics, cloud-based services, and augmented and virtual reality has shifted the paradigm from e-Health to digital health disruption era. As illustrated by Rowlands (2020), seven shifts characterise the 'Digital Health' era (Table 19.1), differentiating Digital Health from the previous e-Health era by the absorption of digital health into people's everyday lives, thinking, and expectations but not merely focusing on technologies and their capabilities. Despite there are more than 90 different definitions for digital health, the AIDH white paper argued that digital health can be defined as health and healthcare in the context of digital societies (Wienert et al., 2022).

Case Studies from Australia

The two case examples from Australia, reflective of the computerisation of General Practice in primary care, and the development and implementation of a national electronic health record, are used to highlight the rationale, importance, policy, and implementation issues reflective of how digital health and technology impact on achieving the healthcare goals in different health system contexts.

Rationale

Digital health has been embraced in Australia based on a long history of need, with the tyranny of distance necessitating the use of innovative delivery methods, and technology to provide and support care across 7.6 million square kilometres of Australia's land mass, populated by just 26 million people. When Reverend John Flynn started the *mantle-of-safety* using a timber and fabric bi-plane named 'Victory' leased by QANTAS, in 1928, what is now called the Royal Flying Doctor Service was born (Royal Flying Doctor Service, n.d.). That same year, Alfred Traeger invented the pedal powered radio, forever transforming the way people communicated in Australia's outback. This technological innovation was an essential foundation for the Royal Flying Doctor Service to connect with people for essential communications and emergency medical assistance (Royal Flying Doctor Service, 2019). This century of innovation in healthcare delivery and support has embraced Australia's willingness to adopt the use of various technology-enabled healthcare services.

Importance

The electronic sharing of patient's information and records that follows their healthcare journey across primary, secondary, and tertiary care can strengthen the continuation of care because patients are at risk of falling out of the system during the transition between different levels of care, practitioners, and service facilities (Australian Commission on Quality and Safety in Health Care, n.d.). The national report on Safety Issues at Transitions of Care highlights the required continued improvement in the compatibility of electronic information systems making it easier for clinicians to have access to patient data and communicate during transitions of care (Australian Commission on Quality and Safety in Health Care, 2017). The launch of the national Personally Controlled Electronic Health Record (later renamed My Health Record) in 2012 in Australia is an example (Federal Register of Legislation, 2012). It was partly driven by the desire to increase consumer participation in their own healthcare and to maintain wellness, by providing personalised health information to each Australian in a summary, electronic, and accessible format. It has enabled health information to be rapidly available to authorised people which improves coordination of care, reduces the risk of healthcare errors, assists practitioners in making faster and more informed healthcare decisions, and improves workflow and management efficiencies for healthcare providers (Department of Health & Aged Care, 2022). Ultimately, it has led to safer patient care and the reduction of waste and duplication of services (de Mesquita & Edwards, 2020).

With eighty per cent of all healthcare transactions in Australia occurring at the primary care level in general medical practices, the imperative to electronically enable General Practice with clinical and practice management systems was prioritised (Dwan et al., 2003). Computerisation in General Practice in Australia has now reached 97% coverage, encouraged and enabled by significant investment and technology uptake, driven by national policy and additional funding provided to general practices via the Australian Government's Practice Incentives Program (PIP) (Vandersman et al., 2020). This included the e-Health Incentive payment which encouraged general practices to keep up to date with digital health and adopt new health technology. Computerisation of GP practices has enabled patients' access to electronic prescriptions, having their pathology and radiology investigation orders and results being generated and sent electronically, as well as accessing medical services via telehealth. Further, the ability to send electronic referrals from primary care to secondary and tertiary care was enabled, and electronic discharge summaries from hospitals and acute care facilities are now able to be sent to the referring primary care general medical practitioner or specialist provider. This has significantly improved communication between different levels of care that is fundamental to the continuity of the services that patients receive, which is particularly important for patients with chronic conditions. A survey of 1000 General Practitioners conducted by the Royal Australian College of General Practitioners in 2021 found that 99% of General Practitioners in Australia were offering telehealth services (Javanparast et al., 2021).

Implementation Issues

Technology-enabled care in Australia has seen a period of intense activity over the last four decades. The journey has been a litany of innovation, success, and challenges, with the story being added to only a daily basis. However, implementation of the digital health initiatives and the adoption of technologies have faced various challenges. Its success is influenced by how prepared the health system and health organisation are in addressing the challenges. These challenges can be placed in three categories as explained in Table 19.2. These key challenges are reflective of the "challenges to help healthcare organisations, health information technology developers, researchers, policymakers, and funders focus their efforts on health information technology–related patient safety" (Sittig et al, 2020, p. 183).

Impact on Achieving the Healthcare Goals in Different Health System Contexts

Digital health uses are many and varied, but all should focus on the delivery of required healthcare services and outcomes based on contextual needs. As part of Australia's response to the global COVID-19 pandemic, the Australian Deputy Chief Medical Officer highlighted that "Digital health innovation has been used to operationalise the nation's pandemic preparedness principles by reducing risk of infection

Table 19.2 Key challenges with health information technology–related patient safety

Categorization of challenges	Key challenges
Design and development challenges	Developing models, methods, and tools to enable risk assessment Developing standard user interface design features and functions Ensuring the safety of software in an interfaced, network-enabled clinical environment Implementing a method for unambiguous patient identification
Implementation and use challenges	Developing and implementing decision support which improves safety Identifying practices to safely manage IT system transitions
Monitoring, evaluation, and optimization challenges	Developing real-time methods to enable automated surveillance and monitoring of system performance and safety Establishing the cultural and legal framework/safe harbor to allow sharing information about hazards and adverse events Developing models and methods for consumers/patients to improve Health IT safety

to both healthcare workers and at-risk patients, sustaining care for chronic and acute health conditions, and supporting the mental health of the population" (Sturgiss et al., 2022, p. 269). The availability of information and communication technologies has enabled and empowered people's access to health information and services electronically, but has presented a challenge to healthcare practitioners and providers alike. Consideration needs to be given as to how to harness the potential value of the increasing volume of patient-generated health data; how to electronically empower people to be more responsible for maintaining their own health, for example, electronically booking and having evidence of required vaccinations. Further, managing patients after discharge from acute care and complying with their rehabilitation regimens can be facilitated through the use of providers' digital clinical and evidence-informed, patient education and wellness information (Smits et al., 2022). With the large variety of digital devices now that can collect and share electronic personal health data, the adoption of relevant digital and governance standards has never been more essential to enhance connectivity and interoperability between the varied healthcare technologies in the digital age.

Case Studies from Hong Kong

Hong Kong has the highest life expectancy worldwide for both female and male since 2010 (Na, 2022). The life expectancies at birth have been raising during the last 50 years, from 67.8 years for males and 75.3 years for females in 1971 to 83.4 years and 87.7 years respectively in 2020 (Centre for Health Protection, 2022). Healthy lifestyles and the city's well-developed infrastructure that provided easy access to health, food, and social services are important contributing factors to prolonged life expectancies (Chung & Marmot, 2020).

The development of digital health initiatives and technologies has been well supported by the Government of the Hong Kong Special Administrative Region (HKSAR) reflected in both the first edition (2017) and second edition (2020) of the 'Smart City Blueprint for Hong Kong'. The Smart City Blueprint strongly supports the development of the infrastructure necessary for a 'Smart City' bringing Hong Kong residents benefits and convenience of using public services. The first blueprint included 76 initiatives under six smart areas of 'Smart Mobility', 'Smart Living', 'Smart Environment', 'Smart People', 'Smart Government', and 'Smart Economy' with successful digital infrastructure projects implemented in Hong Kong (Innovation & Technology Bureau, 2017). The latest blueprint extended the coverage of over 130 initiatives and in particular the use of Innovation and Technology (I&T) in combating COVID-19 under the auspice of 'Smart Living'. Digital health and technology are being implemented with different ubiquitous healthcare devices deployed as a result to tackle the pandemic of COVID-19 (Innovation & Technology Bureau, 2020).

The healthcare system of Hong Kong is characterised by the public/private mix at different levels of care with the majority of the primary care being funded and provided by the private sector and the provisions of secondary care at the hospital level are provided by the public sector of the Hospital Authority (HA) with funding from the Government. The latest strategic plan for 2022–2027 by the HA included the strategic goals of changing the service models towards the provision of 'Smart Care' through the support and commitment of a 'Smart Workforce' and 'Smart Hospitals'. As a result, we have witnessed the development of the infrastructure for digital technology and artificial intelligence (AI) in the hospitals that enable the provision of Smart Care (Hospital Authority, 2021). A specialised IT Innovation Office was set up to facilitate the incubation of technology innovation solutions throughout the whole HA. Under the office, a portal has been launched at https://www.ha.org.hk/innovation/ to serve as a bridge between HA businesses and innovative technologies (Hospital Authority, n.d.). Successful digital health and technology projects and prototypes are being deployed such as the 'HA Go' which is a one-stop mobile platform designed to improve patient experiences in the patient journey. In particular, telemedicine through HA Go was used as a technological tool to battle COVID-19 (South China Morning Post, 2020).

Chinese medicine (CM) is an integral part of Chinese culture in Hong Kong. The Basic Law of Hong Kong Special Administrative Region Article 138 has highlighted the commitment to formulate policies to develop western and traditional Chinese medicine to improve medical and health services. A 'Chinese Medicine Council of Hong Kong' was set up in September 1999 as a statutory body to implement regulatory measures for Chinese medicine (Chinese Medicine Regulatory Office, 2022). A new flagship Chinese medicine hospital with 400 beds covering inpatient and outpatient services is planned to commence services in phases from mid-2025. This Chinese medicine hospital will be the first one of its kind in Hong Kong which is being built by the Government and managed by a non-profit making organisation. Patients will be treated based on a pure Chinese medicine (CM) service or an integrated Chinese-Western Medicine (ICWM) service approach (Health Bureau, 2022). It also serves as a training, education, and research facility and will execute the Government's policy to promote local and world recognition of CM services. This hospital will be an intelligent smart hospital incorporating digital health and technology to provide efficient and effective patient services and healthcare management (Food & Health Bureau, 2019). Advanced IT systems such as patient administration system, enterprise resource planning, CM and WM Pharmacy dispensing system, and other non-clinical patient support systems will be adopted. In particular, a new clinical management system covering both Chinese and Western medicine will be established. This system is compatible with the current territory-wide Electronic Health Record Sharing System (eHRSS) which is the major electronic health record system for all members of the public (Ng et al., 2022). Chinese Medicine at the primary care level has taken a leap step towards digitalisation which is marked by the recent rollout of the Chinese Medicine Information System (CMIS) On-ramp called 'EC Connect'. Chinese medicine clinics in the community are invited to instal the systems at no cost so that they can access patients' online health records as well as share the patients' electronic health records with other practitioners. One of the key features of the system is the adoption of standardised CM terminology to avoid misinterpretation (Chan, 2021).

Competence of Health Services and Information Managers

With the history of digital health being more than half a century old and a rapidly growing digital health workforce globally, the importance of managing and delivering effective and efficient digital technologies and services is consequently high (D'Anza & Pronovost, 2022). In the United Kingdom's National Health Service Topol Review (National Health Service, 2019), addressing how to prepare the healthcare workforce to deliver the digital future, it was predicted that 90% of all jobs will require some element of digital skills within 20 years. There is an increasing range of specialist digital health capabilities and roles across healthcare organisations, for example, chief clinical informatics officer, chief digital health officer, and chief technology officer, as well as a range of digital health lead-roles across the various clinical, administrative, and technical domains. To maximise the benefits of the adoption and the use of digital health, the systems need a specialised workforce that can meet the operational demands of digital health and technologies, as well as health service managers with the capability in leading and managing the transformation of the system, both operationally and strategically (Schreiweis et al, 2019).

A small but growing number of digital health and health informatics competency frameworks have been used to guide education and professional development, as well as providing guidance for career progression in digital health specialties (Nazeha et al, 2020). For example, the Australian Health Informatics Competency Framework

(AHICF) Second Edition (Australasian Institute of Digital Health, 2022) provides a baseline for identifying competencies required for the broader healthcare workforce to perform as a health informatician and includes certification via an online exam that is based on the competencies in the framework. These competencies, across six domains, "apply and contextualise competencies associated with the health sciences, information sciences, information technology, leadership and management, and the social and behavioural sciences, as well as embracing a range of topics that are specialised to health informatics" (Australasian Institute of Digital Health, 2022, p. 2).

A growing body of evidence has argued the importance of investing in developing a competent health service management workforce, including the development of health service managers' understanding of health informatics and digital health, and the capability to effectively scale up and manage (Brice & Almond, 2020; Brommeyer et al., 2021). A recent review confirmed that competencies in the areas of data interpretation and management, project management, engagement of staff and key stakeholders in health informatics design, quality control, and evaluation, and supporting the use of informatics and digital health technology amongst staff, are necessary for health service managers to develop (Brommeyer & Liang, 2022). Competencies required by health service managers continue to evolve as the industry changes, hence, investment in health management workforce development is an ongoing effort.

The need for competency development for health service managers in the digital health space has also been recognised by professional bodies. For example, the Australasian College of Health Service Management (2016) recently revised its health service management competency framework by adding six digital management competencies. These competencies include advocating for the use of digital health solutions to support innovation, quality improvement, research, and health service management; aligning corporate, clinical, and information governance; ensuring digital health solutions meet functional and user requirements; using digital health solutions safely, minimising unintended consequences; using advanced analytics methods and visualisation techniques for information representation; and promoting digital health literacy.

However, the lack of professional recognition and regulation in health management positions provides a limited incentive for health service managers to take on formal management training. Hence the skill uplift of the health service management workforce, appropriate to leading and managing in the digital health era, is no easy task. A holistic approach, with efforts from the system and organisational level in developing the current and future health management workforce, is required. This may include better planning prior to the implementation of digital health initiatives, allowing time to provide targeted training for specific health professional groups including managers, to develop the required capacity. Moreover, the focus must be placed on developing a culture of trust in investing in innovation, which includes adopting well-tested change management principles, including the development of an organisational culture for developing trust in innovation investment. This will then contribute to the development of a supportive team climate that can reduce fear and uncertainty amongst staff in a digitally dynamic environment. This supportive team climate can enable and mobilise system leaders and senior management of the organisations to champion digital health transformation, through demonstrating their strong interest in and a positive attitude towards technology and innovation. In addition, opportunities need to be encouraged in the design of monitoring and evaluation frameworks that measure the impact of the technology, as this enhances the relevance and positive outcomes resulting from the digital changes being evaluated, and broadly communicated, to those who are affected by the changes.

The investment in our workforce must continue, across all healthcare teams and sectors, to ensure that in the era of digital health we can continue to promote evidence-informed decision making in pursuit of quality, safe care, wherever that care is provided. This can be encouraged by harnessing the power of technological advancement and benefitting from the improvements across all levels of care, from better-connected patient care to delivering health improvement, health protection, consumer participation, as well as improvement of health service effectiveness, efficiency, and sustainability.

Conclusion

Health systems need to innovate in order to be sustainable in meeting the growing and evolving healthcare needs of the population that they serve. The adoption of digital health initiatives and technologies has enabled improved quality and continuity of care to be provided which has become more valid after the outbreak of COVID-19 pandemic. Moving beyond the broadly implemented e-Health and Electronic Health Records that focused on fast and safe sharing of patient/service data across different spectrums of care and relevant technologies, Digital Health has been integrated into people's everyday lives, thinking, and expectations. With the ability in improving health service quality, effectiveness, and efficiency which is imperative to achieving "Health for All" WHO global strategy, a holistic approach must be adopted to allow digital health to evolve and healthcare to transform. Such an approach requires political will and investments in ongoing digital health development, and supporting the adoption and implementation at the local levels. It is also critical to strengthen partnerships between health systems, healthcare organisations, health professionals, and tertiary institutions, in developing a health workforce equipped with professionals with specialised digital health competencies and managers who have the capacity in enabling, leading, and managing digital health transformation.

References

Australasian College of Health Service Management. (2016). *Master health service management competency framework*. https://achsm.org.au/Portals/15/documents/education/competency-framework/2020_competency_framework_A4_full_brochure.pdf

Australasian Institute of Digital Health. (2022). *Australian health informatics competency framework: For health informaticians Second Edition*. https://digitalhealth.org.au/wp-content/uploads/2022/06/AHICFCompetencyFramework.pdf

Australian Commission on Quality and Safety in Health Care. (n.d.). *Communicating for safety standard*. https://www.safetyandquality.gov.au/standards/nsqhs-standards/communicating-safety-standard

Australian Commission on Quality and Safety in Health Care. (2017). *Safety issues at transitions of care: Consultation report on perceived pain points relating to clinical information systems*. https://www.safetyandquality.gov.au/sites/default/files/migrated/Safety-issues-at-transitions-of-care-consultation-report.pdf

Federal Register of Legislation. (2012). *My Health Records Act 2012*. Australian Government. https://www.legislation.gov.au/Series/C2012A00063

Brice, S., & Almond, H. (2020). Health professional digital capabilities frameworks: A scoping review. *Journal of Multidisciplinary Healthcare, 13*, 1375–1390. https://doi.org/10.2147/jmdh.s269412

Brommeyer, M., & Liang, Z. (2022). Digital health competencies for health service managers. *Society for Health Administration Programs in Education International Symposium, July 2022*. SHAPE, Townsville.

Brommeyer, M., Mackay, M., Liang, Z. & Balan, P. (2021). Protocol for automated content analysis of corpus to determine informatics competencies amongst health service managers. *Asia Pacific Journal of Health Management, 16*(3), 174–183. https://doi.org/10.24083/apjhm.v16i3.785

Centre for Health Protection. (2022), *Life expectancy at birth (male and female), 1971–2021*. https://www.chp.gov.hk/en/statistics/data/10/27/111.html

Chan, S. H. L. (2021). A step towards digitalisation—Rollout of the Chinese medicine information system (CMIS) on-ramp. *eHealth News, 21*. https://www.ehealth.gov.hk/en/whats-new/ehealth-news/ehealth_news_21/cmis-on-ramp.php

Chinese Medicine Regulatory Office. (2022). *Development of Chinese medicine in Hong Kong*. https://www.cmro.gov.hk/html/eng/about_us/development.html

Chung, R. Y., & Marmot, S. M. (2020), *People in Hong Kong have the longest life expectancy in the world: Some possible explanations. NAM Perspectives*. https://doi.org/10.31478/202001d

D'Anza, B., & Pronovost, P. J. (2022). Digital health: Unlocking value in a post-pandemic world. *Population Health Management, 25*(1), 11–22. https://doi.org/10.1089/pop.2021.0031

de Mesquita, R. C., & Edwards, I. (2020). Systematic literature review of my health record system. *Asia Pacific Journal of Health Management, 15*(1), 14–25. https://doi.org/10.24083/apjhm.v15i1.311

Department of Health and Aged Care. (2022). *Electronic health records*. Australian Government. https://www.health.gov.au/health-topics/health-technologies-and-digital-health/about/electronic-health-records

Dwan, K. M., Western, J. S., Del Mar, C., Western, M. C., & Makkai, T. (2003). Computerisation in Australian general practice. *Australian Family Physician, 32*(3), 180–185. https://search.informit.org/doi/abs/https://doi.org/10.3316/informit.378684542684553

Fatehi, F., Samadbeik, M., & Kazemi, A. (2020). What is digital health? Review of definitions. *Studies in Health Technology and Informatics, 275*, 67–71. https://doi.org/10.3233/shti200696

Food and Health Bureau. (2019). *Clinical services plan for the development of Chinese medicine hospital*. https://www.healthbureau.gov.hk/download/press_and_publications/otherinfo/190900_csp/e_csp.pdf

Health Bureau. (2022). *About Chinese medicine hospital project*. https://www.healthbureau.gov.hk/en/chinese_medicine/about_cmh/positioning.html

Hospital Authority. (n.d.). *Explore, match, transform*. https://innovation.ha.org.hk/
Hospital Authority. (2021). *Strategic plan 2022 – 2027: Towards sustainable healthcare*. https://www.ha.org.hk/haho/ho/ap/HA_StrategicPlan2022-2027_Eng_211216.pdf
Healthcare Information and Management Systems Society. (n.d.-a). *Digital health transformation*. https://www.himss.org/what-we-do-solutions/digital-health-transformation
Healthcare Information and Management Systems Society. (n.d.-b), *Who we are*. https://www.himss.org/who-we-are
Innovation and Technology Bureau. (2017). *Hong Kong Smart City Blueprint*. https://www.smartcity.gov.hk/modules/custom/custom_global_js_css/assets/files/HongKongSmartCityBlueprint(EN).pdf
Innovation and Technology Bureau. (2020). *Hong Kong smart city blueprint 2.0*. https://www.smartcity.gov.hk/modules/custom/custom_global_js_css/assets/files/HKSmartCityBlueprint(ENG)v2.pdf
Javanparast, S., Roeger, L., Kwok, Y., & Reed, R. L. (2021). The experience of Australian general practice patients at high risk of poor health outcomes with telehealth during the COVID-19 pandemic: A qualitative study. *BMC Family Practice, 22*, Article 69. https://doi.org/10.1186/s12875-021-01408-w
Na, E. (2022, June 14). Hongkongers are living longer than ever, but experts flag health problems ahead. *South China Morning Post*. https://www.scmp.com/news/hong-kong/society/article/3181505/hongkongers-are-living-longer-ever-experts-flag-health
National Health Service. (2019). *The Topol Review: Preparing the healthcare workforce to deliver the digital future*. https://topol.hee.nhs.uk/wp-content/uploads/HEE-Topol-Review-2019.pdf
Nazeha, N., Pavagadhi, D., Kyaw, B.M., Car, J., Jimenez, G. & Car, L.T. (2020). A digitally competent health workforce: Scoping review of educational frameworks. *Journal of Medical Internet Research, 22*(11), Article e22706. https://doi.org/10.2196/22706
Ng, F., Briggs, D., & Liu, Y. (2022). Smart health communities: From sick care to health care. In B. Y. F. Fong, & M. C. S. Wong (Eds.), *The Routledge handbook of public health and the community* (pp. 302–312). Routledge. https://doi.org/10.4324/9781003119111-27-31
Rowlands, D. (2020). *What is digital health? And why does it matter?* [White Paper], Australasian Institute of Digital Health. https://digitalhealth.org.au/wp-content/uploads/2020/02/DHWA_WHITEPAPER_2019.pdf
Royal Flying Doctor Service. (n.d.). *John Flynn biography*. https://www.flyingdoctor.org.au/about-the-rfds/history/john-flynn-bio/
Royal Flying Doctor Service. (2019). *How Alfred Traeger gave the outback its voice*. https://www.flyingdoctor.org.au/qld/news/how-alfred-traeger-gave-outback-its-voice/
Schreiweis, B., Pobiruchin, M., Strotbaum, V., Suleder, J., Wiesner, M., & Bergh, B. (2019). Barriers and facilitators to the implementation of eHealth services: Systematic literature analysis. *Journal of Medical Internet Research, 21*(11), Article e14197. https://doi.org/10.2196/14197
South China Morning Post. (2020, July 2). *Coronavirus: Hong Kong's Hospital Authority used IT to fight Covid-19 and stands prepared for future challenges*. https://www.scmp.com/comment/letters/article/3091209/coronavirus-hong-kongs-hospital-authority-used-it-fight-covid-19
Shaw, T., McGregor, D., Brunner, M., Keep, M., Janssen, A., & Barnet, S. (2017). What is eHealth (6)? Development of a conceptual model for eHealth: Qualitative study with key informants. *Journal of Medical Internet Research, 19*(10), Article e8106. https://doi.org/10.2196/jmir.8106
Sittig, D. F., Wright, A., Coiera, E., Magrabi, F., Ratwani, R., Bates, D. W., & Singh, H. (2020). Current challenges in health information technology–related patient safety. *Health Informatics Journal, 26*(1), 181–189. https://doi.org/10.1177/1460458218814893
Smits, M., Kim, C. M., Van Goor, H., & Ludden, G. D. S. (2022). From digital health to digital well-being: Systematic scoping review. *Journal of Medical Internet Research, 24*(4), Article e33787. https://doi.org/10.2196/33787.

Sturgiss, E., Desborough, J., Dykgraaf, S. H., Matenge, S., Dut, G., Davis, S., & Kidd, M. (2022). Digital health to support primary care provision during a global pandemic. *Australian Health Review, 46*(3), 269–272. https://doi.org/10.1071/AH21263

Tabacof, L., Kellner, C., Breyman, E., Dewil, S., Braren, S., Nasr, L., Tosto, J., Cortes, M., & Putrino, D. (2021). Remote patient monitoring for home management of coronavirus disease 2019 in New York: A cross-sectional observational study. *Telemedicine and e-Health, 27*(6), 641–648. https://doi.org/10.1089/tmj.2020.0339

Vandersman, P., Pinto, S. M., Damarell, R., & Tieman, J. (2020). *Health IT in Australian general practice: Opportunities and challenges.* End of Life Directions for Aged Care. https://www.eldac.com.au/Portals/12/Documents/DigitalDashboard/GP%20IT%20integration%20Report_%20Final_V1.1.pdf

Whitehead, M., Dahlgren, G., & Evans, T. (2001). Equity and health sector reforms: Can low-income countries escape the medical poverty trap? *The Lancet, 358*(9284), 833–836. https://doi.org/10.1016/S0140-6736(01)05975-X

World Health Organization. (n.d.), *Global Strategy*. https://www.who.int/health-topics/digital-health#tab=tab_3

World Health Organization. (2021). *Global Strategy on Digital Health 2020–2025*. https://apps.who.int/iris/handle/10665/344249

Wienert, J., Jahnel, T., & Maaß, L. (2022). What are Digital Public Health Interventions? First Steps Toward a Definition and an Intervention Classification Framework. *Journal of Medical Internet Research, 24*(6), Article e31921. https://doi.org/10.2196/31921

Zwi, A. B., & Yach, D. (2002). International health in the 21st century: Trends and challenges. *Social Science & Medicine, 54*(11), 1615–1620. https://doi.org/10.1016/S0277-9536(01)00346-X

Chapter 20
Workplace Wellness and Mental Health Improvement: The Case of Hong Kong

Billy S. H. Ho and Ben Yuk Fai Fong

Abstract Work is an integral and important part of life, but issues in workplace such as increased workloads and blame culture have caught the attention of the general public. In particular, the occurrence of mental health disorders (MHDs) is often associated with psychological hazards and work safety in the workplace. In addition, MHDs can lead to low economic productivity, social exclusion, and stigmatisation, making it more difficult to accomplish health for all in the workplace. There will be some improvement in employees' mental health if they have received early prevention, further treatment, and support in the workplace. Hence, creating a comfortable, friendly, and safe workplace is essential for the health and wellness of employees, in the physical, mental, and social perspectives. This chapter explores measures and strategies for promotion and protection for the well-being and mental health of employees in the workplace, including policy development, personnel involvement, staff organisation, work culture, and equitable distribution of health resources, citing Hong Kong as a case report. There are no substitutes for collaborative efforts among the stakeholders, including policymakers, work agencies, and health professionals, in addressing potential risk factors and achieving health for all.

Keywords Mental health · Mental health disorders · Workplace wellness · Working hours

---

B. S. H. Ho (✉)
School of Professional Education and Executive Development, The Hong Kong Polytechnic University, Hong Kong, China
e-mail: billyho820@gmail.com

B. Y. F. Fong
College of Professional and Continuing Education,
The Hong Kong Polytechnic University, Hong Kong, China

B. Y. F. Fong and W. C. W. Wong (eds.), *Gaps and Actions in Health Improvement from Hong Kong and Beyond*,
https://doi.org/10.1007/978-981-99-4491-0_20

Introduction

The workplace is an irreplaceable part in the achievement of health for all people in their life. People spend an average of one-third of lifetime in the workplace (World Health Organization, 2017). Hence, a comfortable and cheerful work environment and conditions can promote bodily and psychosocial wellness among the employees (Mitchell & Choi, 2018). From the perspective of socio-economic development, the workplace is a vital part for implementation of strategies to address mental health issues (Paterson et al., 2021). Previous studies had demonstrated that employee assistance programmes (EAPs) and public education and mental health campaigns were cost-effective to avoid the aggravation of the symptoms of mental illness (Dimoff & Kelloway, 2013).

Mental health issues in the workplace have caught global attention (World Health Organization, n.d.). An increasing number of workers were reported to suffer from anxiety and depression in the workplace, with approximately 792 million people suffering different degrees of mental health disorders (MHDs) worldwide, accounting for one-tenth of the world population (Dattani et al., 2021). In addition, work-related MHDs are being recognised as the primary causes of disability, higher absenteeism rate, and early retirement throughout the world. Thus, maintaining good mental health at the workplace has become essential not only for the perspective of public health but also for the productivity and competitiveness of the organisations.

In Hong Kong, employee anxiety and depression levels are significant. Over a third (31%) and a quarter (24%) of employees have had anxiety and depressive symptoms at the workplace respectively (Zhu et al., 2017). The City Mental Health Alliance Hong Kong (City Mental Health Alliance Hong Kong, 2020) has found that 27% of employees have experienced different work-related MHDs, higher than the average (22%) in the Asia Pacific region. This reflects that Hong Kong employees are under relatively high psychological stress. Nonetheless, approximately three-quarters of employees with various stages of MHDs do not seek assistance because of the fear of being stigmatised, low awareness of their psychological status, and inadequate resources and services (Lam et al., 2015). EAP remains low in the workplace because most employers do not prioritise employees' mental health and wellness. It is also common that most EAPs and mental health programmes do not meet the needs of workers. Nearly 90 per cent of employees noted that the support for mental health is insufficient and inappropriate in the workplace (City Mental Health Alliance Hong Kong, 2017; Mind HK, 2018).

Work-Related Risk Factors for Health

Long Working Hours

Working hours are an essential determinant of health and mental wellness. Hong Kong is one of the flourishing economies, along with the highest over-working population and most extended working hours in the world. According to the Research Office of the Legislative Council Secretariat (2019), the average weekly hours of work was 44.3, and 37% employees worked 48 h or above weekly, exceeding the international labour standard of a 40-h working week (International Labour Organisation, 2018). In addition, lower-skill workers in some service sectors such as security, elderly homes, and restaurants were expected to serve long working hours. One-third to half of them were required to work at least 60 h a week (Research Office of the Legislative Council Secretariat, 2019). The disproportional work-life imbalance can deteriorate the mental health of people. Not surprisingly, various studies have demonstrated that employees with long working hours will suffer anxiety and depression more easily (Chan et al., 2021; Kim et al., 2016), and increase the risk of social isolation and family conflicts (Lee et al., 2020). On the other hand, excessive working hours can compromise health-seeking behaviours, because employees might lack sufficient time and energy to seek professional, timely, and appropriate help, thus perpetuating the vicious cycle of MHDs in the workplace (Zhu et al., 2017).

Most employers and businesses are less concerned about standard working hours (SWH) because they generally see a reduction in actual working hours as equating to increased labour costs (Hiemer & Andresen, 2019). There is still no law in Hong Kong to regulate working hours (Young, 2019). The Standard Working Hours Committee (SWHC) plans to offer sector-specific working hours guidelines to improve the interests and health of workers. However, the guidelines are not legally binding, and the industry relies on corporate social responsibility (CSR) and attitude of business companies (Legislative Council Panel on Manpower, 2020).

Stigma, Discrimination, and Labelling of MHDs in the Workplace

Stigma, discrimination, and labelling in the workplace are significant barriers to employment for people with MHDs, affecting their workplace relationships and health-seeking behaviour and attitude (Hampson et al., 2020). Unhealthy workplace culture further intensifies social isolation (Zhu et al., 2017), causing the reluctance of workers with MHDs to disclose their health conditions to the employers, and potentially leading to further exacerbation of their conditions (Hampson et al., 2020). In Canada, 77% workers feel uncomfortable talking to their employers about their MHDs for fear of facing discrimination or even dismissal (Canadian Centre for Occupational Health and Safety, n.d.). Similarly, in Hong Kong, discussions about

MHDs are considered an unmentionable taboo in the workplace, and only three-in-ten workers would share their mental health issues with colleagues, 55% respondents mentioned that they experienced stigma in the discussion. In addition, they are scared of the potential disadvantages in career progression, bonus payment, and colleague relationships (City Mental Health Alliance Hong Kong, 2017). Most notably, mental health issues can cause significant externalities on co-workers' psychological conditions in the workplace if they are not handled timely or appropriately, leading to an unhealthy mentally workplace culture (Cottini & Lucifora, 2013).

Employees' Mental Health and Organisational Productivity

The relationships between employees' mental health and organisational productivity are highly correlated. MHDs are significant causes of excessive sick leave absenteeism, increased unemployment, and early retirement (World Health Organization, 2010). The World Federation for Mental Health (World Federation for Mental Health, 2017) has indicated that depression can result in 36 workdays lost per year, reducing organisational productivity and competitiveness. Indeed, the economic loss associated with mental disorders is higher than that of chronic diseases such as cancer and diabetes (Trautmann et al., 2016).

Fatigue affected mental health wellness and on-the-work productivity. Accumulated fatigue and psychological stress in the workplace can present as symptoms of MHDs, including depression and anxiety (Bergefurt et al., 2022; Silva-Costa et al., 2020). People with MHDs are more likely to have difficulties in concentration and handling time pressure or multiple tasks at work, thus affecting the performance. Likewise, sick leaves, frequent time off, and high work disability will result in reduced organisational productivity and competitiveness (Rajgopal, 2010).

Low Employment Rate for People with MHDS

Unstable employment and persistent unemployment are associated with anxiety and depression (Kim et al., 2016; World Health Organization, 2010). Specifically, the stigma and economic hardship associated with unemployment can lead to enormous psychosocial stress, insecurities, and a reduction in self-esteem (Wilson & Finch, 2021). Undoubtedly, employment is beneficial in improving mental health (van der Noordt et al., 2014). Job opportunities allow people to build self-confidence and self-esteem by understanding their work capability and having social contacts at the workplace. Nevertheless, stigma and discrimination are the barriers and have limited the provision and implementation of return-to-work (RTW) programmes in Hong Kong, where employers are not willing to recruit or retain workers with MHDs. People with MHDs remain the highest unemployment rate (8.1%) in the disabilities group, being almost three times the average of the population (Census & Statistics

Department, 2014). In addition, people with MHDs could not receive sufficient social support or employment opportunities from the government, further intensifying their retirement difficulties.

Employee's Mental Health: Challenges

Effect and Impacts of Mental Health Disorders

Excessive psychological stress is the primary risk factor for occupational diseases in the workplace, causing a significantly increased long-term illnesses and absenteeism (World Health Organization, 2017). Global MHDs have risen significantly in recent years, catching worldwide concerns (Marquez & Saxena, 2016). Available evidence indicates that mental health condition of workers has progressively deteriorated in the world. MHDs are among the most important contributors to the global burden of disease and disability, and constitute five out of ten leading causes of disability in most countries in Organisation for Economic Co-operation and Development (Cottini & Lucifora, 2013; Pan American Health Organization, 2019). The increasing demand for worker performance and the high pressure for labour market have imposed increasingly heavy psychological stress on the employees at work (Cottini & Lucifora, 2013). In addition, individuals who work in stressful environments or have prolonged working hours are about four times more likely to develop moderate to severe suicidal ideation than the others (Mitchell & Choi, 2018). In 2015, approximately 14.3% of mortality was contributed to MHDs, accounting for approximately eight million worldwide (Walker et al., 2015). Moreover, the disability and death caused by MHDs can result in social costs of treatment and a significant loss of economic productivity (Marquez & Saxena, 2016). However, the resources for diagnosis, treatment, and support for people with MHDs remain extremely limited in most workplaces (World Health Organization, 2021b). Only 30% of occupational diseases, work-related harm, and injuries are covered by insurance in the world (World Health Organization, 2017).

Gaps of Mental Health Care in the Workplace

Collectivist culture is an essential tradition in Asian countries, where the focus is on organisational performance rather than each individual's needs or desires. Nonetheless, collectivist culture might result in a hierarchical and authoritarian atmosphere in the workplace, leading to significant and long-term work-related pressure and suicidal ideation among workers (Ahn et al., 2020). On the other hand, a management style characterised by authoritarianism will inhibit the voice by employees and is not conducive to building a close and harmonious relationship between superiors and subordinates (Snell et al., 2013). In the Asia Pacific, workers have a profound obedience culture in the workplace. They tactically use obedience to avoid open conflict while receiving better rewards (Bal, 2016). Thus, workers in Asian countries are less likely to express their mental health demands to the line managers or employers. In Hong Kong, 64% employees recognised that their mental status would affect their working efficacy (City Mental Health Alliance Hong Kong, 2019), thereby, weakening the organisational productivity.

Costs of Mental Health Disorders in the Workplace

MHDs can cause a substantial loss in productivity. The economic costs of anxiety and depression were estimated at nearly 1 trillion US dollars per year (World Health Organization, n.d.). More specifically, the total economic loss of MHDs has been estimated at around EUR 600 billion dollars for the European Union (Organisation for Economic Co-operation and Development, n.d.), or at approximately 300 billion dollars for the United States (National Alliance on Mental Illness, n.d.). Furthermore, the Lancet Global Health (2020) estimated that the productivity loss due to poor mental health in the workplace was projected to increase to six trillion by 2030 per year if there was a lack of action to address MHDs. Global studies have shown that workplace health programmes can help reduce approximately 27% absenteeism rate and 26% healthcare cost (World Health Organization, 2017). The collaborative research carried out by the National Opinion Research Center (NORC) at the University of Chicago and National Safety Council demonstrated four times the positive return (HKD31.3) on every US dollar (HKD7.8) of investment in the mental health treatment (National Safety Council, 2021).

In Hong Kong, 77% employees agreed with the positive role of EAPs in addressing mental health issues and emotional-related problems (City Mental Health Alliance Hong Kong, 2019). The total costs associated with MHDs are considerably high, accounting for HKD 5.5 to 12.4 billion yearly, with an average of 55–60 days of presenteeism associated with MHDs per employee yearly (City Mental Health Alliance Hong Kong, 2019). 49% presenteeism occurs among middle-management employees.

The indirect costs, including staff turnover and presenteeism, as well as low morale, and the damage to the reputation and credibility of the organisation, are often underestimated or overlooked (City Mental Health Alliance Hong Kong, 2019). Similarly, the potential socio-economic costs, including the reductions in social trust, workers' self-esteem, and life satisfaction, are far more substantial than the treatment burden (Qin & Hsieh, 2020). The accumulated invisible loss related to employee MHDs is 40 to 90 times higher than the investment in the provision of EAPs. Nonetheless, the amount spent on mental health programmes and EAPs is relatively low, estimated at HKD 130 million per year.

On the other hand, the government and employers paid less attention to RTW programmes for workers with MHDs. Indeed, the resignation of skilled employees with MHDs is equivalent to paying additional time, resources, and costs in recruiting, selection, and training new staff by the company (Xing, 2009). To fully replace a departing employee, new staff generally take 6 to 9 months as an adapting period to become familiar with the new workplace content and culture. At the same time, the workers generally do not pay full attention and responsibility after submitting a resignation and there is usually zero economic output during the turnover period (City Mental Health Alliance Hong Kong, 2019).

Undoubtedly, the successful implementation of mental health interventions such as RTW or EAPs can immensely reduce the company's costs. Despite the growing evidence of the magnitude of MHDs, most employers do not see mental health as a priority in the workplace because of costing consideration.

Government Interventions—The Case of Hong Kong

Government Policies

The integrated legal framework in addressing employees' mental health and workplace safety is not comprehensive in Hong Kong. The Occupational Safety and Health Ordinance ("OSHO") (Cap. 509) ensures that employers put priority on the employees' "safety and physical health, remove the potential hazardous factors to prevent the dangerous occurrence in the workplace". However, the regulation does not put mental health as a priority of the ordinance. Employers are legally obligated to provide compensation, medical care, and vocational rehabilitation to injured employees in occupational accidents under the Employees' Compensation Ordinance (Cap. 282), but the existing ordinance does not cover MHDs nor work-related mental injuries as occupational diseases, failing to effectively protect the mental wellness of employees (Research Office of the Legislative Council Secretariat, 2018). In addition, the discrimination, harassment, and vilification of people with MHDs or ex-MHDs are illegal under the Disability Discrimination Ordinance ("DDO") (Cap. 487). It stipulates that employers are responsible for providing a comfortable and non-discriminatory working environment for employees with MHDs, reducing the likelihood of employees with MHDs being unfriendly treated. Besides, it is illegal if employers refuse to employ, or give low remuneration or unreasonable dismissal based on MHDs (Equal Opportunities Commission, 2022).

Mental Health Workplace Charter

Mental Health Workplace Charter is a joint scheme organised by the Department of Health (DH), the Labour Department (LD), and the Occupational Safety and

Health Council (OSHC). The Charter aims to create a mental health-friendly environment in the workplace and encourage early diagnosis and timely treatment to improve employees' mental well-being. Each chartered organisation can receive the information and support from the scheme for implementation of sustainable and suitable mental health measures to promote workplace mental health improvement. Moreover, the scheme will provide a range of value-added services free of charge, such as Mental Health First Aid programmes to help the organisations in fulfilling the scheme's requirement. Unfortunately, limited free-of-cost activities and grossly inadequate services would weaken the effectiveness of the scheme, particularly for some small and medium-sized enterprises (SMEs) that receive low mental health benefits coverage. Furthermore, the publicity campaigns of the Charter are inadequate, leading to the significantly low participation of signatories in the scheme. Hong Kong has nearly 1.4 million locally registered companies (The Government of the Hong Kong Special Administrative Region, 2021), but only 985 organisations enrolled three years after implementation (Advisory Committee on Mental Health, 2022).

Programmes by Government Departments

For instance, the Selective Placement Division (SPD) of the LD provides various recruitment and incentive programmes to enhance the employment of job seekers with MHDs and employment difficulties, including the "Work Orientation and Placement Scheme" (WOPS) and "Retention Allowance Scheme" (RAS). Employers can receive a maximum allowance of 60,000 from WOPS when employing a person with ex-MHDs, while employees can receive a maximum retention allowance of 9,000 dollars from RAS. Besides, employees with ex-MHDs can participate in the pre-employment training programmes to receive employment counselling and guidance, enhance their relevant job skills, and quickly adapt to the new job requirement (Selective Placement Division of the Labour Department, 2018a, 2018b). OSHC has also provided various seminars, training courses, and publications, with the objective to improve employers' and employees' awareness of the health effects of psychological stress and enhancing the management of workplace stress. Moreover, the Support Programme for Employees with Disabilities (SPED) launched by the Social Welfare Department (SWD) has provided a maximum subsidy of HKD40000 to employees with MHDs for procurement of assistive devices such as computer equipment or work equipment to improve the working efficiency. However, the lack of coordination between different sectors results in the improper allocation of resources. As a result, some mental health services and training are overlapped, causing wastage of some resources, and the service quality may be compromised.

Organisational Interventions in Hong Kong

Employee assistance programmes are employer-sponsored programmes designed to help relieve workers' acute but modifiable health issues. Globally, there are an increasing number of EAP implementation in the workplace (Attridge, 2012). Some studies have mentioned the positive effects of EAP because workers are relieved of psychological stress and return to normal work performance after participating a few times in EAPs (Attridge et al., 2013). In Hong Kong, 77% employees agreed that EAPs have an encouraging role in improving mental health (City Mental Health Alliance Hong Kong, 2019). Unfortunately, 76% organisations do not provide EAPs in Hong Kong. Indeed, the various long-term benefits of implementing EAPs are an area that organisations in Hong Kong can easily ignore. Most employers focus on the initial cost of introducing EAPs rather than the potential invisible costs related to MHDs. More importantly, most employees are generally unwilling to share their mental status in the workplace due to fear of being stigmatised and a lack of adequate information on the resource, weakening their health-seeking behaviours and resulting in the underutilisation of mental health resources in the workplace (City Mental Health Alliance Hong Kong, 2020).

Roles of Policymakers and Organisations

Government

Governments are essential and key contributors to the promotion of the mental health in the workforce, particularly in the early identification, prevention, and timely treatment of MHDs (Food & Health Bureau, 2018). Governments can develop specific policies and legislation in key areas of mental health and integrate mental health programmes into public health policies. Moreover, governments can also support mental health in the workplace by developing legal and monitoring mechanisms to prevent MHD (World Health Organization, 2013). For example, the US government has launched a workplace wellness programme, providing courses, guidance, and materials for businesses and employers to promote mental health and stress management education (Centers for Disease Control & Prevention, 2019). However, most of the mental health guidelines and measures implemented in the workplace lack relevant professional involvement or necessary consultation (Memish et al., 2017). Therefore, the government should regularly measure and monitor the needs, allocate appropriate resources, and promptly adjust psychological services. Moreover, relevant stakeholders and mental health service providers are invited to participate in the planning and preparation of health guidelines, ensuring the actual workplace demands are met (World Health Organization, 2013). In Canada, some companies enhance the early identification, services, and supports for at-risk employees in the workplace after referring and adopting health guidelines (Mental Health Commission of Canada, 2017).

Organisations

Czabała et al. (2011) reviewed 79 studies of organisational mental health interventions and demonstrated that skills training, physical training, and working conditions had multiple positive effects on employees' stress management and mental health status. In Canada, managers and leaders are concerned about employees' mental health status and enhance the availability of mental health resources (Dimoff & Kelloway, 2019). Ahola et al. (2012) found that a 16-h career management programme in Finnish organisations had successfully enhanced employees' seeking-healthcare behaviours and their accessibility to mental health resources, reducing the risk factors for depression and work disability. However, several studies have shown that contact-based workplace training strategies are not practical for employees in obtaining mental health assistance and resource (Moll et al., 2018). Organisations should establish, execute, and disseminate appropriate EAPs and mental health interventions based on the employee's mental health demands. Evidence suggests that a company's awareness of employees' demand for mental health status can be improved through constructive, frank, and open dialogue (Centre for Addiction & Mental Health, 2020). Employers should create a conducive environment for mental wellness and workplace security. Business leaders and employers should increase resources and training for middle management with the skills and knowledge to increase their self-efficacy and responsibility towards mental health issues (LaMontagne et al., 2014).

Recommendations

Government

Development, Implementation, and Enforcement of Standard Working Hours and Prohibition of Forced Overtime

The development, implementation, and enforcement of SWH should be accelerated by the Hong Kong government, while forced overtime should be banned. In the short term, restricting working hours might further aggravate the severity of staff shortage and operating cost of SMEs. Therefore, gradual implementation of SWH enables businesses to adapt and regulate their operational structure and worker flexibility, particularly for some SMEs (Trade & Industry Department, 2022). In 2018,

South Korea announced the SWH legislation and gradually shortened the maximum working hours. The employees were being protected by the law. Employers failing to comply with the rule could result in criminal punishment. The Hong Kong government should conduct collective bargaining and consultations with representatives from the trade and relevant organisations to achieve consensus on flexible working hours, suggested SWH, or other alternatives like labour importation schemes or work sharing (World Health Organization, 2021a). However, Hong Kong companies still exist under the stereotyped concept that longer working hours are equivalent to greater productivity. The government should act as a facilitator to promote the potential benefits and appropriate knowledge of SWH to the public actively.

Cooperation of Employment Services with the Health Sector

The government should promote effective RTW programmes for workers with mild to moderate MHDs to receive timely and appropriate job opportunities. For example, the employment difficulty for people with MHDs could be improved via vocational rehabilitation training and on-the-job training (OJT) schemes (Legislative Council Panel on Welfare Services & Panel on Health Services, 2017). The government can allocate extra resources to SPD for the provision of tailored employment services, assistance, and support to people with MHDs in RTW progress. On the other hand, the government can provide incentives for business leaders and employers to support job seekers with MHDs to RTW. There is evidence that RTW programmes are cost-effective interventions to reduce the influences on the duration of absenteeism and loss of productivity (Noordik et al., 2009). RTW programmes require fewer financial resources to support employees with MHDs' reintegration into the workforce compared with new staff training (Dewa et al., 2021). Besides, RTW interventions can ameliorate the stigmatisation, discrimination, and social marginalisation of workers with MHDs. Given the positive effects on the economy and society, the cooperation of RTW programmes between the health sector and employment services should be encouraged actively by the government in the long term.

Legislation to Improve Occupational Wellness and Work-Related MHDs

Regulations and ordinances should get connected to the international standard. To cite Japan as an instance, Japan passed a law on comprehensive preventive measures against overwork-related diseases in 2014 (Yamauchi et al., 2017). Employees who suffer from MHDs caused by over-working hours and excessive workplace stress could be compensated. Similarly, in Hong Kong, (Cap. 509) ("OSHO") might be necessary to cover mental health as a key component. Additionally, MHDs should be reconsidered as a category of occupational disease and industrial accidents in the Employees' Compensation Ordinance (Cap. 282), ensuring workers suffering from MHDs caused by workplace stress can receive legal compensation and support.

In the Workplace

Promotion and Execution of Workplace Mental Wellness Programmes

The majority of Hong Kong workers expressed that their organisations lack sufficient and appropriate EAPs and mental health programmes. Organisations should strengthen the implementation of workplace mental health interventions. Previous studies demonstrated that conducting a 15-min Body-Mind-Spirit (BMS) training during working hours had a substantial positive effect on cultivating workers' positive awareness and stress management (Ng et al., 2020). Cullen et al. (2018) found that cognitive-behavioural therapy (CBT) interventions had helped strengthen the functional working capabilities of workers with MHDs. Moreover, stress management intervention and psychological training programmes can significantly improve the risk of anxiety and the short-term effects of workplace psychological stress among workers with MHDs (Dalsbø et al., 2013; Huang et al., 2015). Employers should regularly review the EAPs and other mental health services, ensuring these interventions are designed for workers' actual mental health needs and invite involvement of employee.

Creating a Friendly Culture in the Workplace

Since employees with MHDs would not seek help actively, building a culture of trust that helps maintain a healthy and harmonious work environment is essential and advantageous for the workplace. A friendly, respectful, and faithfully organisational management style can help develop a work culture in accepting and supportive of employees struggling with MHDs (Attridge, 2019). Line managers can encourage employees to share their mental status and difficulty. Ultimately, a caring and friendly workplace culture can encourage staff to share their mental problems and help build a sense of belonging and connectedness in the long term (Advisory Committee on Mental Health, n.d.).

Improvement in Workplace Environment

A psychologically safe and supportive work environment has various advantages, including increased productivity and sustainability, as well as the improvement in employee retention and engagement. Conversely, a hostile working environment is highly associated with the prevalence of work-related MHDs (World Health Organization, n.d.). Indoor environmental quality (IEQ) and the prevalence of psychological distress are interrelated and have a significant impact on work performance and productivity (Dunleavy et al., 2020; Mahbob et al., 2011). Therefore, the employer should improve IEQ in the workplace to reduce the psychological stress among employees. Rao et al. (2022) demonstrated that green spaces were crucial in facilitating recovery from psychophysical stress, enhancing office collaboration and organisational cohesion, and reducing the risk of depression and absenteeism. Hence, green spaces should be introduced in the workplace to improve employees' mental health status. Some studies found that a short nap was advantageous in causing lower pressure, higher productivity and morale, and stabler emotion (Hayashi et al., 1999; Silva-Costa et al., 2017; Takahashi et al., 2004). Napping at work was allowed and accepted by employers in Western countries such as America and Spain (Baxter & Kroll-Smith, 2005). In recent years, a growing number of SMEs have implemented a variety of facilities to establish a psychologically healthy workplace.

Health Professionals—Evidence-Based Treatment Guidelines

Clinicians play an integral role in assessing workplace mental health symptoms, providing counselling techniques that facilitate RTW, and combating the stigma associated with mental illness (Dewa et al., 2016). Indeed, improved communication and collaboration among key stakeholders such as employers, employees, and mental healthcare practitioners can effectively drive RTW processes (Tikka et al., 2022). However, employers and management generally lack the training needed for RTW, and discordant relationships between workers and supervisors can reduce the likelihood of achieving the goals of RTW programmes (Jetha et al., 2021). Therefore, healthcare providers should establish communication with employers and allow employees with MHDs to participate in the discussion to realise the workplace demands (Institute for Work & Health, 2019). They should choose appropriate workplace mental health promotion and prevention solutions based on evidence-based treatment guidelines.

Conclusion

Work is a double-edged sword that significantly influences employees' mental health, occupational well-being, and quality of life. Undoubtedly, excessive working hours, increased workloads, and a blame culture have intensified the occurrence of MHDs in the workplace. Additionally, workers with MHDs are more likely to experience increased job pressures and low productivity, which contribute to increased turnover and unemployment rates. Therefore, mental health issues in the workplace will be a continuous challenge for Hong Kong in the future.

More businesses have increased investment in employee mental health. Employers can create an inclusive, transparent, and open work culture in addressing stigma, labelling, and discrimination in the workplace. In addition, improving EAPs utilisation and enhancing supervisor training are recommended for sustainable performance. Creating a comfortable, friendly, and safe workplace is of importance, not only the workers can obtain health improvement, but the businesses can also further strengthen competitiveness and productivity. The whole society can benefit from a healthy workplace because the government cost on mental health is reduced in the long term.

Most notably, there are no substitutes for collaborative efforts among the stakeholders, including policymakers, work agencies, and health professionals, in addressing potential risk factors and achieving health for all. The government and health researchers should eliminate the disagreement between labour and capital with the objective in achieving SWH and maximum working hours implementation to achieve comprehensive workplace wellness and mental health improvement.

References

Advisory Committee on Mental Health. (n.d.). *Workplace Mental Health Guide*. Department of Health. www.joyfulhealthyworkplace.hk/en/pdf/tools/workplace_mental_health_guide_en.pdf

Advisory Committee on Mental Health. (2022, May 31). *Mental Health Workplace Charter—Chartered Signatories (As at 31 May 2022)*. https://www.oshc.org.hk/oshc_data/files/AwardsCampaigns/MentalHealthCharter/MHWC_SignatoriesList.pdf

Ahn, S. H., Lee, Y. J., Jang, E. C., Kwon, S. C., Min, Y. S., & Ryu, S. H. (2020). A study of job stress, suicidal ideation and suicide attempts in display manufacturing workers: A cross-sectional study. *Annals of Occupational and Environmental Medicine, 32*(1), Article e16. https://doi.org/10.35371/aoem.2020.32.e16

Ahola, K., Vuori, J., Toppinen-Tanner, S., Mutanen, P., & Honkonen, T. (2012). Resource-enhancing group intervention against depression at workplace: Who benefits? A randomised controlled study with a 7-month follow-up. *Occupational and Environmental Medicine, 69*(12), 870–876. https://doi.org/10.1136/oemed-2011-100450

Attridge, M. (2012). Employee assistance programs: Evidence and current trends. In R. J. Gatchel, & I. Z. Schultz (Eds.), *Handbook of occupational health and wellness* (pp. 441–467). Springer. https://doi.org/10.1007/978-1-4614-4839-6_21

Attridge, M. (2019). A global perspective on promoting workplace mental health and the role of employee assistance programs. *American Journal of Health Promotion, 33*(4), 622–629. https://doi.org/10.1177/0890117119838101c

Attridge, M., Cahill, T., Granberry, S. W., & Herlihy, P. A. (2013). The National Behavioral Consortium industry profile of external EAP vendors. *Journal of Workplace Behavioral Health, 28*(4), 251–324. https://doi.org/10.1080/15555240.2013.845050

Bal, C. S. (2016). Constituting tactical obedience in the workplace. In C. S. Bal (Ed.), *Production politics and migrant labour regimes* (pp. 79–110). Palgrave Macmillan. https://doi.org/10.1057/978-1-137-54859-7_4

Baxter, V., & Kroll-Smith, S. (2005). Normalizing the workplace nap: Blurring the boundaries between public and private space and time. *Current Sociology, 53*(1), 33–55. https://doi.org/10.1177/0011392105048287

Bergefurt, L., Weijs-Perrée, M., Appel-Meulenbroek, R., & Arentze, T. (2022). The physical office workplace as a resource for mental health—A systematic scoping review. *Building and Environment, 207*, Article 108505. https://doi.org/10.1016/j.buildenv.2021.108505

Canadian Centre for Occupational Health and Safety. (n.d.). *Mental health in the Canadian workplace*. https://www.ccohs.ca/images/products/infographics/download/mentalHealth.jpg

Centre for Addiction and Mental Health. (2020, January). *Workplace mental health: A review and recommendations*. https://www.camh.ca/-/media/files/workplace-mental-health/workplacementalhealth-a-review-and-recommendations-pdf.pdf

Census and Statistics Department. (2014, December). *Special topics report no.62: Persons with disabilities and chronic diseases.* https://www.censtatd.gov.hk/en/data/stat_report/product/B1130121/att/B11301622014XXXXB0100.pdf

Centers for Disease Control and Prevention. (2019, April 10). *Mental health in the workplace.* https://www.cdc.gov/workplacehealthpromotion/tools%20resources/workplace-health/mental-health/index.html

Chan, S. M., Au-Yeung, T. C., Wong, H., Chung, R. Y., & Chung, G. K. (2021). Long working hours, precarious employment and anxiety symptoms among working Chinese population in Hong Kong. *The Psychiatric Quarterly, 92*(4), 1745–1757. https://doi.org/10.1007/s11126-021-09938-3

City Mental Health Alliance Hong Kong. (2017). *Mental health in the workplace: Survey of Hong Kong employees.* https://www.cmhahk.org/docs/research/2017-CMHA-HK-Employee-survey-results-external.pdf?utm_source=website&utm_medium=popup&utm_campaigm=popup_MHW2017

City Mental Health Alliance Hong Kong. (2019, January). *The cost of mental ill health for employers in Hong Kong.* https://www.cmhahk.org/docs/research/2019-Mental-health-in-the-workplace_EN_WEB.pdf?utm_source=website&utm_medium=popup&utm_campaigm=popup_MHW2019

City Mental Health Alliance Hong Kong. (2020, September). *Mental health and wellbeing in the workplace: Survey of APAC employees.* https://www.cmhahk.org/docs/research/CMHA-HK-2020-Mental-Health-&-Wellbeing-in-the-Workplace-Final.pdf?utm_source=website&utm_medium=popup&utm_campaigm=popup_MHW2020

Cottini, E., & Lucifora, C. (2013). Mental health and working conditions in Europe. *ILR Review, 66*(4), 958–988. https://doi.org/10.1177/001979391306600409

Cullen, K. L., Irvin, E., Collie, A., Clay, F., Gensby, U., Jennings, P. A., Hogg-Johnson, S., Kristman, V., Laberge, M., McKenzie, D., Newnam, S., Palagyi, A., Ruseckaite, R., Sheppard, D. M., Shourie, S., Steenstra, I., Van Eerd, D., & Amick, B. C. (2018). Effectiveness of workplace interventions in return-to-work for musculoskeletal, pain-related and mental health conditions: An update of the evidence and messages for practitioners. *Journal of Occupational Rehabilitation, 28*(1), 1–15. https://doi.org/10.1007/s10926-016-9690-x

Czabała, C., Charzyńska, K., & Mroziak, B. (2011). Psychosocial interventions in workplace mental health promotion: An overview. *Health Promotion International, 26*(Suppl_1), i70–i84. https://doi.org/10.1093/heapro/dar050

Dalsbø, T. K., Thuve Dahm, K., Austvoll-Dahlgren, A., Knapstad, M., Gundersen, M., & Merete Reinar, L. (2013). Workplace-based interventions for employees' mental health. *Norwegian Knowledge Centre for the Health Services.* https://www.ncbi.nlm.nih.gov/books/NBK464819/pdf/Bookshelf_NBK464819.pdf

Dattani, S., Ritchie, H., & Roser, M. (2021, August). *Mental health.* Our World in Data. https://ourworldindata.org/mental-health

Dewa, C. S., Hoch, J. S., Loong, D., Trojanowski, L., & Bonato, S. (2021). Evidence for the cost-effectiveness of return-to-work interventions for mental illness related sickness absences: A systematic literature Review. *Journal of Occupational Rehabilitation, 31*(1), 26–40. https://doi.org/10.1007/s10926-020-09904-z

Dewa, C. S., Trojanowski, L., Joosen, M. C., & Bonato, S. (2016). Employer best practice guidelines for the return to work of workers on mental disorder-related disability leave: A systematic review. *Canadian Journal of Psychiatry. Revue Canadienne de Psychiatrie, 61*(3), 176–185. https://doi.org/10.1177/0706743716632515

Dimoff, J. K., & Kelloway, E. K. (2013). Bridging the gap: Workplace mental health research in Canada. *Canadian Psychology/psychologie Canadienne, 54*(4), 203–212. https://doi.org/10.1037/a0034464

Dimoff, J. K., & Kelloway, E. K. (2019). With a little help from my boss: The impact of workplace mental health training on leader behaviors and employee resource utilization. *Journal of Occupational Health Psychology, 24*(1), 4–19. https://doi.org/10.1037/ocp0000126

Dunleavy, G., Bajpai, R., Tonon, A. C., Cheung, K. L., Thach, T. Q., Rykov, Y., Soh, C. K., de Vries, H., Car, J., & Christopoulos, G. (2020). Prevalence of psychological distress and its association with perceived indoor environmental quality and workplace factors in under and aboveground workplaces. *Building and Environment, 175*, 106799. https://doi.org/10.1016/j.buildenv.2020.106799

Equal Opportunities Commission. (2022). *The disability discrimination ordinance and people with mental illness/ex-mental illness.* https://www.eoc.org.hk/en/discrimination-laws/disability-discrimination/faq/the-disability-discrimination-ordinance-and-people-with-a-mental-illness-ex-mental-illness

Food and Health Bureau. (2018, May 1). *Mental health review report.* https://www.healthbureau.gov.hk/download/press_and_publications/otherinfo/180500_mhr/e_mhr_full_report.pdf

Hampson, M. E., Watt, B. D., & Hicks, R. E. (2020). Impacts of stigma and discrimination in the workplace on people living with psychosis. *BMC Psychiatry, 20*, Article 288. https://doi.org/10.1186/s12888-020-02614-z

Hayashi, M., Watanabe, M., & Hori, T. (1999). The effects of a 20 min nap in the mid-afternoon on mood, performance and EEG activity. *Clinical Neurophysiology: Official Journal of the International Federation of Clinical Neurophysiology, 110*(2), 272–279. https://doi.org/10.1016/s1388-2457(98)00003-0

Hiemer, J., & Andresen, M. (2019). "Because work time is life time"—Employees' perceptions of individual overemployment, its causes and its consequences. *Frontiers in Psychology, 10*, Article 1920. https://doi.org/10.3389/fpsyg.2019.01920

Huang, S. L., Li, R. H., Huang, F. Y., & Tang, F. C. (2015). The potential for mindfulness-based intervention in workplace mental health promotion: Results of a randomized controlled trial. *PloS ONE, 10*(9), Article e0138089. https://doi.org/10.1371/journal.pone.0138089

Institute for Work & Health. (2019, May). *Supporting return to work among employees with musculoskeletal or mental health conditions: An evidence-based practical resource.* https://www.iwh.on.ca/tools-and-guides/supporting-return-to-work-among-employees-with-musculoskeletal-or-mental-health-conditions-evidence-based-practical-resource

International Labour Organisation. (2018). *Ensuring decent working time for the future.* https://www.ilo.org/wcmsp5/groups/public/---ed_norm/---relconf/documents/meetingdocument/wcms_618485.pdf

Jetha, A., Le Pouésard, M., Mustard, C., Backman, C., & Gignac, M. (2021). Getting the message right: Evidence-based insights to improve organisational return-to-work communication practices. *Journal of Occupational Rehabilitation, 31*(3), 652–663. https://doi.org/10.1007/s10926-021-09961-y

Kim, W., Park, E. C., Lee, T. H., & Kim, T. H. (2016). Effect of working hours and precarious employment on depressive symptoms in South Korean employees: A longitudinal study. *Occupational and Environmental Medicine, 73*(12), 816–822. https://doi.org/10.1136/oemed-2016-103553

Lam, L. C., Wong, C. S., Wang, M. J., Chan, W. C., Chen, E. Y., Ng, R. M., Hung, S. F., Cheung, E. F., Sham, P. C., Chiu, H. F., Lam, M., Chang, W. C., Lee, E. H., Chiang, T. P., Lau, J. T., van Os, J., Lewis, G., & Bebbington, P. (2015). Prevalence, psychosocial correlates and service utilization of depressive and anxiety disorders in Hong Kong: The Hong Kong Mental Morbidity Survey (HKMMS). *Social Psychiatry and Psychiatric Epidemiology, 50*(9), 1379–1388. https://doi.org/10.1007/s00127-015-1014-5

LaMontagne, A. D., Martin, A., Page, K. M., Reavley, N. J., Noblet, A. J., Milner, A. J., Keegel, T., & Smith, P. M. (2014). Workplace mental health: Developing an integrated intervention approach. *BMC Psychiatry, 14*, Article 131. https://doi.org/10.1186/1471-244X-14-131

Lee, H. E., Kim, I., Kim, H. R., & Kawachi, I. (2020). Association of long working hours with accidents and suicide mortality in Korea. *Scandinavian Journal of Work, Environment and Health, 46*(5), 480–487. https://doi.org/10.5271/sjweh.3890

Legislative Council Panel on Manpower. (2020, May 19). *Latest development in the formulation of sector-specific working hours guidelines and relevant initiatives.* https://www.legco.gov.hk/yr19-20/english/panels/mp/papers/mp20200519cb2-968-5-e.pdf

Legislative Council Panel on Welfare Services and Panel on Health Services. (2017, May 29). *Administration's response to the major views expressed and suggestions raised regarding to community support services for mentally ill and ex-mentally ill persons at the meeting on 29 May 2017.* https://www.legco.gov.hk/yr16-17/english/panels/ltcp/papers/ltcp20170529cb2-1323-1-e.pdf

Mahbob, N. S., Kamaruzzaman, S. N., Salleh, N., & Sulaiman, R. (2011). A correlation studies of indoor environmental quality (IEQ) towards productive workplace. *2nd International Conference on Environmental Science and Technology, 6*, 434–438. http://eprints.um.edu.my/id/eprint/12777

Marquez, P. V., & Saxena, S. (2016). Making mental health a global priority. *Cerebrum.* https://www.ncbi.nlm.nih.gov/pmc/articles/PMC5198754/

Memish, K., Martin, A., Bartlett, L., Dawkins, S., & Sanderson, K. (2017). Workplace mental health: An international review of guidelines. *Preventive Medicine, 101*, 213–222. https://doi.org/10.1016/j.ypmed.2017.03.017

Mental Health Commission of Canada. (2017, October). *Sustaining implementation of the WORKPLACE standard one-year follow-up study with case study research project participants.* https://mentalhealthcommission.ca/wp-content/uploads/2021/09/Workplace_Sustainability_Report_Eng.pdf

Mind HK. (2018, October 10). *Press release: Mind Hong Kong unveils new research ahead of world mental health day.* https://www.mind.org.hk/press-releases/timetochangehkresearch/

Mitchell, S., & Choi, B. (2018, September 13). *Job strain, long work hours, and suicidal thoughts.* Centers for Disease Control and Prevention. https://blogs.cdc.gov/niosh-science-blog/2018/09/13/suicide-prevention/

Moll, S. E., Patten, S., Stuart, H., MacDermid, J. C., & Kirsh, B. (2018). Beyond silence: A randomized, parallel-group trial exploring the impact of workplace mental health literacy training with healthcare employees. *Canadian Journal of Psychiatry. Revue Canadienne de Psychiatrie, 63*(12), 826–833. https://doi.org/10.1177/0706743718766051

National Alliance on Mental Illness. (n.d.). *Health reform & mental illness.* https://www.nami.org/getattachment/Get-Involved/NAMI-National-Convention/Convention-Program-Schedule/Hill-Day-2017/FINAL-Hill-Day-17-Leave-Behind-all-(1).pdf

National Safety Council. (2021, May 13). *New mental health cost calculator shows why investing in mental health is good for business.* https://www.nsc.org/newsroom/new-mental-health-cost-calculator-demonstrates-why

Ng, S. M., Lo, H., Yeung, A., Young, D., Fung, M., & Wang, A. M. (2020). Study protocol of brief daily body-mind-spirit practice for sustainable emotional capacity and work engagement for community mental health workers: A multi-site randomized controlled trial. *Frontiers in Psychology, 11*, Article 1482. https://doi.org/10.3389/fpsyg.2020.01482

Noordik, E., Van Dijk, F. J., Nieuwenhuijsen, K., & Van der Klink, J. J. (2009). Effectiveness and cost-effectiveness of an exposure-based return-to-work programme for patients on sick leave due to common mental disorders: Design of a cluster-randomized controlled trial. *BMC Public Health, 9*, Article 140. https://doi.org/10.1186/1471-2458-9-140

Organisation for Economic Co-operation and Development. (n.d.). *Mental health problems costing Europe heavily.* https://www.oecd.org/newsroom/mental-health-problems-costing-europe-heavily.htm

Pan American Health Organization. (2019, October 2). *Mental health problems are the leading cause of disability worldwide, say experts at PAHO Directing Council side event.* https://www3.paho.org/hq/index.php?option=com_content&view=article&id=15481:mental-health-problems-are-the-leading-cause-of-disability-worldwide-say-experts-at-paho-directing-council-side-event&Itemid=72565&lang=en

Paterson, C., Leduc, C., Maxwell, M., Aust, B., Amann, B. L., Cerga-Pashoja, A., Coppens, E., Couwenbergh, C., O'Connor, C., Arensman, E., & Greiner, B. A. (2021). Evidence for implementation of interventions to promote mental health in the workplace: A systematic scoping review protocol. *Systematic Reviews, 10*, Article 41. https://doi.org/10.1186/s13643-020-01570-9

Qin, X., & Hsieh, C. R. (2020). Understanding and addressing the treatment gap in mental healthcare: Economic perspectives and evidence from China. *Inquiry: A Journal of Medical Care Organization, Provision and Financing, 57*. https://doi.org/10.1177/0046958020950566

Rajgopal, T. (2010). Mental well-being at the workplace. *Indian Journal of Occupational and Environmental Medicine, 14*(3), 63–65. https://doi.org/10.4103/0019-5278.75691

Rao, P., Islary, S., & Natawadkar, K. (2022). Green Space Association with Mental Health and Cognitive Development. In R. A. Castanho, & J. C. Fernández (Eds.), *Urban Green Spaces [Working Title]*. IntechOpen. https://doi.org/10.5772/intechopen.103667

Research Office of the Legislative Council Secretariat. (2018, June 28). *Central employees' compensation system in selected place*. https://www.legco.gov.hk/research-publications/english/1718in12-central-employees-compensation-system-in-selected-places-20180628-e.pdf

Research Office of the Legislative Council Secretariat. (2019, November 8). *Working hours in Hong Kong*. https://www.legco.gov.hk/research-publications/english/1920issh06-working-hours-in-hong-kong-20191108-e.pdf

Selective Placement Division of the Labour Department. (2018a, October 12). *Retention allowance scheme*. https://www2.jobs.gov.hk/isps/WebForm/RAS/Introduction/default.aspx

Selective Placement Division of the Labour Department. (2018b, October 12). *Work orientation and placement scheme (WOPS)*. https://www2.jobs.gov.hk/isps/WebForm/Wops/

Silva-Costa, A., Ferreira, P., Griep, R. H., & Rotenberg, L. (2020). Association between presenteeism, psychosocial aspects of work and common mental disorders among nursing personnel. *International Journal of Environmental Research and Public Health, 17*(18), Article 6758. https://doi.org/10.3390/ijerph17186758

Silva-Costa, A., Griep, R. H., & Rotenberg, L. (2017). Night work and BMI: Is it related to on-shift napping? *Revista de Saude Publica, 51*, 97. https://doi.org/10.11606/S1518-8787.2017051007094

Snell, R. S., Wong, M. M. L., Chak, A. M. K., & Hui, S. S. K. (2013). Representational predicaments at work: How they are experienced and why they may happen. *Asia Pacific Journal of Management, 30*(1), 251–279. https://doi.org/10.1007/s10490-012-9286-8

Takahashi, M., Nakata, A., Haratani, T., Ogawa, Y., & Arito, H. (2004). Post-lunch nap as a worksite intervention to promote alertness on the job. *Ergonomics, 47*(9), 1003–1013. https://doi.org/10.1080/00140130410001686320

The Government of the Hong Kong Special Administrative Region. (2021, January 10). *Companies registry releases statistics for 2020* [Press release]. https://www.info.gov.hk/gia/general/202101/10/P2021010800572.htm

Health, T. L. G. (2020). Mental health matters. *The Lancet, Global Health, 8*(11), e1352. https://doi.org/10.1016/S2214-109X(20)30432-0

Tikka, C., Verbeek, J., Hoving, J. L., & Kunz, R. (2022). Evidence-informed decision about (de-) implementing return-to-work coordination to reduce sick leave: A case study. *Health Research Policy and Systems, 20*, Article 19. https://doi.org/10.1186/s12961-022-00823-4

Trade and Industry Department. (2022). *Support to small and medium enterprises*. https://www.tid.gov.hk/english/smes_industry/smes/smes_content.html

Trautmann, S., Rehm, J., & Wittchen, H. U. (2016). The economic costs of mental disorders: Do our societies react appropriately to the burden of mental disorders? *EMBO Reports, 17*(9), 1245–1249. https://doi.org/10.15252/embr.201642951

van der Noordt, M., IJzelenberg, H., Droomers, M., & Proper, K. I. (2014). Health effects of employment: A systematic review of prospective studies. *Occupational and Environmental Medicine, 71*(10), 730–736. https://doi.org/10.1136/oemed-2013-101891

Walker, E. R., McGee, R. E., & Druss, B. G. (2015). Mortality in mental disorders and global disease burden implications: A systematic review and meta-analysis. *JAMA Psychiatry, 72*(4), 334–341. https://doi.org/10.1001/jamapsychiatry.2014.2502

Wilson, H., & Finch, D. (2021, April 18). Unemployment and mental health. *The Health Foundation.* https://www.health.org.uk/publications/long-reads/unemployment-and-mental-health

World Federation for Mental Health. (2017). *Mental health in the workplace.* https://www.wfmh.global/img/what-we-do/publications/2017-wmhd-report-english.pdf

World Health Organization. (n.d.). *Mental health.* https://www.who.int/health-topics/mental-health#tab=tab_2

World Health Organization. (2010). *Mental health and well-being at the workplace—Protection and inclusion in challenging times.* https://www.euro.who.int/__data/assets/pdf_file/0018/124047/e94345.pdf

World Health Organization. (2013, January 6). *Mental health action plan 2013–2020.* https://www.who.int/publications/i/item/9789241506021

World Health Organization. (2017, November 30). *Protecting workers' health.* https://www.who.int/news-room/fact-sheets/detail/protecting-workers'-health

World Health Organization. (2021a, May 17). *Long working hours increasing deaths from heart disease and stroke: WHO, ILO.* https://www.who.int/news/item/17-05-2021-long-working-hours-increasing-deaths-from-heart-disease-and-stroke-who-ilo

World Health Organization. (2021b). *Mental health atlas 2020.* https://apps.who.int/iris/rest/bitstreams/1376861/retrieve

Xing, J. L. (2009, December). Study on cost control of resignation. *IEEE*, 137–140 https://doi.org/10.1109/ICIII.2009.343

Yamauchi, T., Yoshikawa, T., Takamoto, M., Sasaki, T., Matsumoto, S., Kayashima, K., Takeshima, T., & Takahashi, M. (2017). Overwork-related disorders in Japan: Recent trends and development of a national policy to promote preventive measures. *Industrial Health, 55*(3), 293–302. https://doi.org/10.2486/indhealth.2016-0198

Young, F. Y. (2019). Working conditions of retail industry workers in Hong Kong. *Journal of Asian Development, 5*(2), 41–56. https://doi.org/10.5296/jad.v5i2.14018

Zhu, S., Tse, S., Goodyear-Smith, F., Yuen, W., & Wong, P. W. (2017). Health-related behaviours and mental health in Hong Kong employees. *Occupational Medicine, 67*(1), 26–32. https://doi.org/10.1093/occmed/kqw137

Chapter 21
Active Ageing and Healthy Ageing

Chor Ming Lum

Abstract With increasing life expectancy and its potential economic implication, World Health Organization (WHO) has advocated Active Ageing Policy since the 1990s. In 2000s, more focus is put on Healthy Ageing. Although Hong Kong is leading in league table on Life Expectancy, her older population is not living more healthier than before. Besides, the healthcare system is also much tilted towards hospital-based curative care than to primary and preventive care. Hong Kong Government is not slow in seeing the issue and has looked into policy on Healthy Ageing and development of Primary Healthcare for its Healthy Ageing policy. In this chapter, WHO concepts on Active Ageing and Healthy Ageing will be recapped, followed by an update on health status of older population in Hong Kong. Works in primary care for older adults will be reviewed. These will be discussed with focus on clinical and professional aspects but not from policy, administration, or economic perspective.

Keywords Active ageing · Healthy ageing

Active Ageing

With improvement in sanitation and advancement of medical technologies, life expectancy is extending and there is an increasing number of senior citizens among most countries in the world. Despite this extension of life expectancy, there are concerns that they may not live healthier and that may tax on healthcare and social resources, or that the quality of life among seniors may be compromised. Seeing into the trend, the World Health Organization (WHO) first issued the Brasilia Declaration on Ageing in 1996 (Towards healthy ageing, 1997). It advocates the promotion of mental health and social connections in additional to physical health. To achieve these, maintaining autonomy and independence is essential to maintain good quality of life as one ages. This broad issue of extending needs of an ageing population is

C. M. Lum (✉)
Institute of Ageing, The Chinese University of Hong Kong, Hong Kong, China
e-mail: ccmlum@yahoo.com.hk

B. Y. F. Fong and W. C. W. Wong (eds.), *Gaps and Actions in Health Improvement from Hong Kong and Beyond*,
https://doi.org/10.1007/978-981-99-4491-0_21

conceptualised under Active Ageing in the publication on "Active Ageing: A Policy Framework" (World Health Organization, 2002). "Active Ageing" is defined as a process of optimising opportunities for health, participation, and security in order to enhance quality of life as people age. Accordingly, not only does it refer to physical and mental health as defined by the WHO definition of health, but social connectivity is also equally important. This social connectivity takes place in context of others—friends, work associates, neighbours, and family members. Fundamental to the Declaration, ageing is to be viewed as a developmental issue and older persons are resources for their families, their communities and the economy. Their usually unpaid and unsung contributions are indispensable for development. This is why interdependence as well as intergenerational solidarity are important tenets of active ageing. Determinants of active ageing include health and social services, behavioural and personal factors, environment, social, and economical factors, and are based on recognition of human rights of older people and the UN Principles of independence, participation, dignity care, and self-fulfilment. These are illustrated in Figs. 21.1 and 21.2.

Active Ageing is called upon to addressing the needs of an ageing population with the context of broader social policy. All actions must be intersectoral and take into account the biophysical, social, psychological, economic, and environmental determinants of health. In particular note here is on the three pillars of policy (Fig. 21.2) that are required to support active ageing. Besides health, seniors are encouraged to

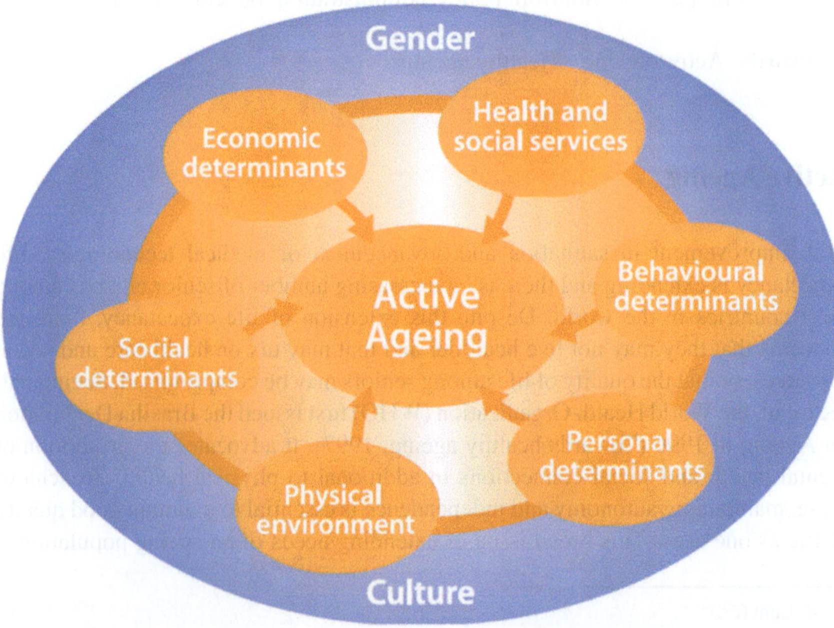

Fig. 21.1 The determinants of Active Ageing. *Source* World Health Organization (2002)

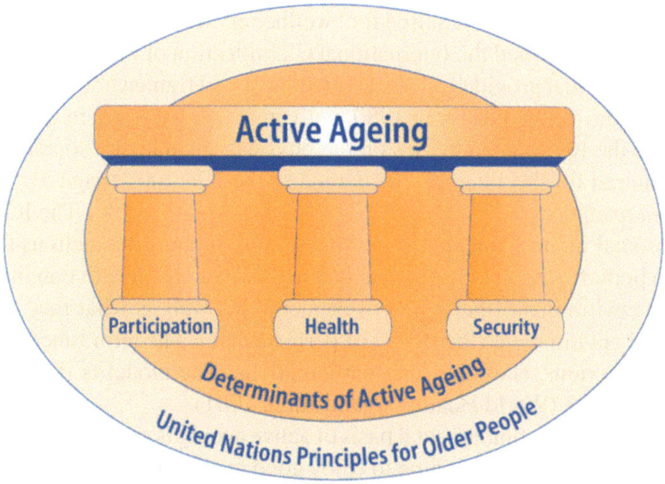

Fig. 21.2 The three pillars of a policy framework for Active Ageing. *Source* World Health Organization (2002)

be active member of a society. Society and environment need to be built on enabling those with special needs to participate as others. Notwithstanding, a good social security system is also required to back up the under-privileged so that they can go beyond basic daily necessity requirement to have reasonable quality of life.

Although there is no hierarchy among the three pillars, the health of seniors plays key role by itself, or in interaction to uphold on active societal participation and to provide a sense of physical security. WHO has particularly highlighted on the needs to promote long-term health and need of focus towards the process of healthy ageing in the framework of active ageing.

Healthy Ageing

Health, as referred by WHO, is not only a state free of disease, but also a state of physical, mental, and social wellbeing. This definition of health and characteristic of a senior person requires further elaboration. Conventionally health was defined as a state free of diseases. Along with the direction, the International Statistics Classification (ICD) of Disease and Related Health Problem (latest version being the ICD-10) is used for collecting data on why a medical consult or procedure is required. For example, a subject may have a numerical measurement of high blood pressure for follow up. This subject is defined as a hypertensive patient because of the label though he or she is functioning as anyone without such a label. Another person may have difficulties in learning mathematics or appreciation of music though she or he is normal in brain structure. There is thus discrepancy between a disease state and that of normal functioning which is required for "wellbeing". To address on the limitation of ICD, WHO first published the International Classification of Functioning, Disability and Health (ICF) that provided a standard language and framework for description of health and health-related issues in 1980, with an updated version in 2001. This ICF supplements the ICD and addresses on the physical, mental, and social functioning that are required for "wellbeing". As quoted in the ICF 2001 (page 3), "*ICD-10 is mainly used to classify causes of death, but ICF classifies health*". The ICF adopts a biopsychosocial model of health and addresses on domains that help us to describe changes in body function and structure that a person with a health condition can do in standard environment (their level of capacity), as well as what they actually do in their usual environment (their level of performance). The term functioning refers to all body functions, activities, and participations. The model is illustrated in the following Fig. 21.3 (World Health Organization, 2001).

As stated above, the fundamental basis of active ageing is on maintaining a healthy state that allows normal functioning to enjoy good quality of life. Over the past half a century, medicine has developed towards specialisation for advancement of knowledge and research. A person is viewed as one run by different systems (e.g. cardiovascular system, neurological system) individually. If a person has any dysfunction, it is often assumed that a single disease from a single system has gone wrong that explains the problems. The fact is that cells of every organ do undergo apoptosis, senescence, or cellular death from insults, though they vary in their rate. At the end, even if there is not a "disease", the organ function will be at a fraction of its peak. While the senior may appear to cope with daily functional demands, its reserves on enhancing the function at time of increased demand will be compromised. This is a

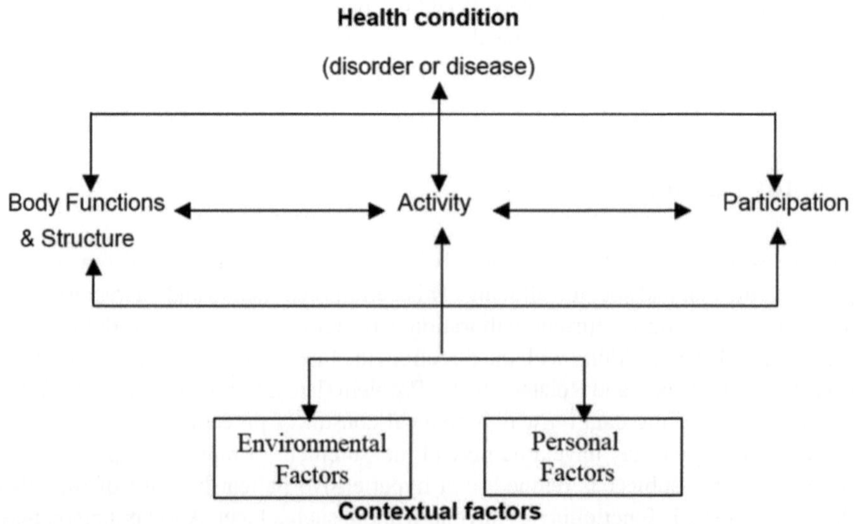

Fig. 21.3 Model of International Classification of Functioning, Disability and Health. *Source* World Health Organization (2001)

state of frailty which is defined as "progressive age-related deterioration in physiological systems that results in extreme vulnerability to stressors and increases the risk of a range of adverse outcomes including care dependence and death" (Beard et al., 2016). To maintain a healthy state, one not only has to consider ways to prevent individual disease, but also means to build up and maintain its reserve (intrinsic capacity). This will be discussed in later section. Health, in the context of a senior, should be considered from the perspective of his or her trajectory of functioning rather than the disease or comorbidity at a single time point (World Health Organization, 2015).

To share characteristics of a senior, adoption of the ICF biopsychosocial model and trajectory of functioning as key determinant of health, WHO (2015) defines *Healthy Ageing as the process of developing and maintaining the functional ability that enables wellbeing in older age.* The key word here is "functioning". This functional ability is an interaction between the environment and individual performance, of which the latter is related to multiple factors that affect one's intrinsic capacity. This relationship is illustrated in Fig. 21.4 (World Health Organization, 2015, p. 28).

In this model, healthy ageing starts from birth with our genetic inheritance. This genetic expression interacts with the behavioural and environmental exposures and shapes our personal characteristics. The interaction among these health characteristics will ultimately determine the intrinsic capacity (reserve capacity) of an individual—that is, the composite of all the physical and mental capacities that an individual can draw on. Intrinsic capacity at any point in time is determined by many factors, including underlying physiological and psychological changes, health-related behaviours, and the presence or absence of diseases (Sadana & Michel, 2019).

While the personal characteristic refers to physical and mental function of an individual, she or he is to live in an environment with participation in activities and

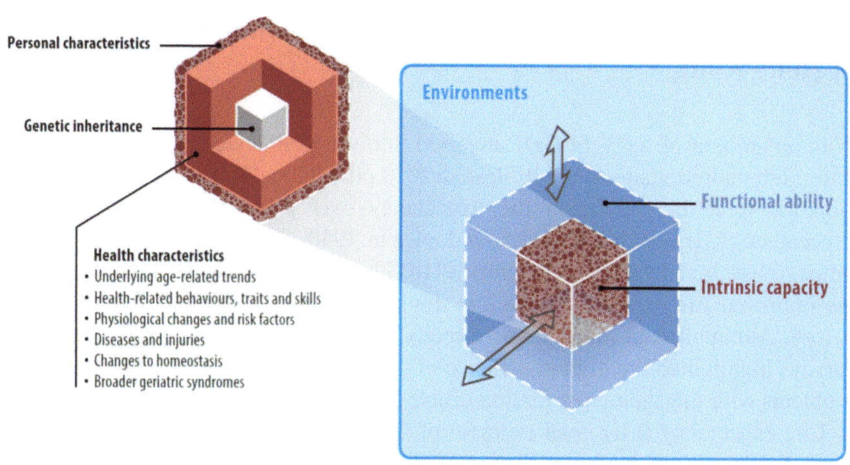

Fig. 21.4 Concept on Intrinsic capacity, Functional ability, and Environment and their interrelationships. *Source* World Health Organization (2015)

interact with others. A person may have limitations in certain functional ability. If the environment is enabling (e.g. barrier free for wheelchair access), he or she may still be able to function well with social participation. This interaction between environment and the individual is the individual's functional ability that draws to the ICF model in Fig. 21.3. At any point in time, an individual may have reserves of functional ability that are not being drawn on. These functional reserves are termed resilience. The healthy ageing model conceptualises resilience as the ability to maintain or improve a level of functional ability in time of adversity. This ability comprises both the intrinsic capacity and environmental components including social networks that can mitigate the deficits.

In summary, healthy ageing refers to the process of developing and maintaining the functional ability that enables wellbeing and life in older age. While wellbeing refers to having good quality of life, death is the universal and ultimate pathway to all. As healthy ageing is considered as a lifelong process, it is to start from birth till its end. That encompasses on both quality of life and quality of dying when the day is to come. While genetic constituent is non-modifiable, behavioural and environmental factors can be modified to maximise intrinsic capacity that builds resilience to adversity. This building of resilience should be viewed as a lifelong process and should not start only late, nor will it be too late to start. Opportunities are also present to re-instate it after episodic transient insults. As biological ageing is universal to all unless one dies before middle age and functional capacity is an interaction between personal capacity and environment, a supportive and enabling physical environment including supportive social network is facilitative to this healthy ageing process. This lifelong course and interaction between environment and personal characteristics towards healthy ageing are best illustrated in Fig. 21.5 (World Health Organization, 2015).

Health Status and Quality of Life Among Senior Population in Hong Kong

With an amount of 5.8% of GDP invested into the healthcare system (as in 2018) (http://hdr.undp.org/sites/default/files/hdr2019.pdf), Hong Kong is proud to champion top three in population life expectancy over past ten years. Overall life expectancy (LE) was at 74.5, 80.5, and 84.9 in 1980, 2000, and 2020 respectively (https://www.macrotrends.net/countries/HKG/hong-kong/life-expectancy). Despite the improved life expectancy, there is doubt if the senior is living healthier than before. Although data may not be directly comparable, surveys from population surveys highlighted the high prevalence of chronic diseases and cognitive or mood problems with the ageing population (Table 21.1).

Life expectancy (LE) is an estimate of survival since birth. As one grows, one surpasses the odds of death at earlier years, and life expectancy at age of 60 is not equal to life expectancy at birth minus 60. Furthermore, life expectancy will be affected by multi-morbidities. As one ages, LE becomes less and less useful as a measurement

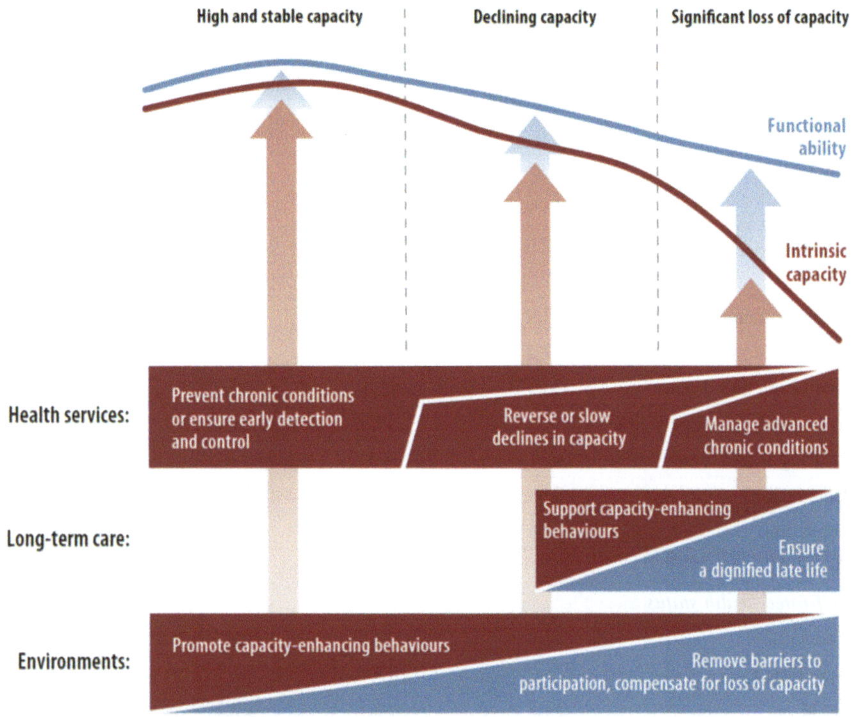

Fig. 21.5 A public-health framework for Healthy Ageing: opportunities for public-health action across the life course. *Source* World Health Organization (2015)

on overall health status or quality of healthcare for seniors. As discussed earlier, health does not refer only to a state free from diseases. Rather it encompasses on a state of bio-psycho-social wellbeing, of which function ability or independence is instrumental to it. Hereby, disability adjusted life years (DALYs) or its converse, i.e. healthy life expectancy will be better surrogate to health status of our senior population. Data from cohorts attending Elderly Health Centre between 2001 and 2012 reviewed more physical limitations among different time cohort of elderly with same age (Yu et al., 2016), with more disability among recent cohorts than previous ones. There is also evidence from population survey that proportion of remaining life in good health without disability has decreased since 1996, indicating a relative expansion of disability (Cheung & Yip, 2010; Table 21.2). These reflect that while we are successful in extending survival life, the quality of it has not been improved concomitantly.

While Hong Kong is monitoring herself for continuous services development in supporting healthy and active ageing, it will be useful to benchmark or compare with other regions and countries for mutual learning. Internationally there is a Global AgeWatch Index (http://www.helpage.org/global-agewatch/) developed by the HelpAge International. It is a multi-dimensional index which assesses key aspects

Table 21.1 Health status among older population in Hong Kong

	2001^	2014–15#		
	Age > 60 (%)	65–74 (%)	75–84 (%)	>85 (%)
Cancer	2.0	3.2	4.7	4.9
CVA	3.5	4.6	7.8	5.7
CHD	15.9	5.6	9.9	12.0
Asthma	10.6	2.4	2.2	1.8
COPD		1.3	1.4	0.4
Hyperlipidemia	17.9	33.6	39.0	26.5
Hypertension	47.2	45.8	64.6	61.2
DM / high blood glucose	20.9	21.0	26.2	22.5
Poor / very poor eye sights	–	11.2	21.0	28.4
Hearing impairment	–	4.6	9.3	18.8
Depression	0.4	1.4	0.7	0.5
Dementia	0.8	0.9	2.3	6.8
Anxiety	–	1.1	0.3	0.3
Self-rated health status				
Excellent	42.8	1.3%	0.4	0.5
Very Good		13.9	9.3	11.0
Good	34.2	36.1	29.3	30.8
Fair	23.0	40.0	45.6	46.4
Poor		8.6	15.5	11.3

Source ^Data extracted from Census and Statistics Department (2001); #Data extracted from Department of Health (2017)

Table 21.2 Life expectancy and disability free life expectancy among older population Hong Kong

Age		Women				Men			
		1996	% of LE	2008	% of LE	1996	% of LE	2008	% of LE
70	LE	16.7		18.5		13.4		14.6	
	DFLE	15.5	91.6	15.5	84.4	12.7	92.9	13.2	90.6
75	LE	13.1		14.3		10.4		11.3	
	DFLE	11.9	89.7	11.6	80.8	9.71	90.5	9.9	87.8
80	LE	9.90		11.0		7.85		8.56	
	DFLE	8.78	86.7	8.32	77.0	7.32	89.4	7.10	83.1

LE: Life Expectancy; DFLE: Disability Free Life Expectancy
Source Data extracted from Cheung and Yip (2010)

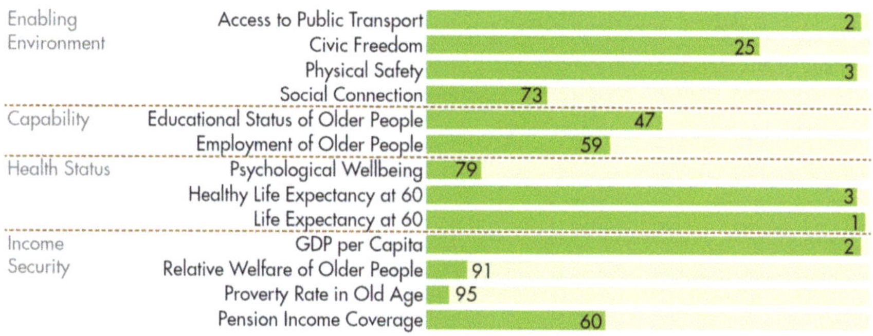

Fig. 21.6 Rankings of Hong Kong among 13 indicators of the Global AgeWatch Index 2014 (out of 97 countries/ territories). *Source* CUHK Jockey Club Institute of Ageing (2014)

of health, economic, and wellbeing of the elderly. Yet Hong Kong is not included in the index for global comparison. Taking reference to the Global AgeWatch Index, an AgeWatch Index for Hong Kong was developed in 2014. Accordingly, Hong Kong ranked 24 among total of 97 participating regions or countries. In the health subscale of the Index, though Hong Kong ranked top three in Healthy Life Expectancy and Life Expectancy at age of 60, she ranked 79 out of 97 in psychological wellbeing, indicating much levy for improvement (Fig. 21.6, CUHK Jockey Club Institute of Ageing, 2014). As in 2016, Hong Kong ranked 11 and 21 in the Health subscale and overall scale out of 97 regions or countries overall.

In 2016, a new tool Hong Kong Elder Quality of Life Index (HKEQOL) was developed. The new tool adopts the four domains from AgeWatch Index but fine tuned on their items. These fine tunes are based on concept of the WHO Age Friendly City (World Health Organization, 2007) that enables Active Ageing and Healthy Ageing, and characteristics of elderly in term of its multi-morbidities state. With reference to the health status domain, three items from AgeWatch Index are revised to include life expectancy at age of 60, elderly hospitalisation utilisation, self-rated health conditions, frailty, mental health, and subjective wellbeing. This revised HKEQOL provides a guide to where we are now, areas where we are proud of, and areas of which efforts are needed to pay on improvement, with ultimate goal on improving QOL of the senior population in Hong Kong. Serial changes in HKEQOL and health status domain of this HKEQOL Index between 2016 and 2020 are shown in Tables 21.3 and 21.4 with data extracted from CUHK Jockey Club Institute of Ageing (2020).

As observed, there was a general trend of improvement in overall QOL between 2016 and 2019. Measured QOL in 2019–2020 might be an exception due to social turmoil in Hong Kong and the start of the COVID-19 pandemic. The overall improvement was attributed to improvement in income security and capability which are more related to domains in Active Ageing. On the other hand, there was a decline in the health status and environment, indicating a need to act on these if Healthy Ageing would be facilitated. Though overall life expectancy had increased over the years,

Table 21.3 HKEQOL score among older population (2016–2020)

Domain in HKEQOL	Scores			
	2016–17 (Baseline)	2017–18	2018–19	2019–20
Income security	25.0	25.19	25.27	24.73
Health status	25.0	24.99	23.85	22.06
Capability	25.0	26.43	27.83	22.82
Enabling environment	25.0	24.37	24.00	23.61
Total score	100.0	100.99	100.95	93.22

Source CUHK Jockey Club Institute of Ageing (2020)

Table 21.4 Health status sub-score from HKEQOL 2016–2020

Indicator within health status in HKEQOL	Scores			
	2016–17 (Baseline)	2017–18	2018–19	2019–20
Life expectancy at 60	4.17	4.17	4.25	4.27
Elderly hospitalization	4.17	4.22	4.09	4.18
Self-rated health condition	4.17	4.08	3.94	3.65
Frailty	4.17	4.37	4.01	3.41
Mental health	4.17	4.02	3.50	2.72
Subjective well-being: life satisfaction	4.17	4.14	4.07	3.82
Sub-total	25	24.99	23.85	22.06

Source CUHK Jockey Club Institute of Ageing (2020)

status on mental health, self-rated health condition, and life satisfaction had shown the reverse. These will be discussed in greater details in later sections. There was also a steady worsening on "Satisfaction with health services" under the Environment domain, which scored 4.17 (baseline), 3.83 (2017–2018) and 3.60 (2018–2019).

Healthy Ageing in Hong Kong

As elucidated at beginning of the chapter, WHO advocates active ageing in preparation of an ageing population. Seniors should be viewed as an asset and a pool of resources. The three pillars on policy frameworks required to support active ageing are having good health, a sense of security, and social involvement or participation. As the latter two involve a wider scope of social policy, it is beyond scope of current discussion. We shall limit our scope on achieving Healthy Ageing in Hong Kong from the professional point of view, challenges and opportunities, and way forward.

Life expectancy in Hong Kong has steadily increased from 67 in 1960, 71.4 in 1970 to 74.7 in 1995. The Hong Kong Government was not slow in recognising special healthcare needs of the senior population. The first geriatrics department in the public hospital system was established in 1971. There was also the need to go from curative medicine to primary care of whole person. In 1997, HKSAR Government, incorporating WHO concept on active ageing, designated "Care for the elderly" as one of its three Strategic Policy Objectives, with the aim of providing the elderly with a sense of security, a sense of belonging, and a feeling of health and worthiness. An Elderly Commission (EC) was established to advise government on the policies and services for the senior population.

Two strategic reports were released. The first report "Report on Healthy Ageing" was published in 2001 (Ad hoc Committee on Healthy Ageing, 2001). The Report, while highlighted on essential philosophies and concepts on Healthy Ageing, also gave policy directions required for Active Ageing. The Report highlighted strategic direction overseas and share the directions in Hong Kong. These directions include:

- *promoting the adoption of a healthy lifestyle from as young as possible to improve the physical and psychosocial wellbeing of an individual;*
- *encouraging personal responsibility while providing support for those in need;*
- *the Government to provide leadership, and work with other stakeholders, such as relevant professional associations, the voluntary agencies and the private sector jointly to promote healthy ageing to the general public;*
- *promoting environmental changes in communities that will facilitate healthy living and "ageing in place" through the design of barrier-free communities, the development of accessible transportation services for persons with frailty and disability, and the development of caring support networks at the community level;*
- *facilitating older persons to continue to take part in community, economic and social activities so as to ensure that they continue to lead an active and interesting life; and*
- *taking steps to promote a positive image of ageing, placing emphasis on the possible contributions older persons can make to their family, the community and society.*

The report then has the foresight on lifelong course on health maintenance, inclusive of all irrespective of their functional capacity and person—environment interactions that are stated at the later WHO guideline. It recommended the Department of Health to take lead at upstream on promoting healthy lifestyle and to emphasise on the importance of early intervention to maintain or restore bodily functions. With reference to Fig. 21.5 on Public-health framework on Healthy Ageing, different government departments and statutory organisations (e.g. Social Welfare Department, Hospital Authority, Housing Authority, Transport Department), and non-government organisations are also called upon to create a supportive environment for those with diminishing functional capacity.

The second report from EC on "Strategic Service Programme Plan" was released in 2017 (Working Group on Elderly Services Programme Plan, 2017). While the first report on Healthy Ageing has focused on upstream health maintenance to maximise or maintain intrinsic capacity for active ageing, this second report outlines different multi-sectoral programme plans to support Ageing in Place and quality of dying when the senior has reduced functional capacity with ultimate aim to achieve care sustainable in current healthcare systems.

Starting from 1998, a total of 18 Elderly Health Centres (EHCs) were established across different districts in Hong Kong to address the multiple health needs of the elderly by providing integrated primary health care services to them. Preventive, promotive, and curative services are provided from a family medicine perspective using a multi-disciplinary team approach. Elders aged 65 or above are eligible for enrolling as members of Elderly Health Centres. Enrolled members are provided with services of health assessment and screening, counselling, health education, and curative treatment at primary care level using a multi-disciplinary team approach and family medicine approach.

With the expansion of medical knowledge and technologies since the 1970s, medical development around the world has focused on disease or curative treatment. Hong Kong has been following through the same path. The government was not slow in recognising the importance of primary healthcare and preventive medicine. A number of healthcare reform consultation documents were released since the establishment of the HKSAR in 1997. These included "Lifelong Investment in Health" (Health & Welfare Bureau, 2001), "Your Health, Your Life" (Food & Health Bureau, 2008), and "My Health, My Choice" (Food & Health Bureau, 2010). In the 2008 consultation document, it held the vision on *"providing (public) with access to lifelong, comprehensive and holistic primary care, with emphasis on health-improving preventive care"*. The consultation document admitted that there was insufficient emphasis on holistic primary care and wellness promotion, limited continuity and integration of care. To enhance primary care, the report recommended to develop basic models for primary care services for reference by both healthcare professionals and individuals, and that a family doctor registry to be built up. Following the consultation document, a Primary Care Office was set up under the former Food and Health Bureau to provide strategic recommendations on enhancing and developing primary care in Hong Kong. At its early phase, the Office developed reference frameworks on management of two common diseases, namely hypertension and diabetes mellitus. It was only in 2011 that a "Hong Kong Reference Framework for Preventive Care for Older Adults in Primary Care Settings" (the Reference Framework)—a framework with reference to a person instead of on disease management (Health Bureau, 2021).

This Reference Framework adopts a combination of population-based life course approach and high-risk individual approach. The population-based life course focuses on health promotion that builds up intrinsic capacity or mitigates behaviours that reduce the intrinsic capacity. Older adults should be advised to keep update on recommended vaccination programme, to keep up with regular exercise, maintain good oral and dental hygiene so that they can have adequate nutrition with wise eating and enjoyment, and enjoy social and leisure activities. They should also avoid ill-health behaviour such as smoking and moderate on alcohol intake. The Reference Framework recommends taking an opportunistic approach to promote these healthy lifestyle behaviours. Although there is a chapter that states that overall health and quality of life may be jeopardised from physical limitation, psychological factors, and limited social connection, little is stated on health promotion towards cognitive and psychological health, and on social participation and engagement into active and meaningful social life and leisure activities.

Besides health promotion, the Framework also lay out areas that an elder should be screened for regularly at 1–3 yearly interval, and opportunistically at every visit—the high-risk individual approach. It should be noted that the recommended screening depends on individual. For those healthy older adults without known chronic disease, a primary prevention approach is adopted whereby one should screen against risk factors for disease development, or early detection of disease. For those who have established conditions, aim of screening is for secondary or tertiary prevention to avoid deterioration or development of complications. There is also a shift of focus from disease screening towards screening on function impairment or disability and supports. This follows the WHO concept on active ageing whereby maintaining disease free state is only a process to allow normal functioning and to enjoy good quality of life. As functional impairment can be from any disease, combination of diseases, or accelerated age-related decline due to non-healthy lifestyle (see Fig. 21.5), it is worthwhile to start from the end, i.e. assess for functional impairment directly. In case there is any evaluation and interventions can be started to restore function or to prevent accelerated decline and to prevent complications. Recommended areas to be screened among different subgroups are summarised in Table 21.5.

As discussed in earlier section, WHO has introduced the concept of intrinsic capacity. With progressive decline in reserve at multiple organs, one may have little resilience to stress when excess demand is required. This state of frailty is defined as "progressive age-related deterioration in physiological systems that results in extreme vulnerability to stressors and increases the risk of a range of adverse outcomes including care dependence and death" (Beard et al., 2016). Multiple studies have shown that living with frailty is associated with higher risk of physical and cognitive decline, increased risk of falls, disability, hospitalisation, institutionalisation and mortality, and increased caregiver burdens (Speechley & Tinetti, 1991; Woo et al., 2006). Though there is great overlap between frailty and physically disability, they are not identical (Woo & Leung, 2014). A person may have disability from a stroke yet he may not be frail. On the other hand, another person may have multiple "trivial" problems in each system of which he can get over to each and each of the individual "trivial" problems, yet in combination and in an integrative model, he can be a frail person. There are three subtypes of frailty—physical frailty that is related to sarcopenia, cognitive frailty relating to dementia, and social frailty that refers to breakdown in social support. Using a FRAIL scale (Morley et al., 2012; Woo et al., 2012) as the measurement tool, a local community study reviewed about 12.5% of seniors age > 65 were frail were 52.4% was pre-frail. Annual survey of the HKEQOL Index showed a worsening trend between 2017 and 2019 (Table 21.4). The important issue is that frailty can be reversed within intensive resistive exercise training and high protein diet (Lee et al., 2014; Yu et al., 2014). WHO (2017) has also emphasised importance of prevention or counteract of frailty for healthy ageing. With the high

Table 21.5 Summary on screening among older adults with different degree of health status

Aspects to be screened	Older adults without chronic disease	Independent older adults with chronic diseases	Older adults with disabilities
Screen/risk assessment for hypertension and DM	√	√	
Screen for hyperlipidemia	√		
Screen for nutrition status (overweight and underweight)	√	√	Assess risk of malnutrition
Screen for cancer (cervical cancer, colorectal cancer)	√		
Screen for functional impairment*	√	√	√ (Opportunistic screening)
Screen/Assess for abilities on self-care and daily livings		√	√
Review on use of medications		√	√
Assess social network and support		√ (social and carer support)	√ (carer stress)

*Functional impairment: hearing, vision, incontinence, falls, dental, depression, dementia, social isolation
Source Health Bureau (2021)

prevalence of frailty or pre-frail, known adverse outcome, availability of simple screening tool and effectiveness of intervention, screen for frailty should be another aspect to be added in the Reference Framework.

Another area of note is that though the Reference Framework has included mood and cognitive assessment and screening for high-risk individual, it has not had enough emphasis on assessment activities or lifestyles for psychological health and social participation or active learning for health at population health promotion level. Poor psychological wellbeing not only affect the social, emotion, and physical wellbeing of older people, but also causes depression with increased risk of suicide. Loneliness is another important factor contributing to poor mental wellbeing of older people (Mushtaq et al., 2014; Sau Po Centre on Ageing, 2018). About 10.1% reported to have loneliness from local population survey (Department of Health, 2017) and 27.9% elderly (age > 65) attending a FM clinic at a district (Zhang et al., 2020). The HKEQOL Index also reflected a worsening of mental wellbeing among senior population through 2017–2019 (Table 21.4) and there was high suicide rate among older population in Hong Kong (HKJC Centre for Suicide Research and Prevention, 2020). Promotion of psychological and social health is another area to develop on.

It is obvious from above Reference Framework on health promotion, assessment, and screening needs to be done at multi-dimensional aspect and needs inter-sectoral collaboration for intervention. Currently, the Primary Care Directory only enlisted medical practitioners, dentists, and Chinese medicine practitioners and there has not had a list of allied health workers in the Directory. It is the aim of the Primary Care Office that through the Reference Framework, to facilitate primary care professionals to collaborate with other professionals to provide coordinated services, and to achieve collaboration and interfacing of service providers in the community through an integrated system. Yet most of the practitioners under the Primary Care Directory are solo practice or in groups without direct support from other disciplines, nor is the provision integrated and collaborated. Seeing the barriers in implementing the suggestions in the Reference Framework and the determination to improve primary care, HKSAR established the first local District Health Centre (DHC) in 2019, with a plan to roll out to each of the 18 districts in Hong Kong. (Details of the DHC can be referred in Chapter 25). Unlike the EHCs, which only allow membership enrolment to those age > 65, there is no age exclusion to enrol criteria to join the DHC. This follows the lifelong health from WHO to build up intrinsic capacity from young or middle age. The establishment of DHCs demonstrates the government's determination to the development of primary care services. Yet the working model and role delineation of DHCs need to be clarified, as well as human resources to its success may need to be addressed. In particular, whether the DHC working model suits the needs of elderly is subject to debate.

In summary, Hong Kong government has taken steps to create a balance between preventive and primary care versus curative hospital care for elderly through the EHCs and the Primary Healthcare Office. Guiding principles of their work follow the WHO Healthy Ageing framework and Elderly Commissioner's Report on Healthy Ageing. There are levies to update on frailty prevention and assessment, and on promotion of psycho-social health with active social participation. It will be valuable to evaluate on uptake rate on recommendations from the Reference Framework among healthcare workers within the Primary Care Directory and to understand facilitators and barriers on its applications. Towards this end, it requires both public (EHCs) and private sectors (healthcare workers within the Primary Care Directory) to work hand in hand to safeguard Healthy Ageing for the senior local population.

References

Ad hoc Committee on Healthy Ageing. (2001). *Report on health ageing*. https://www.elderlycommission.gov.hk/en/library/ROHA.HTM

Beard, J. R., Officer, A., De Carvalho, I. A., Sadana, R., Pot, A. M., Michel, J. P., Lloyd-Sherlock, P., Epping-Jordan, J. E., Peeters, G. G., Mahanani, W. R. & Chatterji, S. (2016). The World report on ageing and health: A policy framework for healthy ageing. *The Lancet*, *387*(10033), 2145–2154. https://doi.org/10.1016/S0140-6736(15)00516-4

Census and Statistics Department. (2001). S*ocial data collected via the general household survey: Special topics—report no. 27*. https://www.censtatd.gov.hk/en/data/stat_report/product/C0000072/att/B11301272001XXXXB0100.pdf

Cheung, K. S. L., & Yip, P. S. F. (2010). Trends in healthy life expectancy in Hong Kong SAR 1996–2008. *European Journal of Ageing, 7*(4), 257–269. https://doi.org/10.1007/s10433-010-0171-3

CUHK Jockey Club Institute of Ageing. (2014). *Report on AgeWatch Index for Hong Kong 2014*. https://www.jcafc.hk/uploads/docs/Report-on-AgeWatch-Index-for-Hong-Kong-2014-(final).pdf

CUHK Jockey Club Institute of Ageing. (2020). *Report on Hong Kong elderly quality of life index incorporating AgeWatch Index for Hong Kong 2019*. https://www.jcafc.hk/uploads/docs/HKEQOL_2019_final_online(v2).pdf

Department of Health. (2017). *Report of population health survey 2014/15*. https://www.chp.gov.hk/files/pdf/dh_phs_2014_15_full_report_eng.pdf

Food and Health Bureau. (2008). *Your health your life: Healthcare reform consultation document*. https://www.healthbureau.gov.hk/beStrong/files/consultation/Condochealth_full_eng.pdf

Food and Health Bureau. (2010). *My health my choice: Healthcare reform second stage consultation document*. https://www.myhealthmychoice.gov.hk/pdf/consultation_full_eng.pdf

Health Bureau. (2021). *Hong Kong reference framework for preventive care for older adults in primary care settings*. https://www.healthbureau.gov.hk/pho/rfs/english/reference_framework/pre_care_for_older_adults.html

Health and Welfare Bureau. (2001) *Lifelong investment in health*. https://www.healthbureau.gov.hk/download/press_and_publications/consultation/HCR/ALL.PDF

Lee, J. S., Auyeung, T. W., Leung, J., Kwok, T., & Woo, J. (2014). Transitions in frailty states among community-living older adults and their associated factors. *Journal of the American Medical Directors Association, 15*(4), 281–286. https://doi.org/10.1016/j.jamda.2013.12.002

Morley, J. E., Malmstrom, T. K., & Miller, D. K. (2012). A simple frailty questionnaire (FRAIL) predicts outcomes in middle aged African Americans. *The Journal of Nutrition, Health & Aging, 16*(7), 601–608. https://doi.org/10.1007/s12603-012-0084-2

Mushtaq, R., Shoib, S., Shah, T., & Mushtaq, S. (2014). Relationship between loneliness, psychiatric disorders and physical health? A review on the psychological aspects of loneliness. *Journal of Clinical and Diagnostic Research*, 8(9), WE01–04. https://doi.org/10.7860/JCDR/2014/10077.4828

Sadana, R., & Michel, J. P. (2019). Healthy ageing: What is it and how to describe it? In J. P. Michel (Ed.), *Prevention of chronic diseases and age-related disability* (pp. 11–24). Springer. https://doi.org/10.1007/978-3-319-96529-1_2

Sau Po Centre on Ageing. (2018). *Best 60s 關注「腦」朋友計劃「無獨耆年」-長者孤獨情緒與精神健康研究結果發佈會* [Best 60s concern "brain" friends programme "No loneliness in senior year" – Results announcement on the elderly loneliness and mental health research]. http://ageing.hku.hk/upload/file/20180510%20Final_HKU.pdf

Speechley, M., & Tinetti, M. (1991). Falls and injuries in frail and vigorous community elderly persons. *Journal of the American Geriatrics Society, 39*(1), 46–52. https://doi.org/10.1111/j.1532-5415.1991.tb05905.x

Towards healthy ageing. (1997). *Health Promotion International, 12*(2), 175–178, https://doi.org/10.1093/heapro/12.2.175

Woo, J., Goggins, W., Sham, A., & Ho, S. C. (2006). Public health significance of the frailty index. *Disability and Rehabilitation, 28*(8), 515–521. https://doi.org/10.1080/09638280500215867

Woo, J., & Leung, J. (2014). Multi-morbidity, dependency, and frailty singly or in combination have different impact on health outcomes. *Age, 36*(2), 923–931. https://doi.org/10.1007/s11357-013-9590-3

Woo, J., Leung, J., & Morley, J. E. (2012). Comparison of frailty indicators based on clinical phenotype and the multiple deficit approach in predicting mortality and physical limitation.

Journal of the American Geriatrics Society, 60(8), 1478–1486. https://doi.org/10.1111/j.1532-5415.2012.04074.x

World Health Organization. (2001). *ICF beginner's guide: Towards a common language for functioning, disability and health.* https://www.who.int/publications/m/item/icf-beginner-s-guide-towards-a-common-language-for-functioning-disability-and-health

World Health Organization. (2002). *Active ageing: A policy framework.* https://apps.who.int/iris/handle/10665/67215

World Health Organization. (2007). *Global age-friendly cities: A guide.* https://apps.who.int/iris/handle/10665/43755

World Health Organization. (2015). World report on ageing and health. https://www.who.int/publications/i/item/9789241565042

World Health Organization. (2017). *WHO clinical consortium on healthy ageing: Topic focus: Frailty and intrinsic capacity: Report of consortium meeting, 1–2 December 2016 in Geneva, Switzerland.* https://apps.who.int/iris/handle/10665/272437

Working Group on Elderly Services Programme Plan. (2017). *Elderly services programme plan.* Elderly Commission https://www.elderlycommission.gov.hk/en/download/library/ESPP_Final_Report_Eng.pdf

Yu, R., Wong, M., Leung, J., Lee, J., Auyeung, T. W., & Woo, J. (2014). Incidence, reversibility, risk factors and the protective effect of high body mass index against sarcopenia in community-dwelling older Chinese adults. *Geriatrics & Gerontology International, 14*(S1), 15–28. https://doi.org/10.1111/ggi.12220

Yu, R., Wong, M., Chang, B., Lai, X., Lum, C. M., Auyeung, T. W., Lee, J., Tsoi, K., Lee, R. & Woo, J. (2016). Trends in activities of daily living disability in a large sample of community-dwelling Chinese older adults in Hong Kong: an age-period-cohort analysis. *BMJ Open, 6*(12), Article e013259. https://bmjopen.bmj.com/content/6/12/e013259

Zhang, D., Sit, R. W. S., Wong, C., Zou, D., Mercer, S. W., Johnston, M. C., & Wong, S. Y. S. (2020). Cohort profile: The prospective study on Chinese elderly with multimorbidity in primary care in Hong Kong. *BMJ Open, 10*(2), Article e027279. https://doi.org/10.1136/bmjopen-2018-027279

Chapter 22
The Future of End-of-Life Care Policy in Hong Kong

Roger Yat-Nork Chung and Derrick Kit-Sing Au

Abstract This chapter is divided into three parts. First, using a socio-ecological model, we highlight the major barriers, issues, and gaps of end-of-life (EOL) care in Hong Kong as identified in the government commissioned report published in 2017. Second, we give an update on the latest developments of EOL care after the commissioned report has been published. Finally, based on the findings from the government commissioned report and the developments thereafter, we reflect on where we think Hong Kong may stand now in terms of its EOL care and how to move forward.

Keywords End-of-life care · Advance care planning · Advance directive · Mental capacity · Palliative care · Do-not-resuscitate · Legislation · Hong Kong · China

Background

Populated by 7.291 million (2022) of predominantly Chinese ethnicity and some ethnic minorities (Census and Statistics Department, 2022a), Hong Kong is a city with a unique socio-political history. In particular, it was a former British colony since 1841 and has become a special administrative region (SAR) of China since 1997. Due to the history of colonial rule, the healthcare system in Hong Kong has some similarities to the United Kingdom (UK). This is a so-called dual track system, comprising a public and a private sector. The public sector is tax-based and historically modelled after the UK National Health Service (lacking however a well-developed primary care arm). In 1990, the Hospital Authority (HA) was established

R. Y.-N. Chung (✉)
JC School of Public Health and Primary Care, CUHK Centre for Bioethics and CUHK Institute of Health Equity, The Chinese University of Hong Kong, Hong Kong, China
e-mail: rychung@cuhk.edu.hk

D. K.-S. Au
CUHK Centre for Bioethics, The Chinese University of Hong Kong, Hong Kong, China
e-mail: ksau@cuhk.edu.hk

B. Y. F. Fong and W. C. W. Wong (eds.), *Gaps and Actions in Health Improvement from Hong Kong and Beyond*,
https://doi.org/10.1007/978-981-99-4491-0_22

through statutory legislation to bring the former government hospitals and NGO-run subvented hospitals under one roof, for management and reform.

During the post-World War II period, we see the rise of Hong Kong as an important global financial hub. Along with this rapid socioeconomic development, Hong Kong has experienced accelerated epidemiologic transition from communicable to non-communicable diseases as the leading causes of death, and its life expectancy at birth has been steadily increasing and overtaken Japan, the traditional champion of the health indicator, since 2010 (The World Bank, n.d.). In 2020, men and women in Hong Kong could live on average for 83.4 years and 87.7 years, respectively (Census and Statistics Department, 2022b). Nevertheless, according to the Economist Intelligence Unit's *Quality of Death Index* in 2015 (The Economist Intelligence Unit, 2015), which measured the quality of end-of-life (EOL) care in five categories (including palliative and healthcare environment, human resources, affordability of care, quality of care, and community engagement), Hong Kong was ranked number 22 in the overall score, behind other developed Asian economies of Taiwan (6), Singapore (12), Japan (14), and South Korea (18), as well as its former sovereignty state, the UK (1). Even though Hong Kong's healthcare system consists of a public and a private sector, and the tax-based public sector is modelled after the UK National Health Service, the situations of EOL care are quite different. For instance, over 90% of deaths in Hong Kong happened in hospitals (Woo et al., 2009), as opposed to 48.5% in the UK (Public Health England, 2018). Moreover, several weaknesses of Hong Kong's EOL care were highlighted in the report, including the lack of compulsory education on the subject in medical training, the lack of legal standing of do-not-resuscitate, and limited understanding of the general public on palliative care. Nevertheless, the relatively short profile of Hong Kong in the report only scratched the surface of the underlying issues.

In 2015, the Food and Health Bureau (FHB) (which is renamed as Health Bureau (HB) since July 2022) of the Hong Kong SAR Government commissioned School of Public Health and Primary Care of the Chinese University of Hong Kong to conduct a three-year research project on the quality of healthcare for the ageing, of which a significant portion was dedicated to identifying the situations, gaps, barriers, and issues in EOL care for older persons with terminal illness or life-limiting conditions. The first author of this chapter was part of the research team of that commissioned study, the final report of which is publicly available (Research Fund Secretariat, n.d.). The major findings were also disseminated through several publications (Chung et al., 2017, 2020, 2021; Threapleton et al., 2017; Wong et al., 2020, 2022). In this chapter, we will first highlight the major barriers, issues, and gaps as identified in the FHB commissioned report, then give an update on the latest developments after the report has been published, and subsequently reflect on where we think Hong Kong may stand now and in the future in terms of its EOL care.

Summary of Barriers, Issues, Gaps of EOL Care in Hong Kong

Using a socio-ecological model (Mcleroy et al., 1988), these barriers, issues, and gaps of EOL care can be summarised in different ecological levels for terminal illness and life-limiting conditions among older persons in Hong Kong.

Policy- and Legal-Level

First and foremost, no overarching policy framework for EOL care exists in Hong Kong, despite the recognition of the importance of quality EOL care by the government. While acknowledging EOL care could be regarded as the final stage of long-term care for people with chronic diseases that become terminal, life-limiting, and irreversible, there is nonetheless no overarching long-term care policy in Hong Kong. The only overarching healthcare policy in Hong Kong is that no one should be denied adequate healthcare due to lack of financial means (GovHK, 2022). In other words, it is a non-denial approach to a service-oriented healthcare, but not one that gives emphasis on assuring the quality of death and dying per se. Moreover, what is considered to be "adequate healthcare" could vary especially in the more complicated cases of EOL care. Therefore, the current overarching healthcare policy alone cannot sufficiently address and cover EOL care cases, where ethical dilemmas are common.

Besides the lack of overarching EOL care policy, there are barriers and gaps with the relevant laws in Hong Kong. In particular, there is an ambiguity in the legal basis for mental incapacity. The *Mental Health Ordinance (Cap. 136) 2022* (HKSAR) was drafted originally for people with mental illness or those who were mentally compromised or handicapped; in other words, no specific provision in the law was provided for persons who were losing their mental capacity due to other reasons and conditions, such as those suffering from a persistent vegetative state, dementia, or in an irreversible coma. No necessary changes have been made even after the Law Reform Commission's proposal for new definitions of mental capacity in 2006 (The Law Reform Commission of Hong Kong, 2006). In effect, the burden of proof of mental capacity lies with the attending clinicians, and this also has direct effect on the validity and applicability of the decisions made in any advance directive (AD) which could only take precedence when the patient who made an AD becomes mentally incapacitated.

Also, there are other existing legislative barriers to AD that must be overcome if Hong Kong decides to put AD into formal legislation. First, the legal requirement for paramedics to "resuscitate" patients as rigidly stipulated by the Fire Services Ordinance (*Fire Services Ordinance (Cap. 95) 2021* (HKSAR)) may come into conflict with any AD or do-not-attempt-cardiopulmonary-resuscitation (DNACPR) decisions. Second, any advance medical decisions may potentially be overridden by the medical practitioner based on the "best interest principle" as stipulated in the Mental Health Ordinance (Cap. 136): "*Where a registered medical practitioner... considers that treatment is necessary and is in the best interests of the mentally incapacitated person, then he may carry out that treatment without the consent of the mentally incapacitated person or that person's guardian (if any) accordingly*" (*Mental Health Ordinance (Cap. 136) 2022* (HKSAR)). Third, the Powers of Attorney Ordinance (Cap. 31) in Hong Kong only allows the appointed attorney, the person delegated with legal authority by the patient, to handle property and financial matters of the patient before and after he/she becomes mentally incapacitated (*Powers of Attorney Ordinance (Cap 31) 2018* (HKSAR)), but not non-financial matters including medical decisions. While keeping this status quo of the powers of attorney will not introduce direct conflict with the potential AD legislation, this potential conflict may still need to be anticipated during the legislature process of AD in preparation for the day when the enduring powers of attorney in Hong Kong is to be extended towards medical decisions on life-sustaining treatments. In fact, the Department of Justice (DoJ) of the Hong Kong Government has launched a two-month long public consultation in 2017 on preparing for a new Continuing Powers of Attorney Bill that extends the powers of attorney towards non-financial matters.

Besides the legislative barriers to AD, the power of guardians in EOL care decisions is also another issue that needs to be addressed. The Mental Health Ordinance (Cap. 136) stipulated that guardians of mentally handicapped or incapacitated persons only have the power to consent to but not refuse, withhold, or withdraw from life-sustaining medical treatments (*Mental Health Ordinance (Cap. 136) 2022* (HKSAR)). However, decisions for patients during their EOL often need to extend beyond consent for medical treatment to include refusal, withholding or withdrawal of futile or unnecessary treatment, tests, or interventions. Therefore, changes in this law with the necessary safeguards are needed to ensure that the appointed guardians can fully perform their role when acting on behalf of their patients during their EOL.

Furthermore, with regard to residential care, the Residential Care Homes (Elderly Persons) Ordinance (Cap. 459) does not require the residential care homes for elderly (RCHEs) to have medical practitioners on staff (Social Welfare Department, 2013). While some higher-level old age homes (e.g. nursing homes) in Hong Kong require medical practitioners to be on staff, this is still a problem because most old age homes in Hong Kong are in fact RCHEs with no such requirement. While these RCHEs could purchase services from visiting medical officers, there is still no requirement for them to visit the RCHEs on a daily basis. As a result, EOL patients who reside in these RCHEs would not receive adequate care in a consistent and regular manner, particularly during non-office hours. Most of the time the staff in these RCHEs would resort to calling emergency ambulances to send the patients off to the Accident and Emergency (A&E) Departments (i.e. emergency rooms), crowding out resources that should otherwise be reserved for acute care, and triggering unnecessary recurring hospitalisations.

Community-Level

At the community level, resources, essential set up, and equipment to facilitate EOL care in the community are very limited. These include easy access to prescription drugs for symptom control, the generally small living space in households, and the generally inadequate knowledge and training of informal caregivers to support EOL care patients. In other words, it is unlikely that EOL patients would receive quality EOL care in the community, and many have to rely on palliative care of the hospitals, which is also limited. Caregiver support services provided by the government's Social Welfare Department (SWD) aim only at training and supporting caregivers to deliver general care for older patients, but not specifically EOL care. This is also reflected in the Economist Intelligence Unit's *Quality of Death Index* report in 2015 (The Economist Intelligence Unit, 2015), where they highlighted that Hong Kong was ranked the lowest at 38 in community engagement relative to other indicators including palliative and healthcare environment (at 28), human resources (at 20), affordability of care (at 18), and quality of care (at 20).

Institutional-Level

While EOL care in the community is at best piecemeal in Hong Kong, EOL patients had to rely on the institutional settings for much of their EOL care. Even in institutional care, there are major gaps and barriers.

First of all, there are inadequate knowledge, training, and resources of EOL care in both the medical and social sectors. The general culture and mindset favour medical intervention of curative nature over palliative care. In a survey of medical practitioners, some perceived palliative care as "giving up" and did not recognise placing symptom control, enhancing quality of life, and respecting patient's autonomy—considered the core function of palliative care—as the heart of the care. The consensus was that the university medical curriculum in Hong Kong emphasised on "curing" instead of "caring for" the patients (Chung et al., 2020). In Hong Kong, EOL care is often delivered by palliative care or geriatric medicine specialists, but the number of specialists is small. As of May 2016, there were about 40 doctors, 300 nurses, and 60 allied health professionals who delivered palliative care for a population with over a million older persons aged 65 or above (Chung et al., 2020; Research Fund Secretariat, n.d.). The coverage of palliative care was low. Even for terminally ill patients, only 64% cancer and 44% end-stage renal patients received palliative care in 2016 (Lo, 2016).

Second, there are inadequate and inappropriate transportation arrangements for EOL care patients in Hong Kong. Many patients with deterioration of medical conditions are admitted to the public hospitals through A&E. While this is not to say that EOL patients should never use A&E care, it could be inappropriate for many of these patients, thereby crowding out the A&E resources for other patients requiring emergency care. When EOL patients present to hospitals, A&E service providers may not have sufficient understanding and coordination to handle them well (Chung et al., 2020). Also, most EOL patients are transported to the A&E via emergency ambulances operated by the Fire Services Department. These ambulances do not transport EOL patients to extended care or sub-acute facilities which could administer the type of care they generally need; commonly, the patients are first handled in the acute setting and then transferred to sub-acute care. Such rigid protocol generates redundancies that could otherwise be avoided if sub-acute ambulatory services could be directly provided. Public hospitals do in fact run a Non-emergency Ambulatory Transfer Service (NEATS) for mobility-disabled patients who are unable to take transportation, but it may take more than two months in advance for booking (Chung et al., 2020). Therefore, in between absolute emergency and two months in advance, there seems to be a huge service gap for those who are diagnosed to be dying but have not reached their last days of life yet.

Third, in the social care sector, there is a conventional understanding that old age homes, including both the RCHEs and the higher-level nursing homes where dying in place is legally permissible, are not suitable settings to facilitate EOL care. This belief was reinforced by the facts that there were inadequate staffing, support, equipment, and resources in these old age homes, especially the RCHEs. Instead, the general notion among their staff was that EOL care should be delivered and death should happen in the hospital settings. Therefore, due to this general notion and actual inadequacy of capacity, it is very common for the old age homes to send these EOL patients to the hospitals, resulting in frequent transfer between these institutions and hospitals. In recent years, non-governmental organisations (NGO) and HA community geriatric assessment service (CGAS), with support from SWD, have piloted EOL care programmes in old age homes (Labour and Welfare Bureau, 2021), the outcomes of which will need to be evaluated.

Fourth, the concepts and practices of advance care planning (ACP) and/or advance directive (AD) were not routinely promoted or recognised across the medical and social care sectors in Hong Kong. HA, managing all public hospitals in Hong Kong, played a leading role in gradually introducing and implementing these tools. Guidance for HA Clinicians on Advance Directives in Adults in HA was first promulgated in 2010 and periodically updated. A comprehensive set of Guidelines on Do-Not-Attempt Cardiopulmonary Resuscitation (DNACPR) was developed in 2014, and comprehensively updated in 2016 and 2020. ACP, on the other hand, had not been actively promoted before 2017, and the set of guidelines was only issued in 2019. Notwithstanding these efforts, the uptake of AD was reportedly low, and the DNACPR form was not widely acknowledged and understood outside of the HA hospital settings, including the old age homes and the Fire Services Department that operated all the emergency ambulances.

Between the medical and social care sectors, there are other issues of inadequate coordination which may disrupt the continuum of care for EOL patients in general. These inadequacies included referral, transfers, information sharing, and access that should be present. For instance, the general notion in the social sector was that it was difficult to access medical records of the patients, and if they were made available, to understand the rationale and appropriateness of the treatments received at the hospital settings. On the other hand, some medical practitioners felt that the medical records were too difficult and complicated for non-medical professionals to fully understand and might be unnecessary for the social care sector. Regardless, this inadequate common understanding and communication might have led to the distrust between the two sectors, which was not conducive of good EOL care.

Fifth, even after death, bereavement, and decedent care were also insufficient. Although HA provided post-death bereavement care to the family of the patients, medical records in the public healthcare information system would be archived after a period following death, thereby discouraging further follow-up and continuity of care. On the other hand, the government department that is traditionally responsible for waste disposal and hygiene, the Food and Environmental Hygiene Department (FEHD), is also in charge of decedent arrangements, including death registration, coroner's investigation in deaths outside of hospitals or nursing homes, cremation/burial arrangements, and licensing of coffin shops and funeral homes. Therefore, more training of the staff at FEHD is needed to enhance dignified care for the decedents.

Intrapersonal- and Interpersonal-Level

Finally, there was a general reluctance and fear of the topics of death and dying, and thus EOL care. Nevertheless, there was age difference in terms of this reluctance—i.e. older people generally felt more willing and likely to engage in conversations about these topics (Chung et al., 2017). This general reluctance made it challenging for healthcare professionals to have discussions with patients and their family members about the issues, thereby reinforcing such conversations as cultural taboo. This culture did not only translate itself to inadequacy of EOL care conversations, it also coupled with another traditional Chinese culture, namely filial piety, to affect the attitude towards EOL care. In particular, it was found that filial piety was commonly interpreted as "doing everything possible and trying the utmost" in terms of curative care to treat the patients in hopes for miracles, despite prognosis of terminal or life-limiting conditions and imminent deaths, as well as the futile and intrusive nature of the treatment that could negatively affect the quality of life of the patients (Chung et al., 2020).

Latest Developments of EOL Care in Hong Kong

There had been further progresses made in EOL care in Hong Kong after the FHB commissioned study. In this section, we will summarise these major developments.

Strategic Service Framework for Palliative Care in the Public Healthcare Sector (2017)

In August 2017, HA issued its "Strategic Service Framework for Palliative Care", which aimed to guide the development of adult and paediatric palliative care services in the next five to ten years (Hospital Authority, 2017). The goal of the framework was to outline the strategies to address existing issues and improve service quality so that all patients with life-threatening and life-limiting conditions and their families/carers could (1) receive timely, coordinated, and holistic palliative care for their physical, psychosocial, and spiritual needs, and (2) be given opportunities to participate in the planning of their care so as to improve, enhance, or slow down the deterioration of their quality of life till the end of their life journey. The framework placed emphasis on the collaboration among different specialties along the care continuum from the hospital to the community settings.

Specifically, the framework outlined four strategic directions for the adult palliative care, including (1) improvement of governance and service organisation with collaboration between the medical and oncology specialists in palliative care, (2) care coordination between palliative care and non-palliative care specialists, (3) enhancement of palliative care in the ambulatory and community settings to reduce unnecessary hospitalisation and (4) performance monitoring for continuous quality improvement. On the other hand, the framework also outlined three strategic directions for the paediatric palliative care rooted in a family-centred approach, namely, to (1) establish territory-wide paediatric palliative care services within the public sector, (2) promote integrated and shared care with the parent teams, and (3) enhance community support for the paediatric patients and their families.

In summary, the framework not only highlights the future service models that HA aspires to deliver, but also calls for a fundamental shift in our care culture by advocating the type of care that goes beyond "saving lives" per se, and helps patients live with comfort, dignity, and peace till the last days of their life journey.

Public Consultation of Legislation on Continuing Powers of Attorney (2017–2018)

Following the 2011 report on "Enduring Powers of Attorney: Personal Care" by the Law Reform Commission of Hong Kong, the Government's DoJ had convened an inter-departmental working group with members from the Labour and Welfare Bureau, the Food and Health Bureau and the SWD, and in December 2017 launched a public consultation on the Continuing Powers of Attorney (CPA) Bill in Hong Kong. In the Law Reform Commission Report, they recommended extending the scope of the Enduring Powers of Attorney (EPA) to cover not only decisions on the financial and property affairs of the donor of such powers, but also decisions on his/her personal care matters, in the event that he/she becomes mentally incapacitated.

DoJ sought to enact the CPA Ordinance to replace the existing Enduring Powers of Attorney Ordinance (Cap. 501) with a new CPA regime, in order to distinguish the two. With the commencement of this new CPA law, new EPAs would no longer be created, but EPAs previously executed would continue to be governed by the Enduring Powers of Attorney Ordinance (Cap. 501). The public consultation ended in April 2018, and the government is considering whether to develop a new CPA law to cover medical decisions in the powers of attorney.

New and Updated Guidelines Related to EOL Care in the Public Healthcare Sector (2019–2020)

As mentioned above, before the end of the FHB commissioned study in 2017, HA had issued guidelines for their clinicians on ADs but not yet on ACP. It was not until June 2019 that HA issued its "HA Guidelines on Advance Care Planning" (Hospital Authority, 2019), which outlined in detail the purpose, initiation, process, scope as well as outcome of the ACP. A standardised ACP form was also introduced, and the follow-up actions needed after the making of the ACP conversation were outlined, including the safekeeping of the form, communication with stakeholders (e.g. community caregivers and the HA Community Geriatric Assessment Team) in the community, special issues to be followed up, review of ACP, signing of DNACPR form if necessary, and the actual application of values, wishes, and preferences documented during the ACP process.

In parallel to the new guidelines on ACP, minor updates were made on the guidelines on DNACPR in September 2020. It should be noted that the DNACPR guidelines, when first issued in 2014, were in itself a major update of the pre-existing do-not-resuscitate guidelines used in HA hospitals since 1998. In 2016, this was further updated with a new addition of a set of guidelines on DNACPR decision-making for non-hospitalised patients, and standardisation of DNACPR forms for all HA hospitals. Further update in 2020 was therefore relatively minor, focusing on aligning categories of applicable conditions for adult patients with AD, minors, and incompetent patients.

Public Consultation of Legislation on Advance Directives and Dying in Place (2019–2020)

Besides the new strategic service framework for palliative care and guidelines related to EOL care in the HA, FHB under the government also conducted a public consultation on legislative proposals on advance directives and dying in place from September 6 to December 19, 2019, after reviewing the recommendations made in the FHB commissioned study report. FHB had received 607 written submissions, which showed clear support on the overall direction of the government's original proposals with opinions on some of the execution details regarding ADs and Coroners Ordinance (Cap 504). According to these responses, FHB then released its consultation report *End-of-life Care: Moving Forward. Legislative Proposals on Advance Directives and Dying in Place* in July 2020 with its final legislative proposals (Food and Health Bureau, 2020).

In terms of ADs, the government proposed that any mentally competent person aged 18 or above could make an AD to refuse life-sustaining treatment, including artificial nutrition and hydration, under pre-specified conditions. They recommended the use of a non-statutory model form covering the pre-specified conditions of terminal illness, persistent vegetative state or a state of irreversible coma, and other end-stage irreversible life-limiting conditions. That means AD not made in any model form should still be accepted given that they are clearly written and not ambiguous. There are also no restrictions as to when a person could make, modify, or revoke an AD, given that the person is mentally competent and not under any undue influence. While the making and modifying of an AD must be in writing, the revocation could be made verbally or in writing. Two witnesses with no interests in the estate of the person of concern must be present in making or modifying an AD, and one of whom must be a medical practitioner who approves that the person has capability to make an AD, and has been informed of the nature and effect of the AD, and the consequences of refusing the treatments as specified in the AD. On the other hand, no witness is required for a written revocation. The AD can be revoked by crossing out and signing on an AD, or tearing/destroying by the person who made the AD or by another person in the presence *and* by direction of the person of concern. For verbal revocation, it requires the presence of at least one witness who has no interests in the estate of the person making the AD, and the presence of a second witness for verbal revocation made by a single family member or carer but not by the person him/herself. Once an AD is made, the primary responsibility of safekeeping the AD and ensuring the original copy be presented to the treatment providers as valid proof shall lie with the person with the AD. A valid AD will only be applicable when the person who suffers from the conditions mentioned above become mentally incompetent of making healthcare decisions.

To facilitate an AD being followed outside the hospital setting, a statutory prescribed DNACPR form is proposed to be used. The original copy will need to be presented to the emergency personnel and/or treatment providers as valid proof of a DNACPR form. The DNACPR form can be used for minors and incompetent adults who do not have an AD and those who have advanced irreversible illnesses, given that CPR is not in the best interests of the patient. It is also proposed that the Electronic Health Recording Sharing shall store the records of ADs and DNACPRs on a voluntary basis. Safeguards will also need to be provided for the treatment providers acting in good faith and with reasonable care. The government would ensure that other relevant legislations, including those of the Fire Services Ordinance (Cap. 95), Mental Health Ordinance (Cap. 136), and the Continuing Powers of Attorney Bill, being proposed but not legislated yet, would not conflict with the administration of

AD. A registered doctor or dentist or an appointed guardian cannot override a valid and applicable AD based on his/her own interpretation of best interests of the patient.

In terms of dying in place, amendments will be made to the Coroners Ordinance to exempt the reporting requirements to the Coroner if a RCHE resident who is diagnosed as having a terminal illness has been attended to by a registered medical practitioner within 14 days prior to his/her death, and that a registered medical practitioner has made a final diagnosis and determined the death as being due to natural causes.

The government intends to introduce the draft bill(s) in this Legislative Council term, which will also be supplemented with stepped-up efforts on public education on EOL care and life and death issues, as well as training and development of various stakeholders, including but not limited to healthcare, elderly care, and emergency rescue workforce. There is so far no public information on whether the legislative initiatives of advance directives and dying in place will take place together with those of continuing powers of attorney, since the two efforts are led respectively by HB and DoJ.

The Future of EOL Care in Hong Kong

In summary, the government commissioned study on EOL care conducted in 2017 had identified various barriers, issues, gaps of EOL care, and made recommendations accordingly. Hong Kong has since then seen several major relevant developments. These include the issuance of the Strategic Service Framework for Palliative Care in the public healthcare sector by HA in 2017, the completion of the public consultation of legislation on continuing powers of attorney in 2018, new and updated guidelines by HA on ACP and DNACPR in the public healthcare sector in 2019 and 2020, and the completion of the public consultation of legislation on advance directives and dying in place by the end of 2019 and the publication of report in 2020. While the strategic service framework and the guidelines in HA can address the gaps and issues at the institutional level, the legislations and law reform if implemented can address those at the legal level.

Although the above-mentioned will be major developments for EOL care in Hong Kong, there are still gaps and issues on other socio-ecological levels that need to be tackled as highlighted by our socio-ecological analysis above. Specifically, more resources and capacity, such as primary care doctors, healthcare professionals trained in palliative care, and training for informal caregivers, accessibility to medical resources, are needed in the community if indeed Hong Kong aspires to head towards the overall direction of dying in place. Likewise, bereavement and decedent care are also not the focus of the recent reform directions. Moreover, more efforts are needed on the intrapersonal- and interpersonal-level in order to address the socio-cultural gaps, issues, and barriers for better EOL care in Hong Kong. The fact that the government recognised the above as gaps and issues and emphasised on increased stepped-up efforts on the non-legal and operational sides of EOL care in their 2020 consultation report is encouraging news to the development of EOL care in Hong Kong. Nevertheless, it is important to acknowledge that there are interactions among these different socio-ecological levels, and any efforts to address these gaps and issues cannot be made in silos since they are interconnected. For example, it is difficult to imagine an increased level of EOL care support and resources at the community level if the concept of ageing and dying in place are not well understood or even disputed by the general public. This brings us back to the point on the absence of an overarching EOL care policy in Hong Kong at the moment, potentially making these efforts and solutions to the gaps and issues of EOL care less integrated, less complementary, and more piecemeal. Therefore, as recommended in the government commissioned study report, an EOL care policy that can be integrated as part of the larger ageing and long-term care policy would be conducive in driving forward changes and institutionalising service integration. These recommendations also align with the findings from another study in Hong Kong in 2019 (Yee et al., 2019).

In moving forward, it is also critical to benchmark the local efforts and solutions to international standards. A scoping review of the international literature was also conducted as part of the government commissioned study which identified important elements of care and implementation barriers and facilitators to inform health system improvements for care of older populations approaching the EOL (Threapleton et al., 2017). These essential components include on a macro-, contextual-level enabling policies and supportive environments; on a meso-, organisation-level, care pathways and models of care, prognostication and assessment of when EOL care discussions should start, ACP and AD, facilities and training for palliative care that shift away from medically oriented care, integrated and multi-disciplinary approach to EOL care, and increased resources to facilitate EOL care; and on a micro-, individual-level, effective communication, staff experience and training, emotional, and/or spiritual support as well as personalised, patient-centred care.

In conclusion, the government will not be able to tackle the numerous gaps, issues, and barriers of EOL care alone, and must co-opt and collaborate with various stakeholders in the community for a concerted and multi-disciplinary effort due to the multi-level and interconnected nature of the problems at hand. It is imperative to capitalise the current momentum to develop a EOL care system that is of international standard, ethical, fair, and sustainable in Hong Kong.

References

Census and Statistics Department. (2022a, August 11). *Mid-year population for 2022*. https://www.censtatd.gov.hk/en/press_release_detail.html?id=5078

Census and Statistics Department. (2022b). *Hong Kong monthly digest of statistics*. https://www.censtatd.gov.hk/en/data/stat_report/product/B1010002/att/B10100022022MM09B0100.pdf

Chung, R. Y., Dong, D., Chau, N. N. S., Chau, P. Y., Yeoh, E. K., & Wong, E. L. (2020). Examining the gaps and issues of end-of-life care among older population through the lens of socioecological model-a multi-method qualitative study of Hong Kong. *International Journal of Environmental Research and Public Health, 17*(14), Article 5072. https://doi.org/10.3390/ijerph17145072

Chung, R. Y., Lai, D. C. K., Hui, A. Y., Chau, P. Y., Wong, E. L., Yeoh, E. K., & Woo, J. (2021). Healthcare inequalities in emergency visits and hospitalisation at the end of life: A study of 395 019 public hospital records. *BMJ Supportive & Palliative Care*. https://doi.org/10.1136/bmjspcare-2020-002800

Chung, R. Y., Wong, E. L., Kiang, N., Chau, P. Y., Lau, J. Y. C., Wong, S. Y., Yeoh, E. K., & Woo, J. W. (2017). Knowledge, attitudes, and preferences of advance decisions, end-of-life care, and place of care and death in Hong Kong. A population-based telephone survey of 1067 adults. *Journal of the American Medical Directors Association, 18*(4), 367.e19–367.e27. https://doi.org/10.1016/j.jamda.2016.12.066

Fire Services Ordinance (Cap. 95) 2021 (HKSAR). https://www.elegislation.gov.hk/hk/cap95!en-zh-Hant-HK.pdf?FILENAME=Consolidated%20version%20for%20the%20Whole%20Chapter.pdf&DOC_TYPE=A&PUBLISHED=true

Food and Health Bureau. (2020). *End-of-life care: Moving forward. Legislative proposals on advance directives and dying in place—Consultation report*. https://www.healthbureau.gov.hk/download/press_and_publications/consultation/190900_eolcare/e_EOL_consultation_report.pdf

GovHK. (2022). *Overview of the health care system in Hong Kong*. https://www.gov.hk/en/residents/health/hosp/overview.htm

Hospital Authority. (2017). *Strategic service framework for palliative care*. https://www.ha.org.hk/haho/ho/ap/PCSSF_1.pdf

Hospital Authority. (2019). *HA guidelines on advance care planning*. https://www.ha.org.hk/haho/ho/psrm/EACPGuidelines.pdf

Labour and Welfare Bureau. (2021). *Administration's response to members' request for information on measures to enhance community and residential care services for the elderly*. https://www.legco.gov.hk/yr20-21/english/panels/ws/papers/ws20210111cb2-936-1-e.pdf

Lo, S. V. (2016). *Enhancing palliative and end of life care services in Hospital Authority*. http://foss.hku.hk/jcecc/wp-content/uploads/2016/01/Dr.-SV-Lo-Palliative-care_2016-January-8_final.pdf

Mcleroy, K. R., Bibeau, D., Steckler, A., & Glanz, K. (1988). An ecological perspective on health promotion programs. *Health Education Quarterly, 15*(4), 351–377. https://doi.org/10.1177/109019818801500401

Mental Health Ordinance (Cap. 136) 2022 (HKSAR). https://www.elegislation.gov.hk/hk/cap136!en-zh-Hant-HK.pdf?FILENAME=Consolidated%20version%20for%20the%20Whole%20Chapter.pdf&DOC_TYPE=A&PUBLISHED=true

Powers of Attorney Ordinance (Cap 31) 2018 (HKSAR). https://www.elegislation.gov.hk/hk/cap31!en-zh-Hant-HK.pdf?FILENAME=Consolidated%20version%20for%20the%20Whole%20Chapter.pdf&DOC_TYPE=A&PUBLISHED=true

Public Health England. (2018). *Statistical commentary: End of life care profiles, February 2018 update*. https://www.gov.uk/government/statistics/end-of-life-care-profiles-february-2018-update/statistical-commentary-end-of-life-care-profiles-february-2018-update

Research Fund Secretariat. (n.d.). *Detail of approved project (Reference no.: Elderly care - CUHK)*. https://rfs2.fhb.gov.hk/app/fundedsearch/projectdetail.xhtml?id=1866

Social Welfare Department. (2013). *Code of practice for residential care homes (Elderly persons)*. https://www.swd.gov.hk/doc/LRB/LORCHE/CodeofPractice_E_201303_201503R5.pdf

The Economist Intelligence Unit. (2015). *The 2015 quality of death index ranking palliative care across the world*. https://impact.economist.com/perspectives/sites/default/files/2015%20EIU%20Quality%20of%20Death%20Index%20Oct%2029%20FINAL.pdf

The Law Reform Commission of Hong Kong. (2006). *Substitute decision-making and advance directives in relation to medical treatment*. https://www.hkreform.gov.hk/en/docs/rdecision-e.pdf

The World Bank. (n.d.). *Life expectancy at birth, total (years)*. Japan, Hong Kong SAR, China. https://data.worldbank.org/indicator/SP.DYN.LE00.IN?locations=JP-HK

Threapleton, D. E., Chung, R. Y., Wong, S. Y. S., Wong, E. L. Y., Kiang, N., Chau, P. Y. K., Woo, J., Chung, V. C. H., & Yeoh, E. K. (2017). Care toward the end of life in older populations and its implementation facilitators and barriers: A scoping review. *Journal of the American Medical Directors Association, 18*(12), 1000-1009.e4. https://doi.org/10.1016/j.jamda.2017.04.010

Wong, E. L., Kiang, N., Chung, R. Y., Lau, J., Chau, P. Y., Wong, S. Y., Woo, J., Chan, E. Y., & Yeoh, E. K. (2020). Quality of palliative and end-of-life care in Hong Kong: Perspectives of healthcare providers. *International Journal of Environmental Research and Public Health, 17*(14), Article 5130. https://doi.org/10.3390/ijerph17145130

Wong, E. L., Lau, J. Y., Chau, P. Y., Chung, R. Y., Wong, S. Y., Woo, J., & Yeoh, E. K. (2022). Caregivers' experience of end-of-life stage elderly patients: Longitudinal qualitative interview. *International Journal of Environmental Research and Public Health, 19*(4), Article 2101. https://doi.org/10.3390/ijerph19042101

Woo, J., Lo, R. S., Lee, J., Cheng, J. O., Lum, C. M., Hui, E., Wong, F., Yeung, F., & Or, K. K. (2009). Improving end-of-life care for non-cancer patients in hospitals: Description of a continuous quality improvement initiative. *Journal of Nursing and Healthcare of Chronic Illness, 1*(3), 237–244. https://doi.org/10.1111/j.1752-9824.2009.01026.x

Yee, H., Ng, T., Lau, C., & Fong, B. (2019). Overview of palliative care service in Hong Kong. *CAHMR Working Paper, 1*(1). http://weblib.cpce-polyu.edu.hk/apps/wps/assets/pdf/cw20190101.pdf

Chapter 23
Promotion of Healthy Lifestyle for Healthy and Safe Cities—The Case of Hong Kong, China

Daphne M. Y. Wu

Abstract Referring to the Zagreb Declaration of World Health Organization, a healthy city should be inclusive, supportive, sensitive and responsive to fulfil the diverse needs and expectations of people of all social groups across the lifespan. A healthy city not only provides the basic necessities for life such as clean air, safe water, sanitation and waste treatment facilities, but also creates conditions and opportunities that encourage, enable, support citizens to adopt healthier lifestyles for sustainability of individuals' health and extension of longevity. People living in a healthy and safe city are free for consuming safe, nutritious and adequate foods to satisfy personal needs, cultural and religious diversities, enjoying social interaction, recreation facilities and easy mobility. This chapter recapitulates the associations among healthy lifestyle behaviours and health outcomes in different life stages. How a healthy and safe city extends its resources endeavouring to help people living there developing healthy lifestyles is discussed. Partnerships among public, private, voluntary and community sectors aiming towards the development of a sustainable healthy and safe city are overviewed. This chapter also enumerates governance for the promotion of healthy lifestyles and challenges came across in the reduction of non-communicable diseases. This chapter conducts a comprehensive overview of concerns and challenges related to building sustainable healthy and safe cities attributable to the implementation of healthy lifestyle.

Keywords Health outcomes · Healthy lifestyles programmes · Sustainability of health · Longevity

---

D. M. Y. Wu (✉)
The University of Hong Kong, Hong Kong, China
e-mail: wudaphne@hku.hk

B. Y. F. Fong and W. C. W. Wong (eds.), *Gaps and Actions in Health Improvement from Hong Kong and Beyond*,
https://doi.org/10.1007/978-981-99-4491-0_23

Healthy Cities

According to Regional Office for Europe (2009), healthy cities are places that engage the whole society and encourage citizens to participate in health decision-making for better health and well-being. The development of healthy cities is to reduce inequalities in health status and access to services, and promote good governance and leadership in the places through multi-sectoral approach. The outcomes are in the pursuit of peace and prosperity. Healthy cities integrate scientific evidence into addressing emerging public health challenges, and aligning with local and international strategies for health and sustainable development with the considerations of own priorities and concerns. The Zagreb Declaration involved five key principles and values to guide for constructing healthy cities (Table 23.1).

Status of Building Healthy City in Hong Kong

The Healthy Cities project was implemented in various administrative districts in the late 1990s in Hong Kong. Of which, Kwai Tsing and Sai Kung Districts, with populations of 489.8 thousand and 4.82.4 thousand in 2022, respectively (Census and Statistics Department, 2022), developed as the pioneering healthy cities. The Hong Kong Government issued "Guidelines for Implementing a Healthy Cities Project" in 2007 (Department of Health, 2007). All 18 administrative districts have now established Healthy Cities projects based on their own environmental, socioeconomic, geographical and public health concerns and issues (Department of Health, 2020a).

The United Nations General Assembly (2015) issued 17 Sustainable Development Goals (SDGs) aiming at ending poverty, reducing inequality and building more peaceful and prosperous societies by 2030. Principally, the SDGs are aligned

Table 23.1 Principles and values of healthy cities

Principles and values	Concepts
Equity	• The right to health for people of all social groups across lifespan
Participation and empowerment	• The right to participate in decision-making that affects health, health care and well-being • The provision of access to opportunities and skills development to empower citizens to become self-sufficient
Working in partnership	• The implementation of integrated approaches and sustainable improvement in health with effective multi-sectoral strategic partnerships
Solidarity and friendship	• The development of the spirit of peace, friendship and solidarity through networking, respect and appreciation of the social and cultural diversity
Sustainable development	• The economic and infrastructural developments are environmentally and socially sustainable for future generations

Source Regional Office for Europe (2009)

with Health Cities. A local non-government network accentuated to prioritise the following five SDGs in Hong Kong (Sustainable Development Solutions Network Hong Kong, n.d.):

Goal 1: End poverty in all its forms everywhere.
Goal 3: Ensure healthy lives and promote well-being for all at all ages.
Goal 4: Ensure inclusive and equitable quality education and promote lifelong learning opportunities for all.
Goal 12: Ensure sustainable consumption and production patterns.
Goal 13: Take urgent action to combat climate change and its impacts.

Healthy Cities strive for continuous improvement and do not end at the accomplishment of health status or outcome. It has been 16 years since the last set of guidelines of developing healthy city was published and the guidelines have not incorporated the element of sustainable development in Hong Kong (Department of Health, 2007, 2020a).

Safe Cities

Development of safe cities also incorporate the sustainability principles of building a more peaceful and prosperous societies. The Economist Intelligent Unit (2021) has issued a safe cities index (SCI) since 2015. The index comprises five pillars: personal, infrastructure, health, digital and environmental security. Hong Kong was ranked eighth with score of 78.6 in 2021 (The Economist Intelligent Unit, 2021).

Undoubtedly digital security is increasing in its importance in recent years. Hong Kong ranked 21st in digital security and ranked 21st in personal security (The Economist Intelligent Unit, 2021). Personal security is mainly considered the risk of citizens vulnerable to crime. One of the indicators in personal security is "Use of data-driven techniques for crime". Cybersecurity threat and crime apparently align with digital security in the current rapid development of digitalisation. In addition, the rapid development of information technology may also jeopardise population health attributable to long sedentary time for online gaming and electronic screen usage.

Healthy and Safe Cities

Hong Kong ranked third in the pillar of health security (The Economist Intelligent Unit, 2021). Healthy and safe issues should be mutually connected as a whole. The output indicators included life expectancy, pandemic performance and preparedness; and issues of mental health (The Economist Intelligent Unit, 2021). The COVID-19 pandemic thrived the medical system on the brink of collapse during the catastrophic outbreak at the fifth wave in Hong Kong in 2022. The healthy security index is also

Table 23.2 Progress of interventions for the prevention of non-communicable diseases and injuries in Hong Kong

Interventions implemented	Interventions yet to be implemented
1. Create a smoke-free city 2. Ban tobacco advertising 3. Reduce speeding 4. Reduce drink driving 5. Increase seat-belt use 6. Prevent opioid-associated overdose deaths 7. Increase motorcycle helmet use 8. Enhance public health data and monitoring systems	1. Tax sugary drinks 2. Set nutrition standards for foods served and sold in public institutions 3. Raise tobacco taxes or levies/fees 4. Regulate food and drink marketing 5. Create healthier restaurant environments 6. Promote active mobility

Source The Partnership for Healthy Cities (n.d.)

considered with relevance to infrastructure in the city (The Economist Intelligent Unit, 2021). Other indicators such as sustainability masterplan, waste management, sustainable energy, waste generation which can be considered as sustainability are taken into account. Hong Kong ranked 27th in the environmental security which was the lowest among all five pillars (The Economist Intelligent Unit, 2021). There is a necessity of uplift the environmental security.

Hong Kong joined the Partnership for Healthy Cities in 2019 (The Government of the Hong Kong Special Administrative Region, 2019a). The partnership network focuses on reduction of factors to fight against non-communicable diseases (NCDs) (The Partnership for Healthy Cities, n.d.). Hong Kong has implemented more than half of the interventions (Table 23.2). All six interventions yet to be implemented may dispose people towards unhealthy lifestyles.

The World Health Organization (2015a) recognised the works of healthy city from Sai Kung and Kwai Tsing Districts. Nevertheless, the World Health Organization (WHO) commented on the challenges of the development of healthy city in Hong Kong due to her high living costs in housing, overcrowding, traffic congestion, air pollution and widening inequities (World Health Organization, 2015a).

Promotion of Healthy Lifestyles for Healthy and Safe Cities

Adoption of healthy lifestyle is crucial for extension of life longevity and facilitates healthy and safe cities development. Hong Kong Government launched "Towards 2025: Strategy and Action Plan to Prevent and Control Non-communicable Diseases in Hong Kong" in 2018 aiming to tackle risk factors of NCDs—unhealthy diet, physical inactivity, tobacco use, harmful use of alcohol (Department of Health, 2018). Hong Kong is also facing a problem of changing in health risk profile with a rapidly ageing population like other developed regions. Childhood and adolescence are critical periods to determine lifelong health. A vicious cycle may be refrained from educating the youth on the concepts of healthy lifestyles. The financial burdens of

NCDs on healthcare systems, productivity, economies and societies are enormous and substantial. Indeed, preventive measures to NCDs can yield substantial financial and health benefits to societies and countries (World Health Organization, 2009, 2018a).

Health Status of Hong Kong Residents

The average life expectancy in Hong Kong is 85.08 years (The World Bank, 2019). Several deranged psycho- and physio-logical conditions are risks for NCDs and premature mortality.

Body Weight

Overweight and obese in childhood and adolescence are likely to remain obese into adulthood. In school year 2018–2019, the detection rates of overweight and obesity of primary and secondary school students were 17.4% and 19.9%, respectively (Centre for Health Protection, 2021a). Despite an overall reduction of the detection rate among primary school students in the school year 2018–2019 (21.4%) as compared with the relevant figures in the school year 2020–2011 (26%), there was an upward trend (19.9%, 2018–2019 vs 18.7%, 2010–2011) among secondary school students. Consistently, the detection rates were higher in boys than in girls during the period (Centre for Health Protection, 2021a). The detection rates of overweight and obesity in school year 2019–2020 were estimated to be higher than in the last survey, which were 23.1% of primary and 21.3% of secondary school students (Centre for Health Protection, 2021a). The Population Health Survey of 2014–2015 (PHS 2014–2015) found that 50.0% of people aged between 15 and 84 were overweight and obese. Of which, higher proportion of males were overweight and obesity (56.9%) than females (43.7%) (Centre for Health Protection, 2017).

Hypertensive Blood Pressure

A study found that 8.2% of boys and 2.2% of girls aged 9–18 years had hypertension in 2014; and 18.2% of boys and 7.7% of girls in the same age group had pre-hypertension (Centre for Health Protection, 2018). The PHS 2014–2015 found that the overall prevalence of hypertension among persons aged 15–84 was 27.7% (Centre for Health Protection, 2017). Nearly half (47.7%), i.e. 13.2% out of 27.7%, had no known history of hypertension. In addition, higher proportion of male (30.1%) were hypertensive than females (25.5%) (Centre for Health Protection, 2017).

Diabetes Mellitus

The PHS 2014–2015 found that the overall prevalence of diabetes among persons aged 15–84 years was 8.4% (Centre for Health Protection, 2017). Over half (53.6%), i.e. 4.5% out of 8.4%, had no known history of diabetes. Similarly, higher proportion of male (10.5%) were diabetic than females (6.4%) (Centre for Health Protection, 2017). Besides, more than 20% of elderly aged 65 years and above are with diabetes. Around 2% of persons under 35 years of age had diagnosed with diabetes. Children and adolescents with diabetes have a five-fold higher risk of death than non-patients of the same age (Hospital Authority, 2022).

Dyslipidaemia

Nearly half (49.5%) of persons aged 15–84 years had hypercholesterolemia (Centre for Health Protection, 2017). Severely, 70.3%, i.e. 34.8% out of 49.5%, had no known history of hypercholesterolaemia. The prevalence of hypercholesterolaemia between males (50.3%) and females (48.8%) was similar (Centre for Health Protection, 2017).

Mental Health

Anxiety disorders (6.9%), oppositional defiant disorder (6.8%), Attention Deficit/ Hyperactivity Disorder (AD/HD) (3.9%), conduct disorder (1.7%), depressive disorders (1.3%) and substance use disorders (1.1%) are the common mental health problems in Hong Kong (Leung et al., 2008). The percentage of mental disorders among Chinese adults aged between 16 and 75 was 13.3% (Food and Health Bureau, 2017). Another survey in 2014 reported that 4.8% of persons aged between 18 and 64 years could be classified as having severe psychological distress (Food and Health Bureau, 2017).

Oral Health

Among 52,300 children aged five years in the Oral Health Survey 2011, around half (50.7%) had tooth decay experience with 92.0% of the affected teeth untreated (Department of Health, 2011). Only 0.4% of 56,000 children aged 12 years had tooth decay experience with 5.4% of the affected tooth untreated. Almost all adults (96.1%) and free-living elderly (99.3%) had various degrees of tooth decay and gum disease. About one-half of free-living elderly had the affected tooth untreated. The oral health status of elderly receiving long-term care services was worse than that of free-living populations (Department of Health, 2011).

Progress of Promotion of Healthy Lifestyle

Hong Kong Government issued two strategic documents in 2008 and 2018 calling for the whole community to promote healthy lifestyles for the prevention and reduction of risk factors of NCDs (Department of Health, 2008, 2018). Five key improvement of population health, through the promotion of healthy start, alcohol free, live well and be active, tobacco free and healthy diet were emphasised (Department of Health, 2018). The documents advocated the importance of taking proactive and multi-sectoral approach to prevent and control NCD risks for better families, healthcare systems, society and economy.

Healthy Eating

Taking low salt or low sodium, adequate amounts of fruit and vegetables, less fat and sugar are considered as healthy eating habits. The PHS 2014–2015 found that the daily mean population intake of salt was 8.8 g in Hong Kong. The proportion of population with daily salt intake higher than the WHO recommended intake, i.e. greater than 5 g per day, was higher among males (90.8%) than females (82.2%). Higher salt intake was found in males (9.8 g) than in females (7.9 g) (Centre for Health Protection, 2017).

Since the school year 2006–2007, "EatSmart@school.hk" Campaign (ESS Campaign) has been launched aiming to tackle the uptrend in childhood obesity and lower risk of diseases associated with eating habits at youth (EatSmart@school.hk, 2020). The "EatSmart School Accreditation Scheme" was launched in the school year 2009–2010, under the ESS Campaign, in order to facilitate schools to set up and implement policy of healthy eating at primary schools, develop a learning environment for healthy eating and cultivate healthy eating habits among school children (EatSmart@school.hk, 2020). Furthermore, the "Salt Reduction Scheme for School Lunches" was launched in the school year 2017–2018 aiming to reduce the sodium level of school lunches. The Department of Health assisted the participating lunch suppliers in assessing the sodium level and amount of sodium reduction in recipes of school lunches. Corresponding guidelines on recipes setting for use in primary and schools were prepared with regular revision (Department of Health, 2022a). Besides, Hong Kong Government set up the Committee on Reduction of Salt and Sugar in Food (CRSS) in 2015 (The Government of the Hong Kong Special Administrative Region, 2015) aiming to achieve WHO recommendation of 30% relative reduction of daily intake of sodium in the mean population by 2025 (World Health Organization, 2020). The CRSS also advocates to reduce sugar intake in foods so as to reduce the risk to obesity and dental caries (The Government of the Hong Kong Special Administrative Region, 2015). Over 500 local food premises joined the CRSS event to offer customers with options of reduced salt and/or sugar in food in 2019 (The Government of the Hong Kong Special Administrative Region, 2019b). Moreover, the "EatSmart Restaurant Star+" Campaign was launched in 2019, with an mobile application to provide information of all EatSmart restaurants in Hong Kong to facilitate consumers perform healthy eating practice (The Government of the Hong Kong Special Administrative Region, 2019c).

Taking less than 3.5 g of potassium per day is also associated with hypertension. Most fruits and vegetables are good sources of potassium. Insufficient consumption of fruits and vegetables is one of leading risk factors of developing obesity and NCDs, such as cardiovascular diseases and certain types of cancers (World Health Organization, 2003). The recent Health Behaviour Survey 2018–2019 reported that 95.6% of persons aged 15 or above consuming inadequate fruits and vegetables (Centre for Health Protection, 2020) with higher proportion of males (97.2%) took inadequate amounts of fruit and vegetables than females (94.1%).

A local online survey found the prevalence of overweight and obesity among children aged 9–13 years tripled, from 7 to 24%, during the pandemic based on the online response by 1,439 parents of kindergarten or primary school students (Faculty of Medicine, 2022). The increase in the prevalence was attributed to children's unhealthy lifestyles, including more sedentary time and unhealthy eating habits such as spending more time on TV or electronic devices while eating (70%); eating more when feeling bored (62%); and eating more snacks that interfered with their appetite for regular meals (59%) (Faculty of Medicine, 2022). More efforts on educating the general public on healthier eating habits post-pandemic are required.

Sufficient Physical Activity

Sedentary time more than 4 h a day is a risk factor for chronic disease, with hazards to health become more apparent over time. The WHO (2018a, 2018b) provides recommendations on the levels of physical activity for people of different age groups and specific needs for staying healthy. In 2011–2012, only 17.7% of the infants spent an hour or more on outdoor activities a day; 51.8% of children, 42.3% of adolescents and 37.1% of adults and the elderly were classified as physically active (Leisure and Cultural Services Department, 2012).

The Government launched the "Healthy Exercise for All" campaign in early 2000s to increase the public interest in exercise and encourage working class to exercise in office (Leisure and Cultural Services Department, 2012). Since 2009, the Sports Ambassador Scheme uses the celebrity effects to arrange athletes to promote sports to the community, schools and corporations and increase public awareness of physical activity (Hong Kong Athletes Career & Education Programme, 2017). During the COVID-19 pandemic, students had to study at home leading to massive reduction of regular walking between home and school, and the amount of school activities

(Faculty of Medicine, 2022). The "School Physical Fitness Award Scheme" promotes physical activities and health-related fitness among primary and secondary students and cultivate the students to maintain moderate physical activity at home (Education Bureau, 2021a). Nevertheless, children's body weights increased due to unhealthy eating habits and more sedentary time on using electronic devices and sleeping (Faculty of Medicine, 2022). Furthermore, 16.8% of Hong Kong adults did not meet the recommended level of physical activity with higher failure percentage of women (18.3%) than men (15.2%) (Centre for Health Protection, 2021b). Comparatively, the Government did not provide the corresponding campaign to encourage adults to keep physically active at home.

Avoidance of Smoking

Smoking of any kinds is a cause to common NCDs; increases the risks of gum disease and oral cancers (Department of Health, 2011); and kills about 8 million people worldwide each year (World Health Organization, 2022a). Electronic cigarettes (e-cigarettes) and heated tobacco products (HTPs) are emerging alternative smoking products (ASPs) in recent years. The ASPs not only result in exposure to second-hand smoke but also lack of evidence to help smokers quit smoking (Hong Kong Council on Smoking and Health, 2022).

The Government amended the law to enlarge pictorial health warnings to occupy 85%, from at least 50%, of the two largest surfaces of cigarette packet (Constitutional and Mainland Affairs Bureau, 2020; Tobacco and Alcohol Control Office, 2022). The smoking prevalence has reduced gradually over decades of anti-tobacco efforts by the Government, from 23.3% in 1982 to 10% in 2017 (Constitutional and Mainland Affairs Bureau, 2020); however, more than half of young respondents used aforementioned emerging ASPs first time due to curiosity (The University of Hong Kong, 2021). The 2018 Policy Address proposed the prohibition of import, promotion, manufacture, sale, or possession for commercial purposes of ASPs (The Government of the Hong Kong Special Administrative Region, 2018a). The law has been effective since April 2022 (Tobacco and Alcohol Control Office, 2022). The "Towards 2025: Strategy and Action Plan for the Prevention and Control of Non-communicable Diseases in Hong Kong" targets to reduce the number of daily smokers to 7.8% by 2025 (Department of Health, 2018), whereas the control of ASPs has yet to set any goal of reduction.

Avoidance of Harmful Use of Drinking

Drinking alcohol is associated with a risk of developing more than 200 diseases (World Health Organization, 2022b). Alcohol consumption also creates mental and behavioural disorders which jeopardise the safety of the city. Being classified as a carcinogen, alcohol increases the risk factors for cancers (World Health Organization, 2022b). Children and adolescents taking alcohol are more likely to develop a higher frequency of drinking and binge drinking at adulthood (The Government of the Hong Kong Special Administrative Region, 2016).

The Government has been regularly monitoring the volume and pattern of alcohol use and figure of hospitalisation due to alcohol use. In 2014–2015, the prevalence of primary 4 to 6 students and secondary school students reported drinking alcohol was 26.0% and 56.8%, respectively (Centre for Health Protection, 2019). In 2015, 43.1% of 2,500 local respondents aged 18 to 64 years reported to have the first taste of alcohol under 18 years old (The Government of the Hong Kong Special Administrative Region, 2016). In 2018–2019, 8.8% of persons aged 15 years or above drinking alcohol on a regular basis with a higher proportion in men (15.0%) than women (3.2%) (Centre for Health Protection, 2019). The estimated total alcohol consumption per capita increased from 2.57 L in 2004 to 2.87 L in 2017 (Centre for Health Protection, 2019). The PHS 2014–2015 found that the prevalence of drinking increased significantly from 33.3% to 61.4% from 2003–2004 to 2014–2015 (Centre for Health Protection, 2019). In 2017, alcohol-related mental and behavioural disorders covered three-quarter (75.2%) of 2,525 hospital admissions in public and private hospitals (Constitutional and Mainland Affairs Bureau, 2020).

The existing preventive measures to reduce harmful use of alcohol to the public include printed health information materials, 24-h education hotline, website as well as electronic publications (Constitutional and Mainland Affairs Bureau, 2020). The "Young and Alcohol Free" campaign fights against underage drinking with multi-sectoral stakeholders including youth and parent groups, schools, healthcare professionals and relevant government units in late 2016 (The Government of the Hong Kong Special Administrative Region, 2016). In late 2017, the "Alcohol Fails" campaign developed with academic and healthcare professionals for public education (Department of Health, 2022b). With effect from 30 November 2018, the sale or supply of liquor to underage in the course of business has been prohibited (The Government of the Hong Kong Special Administrative Region, 2018b).

Mental Health and Sleeping Pattern

Lifestyle behaviours have influences on sleep quality which subsequently is closely correlated with physical and mental health. Insufficient sleep was the main reason cited by children (62.9%) accounting for poor physical health (Leisure and Cultural Services Department, 2012). Playing online games create stimulations to brain and is one of the reasons for insufficient sleep (Leisure and Cultural Services Department, 2012). Nearly two-thirds of children and adolescents aged 10–19 years used electronic devices for more than 2 h a day, significantly longer than the rest of the world (Department of Sports Science and Physical Education, 2018). Only nearly one-third of primary school students met the recommendation of not less than 9 h of sleep per day (Department of Sports Science and Physical Education, 2018).

Besides, sleep deprivation can also increase the risk of being overweight or obese (Lee, 2021). During the pandemic, 40% of children slept more (Faculty of Medicine, 2022). Sleeping more does not guarantee sleeping quality attributed to blue ray stimulation from electronic devices. In the digital era, 90% of children spent more time using electronic devices (Faculty of Medicine, 2022).

Healthy lifestyle and mental health are positively related each other. The conditions of mental health and NCDs are interrelated with each other as they share many mutual risk factors (Stein et al., 2019). A local survey found that 20% of parents of kindergarten and primary school children felt more stressful to handle the situations of child school life, such as child unable to get face-to-face classes, negative emotions by child when reopening of school, or child reluctance to school. There existed a drastic decrease of 35% in child happiness index when parents had high stress levels (Faculty of Medicine, 2022). Another NGO found that nearly three quarters of parents (73.8%) stated having conflicts with children due to children not paying attention to online classes, and more than one-third of them (36.2%) believed the deterioration of the relationship with children during the pandemic (The Hong Kong Lutheran Social Service Office, 2022). The worsening of parent–child relationship attributed to children's academic problems (51.8%); parents' ability of emotional control (44.5%); and work or life stress (40.5%). An insurance company in 2020 found that nearly 20% of 1,000 working persons aged 18–60 years in Hong Kong might attempt to use alcohol or smoking for stress relieve (AXA Hong Kong, 2021). Furthermore, nearly half (47%) of them and one-quarter suffered from high level of pressure in the past six months and several mental health issues, respectively (AXA Hong Kong, 2021).

The Food and Health Bureau (2017) stated that mental health problems among adolescents were associated with authoritarian parenting, low parental warmth and high maternal over-control. Promotion of mental health and prevention mental disorders at early life stage are a crucial moment since up to half of mental disorders in adults developed in early adolescence prior to the age of 14 years. The website "Mental Health@School" has provided information on student mental health since August 2021 (Education Bureau, 2021b). The "Peer Power – Student Gatekeeper Training Programme" has been launched since the school year 2019–2020 (Education Bureau, 2022).

The demand for public psychiatric services has been rising, with the number of patients with mental illness increased from 187,000 in 2011–2012 to over 220,000 in 2015–2016 (Food and Health Bureau, 2017). The Government reaffirmed the importance of strengthening community support for those recovering from mental illness, enhancing capacity of healthcare professionals at the primary care level and developing public–private partnership to provide timely effective services for better mental health (Food and Health Bureau, 2017).

Oral Health

Oral health is also an integral component of health. The oral health must start with prevention and early treatment of dental diseases (Department of Health, 2011). The only accomplishment of the protection of oral health is to visit dentist for regular check up (Department of Health, 2011). A dental care programme is provided for primary school students via provision of oral examination, dental treatment and education of oral healthcare habits, etc. (Department of Health, 2020b). Unfortunately, such dental care programme has yet to extend to secondary school students after request over a decade ago (The Government of the Hong Kong Special Administrative Region, 2007). The "TEENS Teeth Award Scheme" for the secondary school students is developed for oral health promotion (Department of Health, 2022c). The quantity of public oral health services is far from the needs (The Government of the Hong Kong Special Administrative Region, 2022). Currently, the oral health service is dominant in private setting and NGOs in Hong Kong (The Government of the Hong Kong Special Administrative Region, 2022). The most common barrier to access the dental treatments is the financial burden (Yang et al., 2021). Affordable dental services are very limited to adults, unless adults with intellectual disability who are entitled to receive free dental services via "Heathy Teeth Collaboration" (The Government of the Hong Kong Special Administrative Region, 2021b). The Elderly Health Care Vouchers are enough from afar for elderly due to commonly coexistence of various suboptimal health conditions and expensive private dental treatments (The Prince Philip Dental Hospital, n.d.).

Enhancement of Healthy Lifestyle Promotion

One of the Government strategies to promote healthy lifestyle in the community is the strengthening of the prevention-centred primary healthcare system, through the setup of District Health Centres (DHCs) (Legislative Council Panel on Health Services, 2020). Although the development blueprint of public healthcare system shifted from treatment-oriented to prevention-focused, secondary and tertiary prevention services remain available in DHCs.

The first DHC piloted in Kwai Tsing District in 2019 (The Government of the Hong Kong Special Administrative Region, 2019d). Up to June 2022, there were seven DHCs opened (District Health Centre, 2022). The DHC operators cannot impose the charges on DHC clients over the prescribed ceilings set out in the respective tender document since subsidies are received from the Government (The Government of the Hong Kong Special Administrative Region, 2021a). Over HKD 1.9 billion has been spent on the development of DHCs by the Government (*Oriental Daily*, 2022). Generally, DHCs have a total floor area of about 1,000 square metres each. However, the occupancy or usage rates are unsatisfactorily low (*Oriental Daily*, 2022). Since the positioning and resources of the DHCs appear to be overlapped with other community service and health centres, the operation mode of DHCs is being questioned (*Oriental Daily*, 2022). Within limited financial resources, there necessitates to formulate long-term and comprehensive planning in positioning DHCs for promotion and education of healthy lifestyle.

Public–private partnership should integrate with academia so as to implement more effective strategies with evidence supports. For instance, more investigation may be required to identify the correlation between potassium intake and fruit and vegetable intakes so as to formulate strategy on promoting dietary potassium as well as fruit and vegetable intakes. The fitness conditions of population are expected to go downtrend due to the COVID-19 pandemic. It is necessary to strengthen the monitoring of physical fitness and enhance the promotion of exercise coupled with optimisation of policy initiatives on promotion education to populations.

Raising every 10% of prices by tobacco duty would reduce tobacco use by 4% (World Health Organization, 2013). In addition, plain packaging of tobacco products is proven to decrease smoking initiation and increase cessation (World Health Organization, 2019). Certain anti-smoking measures are yet to fully be consistent with WHO's Framework Convention on Tobacco Control. Besides the advocacy movement on avoidance of conventional smoking, the anti-smoking activities should further extend to counteract the access of ASPs by populations. Full implementation of alcohol taxation should be taken into account (Sornpaisarn et al., 2017). Regrettably, the Government waived alcohol taxes on wine and beer since February 2008 (Customs and Excise Department, 2016). The Government should garner a blend of ideas from multi-sectoral parties to launch innovative policy initiatives on anti-smoking and anti-alcohol measures to the internet world targeting those spending lots of times on electronic screens.

Prevention, treatment and care of mental health conditions should be integrated with other NCDs. Currently, mental health services are yet to be available in DHCs (District Health Centre, 2022). Public–private partnership can be further strengthened to provide primary promotion. The Government should prioritise and reconstruct the strategies of health promotion to integrate the mental healthcare and oral health services so as to optimise the overall healthcare service without overlapping service available in the DHCs with other NGOs and healthcare institutions. The coverage of dental treatment should extend to kindergarten pupils and secondary school students (Department of Health, 2011). Development of policy for appropriate and affordable dental services and mental health promotion for public is a matter of urgency.

Since the pandemic, the lifestyle changes of Hong Kong residents may have changed and created chronic downsides on overall health. There is an urge to assess comprehensively the lifestyles, physical fitness, mental health and oral health of Hong Kong residents. The gaps between research findings and knowledge transfer to public needs further narrowing.

Conclusion

Healthy lifestyle improves people's livelihood and is conducive to health and wellness. The Hong Kong Government takes into account of her own socioeconomic, cultural, political and administrative circumstances for healthy and safe city development with unique characteristics and sustainability. The development of NCDs, suboptimal mental health and oral health status are multi-factorial that deserve more attention and target-oriented strategies. Adoption of healthy lifestyles should not only be achieved by individuals, but also rely on sustainable efforts from distinct stakeholders to make the city healthy and safe. The whole-of-government approaches and public–private partnership incorporated with academia should be well consolidated to make strategies effective and outcomes measurable and achievable.

References

AXA Hong Kong. (2021). *AXA Wellness Index 2020*. https://www.axa.com.hk/en/article/axa-wellness-index-2020

Census and Statistics Department. (2022, April 21). *Table 1.1: Land-based non-institutional population by district council district*. https://www.censtatd.gov.hk/en/wbr.html?ecode=B11303012022AN22&scode=150

Centre for Health Protection. (2017). *Report of population health survey 2014/2015*. Department of Health. https://www.chp.gov.hk/files/pdf/dh_phs_2014_15_full_report_eng.pdf

Centre for Health Protection. (2018). *Hypertension: A burning health problem*. Department of Health. https://www.chp.gov.hk/files/pdf/ncd_watch_july_2018.pdf

Centre for Health Protection. (2019). *The toxic truth about alcohol*. Department of Health. https://www.chp.gov.hk/files/pdf/ncd_watch_february_2019.pdf

Centre for Health Protection. (2020). *Report of health behaviour survey 2018/19*. Department of Health. https://www.chp.gov.hk/files/pdf/report_of_health_behaviour_survey_2018_en.pdf

Centre for Health Protection. (2021a). *Overweight and obesity*. https://www.chp.gov.hk/en/statistics/data/10/757/5513.html

Centre for Health Protection. (2021b). *Physical activity and cancer prevention*. Department of Health. https://www.chp.gov.hk/files/pdf/ncd_watch_january_2021.pdf

Constitutional and Mainland Affairs Bureau. (2020). *Fourth report of the Hong Kong Special Administrative Region of the People's Republic of China under the international covenant on economic, social and cultural rights*. https://www.cmab.gov.hk/doc/en/documents/references/papers_reports_others/human_rights/FourthReport_PRC/FullReport-e.pdf

Customs and Excise Department. (2016, February 24). *Types and duty rates*. https://www.customs.gov.hk/en/trade_facilitation/dutiable/types/index.html

Department of Health. (2007). *Building healthy cities—Guidelines for implementing a Healthy Cities Project in Hong Kong*. https://www.chp.gov.hk/files/pdf/building_healthy_cities_guidelines.pdf

Department of Health. (2008). *Promoting health in Hong Kong: A strategic framework for prevention and control of non-communicable diseases*. https://www.change4health.gov.hk/filemanager/common/image/strategic_framework/promoting_health/promoting_health_e.pdf

Department of Health. (2011). *Oral health survey 2011*. https://www.toothclub.gov.hk/en/en_pdf/Oral_Health_Survey_2011/Oral_Health_Survey_2011_WCAG_20141112_(EN_Full).pdf.

Department of Health. (2018). *Towards 2025: Strategy and action plan to prevent and control non-communicable diseases in Hong Kong*. https://www.chp.gov.hk/files/pdf/saptowards2025_fullreport_en.pdf

Department of Health. (2020a). *An overview of healthy cities projects*. https://www.districtcouncils.gov.hk/sk/doc/2020_2023/tc/committee_meetings_doc/EHSWC/18163/EHSWC_2020_P503_EN.pdf

Department of Health. (2020b). *School dental care service*. https://www.schooldental.gov.hk/wsmile/en/aboutus_intro_pamphlet

Department of Health. (2022a). *Nutritional guidelines for children in Hong Kong*. https://www.change4health.gov.hk/en/healthy_diet/guidelines/nutritional/index.html. Last revision date: 29 July 2022.

Department of Health. (2022b). *Alcohol fails*. https://www.change4health.gov.hk/en/alcoholfails/index.html. Last revision date: 29 July 2022.

Department of Health. (2022c). *Target specific oral health promotion programmes*. https://www.toothclub.gov.hk/en/en_home_01_06.html. Last revision date: 25 August 2022.

Department of Sports Science and Physical Education. (2018). *2018 active healthy kids: Hong Kong report card on physical activity for children and youth*. The Chinese University of Hong Kong. https://www.activehealthykids.org/wp-content/uploads/2018/11/hong-kong-report-card-long-form-2018.pdf

District Health Centre. (2022). *Scope of service*. Health Bureau. https://www.dhc.gov.hk/en/healthcare_service_providers.html#scope-of-service

EatSmart@school.hk. (2020). *Background*. https://school.eatsmart.gov.hk/en/content.aspx

Education Bureau (EDB). (2021a). *Physical education—School physical fitness award scheme*. https://www.edb.gov.hk/en/curriculum-development/kla/pe/references_resource/spfas/

Education Bureau (EDB). (2021b). *Prevention of student suicides and promotion of student mental health*. https://www.edb.gov.hk/en/teacher/prevention-of-student-suicides/index.html

Education Bureau (EDB). (2022). *Peer power—Student gatekeeper training programme*. https://mentalhealth.edb.gov.hk/en/support-programmes/peer-power-student-gatekeeper-training-programme.html

Faculty of Medicine. (2022, June 23). *COVID-19 pandemic disrupted the daily lives of schoolchildren in Hong Kong; Proportion of overweight and obese kids more than doubled* (Press release). The Chinese University of Hong Kong. https://www.med.cuhk.edu.hk/press-releases/covid-pandemic-disrupted-the-daily-life-of-schoolchildren-in-hong-kong-the-proportion-of-overweight-and-obese-kids-more-than-doubled

Food and Health Bureau. (2017). *Mental health review report*. https://www.healthbureau.gov.hk/download/press_and_publications/otherinfo/180500_mhr/e_mhr_full_report.pdf

Hong Kong Athletes Career & Education Programme. (2017). *Ambassador recruitment*. http://www.hkacep.org/en/news-centre-detail.php?news_id=27

Hong Kong Council on Smoking and Health. (2022). *"Smoking Hazards 2.0" Health education and publicity programme*. https://www.smokefree.hk/page.php?id=16&lang=en

Hospital Authority. (2022). *Diabetes mellitus*. https://www21.ha.org.hk/smartpatient/SPW/en-us/Disease-Information/Disease/?guid=c73a0386-fe66-42eb-a979-7619ac8359da

Lee, J. (2021, July 8). *Lack of sleep can cause weight gain*? (in Chinese). https://sleep.hku.hk/blog-17-deprived-weight-gain/

Leisure and Cultural Services Department. (2012). *Healthy exercise for all campaign—Physical fitness test for the community*. https://www.lcsd.gov.hk/en/healthy/physical_fitness_test/common/physical_fitness_test/download/SummaryReport_en.pdf

Leung, P. W., Hung, S. F., Ho, T. P., Lee, C. C., Liu, W. S., Tang, C. P., & Kwong, S. L. (2008). Prevalence of DSM-IV disorders in Chinese adolescents and the effects of an impairment criterion: A pilot community study in Hong Kong. *European Child & Adolescent Psychiatry, 17*(7), 452–461. https://doi.org/10.1007/s00787-008-0687-7

Legislative Council Panel on Health Services. (2020). *Development of primary healthcare and "DHC express"*. https://www.legco.gov.hk/yr19-20/english/panels/hs/papers/hs20200110cb2-468-10-e.pdf

Oriental Daily. (2022, July 24). 1.9 billion public funds were wasted by the inaction of the health centre (in Chinese). https://orientaldaily.on.cc/content/%E8%A6%81%E8%81%9E%E6%B8%AF%E8%81%9E/odn-20220724-0724_00174_001/%E5%BA%B7%E5%81%A5%E4%B8%AD%E5%BF%83%E7%84%A1%E4%BD%9C%E7%82%BA--19%E5%84%84%E5%85%AC%E5%B8%91%E6%9E%89%E8%B2%BB

Regional Office for Europe. (2009). *Zagreb declaration for healthy cities: Health and health equity in all local policies*. World Health Organization. https://www.euro.who.int/__data/assets/pdf_file/0015/101076/E92343.pdf

Sornpaisarn, B., Shield, K. D., Österberg, E. & Rehm, J. (2017). *Resource tool on alcohol taxation and pricing policies*. World Health Organization. https://apps.who.int/iris/handle/10665/255795

Stein, D. J., Benjet, C., Gureje, O., Lund, C., Scott, K. M., Poznyak, V., & van Ommeren, M. (2019). Integrating mental health with other non-communicable diseases. *BMJ, 364*, Article l295. https://doi.org/10.1136/bmj.l295

Sustainable Development Solutions Network Hong Kong. (n.d.). *Priorities for SDSN Hong Kong*. https://sdsn-hk.org/en/initiatives/un-sustainable-development-goals-prioritized-sdgs-in-hong-kong

The Economist Intelligent Unit (2021). *Safe cities index 2021*. https://safecities.economist.com/

The Government of the Hong Kong Special Administrative Region. (2007, May 23). *LCQ14: School dental care service* (Press release). https://www.info.gov.hk/gia/general/200705/23/P200705230181.htm

The Government of the Hong Kong Special Administrative Region. (2015, March 13). *Government sets up committee to promote reduction of salt and sugar in food* (Press release). https://www.info.gov.hk/gia/general/201503/13/P201503130749.htm

The Government of the Hong Kong Special Administrative Region. (2016, December 15). *DH launches "Young and Alcohol Free" campaign against underage drinking (with photos)* (Press release). https://www.info.gov.hk/gia/general/201612/15/P2016121500249.htm

The Government of the Hong Kong Special Administrative Region. (2018a, October 10). *Policy address: VI. Improving people's livelihood*. https://www.policyaddress.gov.hk/2018/eng/policy_ch06.html

The Government of the Hong Kong Special Administrative Region. (2018b, November 14). *New legislation to prohibit sale and supply of alcohol to minors in the course of business to commence on November 30 (with photos)* (Press release). https://www.info.gov.hk/gia/general/201811/14/P2018111400281.htm

The Government of the Hong Kong Special Administrative Region. (2019a, December 13). *Hong Kong joins global partnership for healthy cities* (Press release). https://www.info.gov.hk/gia/general/201912/13/P2019121300302.htm

The Government of the Hong Kong Special Administrative Region. (2019b, February 23). *Government promotes reduced salt and sugar diet (with photos)* (Press release). https://www.info.gov.hk/gia/general/201902/23/P2019022200291.htm

The Government of the Hong Kong Special Administrative Region. (2019c, May 2). *Over 1 000 restaurants of EatSmart Restaurant Star + Campaign offer more healthy choices for public (with photos)* (Press release). https://www.info.gov.hk/gia/general/201905/02/P2019050200280.htm

The Government of the Hong Kong Special Administrative Region. (2019d, September 24). *First district health centre officially opens in Hong Kong (with photos/video)* (Press release). https://www.info.gov.hk/gia/general/2019b09/24/P2019092400717.htm

The Government of the Hong Kong Special Administrative Region. (2021a, December 3). *Tenders invited for Tsuen Wan District Health Centre* (Press release). https://www.info.gov.hk/gia/general/202112/03/P2021120300354.htm

The Government of the Hong Kong Special Administrative Region. (2021b, July 16). *Healthy teeth collaboration to continue* (Press release). https://www.info.gov.hk/gia/general/202107/16/P2021071500639.htm

The Government of the Hong Kong Special Administrative Region. (2022, June 22). *LCQ1: Public dental services* (Press release). https://www.info.gov.hk/gia/general/202206/22/P2022062200580.htm

The Hong Kong Lutheran Social Service Office. (2022, August 21). *The results of the "Parent-Child Happiness Index" survey. Children are not focused on online classes and have no intention of learning to play games. More than 5 adults have increased conflicts with their children during the epidemic* (In Chinese: 香港路德會社會服務處公 佈「親子快樂指數」家長調查結果 孩童上網課欠專注 無心向學愛打機 逾5成人疫下與子女衝突增) https://www.hklss.hk/hk/news-center/press-release/1329-20220821-pressrelease

The Partnership for Healthy Cities. (n.d.). *Home page.* https://partnershipforhealthycities.bloomberg.org/

The Prince Philip Dental Hospital. (n.d.). *Schedule of fees for private patients.* Retrieved August 21, 2022, from https://ppdh.org.hk/en/schedule-of-fees/private-patients/

The University of Hong Kong. (2021, April 29). *Use of new tobacco products hits record high among youth smokers, HKU Youth Quitline survey finds.* https://www.med.hku.hk/en/news/press/20210429-youth-quitline-survey-youth-smokers

The World Bank. (2019). *Life expectancy at birth, total (years).* https://data.worldbank.org/indicator/SP.DYN.LE00.IN

Tobacco and Alcohol Control Office. (2022). *Tobacco control legislation.* https://www.taco.gov.hk/t/english/legislation/legislation_asp.html

United Nations. (2015). *Sustainable development goals.* https://www.un.org/sustainabledevelopment/

World Health Organization. (2003). *Fruits and vegetables promotion initiative—Report of the meeting.* https://apps.who.int/iris/bitstream/handle/10665/68395/WHO_NMH_NPH_NNP_0308.pdf?sequence=1&isAllowed=y

World Health Organization. (2009). *Global health risks: Mortality and burden of disease attributable to selected major risks.* https://apps.who.int/iris/bitstream/handle/10665/44203/9789241563871_eng.pdf?sequence=1&isAllowed=y

World Health Organization. (2013). *WHO Report on the Global Tobacco Epidemic 2013: Enforcing bans on tobacco advertising, promotion and sponsorship.* https://apps.who.int/iris/bitstream/handle/10665/85380/9789241505871_eng.pdf?sequence=1

World Health Organization. (2015a). *Health cities: Good health is good politics: Toolkit for local governments to support healthy urban development.* https://apps.who.int/iris/rest/bitstreams/1247033/retrieve

World Health Organization. (2015b). *Guideline: Sugars intake for adults and children.* https://apps.who.int/iris/bitstream/handle/10665/149782/9789241549028_eng.pdf?sequence=1

World Health Organization. (2018a, May 16). *Investing in noncommunicable disease control generates major financial and health gains* (News release). https://www.who.int/news/item/16-05-2018-investing-in-noncommunicable-disease-control-generates-major-financial-and-health-gains

World Health Organization. (2018b, May 18). *WHO plan to eliminate industrially-produced trans-fatty acids from global food supply* (News release). https://www.who.int/news/item/14-05-2018-who-plan-to-eliminate-industrially-produced-trans-fatty-acids-from-global-food-supply

World Health Organization. (2019). *WHO report on the global tobacco epidemic, 2019: Offer help to quit tobacco use.* https://www.who.int/publications/i/item/9789241516204

World Health Organization. (2022a, May 24). *Tobacco.* https://www.who.int/news-room/fact-sheets/detail/tobacco

World Health Organization. (2022b, May 9). *Alcohol.* https://www.who.int/news-room/fact-sheets/detail/alcohol

Yang, S. X., Leung, K., Jiang, C. M., & Lo, E. (2021). Dental care services for older adults in Hong Kong—A shared funding, administration, and provision mode. *Healthcare, 9*(4), Article 390. https://doi.org/10.3390/healthcare9040390

Part IV
Actions in Health In All Policies (HIAP)

Chapter 24
Alleviation of Health Inequity Through Improvement of Health Literacy

Vincent T. S. Law

Abstract The WHO views health systems as all the activities which aim at promoting, restoring, or maintaining health. For the benefit of mankind, WHO's 'Health for All and All for Health' concept serves as strategic, far-reaching, and guiding vision for various stakeholders of health. Government policymakers should take this concept seriously when formulating and implementing health policies, improving health systems, as well as maintaining health equity. To achieve equitable health services, it is also essential for policymakers to consider structural determinants of health such as health system, public policies, resource allocation, cultural and social values, socioeconomic status, gender, and health literacy. Health literacy becomes an important public health goal for alleviating health inequalities within societies. This chapter outlines the equity of health systems and health resources, social determinants of health, definitions, and roles of health literacy, as well as the relationship between health systems, health literacy, and health equity. Policy initiatives, such as improvement of health system, tackling health literacy at multiple levels, sharing of responsibility among stakeholders, formulation of literacy-specific populational policies, as well as strengthening of support for research on health literacy, are recommended.

Keywords Health for all · All for health · Health equity · Health systems · Health literacy

Introduction

Everyone deserves good health because it is important for individuals' well-being and capacity to follow different life plans, as well as its contribution to the prosperity and quality of life (Voigt & Wester, 2015). The World Health Organization

V. T. S. Law (✉)
College of Professional and Continuing Education, The Hong Kong Polytechnic University, Hong Kong, China
e-mail: vincent.law@cpce-polyu.edu.hk

B. Y. F. Fong and W. C. W. Wong (eds.), *Gaps and Actions in Health Improvement from Hong Kong and Beyond*,
https://doi.org/10.1007/978-981-99-4491-0_24

(WHO) has been actively promoting health equity and health for all through multiple initiatives. In 1986, the Ottawa Charter for Health Promotion of the WHO (1986) advocated citizens' participation and self-determination in health-related decisions, and thus aroused self-awareness of health. For the benefit of the whole human race, the WHO (1988) further regards health as a matter of equity and social justice, and called for new approaches, new strategies, and better management of available resources to promote the availability of health advancement to all. Recognising that health systems play a pivotal role in promoting health and maintaining health equity, the WHO (2001) defined health systems as all the activities that the prime goal is to promote, restore, or maintain health. It is imperative to develop the capacity of health systems (public or private) and the public to foster and maintain 'Health for All' for the mankind. The 'Health for All and All for Health' concept plays important and far-reaching roles in guiding the formulation and implementation of health policies, improvement of health systems, as well as the provision of equitable health services by service providers. Health is affected by various social determinants which include age, education, and socioeconomic status (SES). The level of health literacy of citizens affects health equity. Governments should formulate and implement policy initiatives to alleviate the problems of health inequity by improving health literacy.

Equity of Health Systems and Health Resources

Health equity is the absence of preventable or remediable differentiations among various groups of people (Ng et al., 2020). Health inequality can be defined as the variation in health outcomes or the allocation of health factors of the individuals and groups (Kawachi et al., 2002). Although citizens are individually responsible for good or bad health, policymakers, health systems, and health professionals also play important roles. Health equity is related to the structure, effectiveness, and efficiency of health systems which in turn affect the provision and allocation of health resources. Government and healthcare service providers should recognise that equity issues of health system are both multifaceted and sociological in nature (Lv et al., 2020). However, health resources are always scarce and thus policymakers always face an efficiency-equity trade-off of the accomplishment of contesting goals when achieving high quality of health and equitable distribution of health (Mæstad & Norheim, 2012). On the other hand, patients express greater expectations on the health systems for disease treatment which have become increasingly resource-intensive and expensive. Ineffective or inefficient health systems cannot achieve WHO's ideal rule of 'Health for All' (Saboga-Nunes et al., 2019).

Common weaknesses of health systems include inadequate communication skills of professionals, incomprehensible information material, insufficient resources provided by the structures of health facilities, complex access routes, long waiting times for health services (Messer, 2019), as well as failure to provide or maintain equity of health outcomes, utilisation of health services, financing, and allocation of health resources (Lv et al., 2020). If accompanied with poor health policies, weaknesses of health systems may build and further intensify health inequalities among citizens.

From the policy perspectives, questions around health and health policy are high on political agenda over the world (Voigt, 2018). Since fostering equitable health systems is one of the key goals of healthcare reform in many countries (Jervelund et al., 2018), governments need to promote social justice in health so that no one is refused or discriminated to be healthy because of economic and social deprivation (Braveman, 2014). Unfortunately, public policies to alleviate health inequality may sometimes profit those least in need of aiding (Newdick, 2017) but aiding for those most in need is insufficient. When formulating health policy to improve the equity of healthcare system, both the internal structure of health systems and perceived equity by citizens should be gauzed for further improvement (Lv et al., 2020).

Social Determinants of Health

Health is influenced by various economic, political, and social determinants of a society. Based on the conceptual model for action on social determinants of health developed by the WHO (2010), health is affected by many political and social determinants. Structural determinants and social determinants of health equity include governance, public policies, social policies, culture and societal values, socioeconomic status (SES), social class, and educational level. On the other hand, intermediate determinants of health comprise material circumstances, behaviours, biological factors, psychological factors, as well as health systems. Similar determinants affecting health were also discovered by the National Academies of Sciences, Engineering, and Medicine (2017) and such determinants create health inequities. Hence, various factors affect the acquisition, understanding, and sharing of health-related knowledge that contribute to a reasonable level of health literacy.

Health-related justice includes issues such as allocation of healthcare resources, as well as social, economic, and political factors affecting health (Voigt & Wester, 2015). Access to healthcare is only one of the factors that affect people's health outcomes (Voigt & Wester, 2015). Many factors influence care and outcomes, as thus render the task of eradicating health disparities and accomplishing health equity difficult (Williams et al., 2016).

Education and Health

There is no conclusive relationship between education and perceived equity on health. The perceived equity by citizens decreased with age since the older adults were more liable to suffer from a range of diseases (Chatterji et al., 2015) and decreased with education (Lv et al., 2020). Many studies (e.g. Thornton et al., 2016) reported that higher education contributed to better health equity. However, Lv et al. (2020) have shown that perceived equity decreased with education since people with higher education level may be more concerned about their health (Lu et al., 2017). Furthermore, education level is related to health literacy (Van der Heide et al., 2013) and the ability to acquire health information (Sørensen et al., 2012), which guarantees health equity from the standpoint of health outcomes.

Social Class and Health

Importance of global justice has been increasingly recognised and there are increasing questions about health (Voigt, 2018). Although overall standards of health have been improving, health inequalities between rich and poor are also intensifying (Newdick, 2017). Many literatures focus on social inequalities in health, that is inequality in health outcomes among socioeconomic classes (Voigt & Wester, 2015). However, inequity exists at policy, cultural, and social levels. Hence, protection of health may not only be met through the provision of health care but also through public policies that tackle the socially controllable factors affecting health outcomes (Voigt & Wester, 2015). Besides, ethnic minorities suffer from poorer health status and outcomes (e.g. cardiovascular disease, cancer, and others) as compared with the majority of the population (Williams et al., 2016).

Health Inequity

Health has its special status since social equity affects health equity. Healthy choice is the appreciated and easy choice (Gunther et al., 2019). As compared with inequality of other goods, health inequality is morally more disagreeable than those in other goods (Voigt & Wester, 2015). In many economies or regions, high levels of social inequity result in substantial health inequalities (Hancock & Bezold, 2017). Social inequalities in health are not lessening in recent years (Joffe & Mindell, 2004). The influence of health disparities is not restricted to the poor and becomes a universal problem (Blackwell, 2009). Inequalities in population health are reflected in various aspects which include socioeconomic, environmental, cultural, and ethnic differences (Hyyppä, 2010). Information about interventions that could reduce health inequalities is limited (Joffe & Mindell, 2004). People who are more educated and possess socioeconomic resources tend to counter more to health education, thus increasing inequalities (Joffe & Mindell, 2004).

Health Literacy

Definition

The concept of health literacy was originally used in a medical perspective which refers to a patient's capability to comprehend instructions and recommendations by doctors or nurses (Van den Broucke, 2019). From the individual perspective, health literacy evolves and develops over one's life and is not limited to the older adults (Okan et al., 2019). Health literacy is a broad, multifaceted concept (Broder & Carvalho, 2019; Okan et al., 2019) which is a greatly diverse construct with many definitions (Malloy-Weir et al., 2016). There is no consensus about the central construct of health literacy although its field is expanding (Mackert et al., 2015). There is also no unanimously accepted definition while various definitions highlight subtly different aspects (Okan et al., 2019).

Various definitions of health literacy refer it to as a multidimensional, complicated, and heterogeneous concept since they portray different facets of the concept (Sørensen & Pleasant, 2017). Many definitions focus on citizens' participation and interaction in the wider society (Sørensen & Pleasant, 2017). An important definition of health literacy was given by the European Commission (2007) which defined health literacy as the capacity to read, screen, and comprehend health information so as to form sound decisions. Focusing on both individual and social levels, Dodson et al. (2015) defined health literacy as the individual characteristics and social resources necessary for individuals and communities to access, comprehend, appraise, and use information and services to make health-related decisions. Nowadays, health literacy is regarded as an interdisciplinary and multidimensional concept that involves personal knowledge, motivation, and capabilities to access, comprehend, evaluate, and apply health information (Okan et al., 2019).

From the perspectives of formulating and implementing policy initiatives, it is better to have a centrally agreed definition of health literacy. In addition, the 'literacy' component of 'health literacy' has been widely discussed but there is limited discussion of the 'health' element (Saboga-Nunes et al., 2019). Governments and major stakeholders of health are advised to address both the 'health' and 'literacy' elements of health literacy for the benefit of the population and apply the concept to reduce health inequality among citizens.

Nutbeam (2008) classifies health literacy into the functional, interactive, and critical health literacy. First, functional health literacy refers to the fundamental skills in reading and writing needed to function effectively. Second, interactive health literacy is related to advanced cognitive and literacy skills for active participation. Third, critical health literacy refers to more advanced cognitive skills for analysing information to gain better control on life events. Governments should formulate and implement specific initiatives to solve problems related to health literacy in different areas for the benefit of the whole population.

Health Literacy at Various Levels

Health literacy is usually viewed as a personal issue since it is related to knowledge and actions at individual level. However, there is growing empirical evidence that health literacy research is beyond such individual functional level. It plays a role in social support and resources (Sentell et al., 2017). Different environments play a role in the performative aspect of health literacy (Bauer, 2019). The concept of health literacy is still evolving, and it is expected that there are ongoing dynamic changes on all levels (Okan et al., 2019).

At individual level, health literacy is usually viewed as a personal asset. Health literacy can also be viewed as a skill-based process to find and transform information into knowledge and action. This individual nature can be expanded to the societal level since health literacy is about how knowledge enables individuals to uphold and promote their health and be aware of the role of the whole society (Sørensen, 2019). From the population perspective, health literacy does not only serve as a resource for personal health but can also be extended to the whole population as an important resource for population health (Nutbeam, 2008).

At organisational level, organisational health literacy has been rapidly evolving as a research area in recent years since a healthier workforce is more productive (Gunther et al., 2019). The concept can be expanded to the health practice and policy arenas (Farmanova et al., 2018; Lloyd et al., 2018). Organisational health literacy, or health-literate organisations (HLOs), has been gaining importance in various countries such as Australia, Austria, Belgium, Canada, Germany, Italy, New Zealand, and the USA (Pelikan, 2019). The concept of organisational health literacy should be extended to workplaces, schools, and cities (Pelikan, 2019).

Obviously, health literacy is influenced by individual, situational, and societal determinants. It affects health outcomes which are also influenced by various social determinants. From the health perspectives, health literacy influences the use and costs of healthcare, health behaviour, health status, as well as equity (Sørensen et al., 2012). As Kickbusch (2004) views health literacy as a new type of health citizenship, citizens are responsible for their own health and are involved in the social processes that tackle the rudimentary causes of health inequalities. Hence, health literacy is an important element of health equity at individual, community, and national level.

Roles of Health Literacy

Health literacy is multidisciplinary in nature while its information can be located in various health-related databases, such as in education, information sciences, nursing, and communication databases (Okan et al., 2019). This reflects the significance and roles of health literacy in the prevention, promotion, and provision of health. Instrumentally, a reasonable level of health literacy is required to evaluate and decide everyday actions for maintenance or enhancement of quality of life (Okan et al., 2019).

Health literacy takes a vital part in the healthcare system and is one of the indispensable factors to tackle health inequalities. First, it underpins the capacity of health organisations to serve clients. Second, it helps safeguard the health and well-being of citizens at the societal level (Sørensen, 2019). Third, health literacy affects one's ability to make health decisions at home, in the community, and in the political areas (Okan et al., 2019). In addition, health literacy is central in policy decisions regarding the comprehensive range of activities related to health and wellness (Pleasant et al., 2019). The abovementioned various roles of health literacy demonstrate that the health systems and their structures are the pivotal targets for reduction of health literacy and thus improvement of health equity (Okan et al., 2019).

European Experience in Improving Health Literacy

Some European countries have formulated a national policy or devised specific goals about health literacy in their public health targets (Van der Heide et al., 2019). Many policy initiatives were motivated by the first international comparative study on health literacy, that is the European Health Literacy Survey (HLS-EU) in 2011 (Pelikan et al., 2012). The HLS-EU study gauzed the level of health literacy in the general public of eight European countries, including Austria, Bulgaria, Germany, Greece, Ireland, the Netherlands, Poland, and Spain. More European countries hence use the HLS-EU survey instrument to gauze the level of health literacy (Palumbo et al., 2016).

In Europe, the European Commission funded the HEALIT4EU study to get insight into health literacy research and policy (Heijmans et al., 2015). This study performed a literature review of existing knowledge about health literacy interventions in EU member states and evaluated the development of a forecasting model of factors of health literacy using publicly accessible sources.

Government may learn from the European experience in action areas such as supporting health literacy in the society, alignment of values of public goods, placing health literacy on the policy agenda, enhancing evidence-based research on health literacy, as well as fostering adequate capacity for health literacy (Kickbusch et al., 2013).

Patient Participation and Health Literacy

Improvement in health and quality of life requires patients' direct participation in various aspects, such as knowledge, understanding, decision-making, and health literacy as a whole. First of all, patients should be equipped with the necessary knowledge and understanding of disease. Second, patients should be better involved in decision-making and treatment. Third, discrimination against certain patients and population groups should be avoided or reduced (Coulter et al., 2015). Among such involvement, the process of patients' decision-making is equally important as an essential element of health literacy and participation since patients with low health literacy are assumed to be less active, thus need other forms of collaboration with health professionals (Messer, 2019).

Health Literacy and Health Equity

Similar to health promotion, health literacy is also a key element of quality in healthcare (Pelikan, 2019). It is evidenced that health literacy is related to personal health behaviours, health outcomes, use of health services, as well as societal healthcare costs (Kickbusch et al., 2013). Health literacy aids people to make informed decisions related to health. This renders health literacy to become one of the important public goals for reduction of health inequalities within societies (Nutbeam, 2000). Individuals with low health literacy have higher use and suffer from worse outcomes of healthcare services (Brach et al., 2012). Low health literacy casts significant outcomes for the costs of health care (Eichler et al., 2009). Improving health literacy of patients can decrease the demands of health services and offer health education, which help improve the quality of healthcare and lower health gap (Pelikan, 2019).

There is limited literature which address health literacy across the lifespan, especially approaching the end of life (Kondilis, 2019). Related to urban settings in the USA, a systematic review conducted by Chesser et al. (2016) revealed strong associations between low health literacy and poorer health outcomes. A study at South Korea over 1,000 people revealed that social capital could reduce the effect of low health literacy on information resources related to health, efficacy, and behaviours (Kim et al., 2015). Governments should review health policy related to building and upgrading of health literacy over the lifespan of citizens.

Policy to Improve Health Literacy and Alleviate Health Inequity

The 1986 Ottawa Charter (World Health Organization, 1986) stressed on the significance of healthy public policy as a crucial strategy for bettering public health. Public policy is a government action that can be expressed as a law, an order, or a legislation (Sapru, 2017). Public policy is dynamic and complex in nature. It needs collaboration between various policy stakeholders (Khare et al., 2015). While supporting well-being and enabling good health to become pivotal goals in health promotion and policymaking (Maass et al., 2016), the best health protection and a once for all change in the population can be safeguarded in the formulation and implementation of public policies (Joffe & Mindell, 2004).

Improvement of Health System

Since health systems influence the level of health literacy, tackling of limited health literacy of citizens within the health systems becomes an emerging agenda of policymakers, health practitioners, and researchers (Pelikan, 2019). To directly improve health literacy of the public, health systems should not target at single channel but need to formulate and implement policies that enhance health literacy in multiple channels such as written, multimedia, and Internet-based ones (Kickbusch et al., 2013). Governments should also review the balance between the public and private health sectors in terms of utilisation and allocation of resources, so as to streamline resource allocation to boost health literacy of citizens.

Tackling Health Literacy at Multiple Levels

Tackling health literacy issues needs holistic views and multi-level interventions. Other than measuring and improving individual health literacy, government, and practitioners should also measure and improve various types of health literacy which include situational, organisational or systems-specific health literacy (Pelikan, 2019). Major interventions to tackle noncommunicable diseases through health literacy include helping people with lower health literacy, improving capacity of health literacy, as well as enhancing the organisational, government, policy, and system practice (Kickbusch et al., 2013). At the institutional level, institutions such as workplaces, schools, and hospitals can foster and implement appropriate health literacy standards from the policy perspective (Kickbusch et al., 2013). Governments should also develop holistic views on health literacy and tackle its related issues with strategic and effective policy initiatives.

Sharing of Responsibility Among Stakeholders

The responsibility of health literacy rest on multiple stakeholders which include individuals, policymakers, and healthcare professionals (Kickbusch et al., 2013; Mitic & Rootman, 2012). Among them, policymakers and government officials take the most important and final responsibility. Such responsibility also traverses country borders, professions, and jurisdictions (Mitic & Rootman, 2012). However, it is observed that formulation of policy actions to tackle the crisis of health literacy has been slow at all levels (Kickbusch et al., 2013). In addition, from a systems perspective, health literacy demands a systematic approach across various intimate stakeholders of health, such as citizens, organisations, professionals, and government policymakers (Okan et al., 2019). People in the world face problems in getting access to, comprehending, judging, and applying information to manage their health.

To tackle problems of health literacy, collective and orchestrated efforts from all policy stakeholders are required (Okan et al., 2019). On the one hand, policymakers, professionals, and the public should be health-literate (Okan et al., 2019). On the other hand, health literacy at the organisational level, that is organisational health literacy, should not be ignored. As the default formulator and implementer of public policies, government should take the lead, adopt a bottom-up approach on agenda setting and policy formulation, as well as view health equity from a stakeholder approach.

Formulation of Literacy-Specific Populational Policies

The population health status of a country is generally related to the levels of health literacy of the population. Health literacy is not just related to research and clinical practice—governments should exert policy efforts in enhancing health literacy for the whole population (Kickbusch et al., 2013). The WHO report in 2013 advocated actions on policy and strategies to enhance the populational level of health literacy and hence overall health status (Kickbusch et al., 2013).

Governments should set specific health policies to enhance health literacy (Van der Heide et al., 2019). As a goal-setting tactic, governments may set a high level of health literacy as an explicit aim of both health policy and education policy (Kickbusch et al., 2013), so as to achieve better outcomes. Government should also regularly conduct population surveys to assess and monitor health literacy so as to improve accessibility and responsiveness to individuals with lower health literacy (Kickbusch et al., 2013).

Multiple strategies can be employed to improve health literacy: (1) enhancement of health communication via health literacy instruments and guidelines in the settings of healthcare, disease prevention, and health promotion (Vanden Broucke, 2019), (2) enhancement of health education in the population, and (3) fostering and strengthening health literacy-friendly settings to reduce the need for health literacy (Kickbusch et al., 2013).

Strengthening of Support for Research on Health Literacy

One of the important functions of government is to support research. With the help of evidence-based research conducted by academics, think tanks, the healthcare sectors, and political parties, more pragmatic and user-friendly health policies would be formulated. While government itself should also conduct evidence-based research, it may adopt a systems approach which helps study and improve health literacy, and in turn upholds health equity. More research which focus on enhancing the health literacy of health professionals and facilities, as well as their responsiveness, are needed (Messer, 2019).

Conclusion

Health and well-being are important for everyone. The WHO views health systems as all the activities which aim at promoting, restoring or maintaining health. For the benefit of mankind, WHO's 'Health for All and All for Health' concept serves as strategic, far-reaching, and guiding vision for various stakeholders of health. In particular, government policymakers should take this concept seriously when formulating and implementing health policy, improving health systems, as well as maintaining health equity.

The European Commission (2007) defined health literacy as the capacity to read, screen, and comprehend health information in order to form sound decisions. Health literacy becomes an important public health aim for reduction of health inequalities within societies. Since health is affected by various social determinants which include age, education, and socioeconomic status (SES), the level of health literacy among citizens varies. To alleviate the problems of health inequity through improvement of health literacy of citizens, policy initiatives, such as improvement of health system, tackling health literacy at multiple levels, sharing of responsibility among stakeholders, formulation of literacy-specific populational policies, as well as strengthening of support for research on health literacy, are beyond necessary.

References

Bauer, U. (2019). The social embeddedness of health literacy. In O. Okan, U. Bauer, D. Levin-Zamir, P. Pinheiro, & K. Sorensen (Eds.), *International handbook of health literacy: Research, practice and policy across the life-span* (pp. 573–586). Policy Press. https://doi.org/10.51952/9781447344520.ch037

Blackwell, G. A. (2009). Active living research and the movement for healthy communities. *American Journal of Preventive Medicine, 36*(2S), S50–S52. https://doi.org/10.1016/j.amepre.2008.10.004

Brach, C., Keller, D., Hernandez, L.M., Baur, C., Parker, R., Dreyer, B. et al. (2012). *Ten attributes of health literate health care organizations*. https://nam.edu/wp-content/uploads/2015/06/BPH_Ten_HLit_Attributes.pdf

Braveman, P. (2014). What are health disparities and health equity? We need to be clear. *Public Health Reports, 129*(1_suppl 2), 5–8. https://doi.org/10.1177/00333549141291S203

Broder, J., & Carvalho, G. S. (2019). Health literacy of children and adolescents: Conceptual approaches and developmental considerations. In O. Okan, U. Bauer, D. Levin-Zamir, P. Pinheiro, & K. Sorensen (Eds.), *International handbook of health literacy: Research, practice and policy across the life-span* (pp. 39–52). Policy Press. https://doi.org/10.51952/9781447344520.ch003

Chatterji, S., Byles, J., Cutler, D., Seeman, T., & Verdes, E. (2015). Health, functioning, and disability in older adults—Present status and future implications. *Lancet, 385*(9967), 563–575. https://doi.org/10.1016/S0140-6736(14)61462-8

Chesser, A. K., Keene Woods, N., Smothers, K., & Rogers, N. (2016). Health literacy and older adults: A systematic review. *Gerontology & Geriatric Medicine, 2*, 1–13. https://doi.org/10.1177/2333721416630492

Coulter, A., Entwistle, V. A., Eccles, A., Ryan, S., Shepperd, S., & Perera, R. (2015). Personalised care planning for adults with chronic or long-term health conditions. *The Cochrane Database of* Systematic Revie*ws, 2015*(3), Article CD010523. https://doi.org/10.1002/14651858.CD010523.pub2

Dodson, S., Good, S., & Osborne, R. (2015). *Health literacy toolkit for low and of middle-income countries: A series of information sheets to empower communities and strengthen health systems.* World Health Organization. https://apps.who.int/iris/handle/10665/205244

Eichler, K., Wieser, S., & Brügger, U. (2009). The costs of limited health literacy: A systematic review. *International Journal of Public Health, 54*(5), 313–324. https://doi.org/10.1007/s00038-009-0058-2

European Commission. (2007). *Together for health: A strategic approach for the EU 2008–2013.* https://ec.europa.eu/commission/presscorner/detail/en/IP_07_1571

Farmanova, E., Bonneville, L., & Bouchard, L. (2018). Organizational health literacy: Review of theories, frameworks, guides, and implementation issues. *Inquiry: The Journal of Health Care Organization, Provision and Financing, 55*, 1–17. https://doi.org/10.1177/0046958018757848

Gunther, C. E., Peddicord, V., Kozlowski, J., Li, Y., Menture, D., Fabius, R., Frazee, S. G., & Nigro, P. J. (2019). Building a culture of health and well-being at Merck. *Population Health Management, 22*(5), 449–456. https://doi.org/10.1089/pop.2018.0116

Hancock, T., & Bezold, C. (2017). Futures thinking and healthy cities. In E. de Leeuw, & J. Simos (Eds.), *Healthy cities: The theory, policy, and practice of value-based urban planning* (pp. 449–462). Springer. https://doi.org/10.1007/978-1-4939-6694-3_19

Heijmans, M., Uiters, E., Rose, T., Hofsteds, J., Devillé, W., van der Heide, I., Boshuisen, H., & Radenakers, J. (2015). *Study on sound evidence for a better understanding of health literacy in the European Union: Final report*. Publications Office of the European Union. https://data.europa.eu/doi/10.2818/150402

Hyyppä, M. T. (2010). *Healthy ties: Social capital, population health and survival.* Springer. https://doi.org/10.1007/978-90-481-9606-7

Jervelund, S. S., Maltesen, T., Wimmelmann, C. L., Petersen, J. H., & Krasnik, A. (2018). Know where to go: Evidence from a controlled trial of a healthcare system information intervention among immigrants. *BMC Public Health, 18*, Article 863. https://doi.org/10.1186/s12889-018-5741-x

Joffe, M., & Mindell, J. (2004). A tentative step towards healthy public policy. *Journal of Epidemiology & Community Health, 58*, 966–968. https://doi.org/10.1136/jech.2004.023697

Kawachi, I., Subramanian, S. V., & Almeida-Filho, N. (2002). A glossary for health inequalities. *Journal of Epidemiology & Community Health, 56*(9), 647–652. https://doi.org/10.1136/jech.56.9.647

Khare, M. M., Núñez, A. E., & James, B. F. (2015). Coalition for a healthier community: Lessons learned and implications for future work. *Evaluation and Program Planning, 51*, 85–88. https://doi.org/10.1016/j.evalprogplan.2015.01.001

Kickbusch, I. (2004). Health and citizenship: The characteristics of 21st century health. *World Hospitals and Health Services, 40*(4), 12–14. https://www.ihf-fih.org/download_doc_file.php?doc=e5faa10559cc4e9052620d99dcc8ef13

Kickbusch, I., Pelikan, J. M., Apfel, F., & Tsouros, A. (2013). *Health literacy: The solid facts.* World Health Organization. https://apps.who.int/iris/bitstream/handle/10665/128703/e96854.pdf

Kim, Y. C., Lim, J. Y., & Park, K. (2015). Effects of health literacy and social capital on health information Behavior. *Journal of Health Communication, 20*(9), 1084–1094. https://doi.org/10.1080/10810730.2015.1018636

Kondilis, B. K. (2019). A lifespan perspective on health literacy: Ageing and end-of-life issues. In O. Okan, U. Bauer, D. Levin-Zamir, P. Pinheiro, & K. Sorensen (Eds.), *International handbook of health literacy: Research, practice and policy across the life-span* (pp. 633–648). Policy Press. https://doi.org/10.51952/9781447344520.ch041

Lloyd, J. E., Song, H. J., Dennis, S. M., Dunbar, N., Harris, E., & Harris, M. F. (2018). A paucity of strategies for developing health literate organisations: A systematic review. *PloS ONE, 13*(4), Article e0195018. https://doi.org/10.1371/journal.pone.0195018

Lu, J., Lu, Y., Wang, X., Li, X., Linderman, G. C., Wu, C., Cheng, X., Mu, L., Zhang, H., Liu, J., Su, M., Zhao, H., Spatz, E. S., Spertus, J. A., Masoudi, F. A., Krumholz, H. M., & Jiang, L. (2017). Prevalence, awareness, treatment, and control of hypertension in China: Data from 1.7 million adults in a population-based screening study (China PEACE Million Persons Project). *Lancet, 390*(10112), 2549–2558. https://doi.org/10.1016/S0140-6736(17)32478-9

Lv, H., Gu, J. Q., Yuan, X. D., & Miao, Y. D. (2020). Prioritizing the perceived equity of the residents to construct an equitable health care system: Evidence from a national cross-sectional study in China. *BMC Health Services Research, 20*, Article 167. https://doi.org/10.1186/s12913-020-5026-9

Maass, R., Klöckner, C., Lindstrom, B., & Lillefjell, M. (2016). The impact of neighborhood social capital on life satisfaction and self-rated health: A possible pathway for health promotion? *Health & Place, 42*, 120–128. https://doi.org/10.1016/j.healthplace.2016.09.011

Mackert, M., Champlin, S., Su, Z., & Guadagno, M. (2015). The many health literacies: Advancing research or fragmentation? *Health Communication, 30*(12), 1161–1165. https://doi.org/10.1080/10410236.2015.1037422

Mæstad, O., & Norheim, O. F. (2012). A universal preference for equality in health? Reasons to reconsider properties of applied social welfare functions. *Social Science & Medicine, 75*(10), 1836–1843. https://doi.org/10.1016/j.socscimed.2012.07.001

Malloy-Weir, L. J., Charles, C., Gafni, A., & Entwistle, V. (2016). A review of health literacy: Definitions, interpretations, and implications for policy initiatives. *Journal of Public Health Policy, 37*(3), 334–352. https://doi.org/10.1057/jphp.2016.18

Messer, M. (2019). Health literacy and participation in the healthcare of adults: (In)compatible approaches? In O. Okan, U. Bauer, D. Levin-Zamir, P. Pinheiro, & K. Sorensen (Eds.), *International handbook of health literacy: Research, practice and policy across the life-span* (pp. 617–632). Policy Press. https://doi.org/10.51952/9781447344520.ch040

Mitic, W., & Rootman, I. (2012) *An intersectoral approach for improving health literacy for Canada: A discussion paper.* https://phabc.org/wp-content/uploads/2015/09/IntersectoralApproachforHealthLiteracy-FINAL.pdf

National Academies of Sciences, Engineering, and Medicine. (2017). *Communities in action: Pathways to health equity.* The National Academies Press. https://doi.org/10.17226/24624

Newdick, C. (2017). Health equality, social justice and the poverty of autonomy. *Health Economics, Policy and Law, 12*(4), 411–433. https://doi.org/10.1017/S1744133117000093

Ng, T. K. C., Fong, B. Y. F., Fung, M. H. T. (2020). Equity, quality, and gatekeeping. In B. Y. F. Fong, V. T. S. Law, & A. Lee (Eds.), *Primary care revisited: Interdisciplinary perspectives for a new era* (pp. 211–223). Springer. https://doi.org/10.1007/978-981-15-2521-6_13

Nutbeam, D. (2000). Health literacy as a public health goal: A challenge for contemporary health education and communication strategies into the 21st century. *Health Promotion International, 15*(3), 259–267. https://doi.org/10.1093/heapro/15.3.259

Nutbeam, D. (2008). The evolving concept of health literacy. *Social Science & Medicine, 67*(12), 2072–2078. https://doi.org/10.1016/j.socscimed.2008.09.050

Okan, O., Bauer, U., Levin-Zamir, D., Pinheiro, P., & Sorensen, K. (2019). *International handbook of health literacy: Research, practice and policy across the life-span.* Policy Press. https://doi.org/10.51952/9781447344520

Palumbo, R., Annarumma, C., Adinolfi, P., Musella, M., & Piscopo, G. (2016). The Italian health literacy project: Insights from the assessment of health literacy skills in Italy. *Health Policy, 120*(9), 1087–1094. https://doi.org/10.1016/j.healthpol.2016.08.007

Pelikan, J. M. (2019). Health-literate healthcare organisations. In O. Okan, U. Bauer, D. Levin-Zamir, P. Pinheiro, & K. Sorensen (Eds.), *International handbook of health literacy: Research, practice and policy across the life-span* (pp. 539–554). Policy Press. https://doi.org/10.51952/9781447344520.ch035

Pelikan, J. M., Rothlin, F., & Ganahl, K. (2012), *Comparative report on health literacy in eight EU Member States*. http://cpme.dyndns.org:591/adopted/2015/Comparative_report_on_health_literacy_in_eight_EU_member_states.pdf

Pleasant, A., Maish, C., O'Leary, C., & Carmona, R. (2019). Measuring health literacy in adults: An overview and discussion of current tools. In O. Okan, U. Bauer, D. Levin-Zamir, P. Pinheiro, & K. Sorensen (Eds.), *International handbook of health literacy: Research, practice and policy across the life-span* (pp. 67–82). Policy Press. https://doi.org/10.51952/9781447344520.ch005

Saboga-Nunes, L., Bittlingmayer, U. H., & Okan, O. (2019). Salutogenesis and health literacy: The health promotion simplex! In O. Okan, U. Bauer, D. Levin-Zamir, P. Pinheiro, & K. Sorensen (Eds.), *International handbook of health literacy: Research, practice and policy across the life-span* (pp. 649–664). Policy Press. https://doi.org/10.51952/9781447344520.ch042

Sapru, R. (2017). *Public policy: A contemporary perspective*. Sage. https://us.sagepub.com/en-us/nam/public-policy/book257432#description

Sentell, T., Pitt, R., & Buchthal, O. V. (2017). Health literacy in a social context: Review of quantitative evidence. *Health Literacy Research and Practice, 1*(2), e41–e70. https://doi.org/10.3928/24748307-20170427-01

Sørensen, K. (2019). Defining health literacy: Exploring differences and communalities. In O. Okan, U. Bauer, D. Levin-Zamir, P. Pinheiro, & K. Sorensen (Eds.), *International handbook of health literacy: Research, practice and policy across the life-span* (pp. 5–20). Policy Press. https://doi.org/10.51952/9781447344520.ch001

Sørensen, K., & Pleasant, A. (2017). Understanding the conceptual importance of the differences among health literacy definitions. In R. A. Logan, & E. R. Siegel (Eds.), *Health literacy* (pp. 3–14). IOS Press. https://doi.org/10.3233/978-1-61499-790-0-3

Sørensen, K., Van den Broucke, S., Fullam, J., Doyle, G., Pelikan, J., Slonska, Z., Brand, H., & (HLS-EU) Consortium Health Literacy Project European. (2012). Health literacy and public health: A systematic review and integration of definitions and models. *BMC Public Health, 12*, Article 80. https://doi.org/10.1186/1471-2458-12-80

Thornton, R. L., Glover, C. M., Cené, C. W., Glik, D. C., Henderson, J. A., & Williams, D. R. (2016). Evaluating strategies for reducing health disparities by addressing the social determinants of health. *Health Affairs, 35*(8), 1416–1423. https://doi.org/10.1377/hlthaff.2015.1357

Van den Broucke, S. (2019). Capacity building for health literacy. In O. Okan, U. Bauer, D. Levin-Zamir, P. Pinheiro, & K. Sorensen (Eds.), *International handbook of health literacy: Research, practice and policy across the life-span* (pp. 705–719). Policy Press. https://doi.org/10.51952/9781447344520.ch045

Van der Heide, I., Heijmans, M., & Rademakers, J. (2019). Health literacy policies: European perspectives. In O. Okan, U. Bauer, D. Levin-Zamir, P. Pinheiro, & K. Sorensen (Eds.), *International handbook of health literacy: Research, practice and policy across the life-span* (pp. 403–418). Policy Press. https://doi.org/10.51952/9781447344520.ch027

Van der Heide, I., Wang, J., Droomers, M., Spreeuwenberg, P., Rademakers, J., & Uiters, E. (2013). The relationship between health, education, and health literacy: Results from the Dutch adult literacy and life skills survey. *Journal of Health Communication, 18*(Suppl 1), 172–184. https://doi.org/10.1080/10810730.2013.825668

Voigt, K. (2018). Equality, health, and health policy: Introduction. *Les ateliers de l'éthique/The Ethics Forum, 13*(3), 31–37. https://doi.org/10.7202/1061217ar

Voigt, K., & Wester, G. (2015). Relational equality and health. *Social Philosophy and Policy, 31*(2), 204–229. https://doi.org/10.1017/S0265052514000326

Williams, J. S., Walker, R. J., & Egede, L. E. (2016). Achieving equity in an evolving healthcare system: Opportunities and challenges. *The American Journal of the Medical Sciences, 351*(1), 33–43. https://doi.org/10.1016/j.amjms.2015.10.012

World Health Organization. (1986). *The Ottawa Charter for health promotion.* https://www.who.int/publications/i/item/ottawa-charter-for-health-promotion
World Health Organization. (1988). *Health for all—All for health.* https://apps.who.int/iris/bitstream/handle/10665/272516/WH-1988-Jan-Feb-p3-4-eng.pdf
World Health Organization. (2001). *The World health report: 2001: Mental health: New understanding, new hope.* https://apps.who.int/iris/handle/10665/42390
World Health Organization. (2010). *A conceptual framework for action on the social determinants of health.* https://www.who.int/publications/i/item/9789241500852
World Health Organization. (2017). *Promoting health in the SDGs: Report on the 9th Global conference for health promotion, Shanghai, China, 21–24 November 2016: all for health, health for all.* https://www.who.int/publications/i/item/promoting-health-in-the-sdgs

Chapter 25
District Health Care Movement

Will L. H. Leung

Abstract District Health Care Movement is an important process to achieve integrated healthcare delivery through an organised whole-of-society multidisciplinary care approach by effectively and efficiently utilising healthcare resources at the community level, making it more accessible, available, and affordable to address healthcare needs of the community. In the chapter, an overview is provided on the District Health Care Movement from the perspectives of accessibility to health services, primary health care, infrastructure establishment, and team-based participation of healthcare professionals and providers. Putting District Health Care Movement in action, various approaches are discussed with Hong Kong's District Health Centre model and Singapore's Primary Care Network models as illustrations. The challenges and barriers of implementing the District Health Care Movement are addressed. Family Doctors are essential participants of the multidisciplinary care team. A study conducted by the Hong Kong College of Family Physicians in 2021 was to explore Family Doctors' understanding of the District Health Centre model in Hong Kong and to collect opinions from Family Doctors in enabling the primary healthcare team to fulfil the mission and vision of District Health Care Movement. This is an important initiative to fill the existing gaps of the healthcare system in meeting healthcare needs of the community.

Keywords District health · Primary health care · Family physician · Multi-disciplinary care

W. L. H. Leung (✉)
Jockey Club School of Public Health and Primary Care, The Chinese University of Hong Kong, Hong Kong, China
e-mail: lhleung@cuhk.edu.hk

B. Y. F. Fong and W. C. W. Wong (eds.), *Gaps and Actions in Health Improvement from Hong Kong and Beyond*,
https://doi.org/10.1007/978-981-99-4491-0_25

Overview of District Health Care Movement

One of the key elements of "Health for All" is the accessibility to health services. Through a practical unit of "district" with effective coordination among healthcare professionals and community resources in the district, the population of the district could be benefited. A district is an organised unit of local administration of varying size. As a unit, a district is small as compared to a city for healthcare providers to acknowledge the major problems and constraints of bio-psycho-social well-being. The scale of a district is advantageous for inter-sectoral collaborations among various health service providers within a self-contained segment of the health system as a whole (Tarimo, 1991).

Primary health care has been demonstrated to be a highly effective and efficient way to address physical health, mental health, social health, and well-being of individuals, families, and population through a whole-of-society multidisciplinary care approach. The advantages of multidisciplinary integrated care from a clinical perspective are better patient care experiences, better detection of illness, and improvement of overall health outcomes (World Health Organization, 2021). The role of primary care team in chronic disease management had been described in literature as multidisciplinary care teams with clinical and behavioural skills to deliver quality primary care. The participation of community health workers from different disciplines improved chronic disease control parameters through a multi-faceted approach in providing a holistic patient-centred care to patients with various health needs through dynamic care processes (Tan & Earn Lee, 2019).

A district health system is an establishment of infrastructure in the local district which oversees and monitors the delivery of community-based care in the locality. The main functions of district health system include enabling patients with chronic health problems to be managed in primary care with holistic and structured care involving different levels of healthcare personnel, providing more support to primary care providers in managing more patients with chronic health problems effectively and efficiently, and integrating various preventive care measures into the primary care system (Lee, 2019).

For implementation of district-based healthcare movement, teams of competent and experienced healthcare professionals, including medical practitioners, nurses, allied health professionals, pharmacists, dentists, social workers, and other healthcare providers or community working partners, are providing a one-stop comprehensive clinical management, decision-making, and preventive care. This includes primary, secondary, tertiary, and quaternary prevention, in accordance with the philosophy of primary health care at the district level. For effective operations of district-based primary health care, a number of core competencies are ideal for district health system organisations including local health needs knowledge, community engagement, multidisciplinary community-based care team formation with various tiers of healthcare practitioners, professional, and academic expertise in primary care, partnership with hospitals in localities, outreaching capacity, organisation of medical-social welfare-community model to address the bio-psycho-social needs of local population with chronic health conditions, as well as audit and evaluation of organisational processes for continuous quality improvement (Lee & Poon, 2020). Patient engagement through frequent follow-up at the community, active promotion of adherence and compliance to treatment measures, timely adjustment of care plans could be ideally better achieved at district-based health systems as compared with systems heavily depending on secondary or tertiary care.

District Health Care Movement in Action

Globally, decentralisation of healthcare services has been central to the ongoing health sector reforms. Multi-sectoral approach or inter-sectoral collaboration are principles in linking up health provision to other aspects of socioeconomic development that are closely related to health. As compared with the national health system, district health systems focus on community-based care with identification and engagement of key stakeholders in addressing district health needs. District hospitals and primary care facilities provide different levels of care with accessibility at the community level.

Various approaches had been undergoing development for District Health Care Movement such as the traditional primary healthcare model and the collaborative care model with an aim to improve patient experiences, care efficiency, and health outcomes depending on the background epidemiological characteristics and cultural factors such as the overall health status, health indicators, health-seeking behaviour of the community members, self-care capability, health literacy, public acceptance, and operational considerations, such as the existing health models, healthcare financing methodologies, and government policy directions. Innovation and modification of the movement require a strategic approach with elements, such as leadership, culture change, and selecting the right team to fit for the purpose (Chatora & Tumusiime, 2004).

The Hong Kong Experience

In Hong Kong, primary health facilities include public-funded out-patient clinics operated by the Department of Health and Hospital Authority, clinics, health centres, and hospitals in the private sector or run by non-governmental organisations (NGOs), as well as other health service providers in the community. As a milestone of district healthcare movement in Hong Kong, the Government of the Hong Kong Special Administrative Region launched an initiative in setting up District Health Centre (DHC) at each of the districts in the city to strengthen district-based primary healthcare services, to engage medical and health professionals in the community for quality care to improve population health and well-being, to reduce avoidable hospitalisations at secondary and tertiary care settings, and to generate broader social benefits through a multidisciplinary care approach.

The first DHC in Hong Kong commenced operation in September 2019 in the Kwai Tsing District, with a population of 502,400 (6.8% of the Hong Kong population of 7.42 million) (Census and Statistics Department, 2019). In line with DHC's operational mission, the DHC logo consists of a dot in the centre and three crescents symbolising three tiers of person-centred primary healthcare services of the DHC. The outer crescent represents primary prevention for the healthy general public, the middle crescent signals secondary prevention for individuals at high health risk, and the inner crescent refers to tertiary prevention for patients with chronic diseases. The three crescents also represent three key values of the DHC, namely, "district-based", "public–private partnership", and "medical-social collaboration".

The Core Centre of the Kwai Tsing District DHC consisted of an area of 1,500 square metres and five satellite centres located within the district in providing a range of primary healthcare services, including health promotion, disease prevention, chronic disease management, and community rehabilitation (Table 25.1). DHC operator purchases private healthcare services from the district forming a DHC network, comprising of a primary care team in delivering services such as medical consultation, Chinese medicine consultation, physiotherapy, occupational therapy, dietetics, optometry, podiatry, and speech therapy. The DHC operator contracts separately with the network service providers and the Government offers subsidies for the provision of DHC network services. Certain group activities and individual healthcare services provided by nurses, pharmacists, and social workers at the DHC for members are free-of-charge. Individual healthcare services including medical consultation, allied health services, Chinese medicine services, and medical laboratory services require out-of-pocket co-payment by the DHC user. DHCs and DHC Expresses would be established in all the 18 districts of Hong Kong to improve accessibility through a wide geographical coverage in the locality, shifting the emphasis of the healthcare system from treatment-oriented to prevention-focused approach.

Table 25.1 Key functions and features of DHC

Key functions	Key features
A service/resource hub	Community based services
Health promotion	District based services
Disease prevention and screening	Public private partnership
Chronic disease management	Medical social collaboration
Community rehabilitation	Outreach service

The Singapore Experience

In Singapore, various service models and financing mechanisms of its healthcare system had been implemented over the years (Ministry of Health, Singapore, 2022). Effort in building up links and establishing networks between hospitals and local primary care providers with initiatives supporting professional development and integration of public and private healthcare providers to meet increasing chronic disease management needs had been invested by Singapore. A whole-of-government approach in implementing infrastructure, improving service quality, and developing manpower had been important factors to achieve and sustain universal health coverage. There were over a thousand of private clinics, mostly as solo practices, complemented by polyclinics operated by the public sector in supporting a wide range of comprehensive services for chronic disease management, emergency care, diagnostics, disease complication screening, pharmacy services, and preventive care at an affordable rate at the district-based primary care networks. Such model is strategic in promoting care from the hospital to the community. About eighty per cent of primary care services are provided by private practitioners working in solo general practice clinics and multi-physician group practices, while around twenty per cent of such services are delivered by public primary care clinics or polyclinics.

To enhance primary care, the Ministry of Health of Singapore introduced the Primary Care Networks (PCN) scheme to encourage general practitioner clinics in the private sector to organise into networks in supporting holistic and team-based care. Patients receive care through a multi-disciplinary team including doctors, nurses, and primary care coordinators under the scheme for more effective management of their chronic conditions. Patients could access ancillary and support services provided by the PCN, such as diabetic foot and eye screening, to facilitate management of chronic conditions. The PCN scheme is part of the strategic shift to move care beyond the hospital to the community, so that patients can receive effective care closer to home. A strengthened primary care sector could keep the population healthy and manage their chronic conditions holistically within the community (Ministry of Health, Singapore, 2020).

Challenges

Integrated approaches lead to significant synergies in health service delivery. Structural integration of service delivery at the community and primary care levels may result in potential synergy. Intensifying co-ordination of primary healthcare services, empowering patients for patient-centred participatory self-management and health independency, and equipping carers with essential health awareness can be attainable at the district-based health system (Wagner, 2000). The actual implementation of the concept of district-based health system is complex and can be overwhelming. Certain challenges exist in limiting the widespread implementation of District Health Care, including health-seeking behaviour of public, affordability of the public, payment logistics or financial incentives for healthcare providers, regulatory barriers, and segmentation of governance in policy level. Some of the challenges are global ones while certain barriers are specific to local situations. In the modern era, the opportunity in adopting technology solutions, in terms of communication applications, clinical decision support tools, tele-monitoring, and tele-medicine, may be beneficial in complementing existing gaps such as system integration or overcoming challenges such as information dissemination which were less efficiently and effectively performed in the past without the availability of various technological options, which were developed at a rapidly evolving pace.

Family Physicians and the District Health Care Movement

Family Physicians serve a core role in the primary healthcare team of the district health system when delivering a patient-centred whole-person care in the community. A cross-sectional study was conducted by the Hong Kong College of Family Physicians in 2021 to explore Family Physicians' understanding of the DHC in Hong Kong and to gather opinions from them in enabling the District Health Centre and the primary healthcare team to fulfil their mission and vision of District Health Care Movement. Over 300 respondents completed the survey. Around half worked in the public sector and another half worked in the private sector. More than two-third of the respondents knew what the District Health Centre was, although fewer were aware of the objectives of the District Health Centre. In general, participants responded the services provided by the District Health Centre were appropriate despite some barriers were identified by the respondents, including obstacles encountered in clinical practice during chronic disease management, and lack of financial subsidies and allied health support. Nearly eighty per cent of respondents rated the District Health Centre as a useful set up to benefit the general public through a comprehensive care with higher quality services, as alternative options for the public in the community. Regarding the likelihood of using District Health Centre services, such as social work services, cognitive function assessment, fall prevention services, mean scores of respondents working in private sector were statistically lower than those working in the public sector (Leung et al., 2021).

Training is another important domain in equipping healthcare providers to deliver high quality of care of the District Health Care Movement. The survey revealed that most respondents did not enrol in the training funding scheme as some of the Family Physicians perceived there was a lack of need owing to those who were Family Medicine Specialists with adequate depth and breadth of professional clinical training, and the lack of time. In addition to the training funding scheme, there are several programmes in Hong Kong that provide training to primary care doctors such as the Diploma programmes and other post-graduate courses in Family Medicine and primary care. Most respondents viewed that training subsidies offered by the government could be an incentive to encourage more healthcare professionals to enrol in relevant training to support primary healthcare development in the city. The study concluded that District Health Centre was an important initiative to strengthen local district-based primary healthcare services. Most primary care providers found District Health Centre useful. Findings from the survey provided information on areas of improvement to further increase the utilisation of District Health Centre by primary care providers. Implementing academic research or survey findings to practice is crucial to the long-term success of District Health Care Movement with purposeful alignment of successful strategies through evidence-based framework (Leung et al., 2021).

Conclusion

District Health Care Movement is an important initiative in filling the existing gaps of the healthcare system through the delivery of a high quality multi-disciplinary care in the community by a whole-of-society approach. Various societies have had different models and stages of District Health Care Movement in terms of the system, delivery, and degree of participation. Implementing effective District Health Care Movement is a complex process that requires attention to a number of key enablers that are derived from community needs, clinical experiences, academic research, and very importantly, the committed healthcare team with support from the government. Strong commitment at the leadership level with strategic vision would be a key factor for adoption and implementation of the movement. District Health Care Movement shall strive to better co-ordinate and integrate healthcare resources, making it more accessible, available, and affordable to meet healthcare needs of the community.

References

Census and Statistics Department. (2019). *Hong Kong monthly digest of statistics—The profile of Hong Kong population analysed by district council district, 2019.* https://www.statistics.gov.hk/pub/B72009FB2020XXXXB0100.pdf

Chatora, R., & Tumusiime, P. (2004). *Health sector reform and district health systems.* World Health Organization. https://staging.afro.who.int/sites/default/files/2017-06/dsdAFR-DHS-0301_0.pdf

Lee, A. (2019). Family physicians and district health system. *The Hong Kong Practitioner, 41*(3), 57–59. https://www.hkcfp.org.hk/Upload/HK_Practitioner/2019/hkp2019vol41Sep/editorial.html

Lee, A., & Poon, P. K. (2020). District health systems and capacity building. In B. Y. F. Fong, V. T. S. Law, & A. Lee (Eds.), *Primary care revisited: Interdisciplinary perspectives for a new era* (pp. 369–381). Springer. https://doi.org/10.1007/978-981-15-2521-6_23

Leung, W. L. H., Chan, A. C. Y., Chan, D. C. C., Ho, R. Y. F., & Wong, S. Y. S. (2021). Survey on family doctors' perception of the District Health Centre (DHC) in Hong Kong. *The Hong Kong Practitioner, 43*(3), 68–79. https://www.hkcfp.org.hk/Upload/HK_Practitioner/2021/hkp2021vol43Sep/original_article.html

Ministry of Health, Singapore. (2020). *Primary care networks.* https://www.moh.gov.sg/home/our-healthcare-system/healthcare-services-and-facilities/primary-care-networks

Ministry of Health, Singapore. (2022). *Primary healthcare services.* https://www.moh.gov.sg/home/our-healthcare-system/healthcare-services-and-facilities/primary-healthcare-services

Tan, K. B., & Earn Lee, C. (2019). Integration of primary care with hospital services for sustainable universal health coverage in Singapore. *Health Systems & Reform, 5*(1), 18–23. https://doi.org/10.1080/23288604.2018.1543830

Tarimo, E. (1991). *Towards a healthy district: Organizing and managing district health systems based on primary health care.* World Health Organization. https://apps.who.int/iris/bitstream/handle/10665/40785/9241544120.pdf?sequence=1&isAllowed=y

Wagner, E. H. (2000). The role of patient care teams in chronic disease management. *BMJ, 320*(7234), 569–572. https://doi.org/10.1136/bmj.320.7234.569

World Health Organization. (2021). *Primary health care.* https://www.who.int/news-room/fact-sheets/detail/primary-health-care

Chapter 26
Connecting Each Other in Rare Diseases: A Call for Cross-Regional Collaboration

Bun Sheng

Abstract Rare diseases, according to the definition of the European Union, refer to diseases with a population incidence less than 1:2,000. Although individually rare, as a group, they are numerous and affect 4% of the population. More than 80% of these rare diseases are hereditary and many of them have a complicated pathophysiology and lack an effective treatment. In recent years, this pessimistic perspective about rare diseases has been revolutionised through a wider application of molecular genetic diagnostics. Major advancements have been made in rare disease research and an increasing number of innovative therapeutics are now available for commercial use. Despite these technological advancements, the global outlook for rare diseases still faces major challenges, ranging from health inequities within countries or across regions, prioritisation in national healthcare policies, differences in social welfare and health insurance systems, and incentives in rare disease drug development to an individual patient's journey of accessibility to rare disease diagnosis and treatments and unaffordable drug costs. There are multiple obstacles and gaps calling for action and substantial opportunities for improvement. In response to the strong plea from the rare disease population, the 7th Asia-Pacific Economic Cooperation (APEC) High-Level Meeting on Health and the Economy 2017 has set up an initiative for rare diseases and proposed the APEC Action Plan on Rare Disease with the vision that by 2025, APEC member economies will aim to improve the economic and social inclusion of all those affected by rare diseases by addressing barriers to healthcare and social welfare services. Another initiative led by the World Health Organization (WHO) and Rare Diseases International (RDI) is also underway to promote universal health coverage (UHC) for rare diseases through a global collaborative network in rare disease management. On 16 December 2021, the United Nations adopted the first resolution addressing the challenges experienced by persons living with a rare disease and their families. Through these high-level, policy-driven movements, a growing opportunity in cross-regional rare disease collaborations at different levels is seen. It is time for action.

B. Sheng (✉)
Department of Medicine and Geriatrics, Princess Margaret Hospital, Hong Kong, China
e-mail: shengb@ha.org.hk

B. Y. F. Fong and W. C. W. Wong (eds.), *Gaps and Actions in Health Improvement from Hong Kong and Beyond*,
https://doi.org/10.1007/978-981-99-4491-0_26

Keywords Rare disease · Orphan drugs · Universal health coverage

What Is a Rare Disease?

There is no universal definition for a rare disease. As the name implies, rare diseases are health conditions that affect only a small number of people when compared to the prevalent, common diseases that affect the population. Individual rare disease might be neglected in healthcare policies or at the regulatory level given only a small number of patients are affected. However, although each individual disease is rare, it is not uncommon for a person to be affected by a rare disease because more than 6,000 rare diseases have been identified that collectively affect a conservative population of 300 million, or 4% of the world population, which is the paradox of rarity (Nguengang Wakap et al., 2020). With as many as one in 25 citizens suffering from rare diseases, it is obviously a large loophole in national healthcare policy that their medical and social welfare needs are not being adequately addressed.

Under a national healthcare policy for rare diseases, the prevalence of a disease is the most common data that is referred to, and a disease with a prevalence in a country below a certain threshold is defined as rare. This threshold level varies greatly among countries with an official rare disease definition, ranging from 1:1,500 in the US to 1:100,000 in Turkey (Richter et al., 2015). The threshold has no good scientific evidence or universal agreement and the original initiative of having a certain figure, such as that in the US Orphan Drug Act in 1983, is to provide incentives and encouragement for drug development in the field of rare diseases. Under this federal law, a rare disease is defined as any disease affecting less than 200,000 persons or 1:1,500 in the United States (US). In the European Union (EU), the European Commission defines rare diseases as 'life-threatening or chronically debilitating diseases with a low prevalence', and this 'low prevalence' is fewer than 1:2,000. The EU definition is not exclusively based on prevalence; criteria on severity and rarity should both be satisfied for a rare disease designation. The prevalence thresholds for rare disease definitions in the Asian Pacific region are listed in Table 26.1. Apart from a low prevalence, rare diseases also share the characteristics of having a complicated pathophysiology, are progressive, have a debilitating clinical course, and are often life threatening. The majority (80%) are hereditary, and many (70% of hereditary diseases) manifest in childhood. Treatment is only available for a few of these diseases, and most have no cure. These factors combined together distinguish rare diseases as a unique entity that are not integrated into the public healthcare system, and therefore, an alternative, innovative approach should be adopted.

To provide a common reference to facilitate the recognition of rare diseases in healthcare systems, policy development, and the measurement of changes at both local and international levels, the World Health Organization (WHO) and Rare Diseases International (RDI), the largest rare disease patient advocacy organisation formed by a broad representations of national rare disease alliances across the globe, are working together for an internationally recognised operational definition of rare

Table 26.1 Rare disease definitions in Asian Pacific countries/regions

Asian Pacific countries/ regions	Rare disease definition	Remarks
Australia	1:2,000	DOH
China	1:10,000	Unofficial
India	1:2,500	Unofficial
Japan	1:2,500	MHLW
Singapore	1:2,000	MOH
South Korea	1:2,500	MFDS
Taiwan	1:10,000	MHW

Note DOH: Department of Health; MHLW: Ministry of Health, Labour, and Welfare; MOH: Ministry of Health; MFDS: Ministry of Food and Drug Safety; MHW: Ministry of Health and Welfare

diseases (Rare Diseases International, n.d.). The proposed new operational definition will comprise a core definition of rare diseases that is complemented by a descriptive framework, embracing not only the disease characteristics and prevalence but also specific clinical and quality challenges that are faced by patients living with rare diseases. This common reference will help to align national rare disease policies in different healthcare systems and promulgate international collaborations to improve the quality of care under universal health coverage.

An Underprivileged Population of People Living with Rare Diseases

Rare diseases are highly diverse and heterogeneous. Among the more than 6,000 rare diseases that have been identified, 80% are hereditary conditions, and the majority of these hereditary conditions present during childhood. The initial presentation of diseases with childhood onset is often nonspecific, including feeding problems, developmental delays, intellectual disabilities, cognitive regression, seizures, and different forms of neurological symptoms. Some diseases have a characteristic dysmorphic appearance that can be easily recognised, and some children present with acute life-threatening conditions. Diagnosis is often difficult and delayed, and a correct diagnosis may not be achieved even after comprehensive laboratory and imaging studies. Other than the complexity of their disease nature, rare disease patients also suffer from the ignorance or incompetence of medical professionals regarding the disease. Rare diseases are not covered in medical school curriculum and are only presented in short sentences or small print in general medical textbooks. Clinicians can hardly learn about these diseases from clinical practice due to their rarity, fail to recognise the diseases, which leads to delayed or inappropriate investigations, and often provide wrong treatments. It has been a common experience for rare disease patients to undergo a diagnostic odyssey before being correctly diagnosed. However, even with a correct diagnosis, clinicians often do not have the required skills or knowledge to treat these patients, and treatment options, if any, could be very limited.

Many inherited metabolic diseases could be better managed with nutritional interventions. It has been demonstrated that if diagnosed early, appropriate nutritional intervention, with the restriction of certain dietary elements, e.g. phenylalanine restrictions in patients with phenylketonuria whose bodies cannot metabolise the amino acid because of a deficiency of the enzyme phenylalanine hydroxylase, could result in normal growth. For such an intervention to be successful, patients need to learn the different compositions of food elements and be able to perform conversions to fulfil their nutritional needs in their daily dietary preparations. This dietary intervention is unfamiliar to many clinicians and requires dietitians with special training in metabolic diseases to implement advice tailored to the dietary pattern of the country. In addition, with a very restrictive diet, some patients may require nutritional supplements to support their body requirements. These special nutritional products are not readily available in some countries and are usually expensive. For some other diseases, the available treatments are so expensive that the patients or their families would find it hard to afford them if there is no reimbursement from the healthcare authority or medical insurance. Unlike the general public, rare disease patients are often deprived of the right to enjoy an accessible and affordable quality medical service.

Unsurprisingly, under these common themes of challenges, being able to access treatments and therapies that do not yet exist, better coordination of health care, and promoting access to healthcare specialists were the top three priorities identified in a large international survey with rare disease patients regarding their future needs' assessment in 2030 (Dubief et al., 2021). It is a message of urgency to political, academic, and industrial leaders to address the unmet healthcare needs of patients with rare diseases. Patients living with rare diseases are not fighting on their own fronts and sustainable quality health care for rare diseases can only be achieved through multilevel, cross-disciplinary, and international collaborations.

Advancements in Rare Diseases: The Impact of National Rare Disease Policies

The vision of the Sustainable Development Goals is a world in which no one is left behind, including people who suffer from rare diseases. As described by Dr. Tedros Adhanom Ghebreyesus, WHO Director-General, in his statement for Rare Disease Day in 2018, just because a disease affects a small number of people does not make it irrelevant or less important than diseases that affect millions of people (World Health Organization, 2018).

Drug development in rare diseases has unique challenges. Many rare diseases do not have a good animal model in preclinical studies. The prevalence of a rare disease in a country or in a specific ethnic population is usually unknown, the natural history of the disease is often unclear, and treatment effect can be difficult to measure. The design of clinical trials is limited by the small number of eligible patients being recruited, with adverse influences on the validity and generalisability of the observations. All these issues have contributed to the high uncertainty of rare disease research projects and the historic lack of industrial investment in the field of rare diseases. Therefore, despite rapid scientific advancements in the medical field, drug development in the rare disease field has been scarce, and the problem became prominent in the late 1970s. Many different rare disease patient groups and patient advocates emerged, and in the early 1980s in the US, a coalition was formed, which later became the National Organization for Rare Disorders (NORD). The NORD was instrumental in the subsequent enactment of the US Orphan Drug Act in 1983 to encourage drug discovery for rare diseases. Under the Orphan Drug Act, a new drug that targets a disease affecting fewer than 200,000 individuals in the US population could be granted orphan drug designation to enjoy the many incentives for the development of drugs for rare diseases, which includes tax reductions, guidance on clinical trial design, access to research grants to fund drug development, fast-track FDA review and approval, and 7-year marketing exclusivity after a commercial launch.

Many countries followed by developing legislation to provide similar regulatory and economic incentives for developing drugs for rare diseases. This included the formation of the Japanese Ministry of Health, Labour, and Welfare (MHLW) in 1993 and the European Medicines Agency (EMA) in 2000. The FDA and EMA collaborated to harmonise the regulatory process and establish a parallel scientific advice procedure to guide study design and clinical data requirements. It has been noted that 50% of orphan drug submissions to the EMA are now done in parallel to submissions to the FDA (Mariz et al., 2016). These incentives greatly enhanced the development of drugs for rare diseases (Mulberg et al., 2019). There have been over 6,000 orphan drug designations and over 1,000 orphan drug authorisations by the FDA since the Orphan Drug Act was established in 1983 and over 2,200 orphan designations with over 160 authorisations by the EMA since 2000.

Introducing more orphan drugs into commercial markets does not necessarily imply easier patient access to treatments. Countries differ widely in their healthcare budgets with reference to their GDP, structures of national tax and health insurance, and public and private shares of the healthcare market. Many orphan drugs are ultra-expensive, with unclear benefits or limited clinical evidence. Health economics result in a high incremental cost-effectiveness ratio (ICER) that exceeds the usual threshold for reimbursement or health insurance coverage. This unaffordable high cost and the unwillingness to pay have greatly restricted patient access to orphan drugs in many high-income countries, not just in low-income countries. In addition, since the drug price in a region usually refers to the pricing of products in other countries, manufacturers are reluctant to enter new markets at the expense of price reductions to avoid cascading price cuts. In the survey conducted by Dubief et al. (2021), 24% of rare disease patients in Europe did not receive treatment because no drugs were available in their countries, and another 15% did not receive treatment because of unaffordability. Even if a treatment is covered in a healthcare system, the resulting high cost often warrants strict restrictions on treatment eligibility to contain health expenditure, which in turn limits the number of patients who benefit.

As illustrated from the priorities that were identified in the international rare disease patient survey, drug accessibility is only one of the priority concerns. Very few rare diseases have established treatments, and the majority of rare disease patients suffer from a long diagnostic odyssey, lack of medical expertise in clinical care, lack of information, and lack of service coordination to meet their needs. The availability of an effective drug could be life-changing for some patients, but it is not sufficient to change the landscape of rare diseases and does not direct patient-centred medical care to the rare disease population. Many countries have established national action plans, frameworks, or policies regarding rare diseases, and these measures have extended the focus of rare diseases from just medical care to education, social welfare, insurance, etc., touching on every aspect of daily life for rare disease populations (Department of Health and Social Care, 2022; Dharssi et al., 2017; Schieppati et al., 2008; Song et al., 2012). Common themes in these action plans include providing education for and improving awareness of clinicians, applying new genomic technologies in diagnosis, expanding new-born screening programmes for early detection, promoting fast-track evaluations and approvals for orphan drugs, creating reimbursement programmes to improve drug accessibility, developing coordinated care through the establishment of tertiary referral centres or rare disease centres of excellence to nurture expertise, improving quality of care, and supporting research and development of new treatments. It does not matter whether a country is wealthy or economically depleted, these kinds of action plans or roadmaps are indispensable for achieving the goal of universal health coverage (UHC) (World Health Organization, 2014).

Emerging Hopes in the Era of Big Data

Individual rare disease affects a small number of patients, and the actual disease prevalence in a country is often unknown. More patient data are needed to understand the natural history of a disease, spectrum of severity, prognosis, and effects of treatments. Numerous disease registries have been established internationally to collect information regarding specific diseases. These registries can be hosted by academic institutions or collaborate with patient associations, and many are country specific. Although it is important to understand a disease in a country to command the delivery of health care, it could be a waste of data if such information is not integrated into similar registries elsewhere. Efforts have been made to best use the available information by developing registries on a common platform that satisfies the requirements for patient privacy and national legislation restrictions on data security and sharing. One initial effort was RD-Connect, an international community funded by the EU working toward accelerating rare disease research worldwide through the provision of the global RD-Connect Platform, which facilitates research on rare diseases by incorporating databases, patient registries, biobanks, and clinical bioinformatics data into a central resource for researchers worldwide (Thompson et al., 2014). There were some illustrative examples on registries in the RT-Connect approved platform but the overall result was not convincing. One difficulty was the lack of control of the data type to be collected, making the data integration unsuccessful. The academic fields would need to collaborate more on registry designs and data requirements to improve the possibility of cross-national or cross-registry data flow and integration, which could greatly improve our understanding of rare diseases.

Automatic data captured from health informatics systems are another source of big data in the field of rare diseases. Many countries now use electronic healthcare records in their healthcare system to facilitate information transfer and patient management both in primary and secondary health care. In Hong Kong, for example, we are privileged to have a mature and unified electronic patient record system (ePR) that basically captures all clinical activities within the Hospital Authority. However, much information has been idle. It would be a very attractive idea if a registry could be developed through linking the ePR with automatic data capture followed by clearing. Once a patient is identified by ICD coding, the subsequent data on hospitalisation, drug dispensing, clinical attention, imaging studies, rehabilitation service utilisation, etc., could all be extracted through the system and give a good account of the need for health care. Hong Kong is already present in this big data party. Mrs. Carrie Lam, Chief Executive of the Hong Kong Special Administrative Region, announced in her 2019 policy address that the government and the Hospital Authority planned to progressively implement a series of targeted measures, including examining the establishment of databases for individual uncommon disorders to facilitate clinical diagnosis and treatment, deploying resources to promote relevant scientific research and development, and enhancing public awareness of uncommon disorders (The Hong Kong Special Administrative Region of the People's Republic of China, 2019). It was a strong message to the rare disease initiative in Hong Kong.

The International Community

Multilevel, cross-regional collaboration is the key to combating rare diseases. An APEC initiative for rare diseases was set up in the 7th APEC High-Level Meeting on Health and the Economy in 2017 (Asia-Pacific Economic Cooperation, 2017). Under this initiative, the APEC Life Sciences Innovation Forum formed a Rare Disease Network that, through a series of consultations with stakeholders including policymakers, patients, healthcare workers, academies, and industries, developed the APEC Action Plan on Rare Diseases, with the vision that by 2025, APEC member economies will aim to improve the economic and social inclusion of all those affected by rare diseases by addressing barriers to health care and social welfare services. Under the APEC Action Plan, an APEC Life Sciences Innovation Forum was formed, and it adopted a triparty approach engaging governments, academic institutions, industries, and patient consultants in piloting local programmes to drive early access, diagnosis, and treatment in APEC countries. Progress has been made through a series of training workshops to harmonise the health product registration and evaluation, with a vision to accelerate regulatory convergence for medical products in the APEC region as much as possible by 2030 to protect people's safety, make life-saving products available, save public resources, attract investment, mitigate corruption, and improve global standing in the economy of every APEC country. The APEC Action Plan for Rare Diseases is a strong driver of rare disease policy development in the region.

The Global Village for Rare Diseases

Within a country, there are urban cities where sophisticated and complicated medical treatments can be delivered within well-equipped tertiary medical facilities whereas in remote villages only primary health service can be supported. Patients with medical needs that exceed the capacity of the rural clinics are hence diverted to the more appropriate secondary or tertiary facilities to receive treatments. While the majority of basic health care can be addressed locally, the care of more complicated patients can be centralised in facilities with experience and expertise in treating their problems, thus the quality of service could be sustained. This is a very reasonable and logical distribution of medical resources to serve the whole population of the country. Breaking down the country boundary, in the global village, there are well-developed regions (countries) where advanced medical needs for rare diseases could be better addressed and less privileged regions (countries) lacking the required expertise and technology for rare diseases. It is unreasonable that a similar model could not be adopted through cross-regional collaboration for rare diseases—not just for research and clinical trials but for diagnosis, treatment, and continuous medical care. This is the initiative taken by the WHO and RDI to develop a Collaborative Global Network for Rare Diseases under the policy framework of UHC 2019 and the UN Resolution on Addressing the Challenges of Persons Living with a Rare Disease and their Families (United Nations General Assembly, 2019, 2021). It adopts a structured approach of clustering rare diseases by therapeutic areas to be inclusive of all people with rare diseases and leave no one behind. Under the proposal, countries with mixed levels are clustered together to form regional networks, and each nation will develop rare disease national hubs through credentialing. Within the regional network, national hubs connect with each other virtually forming a regional hub, and different regional hubs are connected under a WHO global network. Through these national, regional hubs and global network, training and data collection, research collaborations, virtual consultations, and laboratory support can be developed. Local capacities can be strengthened, and health equity can be reinforced.

The COVID-19 pandemic might have restricted international travel and personal contact but it also boosted the information explosion with innovative IT solutions through webinars, online interactive workshops, better distant learning toolkits, telemedicine, and virtual consultations. Virtual connection with people has never been easier, and there has never been a better time to connect with each other regarding rare diseases.

References

Asia-Pacific Economic Cooperation. (2017). *APEC action plan on rare diseases*. https://www.apec.org/-/media/Satellite/Rare-Diseases/APEC_ActionPlan.pdf

Department of Health and Social Care. (2022). *England rare diseases action plan 2022*. https://www.gov.uk/government/publications/england-rare-diseases-action-plan-2022

Dharssi, S., Wong-Rieger, D., Harold, M., & Terry, S. (2017). Review of 11 national policies for rare diseases in the context of key patient needs. *Orphanet Journal of Rare Diseases, 12*, Article 63. https://doi.org/10.1186/s13023-017-0618-0

Dubief, J., Kole, A., Berjonneau, E., & Courbier, S. (2021). *Rare disease patients' opinion on the future of rare diseases: A rare barometer survey for the rare 2030 foresight study*. EURORDIS-Rare Diseases Europe. https://download2.eurordis.org/rbv/rare2030survey/reports/RARE2030_survey_public_report_en.pdf

Mariz, S., Reese, J. H., Westermark, K., Greene, L., Goto, T., Hoshino, T., Llinares-Garcia, J., & Sepodes, B. (2016). Worldwide collaboration for orphan drug designation. *Nature Reviews Drug Discovery, 15*(6), 440–441.

Mulberg, A. E., Bucci-Rechtweg, C., Giuliano, J., Jacoby, D., Johnson, F. K., Liu, Q., Marsden, D., McGoohan, S., Nelson, R., Patel, N., Romero, K., Sinha, V., Sitaraman, S., Spaltro, J., & Kessler, V. (2019). Regulatory strategies for rare diseases under current global regulatory statutes: A discussion with stakeholders. *Orphanet Journal of Rare Diseases, 14*, Article 36. https://doi.org/10.1186/s13023-019-1017-5

Nguengang Wakap, S., Lambert, D. M., Olry, A., Rodwell, C., Gueydan, C., Lanneau, V., Murphy, D., Le Cam, Y., & Rath, A. (2020). Estimating cumulative point prevalence of rare diseases: Analysis of the Orphanet database. *European Journal of Human Genetics, 28*(2), 165–173. https://doi.org/10.1038/s41431-019-0508-0

Rare Diseases International. (n.d.). *Collaborative global network for rare diseases*. https://www.rarediseasesinternational.org/collaborative-global-network/

Richter, T., Nestler-Parr, S., Babela, R., Khan, Z. M., Tesoro, T., Molsen, E., & Hughes, D. A. (2015). Rare disease terminology and definitions—A systematic global review: Report of the ISPOR rare disease special interest group. *Value in Health, 18*(6), 906–914. https://doi.org/10.1016/j.jval.2015.05.008

Schieppati, A., Henter, J. I., Daina, E., & Aperia, A. (2008). Why rare diseases are an important medical and social issue. *The Lancet, 371*(9629), 2039–2041. https://doi.org/10.1016/S0140-6736(08)60872-7

Song, P., Gao, J., Inagaki, Y., Kokudo, N., & Tang, W. (2012). Rare diseases, orphan drugs, and their regulation in Asia: Current status and future perspectives. *Intractable & Rare Diseases Research, 1*(1), 3–9. https://doi.org/10.5582/irdr.2012.v1.1.3

The Hong Kong Special Administrative Region of the People's Republic of China. (2019). *The Chief Executive's 2019 Policy Address*. https://www.policyaddress.gov.hk/2019/eng/p1.html

Thompson, R., Johnston, L., Taruscio, D., Monaco, L., Béroud, C., Gut, I. G., Hansson, M. G., 't Hoen, P.-B. A., Patrinos, G. P., Dawkins, H., Ensini, M., Zatloukal, K., Koubi, D., Heslop, E., Paschall, J. E., Posada, M., Robinson, P. N., Bushby, K., & Lochmüller, H. (2014). RD-Connect: An integrated platform connecting databases, registries, biobanks and clinical bioinformatics for rare disease research. *Journal of General Internal Medicine, 29*(3), 780–787. https://doi.org/10.1007/s11606-014-2908-8

United Nations General Assembly. (2019, October 18). *Political declaration of the high-level plenary meeting on universal health coverage: Resolution/adopted by the general assembly*. https://digitallibrary.un.org/record/3833350/files/A_RES_74_2-EN.pdf

United Nations General Assembly. (2021, December 16). *Addressing the challenges of persons living with a rare disease and their families: Resolution/adopted by the general assembly*. https://digitallibrary.un.org/record/3953765/files/A_RES_76_132-EN.pdf

World Health Organization. (2014). *Making fair choices on the path to universal health coverage: Final report of the WHO consultative group on equity and universal health coverage*. https://apps.who.int/iris/bitstream/handle/10665/112671/9789241507158_eng.pdf;jsessionid=76B5F12B21531BF62AB0BB7BB0BD100C?sequence=1

World Health Organization. (2018, February 27). *Statement for rare disease day*. https://www.who.int/news/item/27-02-2018-statement-for-rare-disease-day

Chapter 27
Medicalisation in Healthcare

Francesca Quattri

Abstract This chapter provides a theoretical understanding and an overview of the meaning and implications of 'too much too soon' and 'too little too late' medicine, focusing on the medicalised, fear- and risk-based approach to care that seems conducive to practising care defensively. The author will examine an interventionist and risk-based model of care and how it applies to the healthcare system in the UK, the NHS, using examples drawn from the primary, secondary, and tertiary pathways of care, with a particular focus on maternity care. It is shown that an interventionist approach to care does not necessarily lead to high-value care but that it may instead trigger opportunist costs and low-value care. 'Too much medicine' does not create health for all, but it instead creates a gap in health improvements while hindering health equity. Furthermore, with a nuanced approach to the topic, it is argued that the root of a mechanistic approach to care in maternity and healthcare is generated from layers of biased decisions and wrongdoings that include single individuals as well as whole care structures. An alternative model of care will be presented and critically appraised, along with some viable solutions that could be implemented relatively swiftly.

Keywords 'Too much medicine' · Overdiagnosis · Overtreatment · Excessive medicine · Care models · Maternity care · NHS · UK

Definition(s) and Examples of Too Much Medicine

The term 'overdiagnosis' has only recently been acknowledged as a medical term and added as a search word in the US National Library of Medicine (NLM) (Woloshin & Kramer, 2021). Although the meaning of the term is still debatable to date, an official definition has been proposed by two renewed scholars in the Too Much Medicine community. The Too Much Medicine movement includes numerous scholars and

F. Quattri (✉)
Department of Population Health Sciences, University of Leicester, Leicester, UK
e-mail: quattri.francesca@gmail.com

B. Y. F. Fong and W. C. W. Wong (eds.), *Gaps and Actions in Health Improvement from Hong Kong and Beyond*,
https://doi.org/10.1007/978-981-99-4491-0_27

activists around the globe who are studying the effects of excessive healthcare treatments and interventions on different populations and in different medical specialties. They are pushing forward evidence that 'too much medicine' is not a good medical practice, as it may expose patients and clients to unnecessary and avoidable harm and risks.

Woloshin and Kramer's definition of overdiagnosis reads (Woloshin & Kramer, 2021)

> The labelling of a person with a disease or abnormal condition that would not have caused the person harm if left undiscovered, creating new diagnoses by medicalising ordinary life experiences, or expanding existing diagnoses by lowering thresholds or widening criteria without evidence of improved outcomes. Individuals derive no clinical benefit from overdiagnosis, although they may experience physical, psychological, or financial harm.

Overtreatment subjects the patients or clients to unnecessary procedures and treatments following a diagnosis. Overdiagnosis and overtreatment are not correlated concepts, as overdiagnosis does not always lead to overtreatment, although it can trigger it sometimes.

According to the definition above, overdiagnosis is a *dynamic* process. It can involve discovering dormant conditions and ailments which would not have caused any harm if left unfound or untreated. It is a process of creating new conditions, which involves framing states of mind and bodily reactions that are sometimes normal, predictable, or socially acceptable, but which get treated as clinically worthy of attention and cure. Overdiagnosing may be generated by changing the thresholds and criteria for detecting and treating certain diseases, thus increasing the number of people who get labelled as 'patients' and treated as such. While overdiagnosis and overtreatment may exist for various complex reasons, as shown in this chapter, they can lead to a cascade of procedures where the patients are put on 'conveyor belts' of care (Schlachter, 2017).

Scholars seem to agree that 'too much medicine' proves to be cumbersome for single individuals, the healthcare professionals (HCPs), the patients, and healthcare systems at large (Brownlee et al., 2017; McCartney, 2016; Moynihan et al., 2012; Pathirana et al., 2017; Saini et al., 2017). The risks of harm for overtreated patients usually outweigh the benefits of the received care. The clinical staff is under pressure to deliver the best possible care for more patients. In publicly funded healthcare systems, like the National Health Service (NHS), allocating money to care for people who might not need extra clinical attention and intervention can become an issue and generate opportunistic costs.

A Complex Issue with Treatment Discretion

'Too much medicine' does not happen in a vacuum, as it is the response to mechanisms in the care system that need revision. For instance, several authors have framed 'too much medicine' with reference to probabilities or thresholds. Armstrong states that, in the case of overtreatment and overdiagnosis, the associated treatment for an ailment "has a low probability of benefitting the patient" (Armstrong, 2018), thus proving ineffective. Llewelyn argues that "the cut-offs for diagnosis" in 'too much medicine' "are set too low" (Llewelyn, 2021), and that the notions of 'harm' and 'risk' with regard to treatments and diseases lack taxonomy, which leaves the door open to interpretation, exaggeration, and misunderstanding (Llewelyn, 2021). This can apply, for instance, in maternity care, where the labelling of pregnancies as 'high risk' vs 'low risk' are disputed concepts (Kapfhamer et al., 2012; Pearlman, 2006; Symon, 2000). Treadwell et al. (2021) show that overdiagnosis and overtreatment can increase or decrease in medicine depending on how diagnostic thresholds are changed over time. This has been, for instance, the case with Type 2 diabetes. The diagnostic threshold for Type 2 diabetes was reduced from 140 (mg/dL) to 126 (mg/dL) back in the late 1990s, following national recommendations and guidelines. As a result, an additional US population of 1.7 million people became 'new' diabetics in need of care (Fig. 27.1). The rationale for the threshold decrease was that some people, represented in the red window in the graph, showed some early signs of retinal damage from high blood sugar. It was then suggested to treat these people as the rest of the diagnosed Type 2 diabetes patients, despite any lack of evidence that medication would have improved their health over time.

Patients who suffer from certain conditions, including diabetes, cholesterol, or statins, might be overtreated. As Welch and colleagues documented, lowering the diagnostic threshold for cholesterol in the 1990s led to an increase in the number of patients, with 42.6 million new patients put on statins (Welch et al., 2011). This

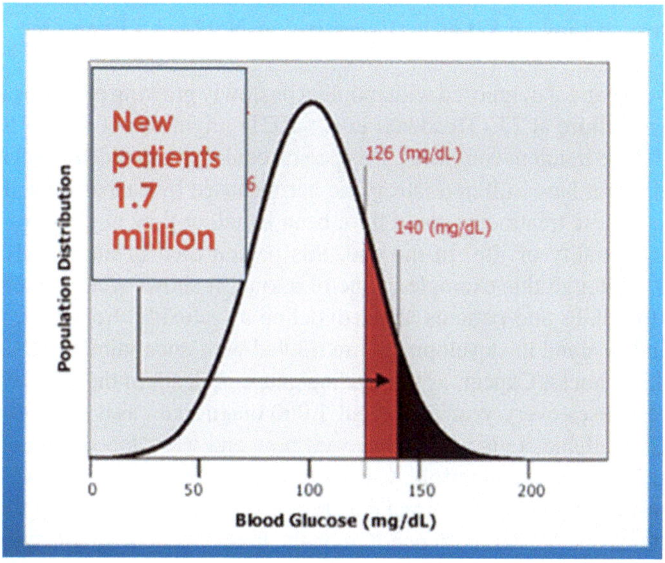

Fig. 27.1 Changes in the diagnostic thresholds for Type 2 diabetes in the late 1990s (*Source* Treadwell et al. 2021)

also applies to psychosomatic conditions, where changes in disease definitions or the creation of new diseases can boost 'too much medicine'. However, some psychosomatic manifestations may happen as a natural, human response to challenging episodes. Hence, not all patients experiencing these moments might need medication or long-term treatments for their symptoms, and not all people who seek help for these symptoms shall be treated as patients.

It is essential to acknowledge that the perception and use of 'too much too soon, too little too late' care can change significantly depending on the level of care given and received, whether it is primary, secondary, or specialist care, which may add confusion to the quest for a single definition of overdiagnosis and overtreatment. Perceptions on 'too much medicine' may also depend on the country's healthcare infrastructure and specific healthcare systems and infrastructures that provide certain kinds of care. For instance, in the United Kingdom (UK), Sajid and colleagues experienced challenges, as NHS practitioners, when discussing or building common diagnostic pathways of care. They noticed that secondary care approaches tend to be dominant in decision-making processes within the NHS. This might project unfairly on the system, where 90% of services are provided in primary care compared to 5% in secondary care. Still, it has been documented that both care pathways present numerous instances of excessive medicine (Brodersen, 2017; Gupta et al., 2020; Kale & Korenstein, 2018; Sajid, 2021), leading to the conclusion that it may eventually rely on the single healthcare practitioners' and patients' discretion to establish what represents and defines 'the best possible care', and to define their tolerance towards risk while exploring treatments and cures.

How to Draw a Line on What Is 'Excessive' or Not?—An Example

A 65-year-old patient diagnosed with indolent or slowly growing prostate cancer who dies of heart failure at 77 (Treadwell et al., 2021) might or not decide to undergo treatment for the indolent condition. This person could have decided to get treated for cancer and might have suffered iatrogenic harm caused by cancer-related interventions or not. These treatments could have been lethal, or they might have worsened this person's quality of life. In the end, this person died of an entirely different reason, and although this example is one of a kind, it shows well how challenging it can be, for HCPs and patients alike, to define a 'valuable' treatment, especially when a condition and its development are riddled with uncertainty and, to a certain extent, unknownness. Cancer, as the leading cause of death in the UK, with around 375,000 new cases every year and about 1,000 diagnosed cases every day (2016–2018; latest available statistics), shows well how and why 'too much medicine' is problematic and how it can unfold. Cancer is a very complex disease, which can be fatal or non-fatal, treatable or untreatable, rare or recurrent, thus calling for different clinical actions and decisions, depending on the kind and the stage of cancer and the patient's preferences. To this day, it is still impossible to apply a one-fit-for-all cure and treatment for this disease, which can exacerbate the quest to try and prevent, cure, eradicate it, or slow it down with the help of more or less aggressive treatments or which might prompt focusing instead on quality of life without seeking any treatment. Podolsky and others claim that treating indolent cancers is ultimately worse for the patients than ignoring them (CEBM Oxford, 2021; Welch, 2010). However, these opinions remain highly debatable, especially given the understandably high emotional toll attached to cancer.

Screenings, which can prevent cancers, can be overly used as well. Screenings provide a good example of how the issue of 'too much medicine' is tangled with other issues, which might not necessarily be related to care and treatment. Scholars have denounced for instance the unfairness in promoting screenings for certain kinds of cancer over others, and the technical inefficiency that screenings entail, eventually impacting on patient safety and disease prevention (Bewley, 2020; Brodersen, 2017; Cassels, 2012; Clarfield, 2010; DeFrank et al., 2015; Katz, 2013; Salerno et al., 2019; Shmerling, 2018; Szabo, 2017). Some screenings might be done inappropriately, as they are done outside Wilson's criteria for screentests (Wilson & Jungner, 1968), potentially leading to overdiagnosis and overtreatment. Recent research shows for instance that 1 in 5 breast cancers detected via mammographic screening in the UK may be overdiagnosed (Bewley, 2020). Treadwell et al. (2021) argue that more than 1 in 3 prostatic cancers detected via PSA screening in the country may also be overdiagnosed. Like any other clinical procedure, screenings can cause or lead to iatrogenic harm or unintentional harm, as demonstrated by thyroid cancer screenings and the booming markets of thyroid removal in South Korea and elsewhere in the world (Ahn et al., 2014; Jegerlehner et al., 2017; Labarge et al., 2018). Opportunistic markets for maternal screenings, such as ultrasound scans for pregnant women, are also on the rise (Howard, 2020).

However, screenings can also save lives, as they can prevent the development of serious ailments, improve the quality of life, and increase life expectancy. The conveyed examples on cancers and screenings have been adopted to provide a glimpse at the evident complexity surrounding the concept of overdiagnosis and overtreatment and the personal and non-personal conflicts that persist behind concepts of 'care' and 'risk' associated to certain diseases. Eventually, it is argued that treatment discretion is advised, as every kind of medical procedure, regardless of its complexity, shall be thoroughly discussed with healthcare professionals, who, together with the patients, shall carefully evaluate their patients' situations, needs, and wishes, as well as the risks and benefits of the procedures. However, as argued in Chapter 6 in this book and by the same author, expectations 'on paper' on the roles and responsibilities of HCPs and patients in decision-making processes do not always match the reality of the job. Realistically, HCPs might not have the means, the time, or the support from the healthcare infrastructure they work for to inform their patients about the best choices thoroughly, and the patients might not have the means, the interest, or the chance of being informed about these procedures, thus allowing instances of overdiagnosis and overtreatment to thrive.

'Too Much Medicine' in Maternity Care

In the UK, maternity care is a complex medical specialty that provides distinct care. While many countries rely primarily on obstetric care and refer to gynaecologists and obstetricians as their prime carers, in the UK, doulas and midwives work alongside obstetricians. Midwives can assist women exclusively, help them give birth in midwifery-led centres, or refer them to obstetric lead units, depending on how well pregnancies progress. Patients can birth in birthing centres, community centres, and hospital wards, or they can be assisted at home. Maternity care staff are long-term providers, caring for mothers and babies, sometimes for a significant amount of time. Maternal care involves many staff and deals with different kinds of clients, as pregnant women can present with all sorts of different, pre-existing, or developing conditions. They can carry unproblematic pregnancies or experience complications before, during and after birth, and in these and similar cases, they may need to be assisted by multidisciplinary teams of primary, secondary and specialist carers, sometimes simultaneously.

There exists "a growing concern" about the impact of 'too much too soon, too little too late' care in maternity care (*The Lancet*, 2016). It has been reported that pain management during childbirth and instrumental deliveries have risen over the years. Scholars in Europe, America, and the UK have recently conducted a multinational cross-sectional study on commonly practised childbirth interventions (Seijmonsberger-Schermers et al., 2020), and they found high percentages in the administration of epidural anaesthesia among nulliparous patients across countries (19.4%), similarly to the use of pharmacological pain relief. The rates of instrumental vaginal deliveries change dramatically across the globe—from 0.7% across multiparous patients in Chile to 7.2% of multiparous patients in England. C-sections remain high across the investigated populations, confirming the 2021 rates reported by the World Health Organization (2021). The authors of the cross-sectional study (Seijmonsberger-Schermers et al., 2020) abstained from investigating the reasons for each country's high or low rates of clinical interventions, as their study's goal was to compare variations of maternity care clinical practices across countries, without insights of possible instances of overdiagnosis or overtreatment.

However, their research provides a comprehensive overview of clinical practices in maternal care that are currently happening across multiple countries, sometimes very different healthcare systems, which have been deemed excessive (Brown, 2007; Murphy, 2001; Orfali, 2012). The rising trends show patterns of care, involving pregnancy and birth, where interventions on births tend to be recurrent, for many, and sometimes not always good, reasons. Hence, it may be reasonable to argue that sometimes, in some circumstances, some healthcare interventions might not be needed, although they are still practised and might be excessive. Indeed, some NHS midwives' and obstetricians' lived experiences of maternal care in the UK reveal instances of 'too much too soon, too little too late' in NHS maternity care (Quattri, 2025). The World Health Organization (World Health Organization, 2021) has raised the flag on increased interventions in maternity care, and it has alerted the international community about the possibility that some practices in maternal care may be excessive and unnecessary (World Health Organization, 2018, 2021).

It has been shown that overdiagnosis and overtreatment are complex phenomena in current society. Scholars seem to agree that 'too much medicine' is pervasive and on the rise (Brownlee et al., 2017; Moynihan, 2012; Moynihan et al., 2008, 2012; Saini et al., 2017), but what are its triggers? The following sections provide an overview.

Triggers of 'Too Much Medicine'

As Thomas (2022) points out, the medicalisation of care and interventionist approaches to care may derive from societal, cultural, political, and economic forces and changes—which can be defined as drivers or triggers of medicalisation and, possibly, overmedicalisation. Lenzer (2012) argues, for instance, that multiple reasons can start overdiagnosis and overtreatment, including fear of medical malpractice lawsuits, lack of medical training, biased research, commercial interests, patients' requests, financial conflicts of guidelines' authors, failure to properly inform patients and share with them the decision-making process. Pathirana and colleagues (2017) have provided a comprehensive oversight of some of these factors and possible solutions, albeit with little evidential support (Fig. 27.2).

However, prescriptive approaches and 'quick fix' solutions to complex issues like overdiagnosis and overtreatment need to be traded carefully. While some factors have been labelled drivers for 'too much medicine' by some authors, it is important to remind that the motivations and the reasons behind each of these alleged triggers remain profoundly personal and contextual. What may look like a driver of 'too much medicine' to somebody might sound like a precautionary, preventative, or even life-saving approach to others. The perceptions of these triggers may change profoundly depending on the patients, the users, and the healthcare professionals involved. For instance, introducing more tests and technology in pregnancy and childbirth has led to more clinical intervention and monitoring. Shall all these interventions be deemed 'excessive'? Some might be as markets exploit the loopholes in the healthcare system for profit (like the case of 'scanxiety' or souvenir scans mentioned above [Howard, 2020]).

Contrarily to Pathirana et al.'s (2017) suggestion that care subjects affecting overdiagnosis and overtreatment could be neatly layered out, as suggested in Fig. 27.2, 'too much medicine' and the factors affecting it might be too complex to be shown in lists. Rather than being concentric to a core, these factors and subjects might probably be best represented in a nested framework, as they are many and intertwined. Also, there needs to be evidence to justify their existence and how much they affect 'too much medicine'.

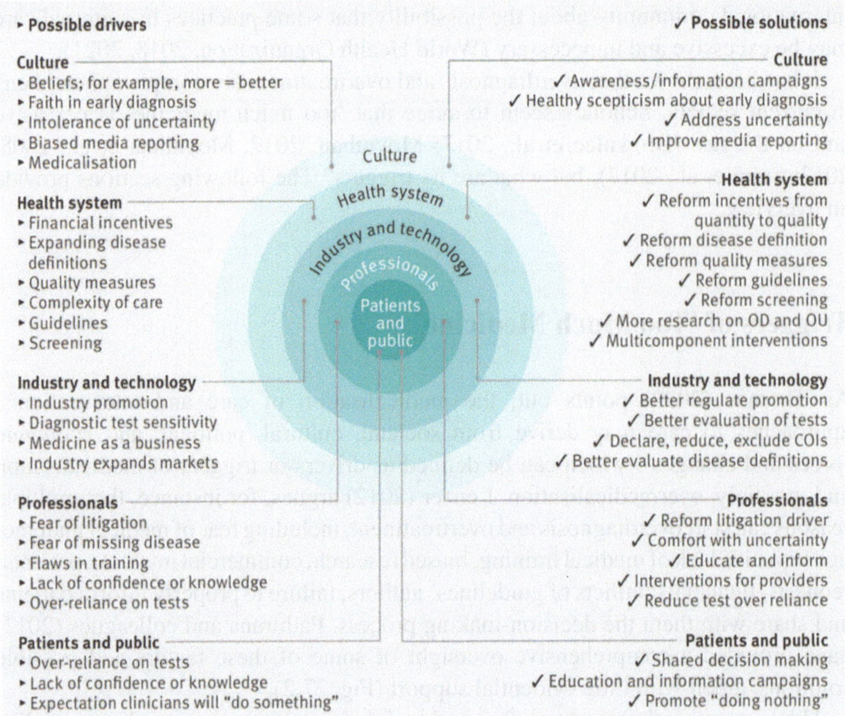

Fig. 27.2 Possible drivers of overdiagnosis and proposed solutions (*Source* Pathirana et al. 2017)

Contextual Care Factors Matter

The context of care in which these drivers operate matters. Drivers of overdiagnosis and overtreatment may be the product of dominating cultures, societal pressures, trends, medical schools, medical training, trusts, units, single individuals, or entire corporations. When analysing them, one cannot escape time and how it affects 'too much medicine'. For instance, the advancement in biotechnologies has profoundly changed the medical profession, and consumer roles and personalised care have gained traction over the years (Conrad, 2007). Drug and advertising regulations have changed, and so have the role and the impact of the Internet on healthcare. Patients and clients are exposed to healthcare matters more than in the past, and some of them might have developed their own opinions on healthcare matters and how they want to be treated (Thomas, 2022). Social media and e-health are also changing healthcare.

Going prescriptively on such care trends by advancing 'quick fixes' may be in vain. Instead, a more sensitised nuanced approach to the topic should be encouraged, where each factor is studied in detail and contextually.

Fear of the Law

Another reason that might motivate HCPs to over-practice medicine, sometimes despite the lack of evidence or benefit, is that they may be worried about the legal, financial, and personal consequences that can happen to them if they do not act according to the expected standards or rules, or if they decide to go with methods and procedures that are not contemplated in healthcare infrastructures' rules and guidelines. They might have perfectly reasonable reasons to practise medicine in a certain way, not least their professional experience and training, and they might be able to back up their medical decisions with evidence, but they might still be fearful to practise 'outside' guidelines. (Positive) defensive medicine refers to clinical choices, sometimes called 'assurance behaviour' practices, that provide little to no value in the patient care but that are performed nonetheless to mitigate or annihilate any possible liability that might happen if adverse events happen (Bourne et al., 2016; Jackson, 2019). With defensive practice, HCPs might, in other words, over-practice or overdiagnose not because it is in their clients' best interests but because they want to avoid criticisms, complaints, civil actions, or even criminal actions against them due to some kind of damage (fatal or non-fatal) that was caused to the patients through their care. Some HCPs may be more worried about medical lawsuits and legal liability than their peers in other specialties. For instance, according to recent data by the NHSR (NHS Resolution, former NHS Litigation Authority), NHS Obstetrics has been for years one of the medical specialties with the highest number of received clinical negligence claims (9% of the total) in the NHS, after Orthopaedic surgery (12%), and A&E (13% of the total received claims). The NHS spends half of the total public money invested in litigation on paying for legal procedures and fees in Obstetrics alone (NHS Resolution, 2019a, 2019b). These data may validate obstetricians' and midwives' fear of legal repercussions if something bad happens to the mothers and their babies.

In reality, the iterative legal and legislative framework, which includes undergoing an investigation, possibly a prosecution, and possibly a trial, is very cumbersome and lengthy for all parties involved, with no guarantee that the damage will be repaid or that the lessons will be learned (Brazier et al., 2016; Brearey-Horne, 2013; Samanta & Samanta, 2021).

Furthermore, HCPs shall not be the only ones to be blamed if something goes awry in clinical care. Clinical decisions are seldom made alone. Medicine, including maternal care, is a teamwork effort exercised within an institutional framework, where several people have a duty of care towards the patients, including clinical leadership and management. Therefore, scholars, prosecutors, and the law have also analysed the possibility of investigating and prosecuting senior management teams in the NHS under the legal framework of corporate manslaughter. However, the legal implications and restrictions of corporate manslaughter and gross negligence manslaughter have significantly limited their applicability and success in healthcare (Brearey-Horne, 2013; Quick, 2010), making the quest for justice harder and the chances of being prosecuted slimmer.

Further Triggers

Besides Pathirana's analysis of triggering factors (Fig. 27.2), there might be other factors, overlooked in the identified triggers in Fig. 27.2, which also affect HCPs' daily practice and are conducive for fostering overdiagnosis and overtreatment. Among them, medical uncertainty and the lack of evidence-based medicine are still predominant topics in healthcare. Uncertainty and unknownness in medicine remain significant hindering factors behind the quest for diagnoses, cures, and treatments, which can lead to 'too much medicine'. Overdiagnosis and overtreatment may also result from the lack or insufficiency of medical evidence-based research. The search for and display of scientific evidence should be a constant in medical and clinical care, yet the lack of robust evidence behind specific tests, procedures, and treatments still haunts medicine these days. In discussion with midwives and obstetricians working for the NHS in the UK (Quattri, 2025), several have expressed their discomfort regarding the lack or very little evidence behind several clinical maternal practices and procedures that maternal staff are required to perform. Several medical and maternity care procedures are conducted out of routine, ancient knowledge, or even personal convictions. Indeed, the Academy of Medical Royal Colleges in the UK has recently identified a list of tests and treatments that shall be suspended from medical practice in various medical specialties, as the evidence of their effectiveness is very little or inexistent. This list includes, for instance, prescribing antibiotics to fight the flu or x-rays for back pain (Campbell, 2014).

Another seemingly overlooked factor in Pathirana et al. (2017) is how a healthcare system, in this case, the NHS, works—so, the context of care, or the model of care which is predominantly applied in a particular healthcare infrastructure at one time.

A Medicalised Model of Care as a Trigger for 'Too Much Medicine'

Is the current NHS healthcare system set to meet the standards of care that it is expected to meet, and are HCPs appropriately trained for and facilitated in their attempt to care for an increasing number of patients showing with multiple complex diseases, as it seems to be the case in current medicine?

Over the years and since its foundation in 1948, the NHS system has experienced the infiltration of several factors which have conflated expenditure. Among them, there is an increased interventionist approach to care, and the penetration in the healthcare framework of several other forces, including the triggers of 'too much medicine' mentioned above (McCartney, 2016). This has, in turn, contributed to the creation of new masses of 'unwell well' people (Department of Health and Social Care, 2021; Mahase, 2021; Porter, 2019).

According to Margaret McCartney, the current NHS model of care is ill-designed to face increasing clinical complexities, as it is (still) designed around the diagnosis and treatment of single diseases at one time, rather than holistic multidisciplinary approaches to care—which would, in turn, require more specialist care and sufficient funding (Porter, 2019). The current healthcare system in the UK relies heavily on guidelines and regulations, which have been framed around how to cure a disease or a condition rather than on how to discontinue these cures (ibid.). This creates an issue for HCPs trying to discontinue treatments for their patients, as discussed later in this chapter.

As a result, the system fosters 'fragmented action in healthcare' (Porter, 2019) and remains unsupportive of continuity of care, including for pregnant people, due to a lack of staff, investment, and infrastructure. Indeed, the latest Ockenden Report 2021 goes as far as to suggest that continuity of care shall be suspended in NHS maternity care until all other elements of care are deemed fit for purpose (Ockenden, 2022).

Implications for the Patients, the HCPs, and the Healthcare System

A medicalised interventionist model of care may be counterintuitive and obstructive for HCPs who wish to avoid 'wasting care'. It may be difficult or even impossible for some to cut off ineffective and unproven tests and therapies. HCPs need to reconcile their patients' priorities, needs, and wishes with their teams' needs and the healthcare system's regulations and requirements, so trade-offs may sometimes not be in their patients' best interests, although this should not be the case.

In maternity care, a medicalised interventionist approach is usually associated with clinical intervention or obstetric care. Consultant obstetricians are expected to take the lead and guide the team, make decisions, perform interventionist clinical procedures, and be assisted by obstetric nurses. In conversation with obstetricians at different levels of their training working for the NHS, including consultant obstetricians, several have criticised these expectations as sometimes too high and have shown concerns about the current model of care (Quattri, upcoming).

An interventionist model of care weighs on individuals and is also unsustainable for the healthcare system in the short and long term. The model is highly technical; it is hard to maintain; it requires human, financial, and technological resources; it generates new populations of sick and unwell people who need to be taken care of; and it lives on expectations that are not always met on the ground, by doctors and patients.

HCPs are expected to have sufficient time to tend to their patients and adequately inform them about healthcare matters, yet the chronic lack of time is a constant component in current healthcare in the UK. The current healthcare system does not seem able to retain employed staff for long periods—as experienced in several trusts and clinics across the country. The British Medical Association released a public statement claiming that the NHS was short of 50,000 staff in 2021 and that this was expected to be one of the worst backlogs of care in the history of the NHS (British Medical Association, 2021). Compared to other European countries, the UK lags behind in the doctor workforce, with just 2.8 doctors every 1,000 patients compared to 3.7 doctors every 1,000 patients on average in the EU (British Medical Association, 2021). Complex care also requires technical skills and competent personnel, yet many specialties, including maternity care, are currently experiencing an exodus of obstetricians and midwives, which COVID-19 has aggravated, leaving the remaining staff strained and stressed. It has been estimated that 30% of maternity staff have stayed away from maternity wards during the pandemic (Dunkley-Bent, 2021), and according to the latest Royal College of Midwives survey, 57% of maternity staff plan to leave the profession indefinitely by 2022 (Royal College of Midwives, 2021).

All these factors foster discontinuity of care for the patients, and increase patients' and clients' mistrust of the current system. Healthcare professionals have also admitted feeling less safe in the care provided to pregnant and birthing people. A survey from the Royal College of Midwives in 2021 revealed that eight in ten midwives felt that the services that they were provided were not up to the required standards, while 83 of the survey participants believed that maternity wards and clinics had insufficient maternity staff to operate safely (Hall, 2021). As a result, national media have reported that women decide to give birth outside guidelines or at home, sometimes despite this being an unoptimal decision. All these and more factors also show that the current standard of care does not fully match the expectations of all its patients.

An unintended collateral consequence of 'too much medicine' can be 'too little, too late care'. The inherent risk of overmedicalisation of care is the generation of new populations of 'unwell well', which will rely on the same system of care, straining existing resources and forcing staff to share the provision of care that they can offer unequally. Underdiagnosis or underintervention is the substandard, sub-quality, low-value, and unsafe care provision that results from this. In conversation with midwives and obstetricians working for the NHS, some talked about 'too little too late care' instances in their working places (Quattri, 2025). While the demand for 'better care' may be endless, the current model of care and its workforce are finite and already stretched. This will, in turn, increase the risk of providing less, worse, or average care to patients and clients.

Alternative Models of Care and Some Viable Solutions

Maternal care is the medical specialty where the shift from a humanistic and holistic approach to a more medicalised, interventionist approach to care is evident. Indeed, as Davis-Floyd explains, three primary care paradigms can apply to maternity care: the technocratic, the humanistic, and the holistic model. The technocratic model resembles the medicalised model of care explained above, but it is brought to the extreme. In this model, the body is studied and treated as a machine ("I have a c-section in room 4.1"). The role of the pregnant person and the birthing parent is almost null. Births are replaced by 'deliveries'. Mothers shall not interfere in the birthing process, and they shall comply with the doctors' and HCPs' advice and decisions. This model of care is prone to mismanagement of care: "*The hospital became the factory, the mother's body became the machine, and the baby became the product of an industrial manufacturing process*" (Davis-Floyd, 2001). Expert Chauvet (2013) argued that this model represents the complete defeat of the birthing person as the prime actor in bringing life to the world, as the task is accomplished either instrumentally or 'performed' by someone else.

The humanistic model humanises the techno-medical approach to birth. It brings compassionate and respectful care to the birthing person as a life-giving individual and the baby as a living creature with its own rights and needs. It fosters maternal bonding and trust between the patient and the caregiver. Clients' needs and wishes are acknowledged and respected; decisions are shared together; patients are properly and fully informed (Davis-Floyd, 2001).

The holistic model of care encompasses the virtues of the humanistic model of care with the openness towards other forms of birthing and healing, including nutritional therapies, Chinese medicine, and birth options. The birthing parent takes the central stage in this model: "*Her labour is uniquely her own. She eats and drinks and moves about at will. She gives birth in place of her choice, attended by the people and the practitioners of her choice. And the practitioner does not respond to the variations in her labour in standardised ways […]. Her intuition will guide her […]*" (Davis-Floyd, 2001).

While the humanistic and holistic models of care are ideal for patients and clients, they may be challenging to preserve and introduce in trusts and clinics across the country due to a conflux of factors. The already existing culture may hinder these models at the institution, together with the already mentioned lack of appropriate staffing levels, appropriate funding, appropriate management of healthcare, and reliance on instrumental and technical assistance (Thomas, 2022). These care models are also complex solutions, sometimes involving large-scale interventions and requiring numerous people's concerted engagement, efforts, and collaboration. Scholars have come forward with smaller (compared to changing an entire model of care), although no less powerful solutions to try and minimise 'too much too soon, too little too late care'. Some of these solutions have already been applied in the UK.

Some alternatives are not necessarily new, as they may already exist but need revalidation. Among them are 'watchful waiting' and 'active surveillance' practices. Watchful waiting in pregnancy consists in taking the time to monitor the patient, particularly birthing people. During birth, the midwife is supposed to sit or stand quietly beside the birthing person and observe or 'watch' the unfolding of the birth and intervene only in cases for which they have been trained. Watchful waiting continues to be taught as a non-invasive, patient-centred practice (Marshall & Raynor, 2020), which seems conducive to fostering the humanistic or holistic models of care mentioned above.

Active surveillance describes a mild interventionist approach to care via monitoring and gradual testing to decide whether further tests and treatments are warranted. It grants more time and flexibility than other interventionist approaches so that matters can be discussed more thoroughly between the HCPs and their clients and help them make thorough decisions.

However, in conversations with midwives and obstetricians (Quattri, 2025), some argued that watchful waiting is not particularly appreciated at their place of work and that staff or management would instead opt for more interventionist approaches. This finding has also been reported by Carlson and Lowe (2014), who claims that in highly collaborative, team-oriented scenarios such as operating theatres or intrapartum settings, watchful waiting can become a challenge as it needs to be discussed and traded off with the rest of the clinical decisions. Hence, this clinical practice is sometimes discarded to avoid conflict.

Deprescribing and the de-implementation of clinical treatments are also ways to tackle overdiagnosis and overtreatment. They both imply taking people off medications and treatments that they no longer need, are no longer adequate for them, or can potentially harm these patients. Deprescribing is not a synonym for "taking people off care". Instead, it means giving "the right medicine, at the right time, to the right patients" (Porter, 2019). In Liverpool, Dr Dan Hawcutt leads deprescribing ward rounds. He is one of the leading experts in the field, trying to achieve a new approach to care in a children's hospital, where some young patients take up to 18 pills a day or more. Deprescribing ward rounds are among the first of its kind in the UK. England is catching up with Australia and Canada, the avant-gardist countries in this relatively new clinical approach, and a UK deprescribing network called EDeN (English Deprescribing Network, www.sps.nhs.uk) has been set up with guidelines on the most overly prescribed medications, including water tablets and sleeping pills. David Alldred, from the University of Leeds, laments that there are currently only a handful of studies and randomised control trials or RCTs that focus on the impact of deprescribing on patients at different stages of care, whereas more efforts and investments shall be put into this matter. This would help parents and patients understand the implications and the benefits of deprescribing, which is often misunderstood, and it will make clinicians more confident in their decision to deprescribe (Porter, 2019).

Another way to improve the quality and quantity of learned intake for HCPs would be to revise how current clinical guidelines, quality assessments, and recommendations are prepared and presented. Greenhalgh and colleagues have, for instance, lamented that the number of clinical guidelines published in the name of evidence-based medicine has now become "unmanageable and unfathomable" (Greenhalgh et al., 2014). James Owen Drife, emeritus professor of OB/GYN, lamented in the BMJ that a friend, a lead of Obstetrics in a hospital in the UK, received "3,825 pages of advice, guidelines, and reports about maternity care" to study and read in just one year or two (Drife, 2010).

In a questionnaire survey conducted among almost 3,000 obstetricians and midwives in two general hospitals in the UK, Mahran and peers found that most of the respondents pleaded for 'user-friendlier' guidelines, which should be shorter and clearer (Mahran et al., 2007). This quest for better-managed learning content could be expanded to other parts of education and training for HCPs, including improving internal communication with staff. Lack of access to up-to-date, clear, and possibly digestible information is an issue for the HCPs and their clients.

Gigerenzer et al. (2009) found much misinformation and misunderstanding of clinical evidence across populations in the UK, Germany, and parts of Europe, and they attributed this to a lack of access to appropriately framed evidence-based knowledge and lacking public healthcare literacy. As a result, the scholars have developed so-called fact sheets on different conditions and diseases, urging HCPs and insurance companies to use them regularly with their clients. These fact sheets are simplified summaries of the latest Cochrane reviews on specific topics (e.g. PSA screening, mammographic screening, or endoscopies), regularly updated with upcoming evidence (Helsana Versicherungen, 2016; Wegwarth & Gigerenzer, 2018). An essential aspect of these summaries is that they do not tell patients and doctors what to do or how to intervene, which was an intentional decision of their authors. Instead, they just present the facts and leave the rest to the professionals to discuss with their patients.

Conclusions

As stated in the 1978 World Health Organization Alma-Ata Declaration of 'Health For All by 2000', health is essential for all people and for human progress. However, more than 40 years after that declaration, most societies and countries have yet to achieve 'health for all'. In the UK and elsewhere, a phenomenon that affects the fair distribution and supply of care to all is 'too much medicine', also known as excessive medicine or overdiagnosis and overtreatment. Scholars seem to agree that the risks of harm in 'too much medicine' instances outweigh the potential and tangible benefits of the received care. The coexistence of 'too much medical' care alongside the proper provision of care to the right patients hinders public efforts to improve healthcare service delivery and to define strategies steering towards 'health for all'.

This chapter analyses the concept of 'too much medicine' focusing on the NHS and the NHS maternity services. It shows that 'too much medicine' remains a complex issue in contemporary medicine, which abounds in every layer of care and medical specialty, and which is triggered by several factors, some of which have been explored in detail. One is the consideration that the way in which healthcare systems operate can also affect 'too much medicine'. A risk-averse and interventionist model of care seems unfit for serving a potentially unlimited number of patients and complex cases, especially if it relies on finite and already stretched human, technical, and financial resources. This model of care cannot guarantee an uncapped provision of care for an increasing number of, among others, 'unwell well' patients, thus making it harder for patients and clients to be given the right amount of care, and to be taken out of care. Several alternatives and viable solutions to this model have been proposed, which have been applied with varying degrees of success.

References

Ahn, H. S., Kim, H. J., & Welch, G. H. (2014). Korea's thyroid-cancer "epidemic"—Screening and overdiagnosis. *The New England Journal of Medicine, 371*(19), 1765–1767. https://doi.org/10.1056/NEJMp1409841

Armstrong, N. (2018). Overdiagnosis and overtreatment as a quality problem: Insights from healthcare improvement research. *BMJ Quality & Safety, 27*(7), 571–574. https://doi.org/10.1136/bmjqs-2017-007571

Bewley, S. (2020, April 14). *Things should never be the same again in the screening world.* The BMJ Opinion. https://blogs.bmj.com/bmj/2020/04/14/susan-bewley-things-should-never-be-the-same-again-in-the-screening-world/

Bourne, T., Vanderhaegen, J., Vranken, R., Wynants, L., De Cock, B., Peters, M., Timmerman, D., Van Calster, B., Jalmbrant, M., & Van Audenhove, C. (2016). Doctors' experiences and their perception of the most stressful aspects of complaints processes in the UK: An analysis of qualitative survey data. *BMJ Open, 6*(7), Article e011711. https://doi.org/10.1136/bmjopen-2016-011711

Brazier, M., Devaney, S., Griffiths, D., Mullock, A., & Quirk, H. (2016). Improving healthcare through the use of 'medical manslaughter'? Facts, fears and the future. *Clinical Risk, 22*(5–6), 88–93. https://doi.org/10.1177/1356262217696623

Brearey-Horne, P. (2013). The Corporate Manslaughter and Corporate Homicide Act 2007 and maternal death: an opportunity to address systemic deficiencies in maternity services? In D. Griffitsh & A. Sanders (Eds.), *Bioethics, medicine and the criminal law* (Vol. 2, pp. 210–226). Cambridge University Press. https://doi.org/10.1017/CBO9781139109376.015

British Medical Association. (2021, September 13). *NHS short of 50,000 doctors heading into winter, BMA research finds* (Press Release). https://www.bma.org.uk/bma-media-centre/nhs-short-of-50-000-doctors-heading-into-winter-bma-research-finds

Brodersen, J. (2017). Overdiagnosis: An unrecognised and growing worldwide problem in healthcare. *Slovenian Journal of Public Health, 56*(3), 147–149. https://doi.org/10.1515/sjph-2017-0019

Brown, H. S., III. (2007). Lawsuit activity, defensive medicine, and small area variation: The case of cesarean sections revisited. *Health Economics, Policy and Law, 2*(3), 285–296. https://doi.org/10.1017/S1744133107004136

Brownlee, S., Chalkidou, K., Doust, J., Elshaug, A., Glasziou, P. P., Health, I., Nagpal, S., Saini, V., Srivastava, D., Chalmers, K., & Korenstein, D. (2017). Evidence for overuse of medical services around the world. *The Lancet, 390*(10090), 156–168. https://doi.org/10.1016/S0140-6736(16)32585-5

Campbell, D. (2014, November 4). NHS wastes £2bn a year on unnecessary or expensive treatments. *The Guardian.* https://www.theguardian.com/society/2014/nov/05/nhs-wastes-over-2-bn-on-unnecessary-treatment

Carlson, N. S., & Lowe, N. K. (2014). A concept analysis of watchful waiting among providers caring for women in labour. *Journal of Advanced Nursing, 70*(3), 511–522. https://doi.org/10.1111/jan.12209

Cassels, A. (2012). *Seeking sickness: Medical screening and the misguided hunt for disease.* Greystone Books. https://greystonebooks.com/collections/alan-cassels/products/seeking-sickness

CEBM Oxford. (2021). *A history of overdiagnosis and lessons to learn* (Video). YouTube. https://youtu.be/Wal-fUOdBXg

Chauvet, E. (Director). (2013). *O renascimento do parto* [The beginning of life] (Documentary). Filmes Fora da Lata.

Clarfield, M. A. (2010). Screening in frail older people: An ounce of prevention or a pound of trouble? *Journal of the American Geriatrics Society, 58*(10), 2016–2021. https://doi.org/10.1111/j.1532-5415.2010.03070.x

Conrad, P. (2007). *The medicalisation of society. On the transformation of human conditions into treatable disorders.* Johns Hopkins University Press.

Davis-Floyd, R. (2001). The technocratic, humanistic, and holistic paradigms of childbirth. *International Journal of Gynaecology & Obstetrics, 75*(S1), S5–S23. https://doi.org/10.1016/S0020-7292(01)00510-0

DeFrank, J. T., Barklay, C., Sheridan, S., Brewer, N. T., Gilliam, M., Moon, A. M., Rearick, W., Ziemer, C., & Harris, R. (2015). The psychological harm of screening: The evidence we have versus the evidence we need. *Journal of General Internal Medicine, 30*(2), 242–248. https://doi.org/10.1007/s11606-014-2996-5

Department of Health and Social Care. (2021). *Good for you, good for us, good for everybody: A plan to reduce overprescribing to make patient care better and safer, support the NHS, and reduce carbon emissions*. https://assets.publishing.service.gov.uk/government/uploads/system/uploads/attachment_data/file/1019475/good-for-you-good-for-us-good-for-everybody.pdf

Drife, J. O. (2010). An avalanche of apple pie: Too many guidelines? *BMJ, 340*(c1208). https://doi.org/10.1136/bmj.c1208

Dunkley-Bent, J. (2021, January 13). *Midwives, maternity and COVID-19* (Keynote address). The London Maternity and Midwifery Festival 2021, London, UK. https://www.maternityandmidwifery.co.uk/midwives-maternity-and-covid-19/

Gigerenzer, G., Mata, J., & Frank, R. (2009). Public knowledge of benefits of breast and prostate cancer screening in Europe. *Journal of the National Cancer Institute, 101*(17), 1216–1220. https://doi.org/10.1093/jnci/djp237

Greenhalgh, T., Howick, J., & Maskrey, N. (2014). Evidence-based medicine: A movement in crisis? *BMJ, 348*, Article g3725. https://doi.org/10.1136/bmj.g3725

Gupta, P., Gupta, M., & Koul, N. (2020). Overdiagnosis and overtreatment; how to deal with too much medicine. *Journal of Family Medicine and Primary Care, 9*(8), 3815–3819. https://doi.org/10.4103/jfmpc.jfmpc_433_20

Hall, J. (2021, June). *Midwifery staff shortages—Have we reached tipping point?* Maternity and Midwifery Forum. https://www.maternityandmidwifery.co.uk/midwifery-staff-shortages-have-we-reached-tipping-point/

Helsana Versicherungen. (2016, May 30). *Referat von Professor Gerd Gigerenzer zu Risiko- und Gesundheitskompetenz* (Lecture by Professor Gerd Gigerenzer on risk and health competence) (Video). https://www.youtube.com/watch?v=imFIcRU6kZ4

Howard, S. (2020). The rise of souvenir scanners: Ultrasonography on the high street. *BMJ, 370*, Article m1321. https://doi.org/10.1136/bmj.m1321

Jackson, E. (2019). *Medical law: Text, cases, and materials* (5th ed.). Oxford University Press. https://doi.org/10.1093/he/9780198825845.001.0001

Jegerlehner, S., Bulliard, J.-L., Aujesky, D., Rodondi, N., Germann, S., Konzelmann, I., Chiolero, A., & NICER Working Group. (2017). Overdiagnosis and overtreatment of thyroid cancer: A population-based temporal trend study. *PLoS ONE, 12*(6), Article e0179387. https://doi.org/10.1371/journal.pone.0179387

Kale, M. S., & Korenstein, D. (2018). Overdiagnosis in primary care: Framing the problem and finding solutions. *BMJ, 362*, Article k2820. https://doi.org/10.1136/bmj.k2820

Kapfhamer, J. D., Menon, S., & Spellecy, R. (2012). The importance of risk tolerance in maternal autonomy. *The American Journal of Bioethnics, 12*(7), 53–54. https://doi.org/10.1080/15265161.2012.680537

Katz, M. H. (2013). Can we stop ordering prostate-specific antigen screening tests? *JAMA Internal Medicine, 173*(10), 847–848. https://doi.org/10.1001/jamainternmed.2013.1164

Labarge, B., Walter, V., Lengerich, E. J., Crist, H., Karamchandani, D., Williams, N., Goldenberg, D., Bann, D. V., & Warrick, J. I. (2018). Evidence of a positive association between malpractice climate and thyroid cancer incidence in the United States. *PLoS ONE, 13*(7), Article e0199862. https://doi.org/10.1371/journal.pone.0199862

Lenzer, J. (2012). Unnecessary care: Are doctors in denial and is profit driven healthcare to blame? *BMJ, 345*, Article e6230. https://doi.org/10.1136/bmj.e6230

Llewelyn, H. (2021, October 19). Group email chat, Google Overdiagnosis Group.

Mahase, E. (2021). Overprescribing: 10% of items dispensed in primary care are inappropriate, review finds. *BMJ, 374*, Article n2338. https://doi.org/10.1136/bmj.n233

Mahran, M. A., Paine, M., & Ewies, A. A. (2007). Maternity guidelines: Aid or hindrance? *Journal of Obstetrics and Gynaecology, 27*(8), 774–780. https://doi.org/10.1080/01443610701667353

Marshall, J., & Raynor, M. (2020). *Myles textbook for midwives* (17th ed.). Elsevier. https://www.elsevier.com/books/myles-textbook-for-midwives/marshall/978-0-7020-7642-8

McCartney, M. (2016). *The state of medicine: Keeping the promise of the NHS*. Pinter & Martin. https://www.pinterandmartin.com/the-state-of-medicine.html

Moynihan, R. N. (2012). Too much medicine, not enough mirth. *BMJ, 345*, Article e7116. https://doi.org/10.1136/bmj.e7116

Moynihan, R. N., Doran, E., & Henry, D. (2008). Disease mongering is now part of the global health debate. *PLoS Medicine, 5*(5), Article e106. https://doi.org/10.1371/journal.pmed.0050106

Moynihan, R. N., Doust, J., & Henry, D. (2012). Preventing overdiagnosis: How to stop harming the healthy. *BMJ, 344*, Article e3502. https://doi.org/10.1136/bmj.e3502

Murphy, J. F. (2001). The relentless rise in caesarean sections. *Irish Medical Journal, 94*(7), 196. http://archive.imj.ie//ViewArticleDetails.aspx?ContentID=1408

NHS Resolution. (2019a). C*linical negligence numbers steady, but rising costs remain a concern.* https://resolution.nhs.uk/2019/07/11/clinical-negligence-numbers-steady-but-rising-costs-remain-a-concern/

NHS Resolution. (2019b). *NHS Resolution annual report and accounts 2018 to 2019*. https://assets.publishing.service.gov.uk/government/uploads/system/uploads/attachment_data/file/824330/NHS_resolution_annual_report_and_accounts_-_web_pdf.pdf

Ockenden, D. (2022). *Findings, conclusions, and essential actions from the independent review of maternity services at the Shrewsbury and Telford Hospital NHS trust*. https://assets.publishing.service.gov.uk/government/uploads/system/uploads/attachment_data/file/1064302/Final-Ockenden-Report-web-accessible.pdf

Orfali, K. (2012). Beyond numbers: The multiple cultural meanings of rising cesarean rates worldwide. *The American Journal of Bioethnics, 12*(7), 54–56. https://doi.org/10.1080/15265161.2012.680544

Pathirana, T., Clark, J., & Moynihan, R. N. (2017). Mapping the drivers of overdiagnosis to potential solutions. *BMJ, 358*, Article j3879. https://doi.org/10.1136/bmj.j3879

Pearlman, M. D. (2006). Patient safety in obstetrics and gynecology: An agenda for the future. *Obstetrics & Gynecology, 108*(5), 1266–1271. https://doi.org/10.1097/01.AOG.0000241096.85499.a8

Porter, M. (2019, July 2). *Inside health: Deprescribing* (Audio podcast). BBC Radio 4. https://www.bbc.co.uk/sounds/play/m0006dmn

Quattri, F. (2025). *The challenges of seeking to avoid overdiagnosis and overtreatment: Exploring defensive medicine* (Unpublished doctoral dissertation). University of Leicester.

Quick, O. (2010). Medicine, mistakes and manslaughter: A criminal combination? *The Cambridge Law Journal, 69*(1), 186–203. https://doi.org/10.1017/S0008197310000231

Royal College of Midwives. (2021). *RCM warns of midwife exodus as maternity staffing crisis grows.* https://www.rcm.org.uk/media-releases/2021/september/rcm-warns-of-midwife-exodus-as-maternity-staffing-crisis-grows/

Saini, V., Garcia-Armesto, S., Klemperer, D., Paris, V., Elshaug, A. G., Brownlee, S., Ioannidis, J. P. A., & Fisher, E. S. (2017). Drivers of poor medical care. *The Lancet, 390*(10090), 178–190. https://doi.org/10.1016/S0140-6736(16)30947-3

Sajid, I. M. (2021). *Presentation of the 'Diagnostic Downshift' paper with Kathleen Frost, Overdiagnosis Google Group, 24th August 2021—virtual event*. Last accessed on 17th September 2021.

Salerno, S., Laghi, A., Cantone, M. C., Sartori, P., Pinto, A., & Frija, G. (2019). Overdiagnosis and overimaging: An ethical issue for radiological protection. *La Radiologia Medica, 124*(8), 714–720. https://doi.org/10.1007/s11547-019-01029-5

Samanta, A., & Samanta, J. (2021). Death caused by negligent medical care: Reconsidering the role of gross negligence manslaughter in the aftermath of Bawa-Garba. *Medical Law International, 21*(4), 293–301. https://doi.org/10.1177/0968533221992838

Schlachter, L. (2017). *Malpractice: A neurosurgeon reveals how our health-care system puts patients at risk.* Skyhorse Publishing. https://www.skyhorsepublishing.com/9781510712591/malpractice/

Seijmonsberger-Schermers, A. E., van den Akker, T., Rydahl, E., Beeckman, K., Bogaerts, A., Binfa, L., Frith, L., Gross, M. M., Misselwitz, B., Hálfdánsdóttir, B., Daly, D., Corcoran, P., Calleja-Agius, J., Calleja, N, Gatt, M., Vika Nilsen, A. B., Declercq, E., Gissler, M., Heino, A., … de Jonge, A. (2020). Variations in use of childbirth interventions in 13 high-income countries: A multinational cross-sectional study. *PLoS Medicine, 17*(5), Article e1003103. https://doi.org/10.1371/journal.pmed.1003103

Shmerling, R. H. (2018, June 28). *Rethinking the screening mammogram* (Short Article). Harvard Health Publishing—Harvard Health Blog. https://www.health.harvard.edu/blog/rethinking-the-screening-mammogram-2018062814151

Symon, A. (2000). Obstetric litigation: Effects on clinical practice. *Gynakologisch-Geburtshilfliche Rundschau, 40*(3–4), 165–171. https://doi.org/10.1159/000053021

Szabo, L. (2017, December 19). Too many older patients get cancer screenings. *The New York Times*. https://www.nytimes.com/2017/12/19/well/live/cancer-screening-tests-seniors-older-patients-harms-overdiagnosis-overtreatment.html

The Lancet. (2016). Maternal health 2016. https://www.thelancet.com/series/maternal-health-2016

Thomas, F. (2022). Medicalisation. In K. Chamberlain & A. Lyons (Eds.), *Routledge international handbook of critical issues in health and illness* (pp. 23–33). Routledge. https://doi.org/10.4324/9781003185215-4

Treadwell, J., Smith, J., & Pathirana, T. (2021, October 19). *An introduction to overdiagnosis* (Webinar presentation). Preventing Overdiagnosis 2021/22 Virtual Programme. https://www.preventingoverdiagnosis.net/2021/Documents/An%20introduction%20to%20Overdiagnosis.pdf

Wegwarth, O., & Gigerenzer, G. (2018). The barrier to informed choice in cancer screening: Statistical illiteracy in physicians and patients. In U. Goerting & A. Mehnert (Eds.), *Psycho-oncology* (pp. 207–221). Springer. https://doi.org/10.1007/978-3-319-64310-6_13

Welch, G. H. (2010). Overdiagnosis in cancer. *Journal of the National Cancer Institute, 102*(9), 605–613. https://doi.org/10.1093/jnci/djq099

Welch, G. H., Schwartz, L. M., & Woloshin, S. (2011). *Overdiagnosed: Making people sick in the pursuit of health.* Beacon Press. http://www.beacon.org/Overdiagnosed-P925.aspx

Wilson, J. M. G., & Jungner, G. (1968). *Principles and practice of screening for disease.* World Health Organization. https://apps.who.int/iris/handle/10665/37650

Woloshin, S., & Kramer, B. (2021). Overdiagnosis: It's official. *BMJ, 375*, Article n2854. https://doi.org/10.1136/bmj.n285

World Health Organization. (2018, February 15). *Individualized, supportive care key to positive childbirth experience, says WHO* (Press release). https://www.who.int/news/item/15-02-2018-individualized-supportive-care-key-to-positive-childbirth-experience-says-who

World Health Organization. (2021, June 16). *Caesarean section rates continue to rise, amid growing inequalities in access.* https://www.who.int/news/item/16-06-2021-caesarean-section-rates-continue-to-rise-amid-growing-inequalities-in-access-who

Chapter 28
Environmental, Social and Governance (ESG) of Listed Companies in the Healthcare Industry of Hong Kong

Tiffany Cheng Han Leung and Shi Xiang You

Abstract The rise of the United Nations Sustainable Development Goals (SDGs), responsible investment and green finance have led to growing Environmental, Social and Governance (ESG) reporting practices over the past few years. ESG reporting is widely adopted to show economic, social, and environmental responsibilities. In Hong Kong, the ESG Reporting Guide (the ESG Guide) was released to regulate ESG reporting. As organisations in the private sector or listed companies in the healthcare industry are critical to realising human society's sustainability, responding to SDG 3. The healthcare industry in Hong Kong is thriving due to the increasing ageing population, strong demand for healthy lifestyles, elevated expectations of healthcare quality, the well-developed financial market and the close connection between Hong Kong and mainland China. It is noteworthy how listed companies in the healthcare industry in Hong Kong had reported their ESG performance. This book chapter provides a general overview of the current ESG reporting practice of the Hong Kong healthcare industry to potential investors and policymakers. Suggestions to improve their ESG performance will be provided at the end.

Keywords Environmental, social and governance · Sustainability · Healthcare

Introduction

In 2015, the United Nations (the UN) put forward the 2030 Agenda for Sustainable Development (the Agenda) to solve the urgent unsustainability issues facing people, the planet, and prosperity. The Agenda proposes 17 Sustainable Development Goals (SDGs) with proposed targets under each SDG, driving widespread and positive

T. C. H. Leung (✉) · S. X. You
Faculty of Business, City University of Macau, Macau, China
e-mail: tiffanyleung@cityu.mo

S. X. You
e-mail: b20092100124@cityu.mo

B. Y. F. Fong and W. C. W. Wong (eds.), *Gaps and Actions in Health Improvement from Hong Kong and Beyond*,
https://doi.org/10.1007/978-981-99-4491-0_28

impacts on the environment and society (Balaisyte et al., 2021). SDG 3 focuses on the health and well-being of human society with thirteen targets (United Nations, 2015). The private sector is integral to the development of SDG 3, of which some businesses in the private sector have already integrated SDG 3 into their operational strategies (Consolandi et al., 2020).

Environmental, Social and Governance (ESG) arises due to responsible investment (Alda, 2021; UN Principles for Responsible Investment, 2020). In response to the increasing environmental and societal issues, such as climate change, modern slavery, and unsustainable production, investors are incorporating ESG factors into their investment decisions (Gianfrate & Peri, 2019). ESG healthcare funds are established as an element of responsible investment in the healthcare business as SDG 3 is realised (Balaisyte et al., 2021). Companies use ESG disclosures to demonstrate their economic, social, and environmental responsibilities. To cope with the worldwide trend of ESG investing and reporting, stock exchanges in developed nations are increasingly publishing ESG reporting recommendations to help listed companies meet stakeholders' ESG performance expectations and attract investment opportunities (Sustainable Stock Exchanges Initiative, 2019).

The Hong Kong Exchanges and Clearing Limited released the Environmental, Social and Governance Reporting Guide (the ESG Guide) in 2011 and revised it in 2019. The ESG Guide consists of mandatory reporting requirements on ESG governance and the 'comply or explain' provisions on listed issuers' environmental and social performance. First, the environmental subject measures listed companies' performance in emissions, use of resources, the impacts of business operations on natural resources, and climate-related risks for the listed companies. Second, the social subject mainly focuses on (i) employment and labour practices, (ii) operating practices in supply chain and product management, (iii) anti-corruption performance and (iv) community involvement. Every aspect consists of general disclosures and key performance indicators (KPIs). The general disclosures require issuers to report their compliance with related laws and regulations. The ESG Guide applies to all listed companies from all sectors on the Main Board and the Growth Enterprise Market (GEM) in the Hong Kong Stock Exchange (Hong Kong Exchanges and Clearing Limited, 2022a).

According to the Hong Kong Trade Development Council (Yim, 2021), life expectancy in Hong Kong is among the highest in the world. Meanwhile, the high life expectancy leads to a large ageing population (Fong et al., 2021). In 2020, health expenditure in Hong Kong increased by up to 203% compared to 2010, which contributes to 6.8% of the Gross Domestic Product (GDP) in Hong Kong (Health Bureau, 2021). Local citizens are expected to maintain healthier lifestyles and to enjoy decent quality healthcare services.

These situations contribute to the prosperity of the healthcare industry in Hong Kong. The healthcare business had 206 listed companies on the HKEX Main Board and GEM at the start of 2022, accounting for approximately 7% of all listed companies. 178 healthcare-related issuers are listed on the Main Board, while the remaining are listed on the GEM. Based on the Hang Seng Industry Classification System, the healthcare industry in Hong Kong consists of two main sectors, namely (i) pharmacy and biotechnology and (ii) medical services and equipment (Hang Seng Indexes Company Limited, 2020). By the beginning of 2022, 116 healthcare companies in the HKEX were cross listed on the Shanghai Stock Exchange (the SHSE) and the Shenzhen Stock Exchange (the SZSE), accounting for over 50% of the total listed companies in the healthcare industry in Hong Kong.

Hong Kong is considered the gateway to the Chinese market for biotech initial public offerings (IPOs). It is now the first and second-largest biotech fundraising hub in Asia and the world, respectively (Hong Kong Exchanges and Clearing Limited, 2020). The healthcare service and equipment sector mainly focus on the household consumer market, providing household products, such as blood pressure monitors. This sector provides products for institutional consumers, such as public and private hospitals, in the buyers' market (Yim, 2021).

Listed companies in the healthcare industry generally outperform other industries in terms of their overall ESG performance and ESG reporting quality (Demir & Min, 2019). First, ESG performance is positively related to corporate financial performance (Brogi & Lagasio, 2019; Xie et al., 2019). Second, the listed healthcare companies need to meet the expectations of multiple stakeholder groups with complicated relationships, including patients, professionals, hospitals, investors and governments (Ananth et al., 2010). In particular, the ESG performance of these companies is related to the well-being and health of human society, so issuers in the healthcare industry should view ESG reporting as a critical strategy to gain a social licence to operate and enhance the corporate brand image and reputation (Demir & Min, 2019). Furthermore, due to its direct connection to health and human well-being, the healthcare industry is intricately linked to SDG 3.

ESG Performance Highlighted in the Healthcare Industry in Hong Kong

Historically, healthcare companies focus more on the social pillar of ESG performance due to its industry characteristics. These companies may benefit by allocating equal attention to the environmental and governance pillars (PwC, 2021a). The following five subsections include emission reduction and waste management, employment and labour practices, product quality and safety, innovations in healthcare services and technologies, and anti-corruption.

Emission Reduction and Waste Management

In the healthcare industry, emission reduction and waste management are top priorities among all environmental performance indicators, but the environmental impacts of healthcare are not well recognised (Lenzen et al., 2020; PwC, 2021a; Thakur &

Ramesh, 2015). Table 28.1 shows that these listed companies need to comply with a number of regulations and laws regarding emission reduction and waste management in both mainland China and Hong Kong.

The adverse impact of climate change and the requirements of the Paris Agreement pose tremendous pressure on all industries, including the healthcare industry. In 2019, the healthcare industry's quantity of carbon dioxide (CO_2) emissions accounted for 4.4% of total CO_2 emissions globally and 5% of total CO_2 emissions in China 2019 (Hensher & McGain, 2020; Pichler et al., 2019).

The initial research on the ESG disclosures of listed healthcare companies on the Main Board of HKEX shows that the greenhouse gas (GHG) emissions mainly come from (i) the consumption of fossil fuels in transportation, (ii) flue gases of coal-fired boilers, (iii) exhaust gases from production and (iv) daily operations. Apart from CO_2, the operations of healthcare companies may generate other GHG emissions, such as sulphur dioxide (SO_2), methane (CH_4) and nitrogen dioxide (NO_2) (Hensher & McGain, 2020; Lenzen et al., 2020). The waste gas treatment process usually goes through three steps: collection, treatment, and disposal. Listed companies avoid direct emissions, which are prohibited by regulations. Some healthcare companies conduct case studies to show how they reduce the quantity of emissions, improve emission management and realise the goal of green operations in their ESG reports.

The World Health Organization (WHO) categorises healthcare waste (HCW) into ten types and requires safe disposal (Ananth et al., 2010; World Health Organization, 2018), accounting for 85% of the total HCW, while the rest of the waste is hazardous. HCW management may negatively impact the environment and public health (Ananth et al., 2010; Thakur & Ramesh, 2015). The ESG Guide requires listed companies to report hazardous and non-hazardous waste separately (Hong Kong Exchanges and Clearing Limited, 2022a). Despite the regulations and laws mentioned in Table 28.1, some healthcare companies establish internal rules on HCW

Table 28.1 Laws and regulations on emission reduction and waste management in mainland China and Hong Kong

Region	Laws and regulations	Enacting time
Mainland China	Water Pollution Prevention and Control Law of the People's Republic of China	1984
	Environmental Protection Law of the People's Republic of China	1989
	Integrated Emission Standard of Air Pollutants GB16297-1996	1996
	Hazardous Chemicals Safety Law of the People's Republic of China (Draft for Comment)	N/A
Hong Kong SAR	Water Pollution Control Ordinance (Cap. 358 of the Laws of Hong Kong)	1980
	Waste Disposal Ordinance (Cap. 354 of the Laws of Hong Kong)	1996
	Waste Disposal (Clinical Waste) (General) Regulation (Cap. 354O of the Laws of Hong Kong)	2010

management to standardise further and optimise the HCW management system. An environmental, health and safety (EHS) committee or team is sometimes responsible for monitoring the disposal of HCW. This technology is critical to reducing and sanitising the HCW (Zhang et al., 2014).

The HKEX provides detailed guidance on calculating related data of KPIs on emissions and waste for listed companies (Hong Kong Exchanges and Clearing Limited, 2022b). Besides, the reporting principles of the ESG Guide mandate issuers to report KPIs using a quantitative approach. The historical data on emissions and HCW must be measurable (Hong Kong Exchanges and Clearing Limited, 2022a). Listed companies sometimes conduct external assurance to ensure accountability and transparency for these quantitative indicators (Machado et al., 2021).

Employment and Labour Practices

The employee group is one of the major stakeholder groups that attach importance to listed companies' ESG performance (Fernandez-Feijoo et al., 2014). Based on the Materiality Map provided by the Sustainability Accounting Standards Board, employee health, safety and well-being are financial materiality in some industries, including the healthcare industry (Consolandi et al., 2020). In Hong Kong, listed companies need to comply with several laws protecting employee rights. Table 28.2 displays these laws and regulations.

Talent is one of the core competencies of healthcare companies, particularly biotech and pharmaceutical companies (Demir & Min, 2019). Drug research and development (R&D) and product innovation necessitate creative abilities. Thus, the listed healthcare companies in Hong Kong disclose how they recruit and retain talent in their ESG disclosure. Concerning human resources, competitive remuneration plans, including salaries and bonuses, attract talents and enhance listed companies' social performance (Kuzey et al., 2021). Some listed companies establish remuneration committees under the board committee to manage remuneration strategies, representing effective communication in ESG engagement (Arayssi et al., 2020).

Apart from remuneration, career development, and employee training are often seen as necessary in the ESG Guide (Hong Kong Exchanges and Clearing Limited, 2022a). Some listed companies offer online and offline courses for employees to learn at any time. The course content is not limited to professional knowledge in healthcare but includes knowledge of industry regulations, analysis of industry frontier and hotspots, and career promotion. Besides, during the COVID-19 pandemic, these companies organised employee training in pandemic response and prevention, helping employees acquire and develop professional skills in an uncertain environment.

Table 28.2 Laws and regulations on employee rights in mainland China and Hong Kong

Region	Laws and regulations	Enacting time
Mainland China	Labour Law of the People's Republic of China	1995
	Provisions on Minimum Wages issued by the Ministry of Labour and Social Security of the People's Republic of China	2004
	Social Insurance Law of the People's Republic of China	2010
Hong Kong SAR	Employment Compensation Ordinance (Cap.282 of the Laws of Hong Kong)	1953
	Employment Ordinance (Cap. 57 of the Laws of Hong Kong)	1968
	Disability Discrimination Ordinance (Cap. 487 of the Laws of Hong Kong)	1996
	Sex Discrimination Ordinance (Cap. 480 of the Laws of Hong Kong)	1996
	Mandatory Provident Fund Schemes Ordinance (Cap. 485 of the Laws of Hong Kong)	1998
	Race Discrimination Ordinance (Cap. 602 of the Laws of Hong Kong)	2008
	Minimum Wage Ordinance (Cap. 608 of the Laws of Hong Kong)	2010

Product Quality and Safety

Product quality and safety are highlighted in the healthcare industry. Listed companies should fulfil their social responsibilities in daily operations and product quality management is one of the most effective strategies (Mehralian et al., 2016). Healthcare equipment is often seen as tangible goods, while healthcare services and technologies are intangible products. Product quality in the healthcare industry could be measured by timeliness, consistency, accuracy, and safety (Edwards et al., 2012; Mosadeghrad, 2014). Edwards et al. (2012) indicate that healthcare product safety requires cooperation and communication with all external stakeholder groups, such as policymakers, health professionals, and the general public (Mehralian et al., 2016; Mosadeghrad, 2014).

Total quality management (TQM) is a common practice adopted in the quality control process (Mehralian et al., 2016). Some companies adopt TQM at all levels of business to ensure they follow quality control standards at all levels. Despite the internal quality control system, some healthcare listed companies in Hong Kong standardise product quality by achieving quality management certification from recognised organisations or authorities, such as the International Organisation for Standardisation (ISO), the Food and Drug Administration (FDA) of the United States, and the European Directorate for the Quality of Medicines (EDQM).

Table 28.3 Regulations and laws related to healthcare product quality in mainland China

Region	Laws and regulations	Enacting time
Mainland China	Pharmaceutical Administration Law of the People's Republic of China	1984
	Product Quality Law of the PRC	1993
	The Measures for the Administration on Adverse Drug Reaction Reporting and Monitoring	2010

Regulations ensure high-quality healthcare service and product safety (World Health Organization, 2017). Table 28.3 shows some regulations related to product safety.

Innovations in Healthcare Services and Technologies

Innovation is critical to listed companies in the healthcare industry in Hong Kong. However, the ESG Guide does not require innovation disclosure. First, for listed companies providing healthcare services and equipment, service innovation refers to a service with new benefits or a new method to deliver existing service realised by customers. A successful service innovation should bring value creation, such as increased efficiency and cost reduction (Berry, 2019). Second, innovation in pharmaceutical and biotechnology companies sometimes refers to the application of a new technology (Zhang & Wu, 2019). The development of information technology and big data contributes to healthcare innovation, and the COVID-19 pandemic accelerates the speed of promotion and application of innovative technologies (PwC, 2021b). In Hong Kong, there are mainly five types of healthcare innovations, namely (i) telehealth, (ii) 3D printing, (iii) robotics, (iv) virtue reality (VR), and (v) biosensors and trackers (Yim, 2021).

First, telehealth provides convenient access to healthcare specialists and services, and 5G technology enables the high-speed internet connection in the telehealth process (Deloitte, 2022). Some companies launched online telehealth platforms, which attracted many users (Yim, 2021). Second, 3D printing is well known for its high dimensional accuracy and is widely adopted to produce healthcare apparatus due to economic benefits and a simplified manufacturing process (Eshkalak et al., 2020). In Hong Kong, the Healthcare Devices Innovation Hub creates a supportive environment for further developing 3D printing technology (Yim, 2021). Third, the emergence of robotics attributes to artificial intelligence and big data. The application of robotics allows accurate diagnosis, productivity, and convenient service delivery (Berry, 2019). Healthcare robotics innovations collaborate with universities and medical centres (Yim, 2021). Fourth, VR is often applied in digital therapeutics (Deloitte, 2022). VR could create an immersive environment for users to overcome pain and anxiety, leading to pain-relief products (Berry, 2019; Deloitte,

2022). Finally, biosensors and trackers are used for healthcare monitoring. Wearable biosensors provide continuous physiological data in real time with biochemical indicators (Kim et al., 2019). This technology is largely developed in both professional and household health monitoring equipment.

Anti-corruption

Generally, a lower level of corruption leads to better ESG performance. The definition of corruption tends to place an emphasis on its illegal or illegitimate nature and economic relationships (Cuervo-Cazurra, 2016). There are two types of corruption, namely individual and institutional corruption. Individual corruption results from the pursuit of personal interests and gains, while institutional corruption is due to institutions' deviation from a particular code of conduct (Sommersguter-Reichmann et al., 2018). It is essential to make a distinction between public corruption and private corruption. Public corruption often occurs when a politician or a civil servant gains additional benefits for a compelling cause (e.g. a contract) or to avoid a lousy cause (e.g. tax avoidance). In contrast, private corruption occurs when the manager of an organisation gains personal income to exchange for personal benefits (e.g. receiving gifts) (Cuervo-Cazurra, 2016). In particular, private corruption appears to be examined in the certain business domains, such as corporate fraud, money laundering, or inside trading (Pontell & Geis, 2007).

In the healthcare industry, corruption generally happens in six forms: (i) bribery in healthcare service delivery, (ii) procurement corruption, (iii) inappropriate market relations; (iv) abusing power; (v) unreasonable reimbursement claims; and (vi) embezzlement of medical equipment and services (Kohler & Dimancesco, 2020; Sommersguter-Reichmann et al., 2018). Corruption causes over 7% of healthcare expenditure loss every year worldwide. With an annual global health expenditure exceeds US$7.5 trillion, corruption in healthcare business may cause about US$500 billion of loss (Transparency International, 2019).

According to Kohler and Dimancesco (2020), healthcare procurement is vulnerable to corruption. Some listed companies in Hong Kong establish internal control to monitor the fair procurement process. For example, some healthcare companies separate procurement payments, inspection and acceptance of procurement, and price negotiation to different responsible parties to prevent potential procurement corruption and give unduly preferential treatment to favoured suppliers.

Improper market relations may lead to antimicrobial resistance. Promotion of healthcare products, particularly pharmaceutical products, will build up loyalty and trigger over medicalisation (Rönnerstrand & Lapuente, 2017). Influential pharmaceutical firms tend to have a risk of bribery, and the discretion of health professions in drug use increases the opportunity for abuse (Vian, 2008).

An effective anti-corruption strategy requires compliance with related regulations, monitoring and revision of the governance structure (Sommersguter-Reichmann et al., 2018). WHO developed Good Governance for Medicines (GGM) programme

Table 28.4 Regulations on anti-corruption from mainland China and Hong Kong

Region	Laws and regulations	Enacting time
Mainland China	Anti-Corruption Law of the People's Republic of China	1980
	Law of the People's Republic of China on Anti-money Laundering	2006
Hong Kong SAR	Prevention of Bribery Ordinance (Cap. 201 of the Laws of Hong Kong)	1971

in 2004, an assessment tool for the pharmaceutical sector to evaluate risks of corruption. The GGM programme adopts both top-down and bottom-up strategies, ensuring anti-corruption is paid attention from all perspectives (United Nations Development Programme, 2015). The HKEX requires issuers to report corruption-related legal cases, corruption prevention measures and necessary anti-corruption training for employees (Hong Kong Exchanges and Clearing Limited, 2022a). Table 28.4 shows some regulations on anti-corruption from mainland China and Hong Kong SAR.

Issues related to healthcare corruption, such as unaffordable drugs, inequality in healthcare service access, and medical malpractice (Sommersguter-Reichmann et al., 2018), could negatively impact on the ESG performance of healthcare companies and misalign with SDG 3 (United Nations, 2015). Besides, corruption in the healthcare industry may cause the siphon of life-saving resources and opacity of new medicine and technology data (Transparency International, 2019). Thus, due diligence is needed to combat corruption in the healthcare industry.

Further Improvement on the ESG Performance

The target 12.6 of SDG 12 encourages companies to integrate sustainability information into ESG reports, using the number of companies issuing ESG disclosures as an indicator (United Nations, 2015). Since there are increasing regulations and guidelines on ESG reporting, the ESG reporting rate is relatively high globally, but the reporting quality varies (KPMG International, 2020). To improve ESG performance and the quality of ESG disclosure, listed companies in Hong Kong could (i) prioritise climate change in their sustainability reports; (ii) enhance ESG governance; and (iii) deepen regional cooperation with mainland China and other countries.

Focusing on Climate Change

KPMG International (2021) and Deloitte (2022) suggest listed companies in the healthcare industry to integrate climate change considerations into corporate strategies, responding to the net-zero goal and the global concern about climate change

(Bui & de Villiers, 2017). The adverse impacts of climate change cause significant disruption to human well-being and the economy (Salas & Jha, 2019; Salas et al., 2020). Climate change brings physical and transition risks for business entities due to the low-carbon economic transition (Task Force on Climate-Related Financial Disclosures, 2017). Hong Kong released the Hong Kong's Climate Action Plan 2030+ and Hong Kong's Climate Action Plan 2050 to show its determination to tackle climate change (Carbon Neutral@HK, 2021; Environment Bureau, 2017). The healthcare sector should lead climate action due to its industry characteristics (Salas et al., 2020). The ESG Guide added reporting provisions on climate change in 2019 to help listed companies evaluate potential risks of climate change to their business operations (Hong Kong Exchanges and Clearing Limited, 2022a). The HKEX encourages listed companies to follow the Task Force on Climate-Related Financial Disclosures for reporting climate-related issues. Furthermore, the HKEX published the Guidance on Climate Disclosures in 2021, requiring all listed businesses to make climate disclosures by 2025 (Hong Kong Exchanges and Clearing Limited, 2021).

Improving ESG Governance

First, listed companies in the healthcare industry can improve governance performance by clearly identifying stakeholder groups and their expectations (KPMG International, 2021). The sustainability of healthcare providers requires comprehensive stakeholder engagement, which drives the sustainability transition of healthcare, rather than focusing on selected stakeholder groups (Mehralian et al., 2016; Pereno & Eriksson, 2020). Table 28.5 shows the stakeholder groups and some major concerns identified in the healthcare industry. Ng and Leung (2020) argued that stakeholder engagement is critical to economic, environmental, and social sustainability, but stakeholder engagement in Hong Kong listed companies is insufficient now.

Second, external assurance allows for more transparent and measurable ESG disclosure. The HKEX also encourages listed companies to seek independent third-party assurance on the ESG data for credibility (Hong Kong Exchanges and Clearing Limited, 2019). According to BDO Hong Kong's (2021) research on the ESG performance of Hong Kong listed companies in the fiscal year 2020, only 5% of the sampled listed companies adopted external assurance on their ESG reports. Among these companies, 44% obtained assurance on selected ESG data, while the remaining sample chose to assure the whole ESG reports (BDO Hong Kong, 2021).

Finally, board involvement enhances the ESG governance structure (BDO Hong Kong, 2021; KPMG International, 2021). The board of directors (the Board) is responsible for setting companies' sustainability strategies (Jizi, 2017). The ESG Guide mandates listed companies to include a board statement to show (i) the board's oversight of the ESG performance, (ii) the ESG governance method and strategy and (iii) how the board achieves the ESG goals. The board statement aims to increase the board engagement level of Hong Kong listed companies (Hong Kong Exchanges and Clearing Limited, 2022a). The mandatory reporting requirement has achieved

Table 28.5 Stakeholders and their concerns in the healthcare industry

Stakeholder groups	Examples of concerns
Customers	• Product R&D and innovation • Data privacy
Government	• Regulatory compliance • Product safety
Investors/ Shareholders	• Financial performance • Risk management
Employees	• Workplace safety • Staff compensation and benefits
Suppliers	• Green supply chain • Business integrity
Community	• Donations and charities • Concern about the public health
Industry associations	• Industry development • Anti-counterfeit medicines

initial success. From 2019 to 2020, the number of companies with board-level ESG commitment and management climbed by 20%, while those with an ESG strategy increased from 36 to 48% of the sample listed companies (BDO Hong Kong, 2021).

Boosting Regional Cooperation

Hong Kong is the ESG investment hub in Asia and the gateway to mainland China's capital market (Financial Services Development Council, 2020, 2021). Thus, Hong Kong ought to leverage these advantages to improve ESG performance and contribute to the healthcare industry. Moreover, Hong Kong is one of the Greater Bay Area (GBA) cities and contributes to the biotech development in this area (Financial Services Development Council, 2021). It connects major research institutions in neighbouring regions to exchange the latest research outcomes and development in the healthcare industry. For example, the Mainland and Hong Kong Closer Economic Partnership Arrangement (CEPA) took effect in 2003, allowing healthcare practitioners in Hong Kong to provide services in mainland China for more than three years (Trade & Industry Department, 2021). The CEPA may provide numerous opportunities for talents and professionals in healthcare service companies, thereby increasing job satisfaction. In mainland China's 14th Five-Year Plan, biopharmaceuticals were prioritised as an industry focus, allowing frequent exchange in healthcare services and research in the GBA (Financial Services Development Council, 2021). Hong Kong and Shenzhen will establish the Hong Kong-Shenzhen Innovation and Technology Park to develop healthcare technologies, share technological knowledge among healthcare professionals, and accelerate the speed of medical products and process innovation in local healthcare companies (Yim, 2021).

Besides, Hong Kong could enhance international health research cooperation (Financial Services Development Council, 2021). For example, in 2017, Clearbridge Medical Group, based in Singapore, established its first centre (the Centre) in Hong Kong as the regional medical hub. The Centre provides healthcare services with advanced technologies cooperating with world-leading research institutions in other countries, including the United States, Japan, and South Korea (InvestHK, 2018).

Concluding Remarks

This chapter provides a general overview of the healthcare industry and its ESG performance in Hong Kong with three main observations.

First, sustainable development has gained increasing concern with some remarkable events over the past years. The UN SDGs were put forward due to unsustainable situations in the environment and society, raising global concern over specific aspects of sustainable development. ESG emerged from increasing responsible investment. Due to the prevalence of ESG investing and ESG financial products, listed companies align with ESG activities. According to the UN SDG 12, listed companies in the private sector are essential drivers for achieving sustainability (United Nations, 2015). Since investors pay more attention to listed companies' ESG performance, the HKEX has developed ESG reporting guidelines.

Second, the healthcare industry in Hong Kong is thriving due to the growing elderly population, strong demand for healthy lifestyles, and grand expectations for healthcare quality. In Hong Kong, the healthcare industry consists of two sectors: (i) pharmaceuticals and biotechnology and (ii) healthcare equipment and services. Hong Kong has a supportive environment for the healthcare industry with its status as a global financial centre and access to mainland China markets.

Third, based on the framework of the ESG Guide, listed companies in the healthcare industry in Hong Kong prioritise certain aspects of ESG performance. Emission reduction and waste management are the top priorities in the environmental pillar. Both emissions and HCW need to be appropriately managed. In the social pillar, issuers are mainly concerned about employment and labour, product safety and quality, innovation, and anti-corruption practices. In particular, employees generally focus on remuneration and career development. Quality control strategies can guarantee healthcare product quality and safety, such as TQM. Innovation is the core competence of the healthcare industry, and five healthcare innovations are dominating in Hong Kong. Anti-corruption contributes to the quality and safety of healthcare services and products and ensures easy access to them.

Finally, there are three suggestions to improve further the ESG performance in the healthcare industry in Hong Kong. First, listed companies could integrate climate-related considerations into their business strategies to make continuous improvement since climate change has been widely recognised as an urgent issue in human society and an ongoing concern in regional development strategies (Carbon Neutral@HK, 2021; Environment Bureau, 2017; United Nations, 2015). Second, healthcare listed issuers can improve their ESG governance structure through stakeholder engagement, external assurance, and board participation (Hong Kong Exchanges and Clearing Limited, 2022a; KPMG International, 2021). Comprehensive stakeholder engagement adds to the materiality of ESG reporting and guarantees stakeholders' interests. External assurance enhances the credibility, accountability, and transparency of ESG disclosure (O'Dwyer & Owen, 2005). Board engagement helps establish an effective internal ESG governance mechanism, reduce information asymmetry, and steer corporate sustainable development (Amran et al., 2014). Third, Hong Kong can strengthen its cooperation in the healthcare sector in mainland China due to Hong Kong's location, market access, and supportive policies of mainland China. Meanwhile, Hong Kong could collect healthcare research outcomes from developed countries and cooperate with leading research institutes, effectively leveraging its financial infrastructure (Financial Services Development Council, 2021). With good ESG performance, listed healthcare companies could provide accessible healthcare products and services for patients, local community, and society at large (United Nations, 2015). Advanced technology may be applied to healthcare treatment and lead to efficient, effective, and safe treatment. All these efforts will lead to the reduction of health risks and accelerate the realisation of SDG 3.

References

Alda, M. (2021). The environmental, social, and governance (ESG) dimension of firms in which social responsible investment (SRI) and conventional pension funds invest: The mainstream SRI and the ESG inclusion. *Journal of Cleaner Production, 298*, Article 126812. https://doi.org/10.1016/j.jclepro.2021.126812

Amran, A., Lee, S. P., & Devi, S. S. (2014). The influence of governance structure and strategic corporate social responsibility toward sustainability reporting quality. *Business Strategy and the Environment, 23*(4), 217–235. https://doi.org/10.1002/bse.1767

Ananth, A. P., Prashanthini, V., & Visvanathan, C. (2010). Healthcare waste management in Asia. *Waste Management, 30*(1), 154–161. https://doi.org/10.1016/j.wasman.2009.07.018

Arayssi, M., Jizi, M., & Tabaja, H. H. (2020). The impact of board composition on the level of ESG disclosures in GCC countries. *Sustainability Accounting, Management and Policy Journal, 11*(1), 137–161. https://doi.org/10.1108/SAMPJ-05-2018-0136

BDO Hong Kong. (2021). *BDO survey: Fourth-year ESG reporting performance survey shows the evolvement in overall ESG involvement of majority listed companies but which remain inadequate to meet the requirements of the Revised Guide* [Press release]. https://www.bdo.com.hk/en-gb/news/2021/bdo-survey-fourth-year-esg-reporting-performance-survey-shows-the-evolvement-in-overall-esg-involve

Berry, L. L. (2019). Service innovation is urgent in healthcare. *AMS Review, 9*(1), 78–92. https://doi.org/10.1007/s13162-019-00135-x

Brogi, M., & Lagasio, V. (2019). Environmental, social, and governance and company profitability: Are financial intermediaries different? *Corporate Social Responsibility and Environmental Management, 26*(3), 576–587. https://doi.org/10.1002/csr.1704

Bui, B., & de Villiers, C. (2017). Business strategies and management accounting in response to climate change risk exposure and regulatory uncertainty. *British Accounting Review, 49*(1), 4–24. https://doi.org/10.1016/j.bar.2016.10.006

Carbon Neutral@HK. (2021). *Hong Kong's Climate Action Plan 2050.* https://www.climateready.gov.hk/files/pdf/CAP2050_booklet_en.pdf

Consolandi, C., Phadke, H., Hawley, J., & Eccles, R. G. (2020). Material ESG outcomes and SDG externalities: Evaluating the health care sector's contribution to the SDGs. *Organization and Environment, 33*(4), 511–533. https://doi.org/10.1177/1086026619899795

Cuervo-Cazurra, A. (2016). Corruption in international business. *Journal of World Business, 51*(1), 35–49. https://doi.org/10.1016/j.jwb.2015.08.015

Deloitte. (2022). *2022 global health care outlook: Are we finally seeing the long-promised transformation?* https://www2.deloitte.com/cn/en/pages/life-sciences-and-healthcare/articles/2022-global-health-care-sector-outlook.html

Demir, M., & Min, M. (2019). Consistencies and discrepancies in corporate social responsibility reporting in the pharmaceutical industry. *Sustainability Accounting, Management and Policy Journal, 10*(2), 333–364. https://doi.org/10.1108/SAMPJ-03-2018-0094

Edwards, B., Hugman, B., Tobin, M., & Whalen, M. (2012). Embedding "Speaking up" into systems for safe healthcare product development and marketing surveillance. *Drug Safety, 35*(4), 265–271. https://doi.org/10.2165/11597860-000000000-00000

Environment Bureau. (2017). *Hong Kong's climate action plan 2030+*. https://www.hkgbc.org.hk/eng/engagement/file/ClimateActionPlanEng.pdf

Eshkalak, S. K., Ghomi, E. R., Dai, Y., Choudhury, D., & Ramakrishna, S. (2020). The role of three-dimensional printing in healthcare and medicine. *Materials & Design, 194*, Article 108940. https://doi.org/10.1016/j.matdes.2020.108940

Fernandez-Feijoo, B., Romero, S., & Ruiz, S. (2014). Effect of stakeholders' pressure on transparency of sustainability reports within the GRI framework. *Journal of Business Ethics, 122*(1), 53–63. https://doi.org/10.1007/s10551-013-1748-5

Financial Services Development Council. (2020). *Hong Kong—Developing into the global ESG investment hub of Asia.* https://www.fsdc.org.hk/media/egvher4d/fsdc_paper_no_44_hong_kong-developing_into_the_global_esg_investment_hub_of_asia_eng.pdf

Financial Services Development Council. (2021). *Fuelling further growth of biotech and healthcare industries: Leveraging Hong Kong's financial infrastructure.* https://www.fsdc.org.hk/media/c2cpcpld/20211115-fsdc-research-report-healthcare-financing_en.pdf

Fong, B. Y. F., Law, V. T. S., Leung, T. C. H., Lo, M. F., Ng, T. K. C., & Yee, H. H. L. (2021). Sustainable development goal 3: Health and well-being of ageing in Hong Kong. *Routledge.* https://doi.org/10.4324/9781003220169

Gianfrate, G., & Peri, M. (2019). The green advantage: Exploring the convenience of issuing green bonds. *Journal of Cleaner Production, 219*, 127–135. https://doi.org/10.1016/j.jclepro.2019.02.022

Hang Seng Indexes Company Limited. (2020). *Hang seng industry classification system.* https://www.hsi.com.hk/static/uploads/contents/en/dl_centre/brochures/B_HSICSe.pdf

Health Bureau. (2021). *Hong Kong's domestic health accounts (DHA).* https://www.healthbureau.gov.hk/statistics/download/dha/en/dha_summary_report_1920.pdf

Hensher, M., & McGain, F. (2020). Health care sustainability metrics: Building a safer, low-carbon health system. *Health Affairs, 39*(12), 2080–2087. https://doi.org/10.1377/hlthaff.2020.01103

Hong Kong Exchanges and Clearing Limited. (2019). *Consultation conclusion: Review of the environmental, social and governance reporting guide and related listing rules.* https://www.hkex.com.hk/-/media/HKEX-Market/News/Market-Consultations/2016-Present/May-2019-Review-of-ESG-Guide/Conclusions-(December-2019)/cp201905cc.pdf?la=en

Hong Kong Exchanges and Clearing Limited. (2020). *HKEX in biotech: Connecting the healthcare industry.* https://www.hkex.com.hk/-/media/HKEX-Market/Join-Our-Markets/IPO/Biotech-Newsletter/HKEXBIOTECH_Newsletter_issue4_eng.pdf

Hong Kong Exchanges and Clearing Limited. (2021). *Guidance on climate disclosures.* https://www.hkex.com.hk/-/media/HKEX-Market/Listing/Rules-and-Guidance/Environmental-Social-and-Governance/Exchanges-guidance-materials-on-ESG/guidance_climate_disclosures.pdf?la=en

Hong Kong Exchanges and Clearing Limited. (2022a). *Appendix 27: Environmental, social and governance reporting guide*. https://en-rules.hkex.com.hk/pdf-manipulate?/sites/default/files/net_file_store/HKEX4476_3841_VER18584.pdf

Hong Kong Exchanges and Clearing Limited. (2022b). *How to prepare an ESG report*. https://www.hkex.com.hk/-/media/HKEX-Market/Listing/Rules-and-Guidance/Environmental-Social-and-Governance/Exchanges-guidance-materials-on-ESG/app2_envirokpis.pdf

InvestHK. (2018). *Singapore-based medical group opens first medical centre in Hong Kong*. https://www.investhk.gov.hk/en/news/singapore-based-medical-group-opens-first-medical-centre-hong-kong.html

Jizi, M. (2017). The influence of board composition on sustainable development disclosure. *Business Strategy and the Environment, 26*(5), 640–655. https://doi.org/10.1002/bse.1943

Kim, J., Campbell, A. S., de Ávila, B. E. F., & Wang, J. (2019). Wearable biosensors for healthcare monitoring. *Nature Biotechnology, 37*(4), 389–406. https://doi.org/10.1038/s41587-019-0045-y

Kohler, J. C., & Dimancesco, D. (2020). The risk of corruption in public pharmaceutical procurement: How anti-corruption, transparency and accountability measures may reduce this risk. *Global Health Action, 13*, Article 1694745. https://doi.org/10.1080/16549716.2019.1694745

KPMG International. (2020). *The time has come: The KPMG survey of sustainability reporting 2020*. https://assets.kpmg/content/dam/kpmg/xx/pdf/2020/11/the-time-has-come.pdf

KPMG International. (2021). *ESG reporting in healthcare: Driving a connection to health outcomes*. https://info.kpmg.us/content/dam/info/en/news-perspectives/pdf/2021/ESG%20Healthcare%20slipsheet.pdf

Kuzey, C., Uyar, A., Nizaeva, M., & Karaman, A. S. (2021). CSR performance and firm performance in the tourism, healthcare, and financial sectors: Do metrics and CSR committees matter? *Journal of Cleaner Production, 319*, Article 128802. https://doi.org/10.1016/j.jclepro.2021.128802

Lenzen, M., Malik, A., Li, M., Fry, J., Weisz, H., Pichler, P.-P., Chaves, L. S. M., Capon, A., & Pencheon, D. (2020). The environmental footprint of health care: A global assessment. *The Lancet Planetary Health, 4*(7), e271–e279. https://doi.org/10.1016/S2542-5196(20)30121-2

Machado, B. A. A., Dias, L. C. P., & Fonseca, A. (2021). Transparency of materiality analysis in GRI-based sustainability reports. *Corporate Social Responsibility and Environmental Management, 28*(2), 570–580. https://doi.org/10.1002/csr.2066

Mehralian, G., Nazari, J. A., Zarei, L., & Rasekh, H. R. (2016). The effects of corporate social responsibility on organizational performance in the Iranian pharmaceutical industry: The mediating role of TQM. *Journal of Cleaner Production, 135*, 689–698. https://doi.org/10.1016/j.jclepro.2016.06.116

Mosadeghrad, A. M. (2014). Factors influencing healthcare service quality. *International Journal of Health Policy and Management, 3*(2), 77–89. https://doi.org/10.15171/ijhpm.2014.65

Balaisyte, J., Nair, N., & Mahmood, R. (2021). *MSCI ESG healthcare funds and SDG 3*. MSCI. https://support.msci.com/documents/10199/c192c240-9e89-5af7-a3c1-060eb6cf0639

Ng, A. W., & Leung, T. C. H. (2020). Relevance of SEA to a global financial centre under one country two systems: Engaging stakeholders for sustainability and climate change. *Social and Environmental Accountability Journal, 40*(2), 140–148. https://doi.org/10.1080/0969160X.2020.1776625

O'Dwyer, B., & Owen, D. L. (2005). Assurance statement practice in environmental, social and sustainability reporting: A critical evaluation. *British Accounting Review, 37*(2), 205–229. https://doi.org/10.1016/j.bar.2005.01.005

Pereno, A., & Eriksson, D. (2020). A multi-stakeholder perspective on sustainable healthcare: From 2030 onwards. *Futures, 122*, Article 102605. https://doi.org/10.1016/j.futures.2020.102605

Pichler, P.-P., Jaccard, I. S., Weisz, U., & Weisz, H. (2019). International comparison of health care carbon footprints. *Environmental Research Letters, 14*(6), Article 064004. https://doi.org/10.1088/1748-9326/ab19e1

Pontell, H. N., & Geis, G. L. (2007). *International handbook of write-collar and corporate crime*. Springer. https://doi.org/10.1007/978-0-387-34111-8

PwC. (2021a). *ESG for healthcare organizations: What's right for the world is good for business*. https://www.pwc.com/us/en/industries/health-industries/library/assets/pwc-esg-health-insights-health-org.pdf
PwC. (2021b). *Global top health industry issues 2021: Innovation fuelled by digital capabilities*. https://www.pwc.com/gx/en/healthcare/pdf/pwc-global-top-health-industry-issues-2021.pdf
Rönnerstrand, B., & Lapuente, V. (2017). Corruption and use of antibiotics in regions of Europe. *Health Policy, 121*(3), 250–256. https://doi.org/10.1016/j.healthpol.2016.12.010
Salas, R. N., & Jha, A. K. (2019). Climate change threatens the achievement of effective universal healthcare. *BMJ, 366*, Article l5302. https://doi.org/10.1136/bmj.l5302
Salas, R. N., Maibach, E., Pencheon, D., Watts, N., & Frumkin, H. (2020). A pathway to net zero emissions for healthcare. *BMJ, 371*, Article m3785. https://doi.org/10.1136/bmj.m3785
Sommersguter-Reichmann, M., Wild, C., Stepan, A., Reichmann, G., & Fried, A. (2018). Individual and institutional corruption in European and US healthcare: Overview and link of various corruption typologies. *Applied Health Economics and Health Policy, 16*(3), 289–302. https://doi.org/10.1007/s40258-018-0386-6
Sustainable Stock Exchanges Initiative. (2019). *Stock exchange database*. https://sseinitiative.org/exchanges-filter-search/
Task Force on Climate-Related Financial Disclosures. (2017). *Recommendations of the task force on climate-related financial disclosures*. https://assets.bbhub.io/company/sites/60/2021/10/FINAL-2017-TCFD-Report.pdf
Thakur, V., & Ramesh, A. (2015). Healthcare waste management research: A structured analysis and review (2005–2014). *Waste Management and Research, 33*(10), 855–870. https://doi.org/10.1177/0734242x15594248
Trade and Industry Department. (2021). *Mainland and Hong Kong closer economic partnership arrangement*. https://www.tid.gov.hk/english/cepa/
Transparency International. (2019). *The ignored pandemic: How corruption in healthcare service delivery threatens universal health coverage*. https://ti-health.org/wp-content/uploads/2019/03/IgnoredPandemic-WEB-v2.pdf
United Nations. (2015). *Transforming our world: The 2030 agenda for sustainable development*. https://sdgs.un.org/sites/default/files/publications/21252030%20Agenda%20for%20Sustainable%20Development%20web.pdf
United Nations Development Programme. (2015). *Fighting corruption in the health sector*. https://www.undp.org/publications/fighting-corruption-health-sector
UN Principles for Responsible Investment. (2020). *Principles for responsible investment: An investor initiativein partnership with unep finance initiative and the un global compact*. https://www.unpri.org/download?ac=10948
Vian, T. (2008). Review of corruption in the health sector: Theory, methods and interventions. *Health Policy and Planning, 23*(2), 83–94. https://doi.org/10.1093/heapol/czm048
World Health Organization. (2017). *WHO global model regulatory framework for medical devices including in vitro diagnostic medical devices: WHO Medical device technical series*. https://apps.who.int/iris/rest/bitstreams/1083399/retrieve
World Health Organization. (2018, February 8). *Health-care waste*. https://www.who.int/news-room/fact-sheets/detail/health-care-waste
Xie, J., Nozawa, W., Yagi, M., Fujii, H., & Managi, S. (2019). Do environmental, social, and governance activities improve corporate financial performance? *Business Strategy and the Environment, 28*(2), 286–300. https://doi.org/10.1002/bse.2224
Yim, S. (2021). Biotechnology, medical & healthcare industry in Hong Kong. *Hong Kong Trade Development Council Research*. https://research.hktdc.com/en/article/MzEzOTQ1MjMz
Zhang, F., & Wu, F. (2019). Rethinking the city and innovation: A political economic view from China's biotech. *Cities, 85*, 150–155. https://doi.org/10.1016/j.cities.2018.09.003
Zhang, X. H., Ogunseitan, O. A., Xu, M. J., & Chen, M. J. (2014). Healthcare waste management policy assessment in China. *Advanced Materials Research, 878*, 594–599. https://doi.org/10.4028/www.scientific.net/AMR.878.594

Chapter 29
Effect of Offering Organisational Supports to Employees with Responsibilities for Elderly Family Members: Evidence from China

Bowen Dong

Abstract In China, the significant proportion of the ageing population leads to a rising need for eldercare provision that resulted in disruptions, such as making and receiving calls related to eldercare and temporary leave for caregiving, for their working relatives. This phenomenon poses a challenge for organisational decision-makers, on how to support stressful employees who are struggling to strike a balance between full-time employment and eldercare provision for the family. To address this issue, four in-depth interviews were conducted in China, which identified extant policy-based and non-policy-based supports that were being offered in modern organisations. Based on thematic analysis, employees with eldercare responsibilities acknowledged the value of flexible work arrangements (e.g. flextime and flex-place) and expected more flexible options (e.g. more paid leave) to be provided to reduce strain as it helped employees to better reconcile eldercare with employment. They also expressed uncertainty concerning the effectiveness of family-friendly policies in consideration of the difficulty in negotiating the work and eldercare domains. Resource availability and strategic direction hence influenced an organisation's decision on whether flexible practices should be adopted. These findings could provide some implications to policymakers and organisational practitioners.

Keywords Eldercare · Human resources policies · Non-policy-based supports · Organisational supports

B. Dong (✉)
Faculty of Business, City University of Macau, Macau, China
e-mail: bwdong@cityu.mo

B. Y. F. Fong and W. C. W. Wong (eds.), *Gaps and Actions in Health Improvement from Hong Kong and Beyond*,
https://doi.org/10.1007/978-981-99-4491-0_29

Introduction

With the rapidly expanding ageing population all over the world, pronounced challenges for modern organisations have emerged: employees suffering from a rising need to care for their older family members, which leads to physical and psychological strain, and hence increases absenteeism (Kim et al., 2013). Both practitioners and scholars have addressed this issue and explored how human resources management (HRM) practices in organisations can help employees to better manage the balance between full-time employment and family responsibilities (Montez et al., 2014).

Seeking for effective HRM practices to reconcile work and family roles, a burgeoning body of literature notes the necessity to focus on eldercare, a responsibility that differs from other caregiving roles and creates more stress from work and family. On one hand, the dependence and care needs of elders increase with age, which places a heavy burden on caregivers (Murphy & Cross, 2021). On the other hand, the onset and duration of eldercare duties tend to be quite unpredictable, making it almost impossible for employees to plan for required leave (Clancy et al., 2020). Currently, work-family balance practices are generally designed for all employees, regardless of the type of care responsibility, and few studies have investigated differing value of organisational practices and their effects on employees with eldercare responsibilities, thus limiting our understanding of how to help employees reconcile eldercare with work.

To fill the gap in the research and examine the rising needs of employees with eldercare responsibilities, this chapter presents four case studies conducted in China, a developing country that has become an ageing society. Several implications are offered to the eldercare literature and managerial practice. First, this chapter describes what types of formal and informal practices modern organisations in China have provided to reduce strain experienced by caregivers. Second, it further delineates how employees perceive the value of these formal and informal practices. Finally, it identifies the three factors that affect managers' decisions on what types of organisational practices should be implemented.

Defining Eldercare Responsibility

Eldercare refers to "informal care of the elderly by family and friends" (Smith, 2004, p. 353). It can be conceptualised as a dynamic process that evolves with the care recipient's condition: short-term caregiving after an injury or surgical procedure or long-term caregiving after a permanent physical or cognitive decline (Calvano, 2013). More precisely, eldercare can be divided into three aspects based on the tasks that caregivers undertake: personal and health care (e.g. administering medications), instrumental activities of daily living (e.g. meal preparation), and eldercare management (e.g. socio-emotional support) (Murphy & Cross, 2021). It addresses a combination of needs in terms of psychology, medical treatment, and finance.

With increasing life expectancy comes, there is a rising need for younger generations to care for older family members. This pushes employees to redefine the domains of work and family and requires them to seek for a new work-family balance. As they negotiate their roles, employees are found to suffer from psychological, physical, and financial strains that may result in burnout and fatigue in the workplace, with a negative effect on job performance (Kim et al., 2013; Matthews et al., 2014).

Organisational Practices for Managing Work-Family Balance

Among various studies on work-family balance, there is a consensus that corporate-level support with available resources provision can be an effective way in helping employees to manage the strain, given that employees have finite resources for which both work and family compete (Clancy et al., 2020; Liao et al., 2019). Based on the job demand/resources model, the extant literature identifies diverse work-life balance policies implemented in modern organisations, such as paid leave, compressed hours, remote/home-working, and flexible working hours (Murphy & Cross, 2021). Paid leave and compressed hours support employees who leave their employment temporarily to resolve short-term and urgent family issues, while remote/home-working and flexible working hours can be a sustainable option for employees who take on family responsibilities (e.g. eldercare) and job duties simultaneously.

In addition to policy-based supports, the extant literature also sheds light on various nonpolicy-based supports that help employees manage the work/family interface. Supervisor behaviours pertaining to employee support (e.g. adjusting work assignments to satisfy employees' need, and sharing ideas or advice with employees) create group norms and climates that regulate group behaviours regarding the use of group and organisational resources (Breaugh & Frye, 2008). For example, in a supportive workplace, employees are at ease to use formal supports to care for family members. Even though work interruptions occur, supervisors are found to hold a positive perception regarding caregivers' job performance (Kim et al., 2013). In addition, this informal support can form emotional connections between caregivers and supervisors, and in turn positively affects their work commitment, even when caregivers experience high levels of work stress (Peng et al., 2020).

While numerous family-friendly practices have been identified in the literature, few of them are specifically designed for employees with eldercare responsibilities, raising a question as to their effectiveness in helping employees manage their strain relevant to the work-eldercare balance (Gordon et al., 2012; Henle et al., 2020). A recent study (Peng et al., 2020) provides evidence that family-supportive supervision may not function as well as dedicated eldercare-supportive supervision for employees with a high caregiver burden. Therefore, there is a call for studies to understand how to best reduce strains that impact employees with eldercare responsibilities and what affects organisational decision-makers to implement policy-and non-policy-based supports that seem to be helpful in managing the work-eldercare balance (Clancy et al., 2020).

Case Studies

The study was conducted during February and March 2022 in China, a developing country with an ageing society and a strong cultural context in which people have an obligation to care for their family members. An inductive research logic is employed to provide rich descriptions and advance the understanding of the value of organisational supports for caregivers. Multiple case study method was adopted to broaden the exploration of our research questions and theoretical elaboration (Eisenhardt & Graebner, 2007).

Nine eligible individuals were identified from the author's personal network and received interview invitations via email and WeChat (the most widely used communication tool in China). Five agreed to participate in this study. Based on a review of the extant literature on eldercare and HRM, a sequence of questions was developed and sent to participants through WeChat. The interview protocol centres on (1) policy-based supports associated with family and eldercare in the participant's organisation; (2) non-policy-based supports in his/her work group; and (3) perceptions of these organisational supports. A semi-structured interview was then conducted by telephone due to travel restrictions from the COVID-19 pandemic. One of the participants missed the interview appointment due to personal affairs and responded to the survey questions through texting. Although answers to the questions during the texting were informative and detailed, the reliability of the process could be an issue. Therefore, only four cases were finally retained in this study. With the participants' approval, the four interviews were tape-recorded to avoid potential memory bias for subsequent data analysis procedures. After interview transcripts were coded, follow-up queries were conducted to examine and enrich the data until no new information emerged (theoretical saturation). Each interview lasted approximately 25–60 min. The background information of the participants is shown in Table 29.1.

To conduct the thematic analysis, a HRM professional was invited to read the interview transcript and develop narratives for each case independently from the author. Comparison and confirmation of results were adopted at each step to ensure validity and reliability in the coding procedure. The narratives illustrate the kinds of support that were provided in the organisations, how this support works for caregivers, and participants' perception of their value for employees. These practices were grouped into three specific types: work arrangement, form of leave, and period of time off. First-order categories were further aggregated into two higher-order codes: policy-based and non-policy-based supports. For each type of practice, the suitability of organisational supports was then evaluated based on participants' perceptions.

Table 29.1 Demographic information of participants

Participant	Age	Gender	Employment sector	Position	Care recipient	Support from other family members
1	28	Male	Internet industry Small private enterprise Data analysis	Department Manager	Father, mother	None
2	31	Male	Internet industry Large public enterprise Operations management	Operations Manager	Father, mother	None
3	44	Male	Petrochemical industry Large state-owned enterprise Technical specialist	Vice President	Father, mother	Support from siblings
4	56	Female	Banking industry Large state-owned enterprise Accounting	Sales Manager	Father, mother	Support from siblings

Case 1: Online Commerce Company

Participant 1 worked as a senior manager in the data analysis centre under a small-size private company. This company, with a good cash flow, was acknowledged as the only one in the internet industry that paid each employee weekly at a high salary and gave RMB (Chinese dollars) 666 to employees' parents for each festival.

Work-Family Balance Practices Within the Organisation

Once a month, employees could apply to leave the workplace for two hours for any reason. If employees needed to care for their family members for a short period, they were encouraged to use unpaid leave (maximum amount of leave is 3 days) or annual leave (maximum amount of leave is 15 days). Leave for a longer period (more than 15 days) required permission from the direct supervisor, otherwise, it would be recorded as absenteeism. Noteworthily, the workplace culture in this company was competitive rather than supportive. The office hours were from 10:00 a.m. to 7:00 p.m., but most employees left the office after 9:00 p.m. Everyone seemed to be busying himself/herself with work tasks and were provided with no more support as caregivers than basic socio-emotional support (e.g. prayers and words of encouragement). Therefore, most employees were hesitant to use existing supportive benefits for family issues because of fearing possible penalties such as negative career consequences and ostracism.

Perceptions of Organisational Practices

The two-hour temporary leave was quite a valuable assistance for handling sudden needs for caregiving, but unpaid or annual leave for short-term or long-term care might not decrease work-related strain since employees suffered a loss of wage and opportunities for recognition from supervisors. In this company, there was no specific set of competencies required for completing work tasks, and the high salary made it easy to access highly qualified employees in the labour market. In such a competitive environment, employees needed to manage the conflicts of full-time employment and eldercare provision by themselves.

Case 2: Internet Technology Company

Participant 2 worked as an operations manager in a large-scale public company established in 1997. Not only being a top-tier company in mobile games, online music content communities, and global e-commerce platform, the company was also well-known for creating work time flexibility and autonomy for employees. For example, the office hours began from 9:30 a.m., but when employees come into the office was largely their individual preference.

Work-Family Balance Practices Within the Organisation

First, paid leave, for a maximum period of 10 days, was provided for all employees to use at any time in a year, and employees could apply to use their current and future annual leave in advance as an extension. Second, remote/home-working for a given period was readily permitted by the HR office and supervisors if employees needed to care for older family members. Participant 2 stated, as an example, that his colleague was allowed to work in his home city for one week and came to the office every other week. Third, the company also provided welfare programmes to employees. For example, the staff union purchased health insurance for employees' parents and provided financial support for parents' medical treatment. In terms of non-policy-based support, socio-emotional support (e.g. sharing ideas or advice with employees) had been continuously provided to caregivers. In addition, supervisors and colleagues attended to participants' eldercare-related needs (e.g. adjust work arrangement) and assistance in completing associated work tasks.

Perceptions of Organisational Practices

The company had numerous flexible options for employees to satisfy the demands of eldercare, facilitating the negotiation between the domains of work and eldercare. As Participant 2 illustrated, the remote/home-working provided employees with the necessary autonomy to reconcile eldercare with work responsibilities. However, it was also noted that while these flexible work arrangements could be effective for improving employee productivity, they might also increase costs of time and efforts to coordinate the work.

Case 3: Integrated Energy and Chemical Company

Participant 3, who had worked for a large state-owned company in the past 25 years, was appointed as the vice president of a subsidiary this year. In the subsidiary, most employees were technicians and had access to the same policies as in the parent company. For example, the office hours were restricted to 9:00 a.m. to 5:00 p.m. However, Participant 3 still attended to the design of flexible HR practices for the technicians.

Work-Family Balance Practices Within the Organisation

A flexible work arrangement policy was adopted in the company. Employees who were in charge of regular preventative maintenance and emergency maintenance, usually performed at night, could leave the office and cared for their family members in the daytime. For temporary leave, employees were not required to get permission from supervisors and could take leave at any time as long as a new work schedule was arranged. For a longer time off, taking annual leave was suggested. Remote/home-working for a given period was another flexible option for caregivers.

In such a supportive workplace, colleagues not only provided emotional support (e.g. prayers and words of encouragement) to caregivers, but also assisted caregivers in coping with work-related stress (e.g. help to complete work on time), particularly when they had difficulty in balancing the competing demands of eldercare and work. Furthermore, supervisors were encouraged to use their network resources to help employees seek medical treatment and organise colleagues to help with caregiving.

Perceptions on Organisational Practices

Based on the HR feedback, benefits such as flexible work arrangements reduced employees' work-related strains and the likelihood of absenteeism. However, the flexibility also resulted in some disruptions at work, though most of these could be solved with non-policy-based supports from supervisors and colleagues. The family-friendliness of an organisation could have a positive impact by enhancing a caregiver's commitment to the organisation and reducing turnover-related costs.

Case 4: Commercial Bank

Participant 4 worked in a large state-owned company in the banking industry. In her almost 25 years on the job, Participant 4 had risen through the ranks of the sales department from a teller to the manager. Her long tenure had allowed her to witness the development of Human Resource practices in this company, which was a highly structured organisation with strict HR policies. For each employee, the company kept a manual timekeeping record of days he/she was late or absent, and it was posted online to immediate supervisors and colleagues each month. There was also a complex procedure for employee leave.

Work-Family Balance Practices Within the Organisation

For temporary leave (the maximum amount of unpaid leave was 3 days per quarter and 7 days per year), an employee had to apply at least half a day in advance and get the permission from different supervisors depending on the length of time off. For 1-day leave, approval was obtained from the department manager; for 1- to 3-day leave, approval was obtained from the sub-branch manager, and for leaves of more than 3 days, approval could only be granted through the discussion among the top management team. Caregivers could apply for financial assistance (RMB 2,000–10,000) from the company's staff union. Non-policy-based supports relied on the benevolence of supervisors and some departments did provide socio-emotional support, such as information sharing and caring visits, while others did not.

Perceptions of Organisational Practices

The discipline of the workplace was strict, and there was little or no flexibility over the daily work schedule of employees. The established rules and policies encouraged employees to deal with eldercare needs during off-work hours or to use unpaid leave and annual leave. When these practices were performance-oriented and managing the risks of poor coordination, Participant 4, as a department manager, was worried about the impact on employee turnover and thought that more assistance should be provided for employees to deal with physical, psychological, and financial strain associated with eldercare.

Findings and Discussion

The thematic analysis presented several organisational supports, both policy-based and non-policy-based, that might be helpful for employees in eldercare provision. Policy-based practices included flexible working hours, temporary leave, annual leave, remote/home-working, and employee assistance programmes, while non-policy-based supports included socio-emotional support, caregiving, and financial assistance, and were strongly related with the actions of supervisors and colleagues. The detailed descriptions of each type of practice are shown in Table 29.2. While numerous organisational supports have been provided to reduce the employees' strain in an attempt to balance the demand of work and family, it raises concerns in the Chinese context about the value of these organisational support to employees with eldercare responsibilities and the factors that affect the decision on whether to make these supports available to employees.

Value of Organisational Supports to Caregivers

Modern organisations view flexibility as valuable resources that can buffer the negative effects of work demands on employee health and implement organisational practices such as designing policies and cultivating supportive culture to aid employees in meeting their needs to care for family members. For caregivers, the higher the level of autonomy associated with the work role, the more permeable the boundaries between elder caregiving and work become (Clark, 2000). Practices like flextime and flexplace allow employees to effectively reconcile eldercare and work responsibilities, leading to an increase in employee job satisfaction and commitment to the organisation. Participant 2 is a case in point. He stated that he enjoyed the benefits of flexibility his organisation allowed and could not imagine working for other companies.

In addition, participants noted that broadening non-policy-based practices (e.g. socio-emotional support, caregiving, and financial assistance) also delivered great support to them. As Participant 3 stated, he could not handle it without the selfless help from his colleagues. Such practices are a manifestation of an organisational culture that shapes group norms and expectations regarding the usage of benefits. Within a competitive working environment, potential penalties from taking leave, such as lower wages and reduced chance of promotion, may prevent employees from availing themselves of work-family balance policies even if they are offered. Organisations that implement non-policy-based practices, such as assistance in seeking medical treatment, foster a culture that can facilitate employee gratitude, which from a social exchange perspective leads to increased obligation to repay supervisors with more effort in the completion of work tasks.

Table 29.2 Overview of organisational practices and their value to caregivers

Organisational practices related to caregivers	Description	Evidence of use among participants' companies	Perception of participants	Value to the caregivers
Policy-based supports				
Flexible working hours	Allows employees to allocate their work hours to caregiving based on their personal needs.	Employees can arrive at the office after 10 a.m. and leave based on personal need. (Case 2) If employees can finish their tasks in time, there is no strict schedule for starting and finishing hours, especially for technical employees who needs to perform maintenance at night. (Case 3)	A sustainable option for employees to deal with long-term caregiving issues, but the flextime presents some difficulties for supervisors, such as scheduling work among a team.	High
Temporary leave	Employees can leave their employment immediately for urgent reasons. The period can last for several days without penalty.	Employees can decide when to take 10 day paid leave. It is extra day off and not included in annual leave. (Case 2)	This form of leave satisfies the need for sudden caregiving. If caregivers can arrange their tasks well, it can be suitable to caregivers.	High
Annual leave	Employees can only use annual leave (normally 10–15 days, based on tenure) for caregiving; otherwise they incur penalties.	If employees cannot undertake tasks in the workplace due to personal affairs, they must apply for annual leave; otherwise they will be fined. (Cases 1 and 4)	This is not a priority option for caregivers because it means that they use their own holiday and annual leave entitlements to cover care requirements. However, it can benefit organisations.	Medium

(continued)

Table 29.2 (continued)

Organisational practices related to caregivers	Description	Evidence of use among participants' companies	Perception of participants	Value to the caregivers
Remote/ home-working	Allows employees to perform their roles from home or remotely if possible.	A colleague in the participant's department was permitted to work in his home city for one week and come to the office every other week. If someone is restricted from working due to COVID-19, remote working is strongly supported. (Case 2)	Employees can undertake their work and caregiving roles at the same time. But currently, this option is only provided in specific industries and occupations, such as programmers in the tech sector.	High
Employee assistance program	Provides benefits to employee's parents or supportive services for employees to take care of their parents.	For each festival, employees' parents will get RMB 666 as a gift. (Case 1) Free insurance is provided for parents. (Case 2) The labour union can provide financial support for medical treatment. (Cases 2, 3 and 4)	Helpful for employees to provide high-quality care, but it may be no helpful in reconciling eldercare and employment.	Medium
Non-policy-based supports				
Socio-emotional support	Shapes a supportive climate in which supervisors provide information, advice and emotional support to help caregivers.	Supervisors and colleagues concern about caregivers' mental and physical state. They generally lend a hand to caregivers in completing tasks. (Cases 1, 2, 3 and 4)	The cohesive and friendly climate can form a strong tie between caregivers and colleagues, even though some socio-emotional supports may not be helpful for the caregivers.	Medium/ high
Caregiving and financial assistance	Supervisors and colleagues share their financial or network resources with caregivers to coordinate care.	Supervisors help arrange the best medical treatment available. Colleagues provide financial assistance (Case 1, 2, 3, 4) and unpaid care to care recipients. (Case 3)	Very helpful. Caregivers may feel gratitude and consequently feel stronger commitment to their work group and organization.	High

Factors that Affect Organisational Decision to Implement Flexible Practices

While increasing empirical literature highlights the win–win outcomes work-life balance practices create for both individuals, e.g. increases in well-being (Pei et al., 2017) and organisations, e.g. building organisational image and reputation (Barnes et al., 2016), some of the participants expressed uncertainty concerning the effectiveness of family-friendly policies and whether the benefits could outweigh the costs. This concern is supported by the literature, which has shown that taking advantage of flextime and flexplace can be interpreted as a signal of being "always on", as there may be difficulties in negotiating the work and eldercare domains and otherwise increases work-family conflict and associated strain (Schooreel & Verbruggen, 2016). Some organisations may also promote work-life balance practices for a positive external image yet take strategic actions to prevent their usage by employees (Perrigino et al., 2018). As shown in Case 4, some organisations design a complex procedure to shift away from family-friendly practices, forcing employees to use off-work hours and leave that is guaranteed by law like annual leave to manage their eldercare responsibilities.

The aforementioned four cases show that resource availability and strategic orientation have a significant impact on the decisions managers make in response to an employee's need for workplace flexibility for eldercare. First, managers may regard policies of providing flexibility as an unnecessary expense for organisational survival. Direct benefits given to employees with eldercare responsibilities (e.g. financial assistance in Case 2 and Case 4) are also unlikely to be affordable if the organisation is under financial stress. Second, as illustrated in Cases 1 and 2, technology-oriented companies that seek innovation as a strategy prefer to implement employee-centred management that provides flexible work arrangements and a variety of informal supports. A high level of organisational autonomy has been found to be highly related to job creativity (Liu et al., 2011), which could, in turn, build competitive advantage for technology-oriented companies.

Health for All and Health in All Policies

Today, individuals have multiple roles in aspects such as work and eldercare. When personal resources (e.g. energy, time, money) could not fully satisfy the total demands of work expectation and eldercare provision, individuals are likely to suffer from physical, emotional, and even financial strain, thereby resulting in some personal health issues, such as depression and somatic symptoms (Clancy et al., 2020; Shifrin & Michel, 2022). While there are existing legal protections to safeguard employees from long time work and heavy duties, organisations nowadays could play a more important and direct role to help employees manage job-related stress and ensure their health by implementing HRM policies and offering supporting practices.

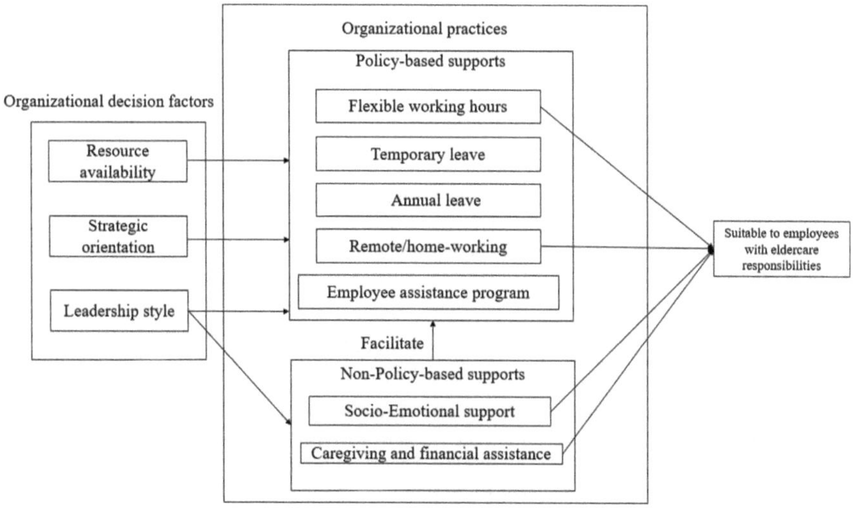

Fig. 29.1 The suitability of organisational practices

As shown in Fig. 29.1, this chapter focuses on the Chinese context, comparing and illustrating alternative policies (e.g. unpaid leave), flexible work arrangements (e.g. flextime and flexplace), and non-policy-based supports (e.g. creating a supportive culture) that could be more accessible for employees to take care of their elderly family members. If caregivers have these boundary-spanning resources in the form of organisational supports, they are likely to succeed in accommodating demands of job responsibilities with eldercare responsibilities, so as to deal with eldercare needs, for which onset and duration are unpredictable, and avoid work-related costs (e.g. a loss of wage).

The findings suggest that workplace flexibility in a supportive workplace culture could foster employee health in general and satisfy the demand for taking care of elderly family members. However, it should be noted that the strategy of flexibility should be well designed and personalised, otherwise, the signal of workplace flexibility (being "always on") may render caregivers to experience more physical and mental stress from the extrinsic (e.g. few career promotion) and social penalties (e.g. stigmatisation). Managers should evaluate the feasibility of flexibility with reference to the daily operations and organisational development based on resource availability and strategic orientation. In addition, managers should continuously seek to design innovative practices that encourage employees to form strong as well as less formal, emotional, and social connections with the organisation.

References

Barnes, C. M., Jiang, K., & Lepak, D. P. (2016). Sabotaging the benefits of our own human capital: Work unit characteristics and sleep. *Journal of Applied Psychology, 101*(2), 209–221. https://doi.org/10.1037/apl0000042

Breaugh, J. A., & Frye, N. K. (2008). Work-family conflict: The importance of family-friendly employment practices and family-supportive supervisors. *Journal of Business and Psychology, 22*(4), 345–353. https://doi.org/10.1007/s10869-008-9081-1

Calvano, L. (2013). Tug of war: Caring for our elders while remaining productive at work. *Academy of Management Perspectives, 27*(3), 204–218. https://doi.org/10.5465/amp.2012.0095

Clancy, R. L., Fisher, G. G., Daigle, K. L., Henle, C. A., McCarthy, J., & Fruhauf, C. A. (2020). Eldercare and work among informal caregivers: A multidisciplinary review and recommendations for future research. *Journal of Business and Psychology, 35*(1), 9–27. https://doi.org/10.1007/s10869-018-9612-3

Clark, S. C. (2000). Work/family border theory: A new theory of work/family balance. *Human Relations, 53*(6), 747–770. https://doi.org/10.1177/0018726700536001

Eisenhardt, K. M., & Graebner, M. E. (2007). Theory building from cases: Opportunities and challenges. *Academy of Management Journal, 50*(1), 25–32. https://doi.org/10.5465/amj.2007.24160888

Gordon, J. R., Pruchno, R. A., Wilson-Genderson, M., Murphy, W. M., & Rose, M. (2012). Balancing caregiving and work: Role conflict and role strain dynamics. *Journal of Family Issues, 33*(5), 662–689. https://doi.org/10.1177/0192513X11425322

Henle, C. A., Fisher, G. G., McCarthy, J., Prince, M. A., Mattingly, V. P., & Clancy, R. L. (2020). Eldercare and childcare: How does caregiving responsibility affect job discrimination? *Journal of Business and Psychology, 35*(1), 59–83. https://doi.org/10.1007/s10869-019-09618-x

Kim, J., Ingersoll-Dayton, B., & Kwak, M. (2013). Balancing eldercare and employment: The role of work interruptions and supportive employers. *Journal of Applied Gerontology, 32*(3), 347–369. https://doi.org/10.1177/0733464811423647

Liao, E. Y., Lau, V. P., Hui, R. T. Y., & Kong, K. H. (2019). A resource-based perspective on work-family conflict: Meta-analytical findings. *Career Development International, 24*(1), 37–73. https://doi.org/10.1108/CDI-12-2017-0236

Liu, D., Chen, X. P., & Yao, X. (2011). From autonomy to creativity: A multilevel investigation of the mediating role of harmonious passion. *Journal of Applied Psychology, 96*(2), 294–309. https://doi.org/10.1037/a0021294

Matthews, R. A., Mills, M. J., Trout, R. C., & English, L. (2014). Family-supportive supervisor behaviors, work engagement, and subjective well-being: A contextually dependent mediated process. *Journal of Occupational Health Psychology, 19*(2), 168–181. https://doi.org/10.1037/a0036012

Montez, J. K., Sabbath, E., Glymour, M. M., & Berkman, L. F. (2014). Trends in work–family context among US women by education level, 1976 to 2011. *Population Research and Policy Review, 33*(5), 629–648. https://doi.org/10.1007/s11113-013-9315-4

Murphy, C., & Cross, C. (2021). Blurred lines: Work, eldercare and HRM. *The International Journal of Human Resource Management, 32*(7), 1460–1485. https://doi.org/10.1080/09585192.2018.1528470

Pei, X., Luo, H., Lin, Z., Keating, N., & Fast, J. (2017). The impact of eldercare on adult children's health and employment in transitional China. *Journal of Cross-Cultural Gerontology, 32*(3), 357–372. https://doi.org/10.1007/s10823-017-9330-8

Peng, Y., Xu, X., Matthews, R., & Ma, J. (2020). One size fits all? Contextualizing family-supportive supervision to help employees with eldercare responsibilities. *Journal of Occupational Health Psychology, 25*(5), 368–383. https://doi.org/10.1037/ocp0000237

Perrigino, M. B., Dunford, B. B., & Wilson, K. S. (2018). Work–family backlash: The "dark side" of work–life balance (WLB) policies. *Academy of Management Annals, 12*(2), 600–630. https://doi.org/10.5465/annals.2016.0077

Schooreel, T., & Verbruggen, M. (2016). Use of family-friendly work arrangements and work–family conflict: Crossover effects in dual-earner couples. *Journal of Occupational Health Psychology, 21*(1), 119–132. https://doi.org/10.1037/a0039669

Shifrin, N. V., & Michel, J. S. (2022). Flexible work arrangements and employee health: A meta-analytic review. *Work & Stress, 36*(1), 60–85. https://doi.org/10.1080/02678373.2021.1936287

Smith, P. R. (2004). Elder care, gender, and work: The work–family issue of the 21st century. *Berkeley Journal of Employment and Labor Law, 25*(2), 351–399. http://www.jstor.org/stable/24052201

Chapter 30
Action in Policies: WHO Framework Convention on Tobacco Control

Simpson S. C. Tam and Ben Yuk Fai Fong

Abstract Marking a milestone for the war against smoking, the World Health Organisation Framework Convention on Tobacco Control came into force in 2005. The social risk of adolescents and the emergence of e-cigarettes pose a significant threat these days. The World Health Organisation endorses a multi-sectoral approach, in which the Health in All Policy may shed light on the way to a smoke-free community. This involves a top-down reform, including institutional changes and an integrated approach from multiple policy bureaux and local councils. The chapter proposes a red-light district model in managing tobacco, in which the government tightly regulates the right of use and access to tobacco products while realising its unhealthy nature. The health authority should learn from oversea practices, formulate their own policy and long-term roadmap, and ultimately progress towards a 'zero smoke-free city', or tobacco endgame, in maximising the social benefit, and physical and mental well-being.

Keywords Tobacco control · E-cigarettes · Smoke-free city · Red-light district · Policy implementation

Introduction to the Framework Convention on Tobacco Control

The global world has long endeavoured towards the elimination of smoking. The first multilateral consensus on tobacco control was only established to arrive in 2003. At the 56th World Health Assembly held in Geneva, Switzerland, the World Health Organisation (WHO) adopted the Framework Convention on Tobacco Control

S. S. C. Tam (✉)
School of Clinical Medicine, University of Cambridge, Cambridge, UK
e-mail: sct55@cam.ac.uk

B. Y. F. Fong
The Hong Kong Polytechnic University, Hong Kong, China

B. Y. F. Fong and W. C. W. Wong (eds.), *Gaps and Actions in Health Improvement from Hong Kong and Beyond*,
https://doi.org/10.1007/978-981-99-4491-0_30

(FCTC), which is the treaty setting the standards for parties to regulate the production, sale and distribution of tobacco, on 21 May 2003. The treaty subsequently came into force on 27 February 2005. It has reached 168 signatories and is legally binding in 182 ratifying parties. It lays out tax measures, protection from exposure to tobacco smoke, regulation of the contents, restriction on product disclosure and advertisement, and prohibition of sales to minors.

The WHO Report on the Global Tobacco Epidemic in 2008 established the MPOWER package—a collection of six proven and high-impact measures—to offer practical guidelines to help countries and honour the promise of FCTC . The general directions include Monitoring tobacco use and prevention policies, Protecting people from tobacco smoke, Offering help to quit tobacco use, Warning about the dangers of tobacco, Enforcing bans on tobacco advertising, promotion and sponsorship, and Raising taxes on tobacco. In addition, the WHO issued *The Protocol to Eliminate Illicit Trade in Tobacco Products*, adopted by consensus at the fifth session of the Conference of the Parties to WHO FCTC in 2012. In addressing *Article 15* of the FCTC, it offered the practical guideline for countering illicit trade and strengthening legal aspects of multilateral health collaboration.

The most common practice is to apply economic theory to internalise the externality through imposing an indirect tax—specific or ad valorem—to reflect the full externality of consumption. However, the effect of taxation could be unequal within a society (Alghamdi et al., 2020). Over the years, politicians and public health researchers should ponder complementary and further effective strategies to fight for an even lower smoking rate or potentially tobacco endgame.

Current Obstacles and Challenges

Youth and Tobacco

The proportion of daily cigarette smokers initiating smoking from the age of 18 to 23 has increased gradually over the past two decades in the United States (US; Barrington-Trimis et al., 2020). It simply highlights the importance of restricting tobacco consumption access earlier on in life. As the cigarette contains a substantial amount of nicotine, it could be a struggle to quit once the adolescent becomes addicted to it. The phenomenon that adolescents being vulnerable to social influences cannot be neglected, mainly because adolescents are susceptible to impulsive behaviours (Kim & Lee, 2011). Understanding social networks could be important since 61.1% of individuals who ever smoked reported having initiated smoking because of peer influence (Muttarak et al., 2013). Given the theory of social connection and understanding of group pressure, policymakers should be mindful of the structural characteristics of youth smokers, who tend to possess lower educational attainment where those homogenous peers tend to group (Valente & Pitts, 2017), in order to formulate targeted actions.

In the United States, the adolescent smoking rate among ethnicities varies greatly. The White population tends to have significantly higher smoking rates than Hispanics and Blacks. The smoking rate among the White population is 25%, while the rate in Black and Hispanics is 16% and 6%, respectively (Amin & Lhila, 2016). The racial differences are influenced by multiple factors, including, but not limited to, friends' smoking habits, social pressure, parental smoking norm and cigarette availability at home. Hence, policymakers should consider how the neighbourhood and study environment may affect the take-up rate in early adulthood.

E-cigarettes

E-cigarettes (EC) have gradually gained popularity since the beginning of the millennium. From 2012 to 2018, the prevalence of current smoking dropped from 45.4 to 31.5%, and meanwhile, the use of EC increased by 2.3% among men and 0.6% among women in Estonia (Reile & Pärna, 2020). The prevalence of EC use was statistically significantly higher among ex-smokers. It can be argued as an alternative to conventional tobacco products but can also be considered as the hindrance in keeping citizens entirely away from tobacco-related products. Scientists have gathered evidence of the harmful nature of EC (Heldt et al., 2020). Beyond the individual level, active EC consumers and bystanders might be exposed to similar lung function changes and nicotinic impact levels (Flouris et al., 2013).

The notorious marketing tactic of conventional tobacco products used decades ago was replicated these days for EC. It is of significant public health concern that over 70% of US adolescents reported exposure to EC advertisements over the past month, and this may play an influential role in propelling susceptible youth to attempt appealing products (Chen-Sankey et al., 2019), which indeed contradicted the principle of *Article 13* of FCTC. For instance, guests attending the World Vapor Expo 2017 were permitted to enter the venue without age verification and were encouraged to attempt new flavours under the promotion by attractive young women hired by vendors targeting adolescents (Ziyad & Mohammad, 2018). The distribution of sweets appealing to youth during the promotion of EC products contradicted *Article 16* of FCTC, undermining the decade-long effort to eliminate tobacco products gradually.

Policy Implementation

Health in All Policy on Smoking

The general direction of Health in All Policy (HiAP), as built on the Declaration of Alma-Ata (1978), the Ottawa Charter for Health Promotion (1986) and the Adelaide Statement on Health in All Policies (2010), is inclusive and emphasises community care delivery. The HiAP adopts a multi-sectoral approach when considering the health implications of decisions, identifying synergies and ameliorating detrimental health consequences to enhance population health and equity, highlighting the effectiveness of public policy as well as the determinants of health and well-being. The Framingham Heart Study discovered that the cluster of smokers within the social network ceased smoking approximately in concert, according to the diagram generated by the statistics of all reported relationships in Framingham (Christakis & Fowler, 2008). In comparison, the remaining smokers tend to live on the peripheral of a social, but not geographical, network. A collective effort, such as a small, focused smoker support group, was suggested to promote effective targeting and intervention. Collaboration on an institutional level also plays a pivotal role.

The study of cigarette cessation is broad, ranging from primary to secondary care and from taxation policy to law enforcement. The involvement of all relevant departments has demonstrated to be effective in achieving the policy objective. The run-through by various policy bureaux, departments or ministries enables stakeholders to view their goals and gauge their interests hence designing a more effective and comprehensive policy. Innovative thought and governmental procedure should be installed in the policymaking process. For instance, the use of the HiAP strategy by the South Australian Government in launching the Healthy Weight Project did not restrict the work to any seemingly highly relevant departments. It turned out that ten departments and divisions contributed to the 'Eat Well Be Active Strategy for South Australia 2011' and oversaw policy areas, such as national park management, food possessing, building design standards and transportation (Newman et al., 2014). In the context of Hong Kong, the Policy Committee, chaired by the Chief Secretary of Administration, is responsible for ironing out and resolving any cross-bureau and cross-departmental issues and benefiting the committee at large.

The entry into European Union (EU) informed a different story for Finland in the 1990s. The introduction and execution of the anti-smoking policy were puzzling, as with tariff policy, trade liberalisation and cross-border advertisement. At that time, it was not a unanimous decision to prioritise health concerns over economic prosperity in the EU-level work. When Finland held the presidency in 2006, the HiAP policy was since incorporated into the mainstream idea. The ultimate goal was to improve evidence-based policymaking by drawing connections between policies and interventions and risk factors of health, in which health outcomes would hopefully be much more informative for principal officials (Ollila et al., 2006). To start with, the government highlighted high-risk citizens who would likely turn into smoking and provided structured therapy by a trained practitioner working in conjunction with primary care physician. It has successfully delivered smoking cessation for people with, say, severe mental illness (Gilbody et al., 2019). Multi-faceted approaches tailored to deprived smokers are pivotal in driving towards cessation and bringing down health inequalities (Kock et al., 2019), like brief counselling sessions focused on cessation goals and beliefs (Christiansen et al., 2015). In short, public health experts should embrace a forward-looking and all-inclusive vision to oversee other policy work, alongside the existing tobacco control effort, in managing the risk factor of tobacco uptake.

Health impact assessment (HIA) is an integrative evaluation of factors, including risk, environmental impact, strategic environmental protection, and social and economic impacts (Mindell & Joffe, 2003). A core component of HIA is to gauge to what extent each group and sub-group of the population would be affected the most (Melkas, 2013). Denmark further developed the 'Dynamic Modelling in Health Impact Assessment' (DYNAMO-HIA) with quantifiable data. Adapted to the population of Copenhagen, Denmark, the DYNAMO-HIA supported the combined intervention targeting the initiation at adolescence and cessation and re-initiation during adulthood (Holm et al., 2014). The upside of this projection method is its dynamic nature and multistate structure, taking differential smoking rates and smoking disease outcomes and mortality. A similar study was conducted in the Netherlands which found that population-wide intervention has the most remarkable effect on public health (Kulik et al., 2012). The DYNAMO-HIA has high applicability worldwide, synthesising existing data and statistics of individual countries and comparing the outcomes of different smoking interventions. In 2006, the European Council called for full implementation of the HiAP and actions at the EU and its member states. While the EU sought the possibilities in fulfilling legal obligations on reporting health implications of a community project, all Member States should explore pre-requisites for implementing HiAP in the local context, taking the legal support, organisation structure and procedures into account (Ollila et al., 2006). It is also important to stress that citizens' involvement is as critical as a national directive amidst the long-standing war against tobacco.

Integrated Approach in Local Councils

Generally speaking, the local district council, or any agency overseeing the welfare of a community, should strive to improve community well-being and facilitates local support services. Depending on the political context, the local representatives tend to understand the local situation better and hence are expected to know the priorities of local needs. The practice of HiAP should comprise extensive consultation and opinions of a broad range of stakeholders, in which the local council should be in a more capable position in channelling the explanation of policy and implementing the guidelines on a down-to-earth basis.

An 11-year-long longitudinal study of 1,190 participants identified smoking as a risk factor and found heavy smokers were four times more likely to suffer from depression (Klungsøyr et al., 2006). At the local level, the HiAP should favour a multi-faceted, yet not compartmentalised, approach. The delivery of smoking cessation services can also consider other health aspects, such as mental health status. Adequate counselling services, such as self-monitoring, social support and relaxation, should help improve mental health and keep citizens away from smoking and potentially drug abuse. Motivation enhancement techniques strive to decrease ambivalence and clarify the direction of change. It reinforces the 'quit' behaviour and drives the entire smoking cessation process, preventing the vicious cycle of quitting and re-joining.

In addition, the effective training for healthcare professionals will boost the capability to identify target patients and confidence in introducing therapy with the updated skills and knowledge. Not only should the scope of training cover existing medical staff, but smoking cessation and training should also extend to the future generation of healthcare practitioners. A national survey among medical schools in the United Kingdom (UK) found that only a third offered practical skills training, including workshops in artificial (i.e. role play) or clinical settings (Raupach et al., 2015). With that said, there is much work to do to equip medical students with general knowledge of smoking cessation support and therapy options.

Financial and political support from the central government is as essential as training for medical staff. In the UK, the reshuffle of duties shifted the responsibility of public health management from politically impartial NHS to local authorities governed by locally elected councillors. While the public health specialists may face scrutiny from politically elected representatives, the NICE guideline may find its role in safeguarding the evidence-based framework and addressing local issues. The UK Government announced a surprising £200 million (6.7%) cut in public health expenditure in July 2015, with further reduction in real terms value over the next few years to slightly below £3 billion in 2020–2021 (House of Commons Health Select Committee, 2016). It inevitably reflected in weaker tobacco control work, with a cut of 25% of local authorities in 2015 and 45% in the following year (Anderson et al., 2018). Political involvement interferes with public health professionals' priorities and poses a risk of undermining evidence-based medicine due to explicit or implicit political agendas. Thereby, the financial support has to be stable and political involvement should be minimised wherever possible, alongside a robust system to support long-term ambition.

A separate yet similar strategy should be adopted in nations with a vibrant private healthcare sector. A comprehensive, barrier-free and widely promoted smoking cessation treatment under insurance coverage increases the adoption of treatment services and hence higher success rates (U.S. Department of Health and Human Services, 2020). The cessation treatments are generally clinically effective and highly cost-effective (Tobacco Use and Dependence Guideline Panel, 2008). According to Section 1001 of the Patient Protection and Affordable Care Act, colloquially known as Obamacare, it required most private health plans to cover clinical prevention services, including tobacco cessation interventions in the United States. While the Medicare (primarily for the elderly by the federal government) covers up to 8 face-to-face visits in 12 months, all states should cover at least some treatments for insured persons under Medicaid (mainly for people with low income supported by federal and state governments), but this practice varies by states. Employers were also encouraged to include the coverage of cessation services during negotiation with private health insurers, especially when heavy smoking could be associated with social support and psychosocial work environment, as revealed in the 16-year-long longitudinal study by Dobson et al. (2018).

The proximity of cigarette or EC vendors to education institutions should fall under the scope of the regulation (Giovenco et al., 2016), referring to the precedent exemplar policy in St Helens, UK, in drawing exclusion zone of new hot food take-aways within 400 m of schools (St. Helens Council, 2011). The urban planning and vendor license application process also implies restricting access to the demerit goods from school-aged teenagers. The ideal outcome is to hinder school-aged adolescents' access to cigarette or EC retailers. With that said, the work on smoking cessation should extend beyond the health authority and that should include urban planning agencies and consultation of wider stakeholders in the community.

Way Forward

Lesson from the Management of Red-Light District

The decriminalisation and legalisation of prostitution have been a controversial topic worldwide, partly spurred by the formation of the Red-Light District in Amsterdam, which is recognised as one of the oldest areas for visible and legal prostitution. Amsterdam is widely recognised as a vibrant city that creates much room for studies into sexuality and urban planning. Similar policy implementation may suggest how the tobacco control policy may move forward. The government is mindful of the controversial nature of the prostitution business and the fact that it carries negative externality of consumption—the spread of sexually transmitted diseases, unexpected pregnancy and other risky behaviour. In the context of historical background, it is virtually impossible to ban the business completely. Otherwise, this may flourish everywhere, and it becomes harder to regulate. The so-called regulated tolerance is the current regulatory approach to prostitution (Aalbers & Sabat, 2012), where the local council legalises prostitution and brothels.

The implementation of the red-light district-like policy can be dissected into two aspects, the point-of-use and the point-of-sale. For instance, Hong Kong outlawed smoking initially in shopping centres, subsequently in indoor workspace, karaoke establishments and bars, and more recently bus interchanges and adjoining facilities. Eventually, the restriction area can gradually expand and ultimately until a point where the area of use is restricted to a certain area, as part of the orderly progress towards a smoke-free city. On the flip side, the point-of-sale may face challenging practical constraints, and the tobacco product can be sold in the black market elsewhere. For example, the Therapeutic Goods Administration of the Department of Health and Aged Care in Australia incorporated nicotine vaping products, such as nicotine ECs, nicotine pods and liquid nicotine, in Schedule 4 medicines only available via prescription from 1 October 2021. It was illegal for retailers to sell nicotine vaping products. The Royal Australian College of General Practitioners (2021) updated the guideline on nicotinic products that would only recommend nicotinic vaping products with pre-specified concentration when the first-line therapy (the combination of pharmacotherapy and behavioural support) was unsuccessful, and patient remained to be determined to quit smoking. The prescriber, who is likely to be an Australian registered medical practitioner, has to apply to become an Authorised Prescriber to prescribe unapproved nicotine vaping products without further applications or permissions. In Hong Kong, the retail activity of EC was completely outlawed to strictly eliminate all point-of-sale. The proposal, based on the 'red-light district' policy, was to offer some room for remaining smokers in terms of the right to use and purchase before the full elimination of tobacco products in a smoke-free community. There is limited practice on district-based cigarette control and no conclusive evidence on its effectiveness; however, there have been signs and progress on restricting the use and managing access in the same vein as the red-light district and towards the pathway of transforming into a smoke-free society.

In dealing with tobacco, governments are expected to be well aware of its demerit nature, especially regarding health. Despite the strict rule in Bhutan, there have been multiple reports that the retail activity of cigarettes remains active (Kuensel Newspaper, 2009). Rather than outlawing the tobacco product, the government should introduce an active licensing system to regulate the number of stalls allowed to sell legally, considering the precedent example of the red-light district. In addition, there should be a quota of cigarettes each person can buy over a certain period, promoting responsible smoking behaviour. A record of tobacco product sales may be set up to enable the government to monitor its use, adopt targeted approaches and support the research on smoking cessation. Instead of an abrupt switch to a smoke-free city, this approach offers a gentle transition under the stringent regulatory regime.

Zero-Smoking Living Place

Tobacco Endgame

The phrase 'tobacco endgame' should be generally defined as the termination of consumption of processed nicotine-rich leaves and the smoking and chewing behaviour. McDaniel et al. (2016) postulated a set of integrative endgame strategies: that comprised product-focused, user-focused, supply-focused and institutional-focused strategies. Most current strategies are ad hoc and moderate, lacking a well-written road map and merely foreseeing the identifiable endpoint. Unless there is a novel direction with a complete and irreversible endgame, the public health authority will be in a cat and mouse game against the tobacco industry and its vested interests.

Smoker license is a user-focused strategy, consisting of setting daily quota and financial incentives for permanent license surrender. Establishing a national database ensures efficient communication and accurate tracking of smoking cessation behaviour, in addition to the benefit of longitudinal regional monitoring of tobacco sales. It is not uncommon that health practitioners face difficulty with patients under-reporting cigarette consumption (Stuber & Galea, 2009). The centralised reporting system, alongside data sharing with doctors and nurses, may offer a solution to the long-standing mistrust problem in accurately reporting average cigarette consumption. The licensing system should be able to alert current smokers that tobacco is not a simple confectionery in a supermarket but possesses harmful health effects.

United Kingdom

The government laid out a smoke-free objective by 2030, in which below 5% of the population would consume cigarettes. The Office for Health Improvement and Disparities published an independent report and proposed the gradual increase in the legal age of sale until no one can purchase tobacco products, similar to the Russian permanent ban on selling cigarettes to people born in and after 2014. It also identified a critical issue in implementing the national pledge, indicating the disparity in smoking cessation between fortunate and deprived communities. In fact, Office for Health Improvement and Disparities (2022) proposed a system change and revision of the critical role of the NHS and the importance of collaboration. The mobilisation of a multi-sectorial alliance involving NHS, local authorities, primary care providers and voluntary organisations should promote smoke-free actions and disseminate down-to-earth smoking reduction services. The 'place-based partnerships' incorporate the support of pharmacists, ensuring at least one high-street pharmacy provides pharmacotherapy and skilled behavioural support. GPs and other trained healthcare professionals can jointly provide cessation support services to maximise service delivery.

New Zealand

The Ministry of Health published the Smokefree 2025 Action Plan in 2021, which outlined three outcomes and six focus areas. The most striking directive is the vision of a smoke-free population by banning all sales of tobacco from next year to anyone who was born after 2008 and cutting down the number of shops selling tobacco from 8000 to 500 by 2024 (Dyer, 2021), a step closer to the ultimate tobacco regulation—completely banning all sales. The Action Plan also strives to reduce the addiction and availability of smoked tobacco products while offering more evidence-based stop-smoking services. The legislation's amendments intend to strike a balance between limiting the uptake among youngsters and assisting people in switching to a less harmful product. The Smoke-free Environments and Regulated Products (Vaping) Amendment 2020 came into force on 11 November 2020; the execution is phased in over 15 months. Vaping is restricted in certain places and only be sold by licensed retailers. Any advertisement is prohibited, while the manufacturers, importers and

Specialist Cape Retailers are obliged to submit annual reports and return under the new legislation. This triggered the formation of self-help vaper community support group and offered alternative cessation advice to smokers by converting them to vaping (Fraser et al., 2018), as part of the multi-sectoral approach. As part of the long-term plan, the government has imposed a lifetime ban on individuals aged 14 or below from purchasing cigarettes from 2027 (Kaye, 2021). In the same vein, Malaysia has also issued an endgame strategy to ban the right to purchase tobacco products for those born after 2005 (Das, 2022).

Hong Kong

Smoking has been prohibited in indoor areas of all restaurant premises, public indoor places and workplaces since the amendment and enforcement of the Smoking (Public Health) Ordinance in 2007. A further amendment in 2021 banned the retail activity of ECs in a bid for tobacco endgame, suppressing its popularity and promoting positive health and well-being, which is a promising start in phasing out the tobacco-related products completely. The government has laid out an ambition to reduce smoking prevalence to 7.8% by 2025 in the *Towards 2025: Strategy and Action Plan to Prevent and Control Non-communicable Diseases in Hong Kong*. Three major areas of work were identified: a comprehensive review of the current legislation, enhancing smoking cessation services and promoting a smoke-free society. The adolescents' smoking rate has remained comparatively low. The Primary Care Office of the Department of Health has initiated a Pilot Public–Private Partnership Programme on Smoking Cessation to encourage private practitioners to attempt smoking cessation therapy during consultation. With reference to HIA and DYNAMO-HIA, the government, the newly reformed Health Bureau, in particular, should embrace and adopt the HiAP approach not restricted by the bureaucratic segmentation of work division. For instance, the Education Bureau should be responsible for school education, the Home and Youth Affairs Bureau is in charge of local support and cessation service coordination, the Development Bureau steers urban planning and restricting the point-of-sale and Security Bureau is accountable for surveillance and law enforcement. With the Steering Committee on Primary Healthcare Development, the community is observing the shift of the bulk of health care from hospitals to local clinics, in which the general practitioner should act as the first point of call and work closely with other smoking cessation clinics.

Conclusion

During the COVID-19 pandemic, many elective surgeries and non-urgent treatments have been postponed, including the smoking cessation service in Hong Kong and beyond. Citizens cannot receive appropriate advice and obtain nicotine replacement therapy at the time of treatment. This weakens the effort in the fight against tobacco products. In addition to that, prominent challenges these days include the social risk for adolescents and the attractiveness of EC. The world spent decades, if not a century, to fully realise the appalling consequences of conventional tobacco products and draw multilateral efforts in combatting the tobacco pandemic. The primary objective of the HiAP policy is to consider tobacco control as a broader societal issue, instead of a stand-alone subject, and strengthen smoking cessation service through the support from the local council or authority. The lesson of the Red-Light District management can be learnt, especially in the restriction of point-of-use and the point-of-sale. While recognising the hideous essence of the industry, it is suggested that the government can learn from other jurisdictions, impose stringent restrictions for tobacco products to protect citizens, design a long-term strategic plan based on local circumstances and encourage cessation on the pathway towards tobacco endgame—i.e. a smoke-free population.

Acknowledgements The authors wish to express their heartfelt gratitude to Professor Martin Roland CBE for his advice, review and support throughout the chapter writing. Our sincere thanks are due to Mr Sam Hui for his guidance, encouragement and particularly the suggestion on the Red-Light District management policy.

References

Aalbers, M. B., & Sabat, M. (2012). Re-making a landscape of prostitution: The Amsterdam red light district. *City, 16*(1–2), 112–128. https://doi.org/10.1080/13604813.2012.662372

Alghamdi, A., Fallatah, A., Okal, F., Felemban, T., Eldigire, M., & Almodaimegh, H. (2020). Smoking behaviour after enforcement of a 100% tax on tobacco products in Saudi Arabia: A cross-sectional study. *Eastern Mediterranean Health Journal, 26*(1), 39–46. https://doi.org/10.26719/2020.26.1.39

Amin, V., & Lhila, A. (2016). Decomposing racial differences in adolescent smoking in the U.S. *Economics & Human Biology, 22*, 161–176. https://doi.org/10.1016/j.ehb.2016.05.001

Anderson, W. J., Cheeseman, H., & Butterworth, G. (2018). Political priorities and public health services in English local authorities: The case of tobacco control and smoking cessation services. *Journal of Public Health, 40*(3), e269–e274. https://doi.org/10.1093/pubmed/fdx143

Barrington-Trimis, J. L., Braymiller, J. L., Unger, J. B., McConnell, R., Stokes, A., Leventhal, A. M., Sargent, J. D., Samet, J. M., & Goodwin, R. D. (2020). Trends in the age of cigarette smoking initiation among young adults in the US from 2002 to 2018. *JAMA Network Open, 3*(10), Article e2019022. https://doi.org/10.1001/jamanetworkopen.2020.19022

Chen-Sankey, J. C., Unger, J. B., Bansal-Travers, M., Niederdeppe, J., Bernat, E., & Choi, K. (2019). E-cigarette marketing exposure and subsequent experimentation among youth and young adults. *Pediatrics, 144*(5), Article e20191119. https://doi.org/10.1542/peds.2019-1119

Christakis, N. A., & Fowler, J. H. (2008). The collective dynamics of smoking in a large social network. *New England Journal of Medicine, 358*(21), 2249–2258. https://doi.org/10.1056/NEJMsa0706154

Christiansen, B. A., Reeder, K. M., TerBeek, E. G., Fiore, M. C., & Baker, T. B. (2015). Motivating low socioeconomic status smokers to accept evidence-based smoking cessation treatment: A brief intervention for the community agency setting. *Nicotine & Tobacco Research, 17*(8), 1002–1011. https://doi.org/10.1093/ntr/ntu345

Das, M. (2022). Malaysia to ban tobacco sales to people born after 2005. *The Lancet Oncology, 23*(3), 331. https://doi.org/10.1016/S1470-2045(22)00067-5

Dobson, K. G., Gilbert-Ouimet, M., Mustard, C. A., & Smith, P. M. (2018). Association between dimensions of the psychosocial and physical work environment and latent smoking trajectories: A 16-year cohort study of the Canadian workforce. *Occupational and Environmental Medicine, 75*(11), 814–821. https://doi.org/10.1136/oemed-2018-105138

Dyer, O. (2021). New Zealand plans to outlaw tobacco sales to citizens born after 2008. *BMJ, 375*, Article n3057. https://doi.org/10.1136/BMJ.N3057

Flouris, A. D., Chorti, M. S., Poulianiti, K. P., Jamurtas, A. Z., Kostikas, K., Tzatzarakis, M. N., Hayes, A. W., Tsatsakis, A. M., & Koutedakis, Y. (2013). Acute impact of active and passive electronic cigarette smoking on serum cotinine and lung function. *Inhalation Toxicology, 25*(2), 91–101. https://doi.org/10.3109/08958378.2012.758197

Fraser, T., Glover, M., & Truman, P. (2018). Government and public health responses to e-cigarettes in New Zealand: vapers' perspectives. *Harm Reduction Journal, 15*, Article 13. https://doi.org/10.1186/S12954-018-0219-9

Gilbody, S., Peckham, E., Bailey, D., Arundel, C., Heron, P., Crosland, S., Fairhurst, C., Hewitt, C., Li, J., Parrott, S., Bradshaw, T., Horspool, M., Hughes, E., Hughes, T., Ker, S., Leahy, M., McCloud, T., Osborn, D., Reilly, J., … Vickers, C. (2019). Smoking cessation for people with severe mental illness (SCIMITAR+): A pragmatic randomised controlled trial. *The Lancet Psychiatry, 6*(5), 379–390. https://doi.org/10.1016/S2215-0366(19)30047-1

Giovenco, D. P., Casseus, M., Duncan, D. T., Coups, E. J., Lewis, M. J., & Delnevo, C. D. (2016). Association between electronic cigarette marketing near schools and e-cigarette use among youth. *Journal of Adolescent Health, 59*(6), 627–634. https://doi.org/10.1016/j.jadohealth.2016.08.007

Heldt, N. A., Seliga, A., Winfield, M., Gajghate, S., Reichenbach, N., Yu, X., Rom, S., Tenneti, A., May, D., Gregory, B. D., & Persidsky, Y. (2020). Electronic cigarette exposure disrupts blood-brain barrier integrity and promotes neuroinflammation. *Brain, Behavior, and Immunity, 88*, 363–380. https://doi.org/10.1016/j.bbi.2020.03.034

Holm, A. L., Brønnum-Hansen, H., Robinson, K. M., & Diderichsen, F. (2014). Assessment of health impacts of decreased smoking prevalence in Copenhagen: Application of the DYNAMO-HIA model. *Scandinavian Journal of Public Health, 42*(5), 409–416. https://doi.org/10.1177/1403494814530048

House of Commons Health Select Committee. (2016). *Public health post-2013: Second report of session 2016–17*. https://publications.parliament.uk/pa/cm201617/cmselect/cmhealth/140/140.pdf

Kaye, B. (2021, December 9). Explainer: How will New Zealand's lifetime ban on cigarette sales work? *Reuters*. https://www.reuters.com/world/asia-pacific/how-will-new-zealands-lifetime-ban-cigarette-sales-work-2021-12-09/

Kim, S., & Lee, D. (2011). Prefrontal cortex and impulsive decision making. *Biological Psychiatry, 69*(12), 1140–1146. https://doi.org/10.1016/j.biopsych.2010.07.005

Klungsøyr, O., Nygård, J. F., Sørensen, T., & Sandanger, I. (2006). Cigarette smoking and incidence of first depressive episode: An 11-year, population-based follow-up study. *American Journal of Epidemiology, 163*(5), 421–432. https://doi.org/10.1093/aje/kwj058

Kock, L., Brown, J., Hiscock, R., Tattan-Birch, H., Smith, C., & Shahab, L. (2019). Individual-level behavioural smoking cessation interventions tailored for disadvantaged socioeconomic position: A systematic review and meta-regression. *The Lancet Public Health, 4*(12), e628–e644. https://doi.org/10.1016/S2468-2667(19)30220-8

Kuensel Newspaper. (2009, March 19). The lucrative lure of a black market. *Kuensel Online*.

Kulik, M. C., Nusselder, W. J., Boshuizen, H. C., Lhachimi, S. K., Fernández, E., Baili, P., Bennett, K., Mackenbach, J. P., & Smit, H. A. (2012). Comparison of tobacco control scenarios: Quantifying estimates of long-term health impact using the DYNAMO-HIA modeling tool. *PLoS ONE, 7*(2), Article e32363. https://doi.org/10.1371/journal.pone.0032363

McDaniel, P. A., Smith, E. A., & Malone, R. E. (2016). The tobacco endgame: A qualitative review and synthesis. *Tobacco Control, 25*(5), 594–604. https://doi.org/10.1136/tobaccocontrol-2015-052356

Melkas, T. (2013). Health in all policies as a priority in Finnish health policy: A case study on national health policy development. *Scandinavian Journal of Public Health, 41*(Suppl. 11), 3–28. https://doi.org/10.1177/1403494812472296

Mindell, J., & Joffe, M. (2003). Health impact assessment in relation to other forms of impact assessment. *Journal of Public Health, 25*(2), 107–112. https://doi.org/10.1093/pubmed/fdg024

Muttarak, R., Gallus, S., Franchi, M., Faggiano, F., Pacifici, R., Colombo, P., & la Vecchia, C. (2013). Why do smokers start? *European Journal of Cancer Prevention, 22*(2), 181–186. https://doi.org/10.1097/CEJ.0b013e32835645fa

Newman, L., Ludford, I., Williams, C., & Herriot, M. (2014). Applying health in all policies to obesity in South Australia. *Health Promotion International, 31*(1), 44–58. https://doi.org/10.1093/heapro/dau064

Office for Health Improvement and Disparities. (2022). *The Khan review: Making smoking obsolete.* https://www.gov.uk/government/publications/the-khan-review-making-smoking-obsolete

Ollila, E., Ståhl, T., Wismar, M., Lahtinen, E., Melkas, T., & Leppo, K. (2006). *Health in all policies in the European Union and its member states.* https://ec.europa.eu/health/ph_projects/2005/action1/docs/2005_1_18_frep_a4_en.pdf

Raupach, T., Al-Harbi, G., McNeill, A., Bobak, A., & McEwen, A. (2015). Smoking cessation education and training in U.K. medical schools: A national survey. *Nicotine & Tobacco Research, 17*(3), 372–375. https://doi.org/10.1093/ntr/ntu199

Reile, R., & Pärna, K. (2020). E-cigarette use by smoking status in Estonia, 2012–2018. *International Journal of Environmental Research and Public Health, 17*(2), Article 519. https://doi.org/10.3390/ijerph17020519

Royal Australian College of General Practitioners. (2021). *Supporting smoking cessation: A guide for health professionals.* https://www.racgp.org.au/clinical-resources/clinical-guidelines/key-racgp-guidelines/view-all-racgp-guidelines/supporting-smoking-cessation

St. Helens Council. (2011). *Local development framework: Supplementary planning document hot food takeaways.* https://www.sthelens.gov.uk/media/2403/Hot-Food-Takeaway-June-2011/pdf/Hot_Food_Takeaway_SPD_2011.pdf?m=637800928394500000

Stuber, J., & Galea, S. (2009). Who conceals their smoking status from their health care provider? *Nicotine & Tobacco Research, 11*(3), 303–307. https://doi.org/10.1093/ntr/ntn024

Tobacco Use and Dependence Guideline Panel. (2008). *Treating tobacco use and dependence: 2008 update—Clinical practice guideline.* https://www.ahrq.gov/sites/default/files/wysiwyg/professionals/clinicians-providers/guidelines-recommendations/tobacco/clinicians/update/treating_tobacco_use08.pdf

U.S. Department of Health and Human Services. (2020). *Smoking cessation: A report of the surgeon general.* https://www.hhs.gov/sites/default/files/2020-cessation-sgr-full-report.pdf

Valente, T. W., & Pitts, S. R. (2017). An appraisal of social network theory and analysis as applied to public health: Challenges and opportunities. *Annual Review of Public Health, 38*(1), 103–118. https://doi.org/10.1146/annurev-publhealth-031816-044528

Ziyad, B. T., & Mohammad, E. K. (2018). World Vapor Expo 2017: E-cigarette marketing tactics. *Tobacco Control, 27*(e1), E81–E82. https://doi.org/10.1136/TOBACCOCONTROL-2017-054128

Chapter 31
Experiences in Working at Residential Care Home for the Elderly: Voices from Health Care Workers

Sui Yu Yau, Linda Yin King Lee, Siu Yin Li, Shixin Huang, Sin Ping Law, Sze Ki Lai, Janet Lok Chun Lee, and Suet Lai Wong

Abstract With the ageing population worldwide, there is a massive demand for residential care homes for the elderly (RCHEs). Health care workers work closely with the older adults by providing basic care such as feeding, bathing, changing napkins, or assisting with activities of daily living. According to various reports and statistics, the turnover rate of health care workers is extremely high due to the "dirty work" nature, irregular working hours, lack of resources and support from employers or government, "ageing" of health care workers, etc. Research reported that the low social and occupational status, socially stigmatised, marginalised, and the social process of boundary-making also contributed to the high turnover rate of health care workers in the field. Thus, this chapter aims to uncover the voices from

S. Y. Yau · L. Y. K. Lee · S. Y. Li · S. P. Law · S. K. Lai · S. L. Wong (✉)
School of Nursing and Health Studies, Hong Kong Metropolitan University, Hong Kong, China
e-mail: laiwong7271@gmail.com

S. Y. Yau
e-mail: isyyau@hkmu.edu.hk

L. Y. K. Lee
e-mail: yklee@hkmu.edu.hk

S. Y. Li
e-mail: siyli@hkmu.edu.hk

S. P. Law
e-mail: ssplaw@hkmu.edu.hk

S. K. Lai
e-mail: sklai@hkmu.edu.hk

S. Huang
Department of Sociology and Social Policy, Lingnan University, Hong Kong, China
e-mail: shixinhuang@ln.edu.hk

J. L. C. Lee
Department of Rehabilitation Sciences, The Hong Kong Polytechnic University, Hong Kong, China
e-mail: lcjlee@polyu.edu.hk

B. Y. F. Fong and W. C. W. Wong (eds.), *Gaps and Actions in Health Improvement from Hong Kong and Beyond*,
https://doi.org/10.1007/978-981-99-4491-0_31

health care workers' perspectives in order to understand their immediate needs for benefit from new insights. RCHEs policymakers would also gain important practical implications generated from the analysis results for developing policy initiatives to recruit and retain RCHEs workers.

Keywords Health care workers · Working experiences · Residential care home · Older adults

Introduction

It is challenging to recruit and retain health care workers (HCWs) at residential care homes for the elderly (RCHEs) to assist and promote the daily living activity needs of the frail ageing population in developed countries. There is an ongoing social stigmatisation of the provision of "dirty work" at RCHEs, such as feeding, bathing, toileting, changing napkins, making beds, and housekeeping, rather than recognising the competence of health care (Fisher & Kang, 2013). The previous investigation of RCHEs working conditions as "dirty work" was driven by analytics or top-down perspectives resulting from the lack of voices from HCWs' perspectives (Yau et al., 2022), leading to a high turnover rate.

HCWs are frontline health care personnel who play prominent roles in the lives of those who are unable to care for themselves. HCWs work majorly in long-term residential care settings, called care and attention homes, nursing homes, or infirmary units. The use of residential care services aims to (1) provide residential care and facilities for those who are unable to live at home; (2) promote and maintain the health of older adults at optimal levels and assist them with their varying daily personal care needs; and (3) fulfil the social and recreational needs of the older adults at RCHEs (Social Welfare Department, 2021).

The residential care workforce is hierarchical in general linking to economic sustainability. In Hong Kong, for instance, there is a clear division of labour regulated by the Social Welfare Department (2021) from top to bottom levels, including home managers, registered nurses, enrolled nurses, physiotherapists, health workers, care workers, and ancillary workers. Most of the hands-on care is provided by frontline health care workers, while enrolled nurses and registered nurses offer a lesser extent. The role of the registered nurse has become mainly supervisory. Health workers are regulated and licensed by the Social Welfare Department (2021) after a minimum of 200 hours of formal training. Care workers, in Hong Kong and other developed countries, are unregulated workers with or without proper training who operate under various job titles such as personal care assistants, personal care workers, and nurse assistants (Aerschot et al., 2021). This chapter uses the term health care workers (HCWs) for consistency to refer to care workers who work at RCHEs.

The demand for frontline HCWs working at RCHEs soars rapidly due to the global ageing population and a decline of family caregivers from the development of nuclear or single families (Jacobsen et al., 2018). The role of HCWs in the quality and safety of care will be even more essential that prompting us to answer the following two research questions from a bottom-up approach: (1) What do HCWs express about their meanings of RCHEs work? (2) Is it impossible for the "dirty work" metaphor to impact HCWs positively? The chapter presents an integrative literature review for summarising, analysing, and synthesising eligible studies (Kable et al., 2012) in order to answer these two questions.

Review and Findings

The integrated review aims to identify the perceptions and impact of the "dirty work" metaphor as reflected by HCWs' working experiences at RCHEs to inform better policy on their recruitment and retainment of HCW. The integrated method was adopted to synthesise various streams of literature to generate new knowledge answering the pre-set research questions (Kable et al., 2012). At the initial stage, multiple databases, including CINAHL, ERIC, LWW Nursing and Health Professions Premier Collection, Web of Science, and SAGE Journals, were used to search the relevant articles. Five broad search categories were used: health care workers, experiences, voices, residential care, and older adults/elderly. The keywords within each category were searched separately and then dug in combination with filters for refinement on health care service science from 2012 to 2022. Duplicate publications were eliminated among multiple databases. Lastly, a manual search of the reference lists from the eligible articles was conducted. Inclusion criteria for the article selection were as follows: (1) The search was limited to articles published in English between the years 2012 and 2022; (2) the study had to identify the meanings of RCHEs work reflected by HCWs' working at RCHEs; (3) the manuscripts should be in full text primarily and peer-reviewed. Editorials, conference abstracts, unpublished dissertations, and studies only outlined the strategies to improve the policies of RCHEs were excluded.

A total of 24 articles were retrieved in the initial search. The articles were then screened for relevance by an in-depth review of abstracts. Eventually, 7 out of the 24 articles met the inclusion criteria. Of the 7 articles retained, 4 used explorative and descriptive qualitative research design, 2 used mixed methods, and 1 used survey methods. 5 out of 7 reviewed studies were conducted in Canada (Baines & Daly, 2021; Banerjee et al., 2012, 2015, 2021; Braedley et al., 2018), and two remained studies were conducted in Nordic countries (Elstad & Vabo, 2021) and China (Wei et al., 2015). The majority of the participants in the included studies were females in middle age. The process of analysis and synthesis began explicitly with data extraction presented in Table 31.1 to identify what HCWs had said about their meanings of RCHEs work.

Table 31.1 Characteristics of reviewed studies and identified RCHEs work meanings reflected by HCWs

Citation (year)	Country	Study design	Context	Identified RCHEs work meanings
Baines and Daly (2021)	Canada	Mixed methods	Long-term residential care homes in Ontario	They removed the dignity from the care act whenever they had too much to do in a very time-limited environment
Banerjee et al. (2015)	Canada	Explorative and descriptive methods	Long-term residential care homes in British Columbia	They lose after subcontracting
Banerjee et al. (2012)	Canada	Explorative and descriptive methods	Long-term residential care homes in British Columbia	They desired to be cultivating trust in their capacity to solve problems in a working environment
Banerjee et al. (2021)	Canada	Mixed methods	Long-term residential care homes in British Columbia	They perceived their work was routinized, task-based manners, and they had insufficient time emphasis on the relational dimensions of care made it challenging to accomplish the quality care during working hours
Braedley et al. (2018)	Canada	Explorative and descriptive methods	Long-term residential care homes in British Columbia	They received psychological benefits from providing care. However, they were often required to cope individually with the worsened working environment
Elstad and Vabo (2021)	Nordic countries	Survey	Frontline eldercare workers in Denmark, Finland, Norway, and Sweden (N = 3677)	They reflected their recognition was strongly associated with their consideration to quit
Wei et al. (2015)	China	Explorative and descriptive methods	One public and one private nursing home in Fuzhou city, Fujian province, China	They revealed their working experience in both positive and negative aspects of nursing homes

HCWs Express Their Meanings of RCHEs Work

With the increasing longevity of the frail old-olds, long-term residential care home services should be provided efficiently and sufficiently with the required ancillary workforces (Baines & Daly, 2021; Banerjee et al., 2015). According to these literature, there are three operational meanings that HCWs attributed to their care work in RCHEs, including (1) nature of routinised, task-based dirty works plus individualised relational care (Banerjee et al., 2021; Wei et al., 2015); (2) roles of direct care providers and assistant for anyone within a team (Banerjee et al., 2015); and (3) responsibilities for human safety and dignity rights with compassions (Banerjee et al., 2012; Wei et al., 2015).

HCWs received optimal occupational training to provide direct care and obtained favourable psychological benefits and appreciation from care recipients and teammates (Braedley et al., 2018). However, the findings revealed that the quitting of HCWs was widespread after the subcontracting occurrence in the field (Banerjee et al., 2015). The lack of recognition and support from the society and managers, respectively, was also strongly related to their resignation (Banerjee et al., 2012, 2015; Elstad & Vabo, 2021).

Key Impacts of "Dirty Work" Metaphor

Content analysis was employed to determine the presence of reflective words, themes, or concepts (Silarova et al., 2022) from data extraction to quantify and analyse the positive and negative impact of "dirty work" metaphor on HCWs, with exemplars in Table 31.2. The metaphor of "dirty work" perceived by HCWs included the characteristic of caring tasks at RCHEs and the supervision from the environment contributing to the work completion (Baines & Daly, 2021; Banerjee et al., 2012, 2015, 2021; Braedley et al., 2018; Elstad & Vabo, 2021; Wei et al., 2015). HCWs' reflections on dirty work from the literature could be divided into three main themes: (1) intrapersonal, (2) interpersonal, and (3) job performance, with six subthemes illustrating both positive and negative vital impacts on HCWs listed in Table 31.2.

Discussion

The integrated review aims to reveal the meaning of "dirty work" and its impacts on HCWs who are at the frontline position to provide direct care at RCHEs. The dirty work implied positively workable care leading to job satisfaction and sustainable therapeutic relationships with residents at RCHEs. The HCWs' beliefs on providing care to the older adults also motivated them to engage in caring energetically (Elstad & Vabo, 2021; Wei et al., 2015). In contrast, the lack of facilitation and supervision

Table 31.2 Key impacts of dirty work metaphor and examples reflected by HCWs

		Positive impacts		Negative impacts	
Key impacts	Subthemes	Description	Examples	Description	Examples
Interpersonal level	Work meanings	The promising characteristics of "dirty work" sustained care relationships with residents and felt a sense of meaning in the work	Felt achievement, companionship, happy from care recipients and workmates (Elstad & Vabo, 2021; Wei et al., 2015)	Job stress induced due to the worst and unfair working environments	Cope with difficulties such as insufficient staffing and immoral situations individually (Banerjee et al., 2015)
	Communication with managers	An authentic communication environment generated safety and trust	Able to reveal difficult situations honestly and trace out problem-solving (Banerjee et al., 2012)	It is a challenging process with tensions between managers and HCWs	HCWs' bitter expressions shocked some managers/a tension between scheduling meetings regularly to ensure diverse participation (Banerjee et al., 2012)
	Recognition	Cultivating trust in the team to innovate	It is the time taken from their personal lives and paid back only in the form of human relationships (i.e., unpaid overtime to complete care work) (Baines & Daly, 2021)	Lost of recognition at the societal level, exemplified by leaders, mass media and the general public	Experiences of sexism and hierarchies of knowledge (Banerjee et al., 2021)
Job performance level	Task priority	Relational care required more time to accomplish except for a higher priority case by case	Vulnerable residents and their families require attentive, careful support (Braedley et al., 2018)	Little decision-making autonomy/little flexibility in organizing their work orders with a tight schedule	Assembly care line outside at the bathroom/the avalanche of paperwork at stations (Banerjee et al., 2021)
	Task compliance	Tasks triaging became drawing supervisors' attention	Dirty work and Documentation (Baines & Daly, 2021)	Faux compliance with rules	Engaging in relational care when they felt that residents' needs were being ignored (Baines & Daly, 2021)
	Work capacity	Able to deal with relational care	Changed and managed dementia patients' minds and emotions after offering kindness (Wei et al., 2015)	Low control in the working environment	Task difficulties related to time pressures, staffing, and autonomy to meet residents' preferences (Braedley et al., 2018)

in the working environment was the stressful reason HCWs could not tolerate and consider quitting individually (Banerjee et al., 2015).

Limited studies had been conducted in North America, Nordic countries, or China to let HCWs voice out their experiences. Elstad and Vabo (2021) reported that two-fifths of HCWs ($n = 3677$) had considered leaving their jobs in the NORDCARE survey conducted in four Nordic countries, including Denmark, Finland, Norway, and Sweden. About 93 to 97% of respondents among these four countries were female; the median age of respondents ranged from 43 to 53. HCWs were required to provide the so-called dirty works. They were also required to collect vital signs, record and report residents' conditions, carry out the care plans, and assist other team members. Their intentions of leaving the job were significantly and consistently associated with the lack of supervisor support at work and recognition from the society (Elstad & Vabo, 2021).

Communication with managers could be enhanced and facilitated by an authentic and safe environment to encourage honest dialogues incorporated in regular hand-over or conference staff meetings (Banerjee et al., 2012). Yet, there were inconsistent meeting schedules due to no time or space squeezed out of the busy working environment. The communication disruption could occur when the managers could not listen to and motivate the diverse participation (Banerjee et al., 2012).

The social process of boundary-making substantially contributed to the leaving of HCWs in the field. Within a team's positive recognition, the loyalty and devotion of HCWs were recognised with outstanding performance when it was time taken from care workers' personal lives and paid back only in the form of human relationships by unpaid overtime to complete care work (Baines & Daly, 2021). In contrast to the negative societal level, the hierarchy of knowledge and the sexism put the majority of female HCWs in a marginalised and lower social and occupational status with stigmatisation (Banerjee et al., 2021).

Evidence suggests that the majority of HCWs were female, who were vulnerable at the bottom of the organisational hierarchy with less autonomy to handle the deteriorating working environment leading to high turnover (Gao et al., 2015; Jacobsen et al., 2018). RCHEs' dirty work is feminised and devalued because the society assumes women's natural abilities to care for family and makes them ideal for the care work in the subordinated place, which is usually considered unskilled or low skilled (Armstrong, 2018).

In addition to being the primary physical carer at RCHEs, female HCWs were often the primary providers of social and emotional support for older adult residents and the assistant role to be all rounded (Wei et al., 2015). Based on the residential care workforce hierarchy, HCWs complied with the task hierarchy allocated by supervisors regarding conducting "dirty work" and paperwork reporting significantly. However, HCWs were struggling for faux compliance with rules when they felt residents should be addressed by needs of relational care, which was time-consuming to accomplish subsequently during staff shortage. Moreover, HCWs perceived that completing relational care might not draw the supervisor's attention as those care usually should be assigned to qualified and professional staff. HCWs might also take care of those relational care during staff shortages upon their routinised tasks (Wei et al., 2015).

Implications and Policies

The social stigmatisation of "dirty work" is not the only factor leading to HCWs' turnover (Fjaer & Vabo, 2013; Hjelmar & Rostgaard, 2020; Simmons et al., 2021), and HCWs express that their working experiences are rewardful where they are happy to establish care relations with residents (Wei et al., 2015). The deteriorating working environment linking to resource reallocation in neoliberalism and organisational reforms should be addressed to recruit and retain HCWs (Daly & Szebehely, 2012; Daly et al., 2016; Read & Fenge, 2019).

With specific criteria of universal health coverage, it might be an unattainable goal reserved for the developed countries as found in the integrated review. RCHEs' service model adhering to the economic sustainability and regulated activities at basic care and interventions has been threaten the autonomy of staff (Baines & Daly, 2021; Strandell, 2020; Trydegard, 2012). HCWs have reflected their job stress and always struggle from task priority, task compliance and work capacity at RHCEs. Three subthemes reflecting job performance level related to HCWs' roles and responsibilities at RCHEs. As the direct care providers and assistants within a team, HCWs were willing to perform the higher priority of relational care out of the list of routinised and task-based dirty work when necessary (Braedley et al., 2018). There was little decision-making autonomy and flexibility for the assistant role in a team to organise the task priority meeting a tight schedule (Banerjee et al., 2021).

The work capacity was highly related to HCWs' responsibilities for a human who was the care recipients living in RCHEs. HCWs respected residents' right to safe care and dignity at RCHEs consequently so that HCWs reflected they could deal with parts of the relational care in some challenging situations with the accumulation of working experiences and the sustainable relationships with care recipients (Wei et al., 2015). However, HCWs experienced lower control in the working environment, frequently leading to unmatched care recipients' preferences (Braedley et al., 2018). With this view, key considerations are generated for the workforce, practitioners, and vital practical implications for policymakers.

Firstly, researcher should explore and revitalise the meanings of care work with its characteristic and context to minimise social stigmatisation in society. Personal care work should be essential and equitable access under the provision of universal health coverage for those who are eligible to live in RCHEs. Therefore, the workforce in the field is able to enhance the better working environment such as staffing, training needs, and benefits to expect a significant improvement in recruitment and retainment of HCEs immediately. Secondly, the existing female HCWs should be empowered and equipped regularly with up-to-date training to increase their ability and confidence to control their work at RCHEs. Since the review found that the management team had spent less time to communicate with HCWs, thus, the management team should cultivate an authentic communication channel to engage HCWs' and teams' participation for improvement. Lastly, researcher should extent and expand the feasibility of RCHEs' service model to inform policymakers. Every region/country is unique in finding its pathway towards universal health coverage, considering its contextual strengths and weaknesses via evidenced-based practice.

Acknowledgements The work described in this paper was fully supported by a grant from the Research Grants Council of HKSAR, China [RGC: UGC/FDS16/M12/20].

References

Aerschot, L. V., Puthenparambil, J. M., & Olakivi, A. (2021). Psychophysical burden and lack of support: Reasons for care workers' intentions to leave their work in the Nordic countries. *International Journal of Social Welfare, 31*(3), 333–346. https://doi.org/10.1111/ijsw.12520

Armstrong, P. (2018). Balancing the tension in long-term residential care. *Ageing International, 43*, 74–90. https://doi.org/10.1007/s12126-017-9284-8

Baines, D., & Daly, T. (2021). Borrowed time and solidarity: The multi-scalar politics of time and gendered care work. *Social Politics, 28*(2), 385–404. https://doi.org/10.1093/sp/jxz017

Banerjee, A., Armstrong, P., Daly, T., Armstrong, H., & Braedley, S. (2015). "Careworkers don't have a voice": Epistemological violence in residential care for older people. *Journal of Aging Studies, 33*, 28–36. https://doi.org/10.1016/j.jaging.2015.02.005

Banerjee, A., Daly, T., Armstrong, P., Szebehely, M., Armstrong, H., & Lafrance, S. (2012). Structural violence in long-term, residential care for older people: Comparing Canada and Scandinavia. *Social Science & Medicine, 74*, 390–398. https://doi.org/10.1016/j.socscimed.2011.10.037

Banerjee, A., McGregor, M., Ponder, S., & Longhurst, A. (2021). Long-term care facility workers' perceptions of the impact of subcontracting on their conditions of work and the quality of care: A qualitative study in British Columbia. *Canadian Journal on Aging, 41*(2), 264–272. https://doi.org/10.1017/s071498082100012x

Braedley, S., Owusu, P., Przednowek, A., & Armstrong, P. (2018). We're told, 'Suck it up:' Long-term care workers' psychological health and safety. *Ageing International, 43*, 91–109. https://doi.org/10.1007/s12126-017-9288-4

Daly, T., Struthers, J., Muller, B., Taylor, D., Goldmann, M., Doupe, M., & Jacobsen, F. F. (2016). Prescriptive or interpretive regulation at the frontlines of care work in the "Three worlds" of Canada, Germany and Norway. *Labour/le Travail, 77*, 37–71. https://doi.org/10.1353/llt.2016.0029

Daly, T., & Szebehely, M. (2012). Unheard voices, unmapped terrain care work in long-term residential care for older people in Canada and Sweden. *International Journal of Social Welfare, 21*(2), 139–148. https://doi.org/10.1111/j.1468-2397.2011.00806.x

Elstad, J. I., & Vabo, M. (2021). Lack of recognition at the societal level heightens turn over considerations among Nordic eldercare workers: A quantitative analysis of survey data. *BMC Health Services Research, 21*, Article 747. https://doi.org/10.1186/s12913-021-06734-4

Fisher, L. T., & Kang, M. (2013). Reinventing dirty work: Immigrant women in nursing homes. In N. Flores-Gonzalez, A. R. Guevarra, M. Toro-Morn, & G. Chang (Eds.), *Immigrant women*

workers in the neoliberal age (pp. 164–185). University of Illinois Press. https://doi.org/10.5406/illinois/9780252037573.003.0010
Fjaer, E. G., & Vabo, M. (2013). Shaping social situations: A hidden aspect of care work in nursing homes. *Journal of Aging Studies, 27*(4), 419–427. https://doi.org/10.1016/j.jaging.2013.10.002
Gao, F., Tilse, C., Wilson, J., Tuckett, A., & Newcombe, P. (2015). Perceptions and employment intentions among aged care nurses and nursing assistants from diverse cultural backgrounds: A qualitative interview study. *Journal of Aging Studies, 35*, 111–122. https://doi.org/10.1016/j.jaging.2015.08.006
Hjelmar, U., & Rostgaard, T. (2020). Supplemental home care and topping-up: A shift from service universalism towards a new and privatised public service model? *International Journal of Social Welfare, 29*(2), 118–128. https://doi.org/10.1111/ijsw.12390
Jacobsen, F. F., Day, S., Laxer, K., Lloyd, L., Goldmann, M., Szhebehely, M., Choiniere, J. A., & Rosenau, P. V. (2018). Job autonomy of long-term residential care assistive personnel: A six country comparison. *Ageing International, 43*, 4–19. https://doi.org/10.1007/s12126-017-9291-9
Kable, A. K., Pich, J., & Maslin-Prothero, S. E. (2012). A structured approach to documenting a search strategy for publication: A 12 step guideline for authors. *Nurse Education Today, 32*(8), 878–886. https://doi.org/10.1016/j.nedt.2012.02.022
Read, R., & Fenge, L.-A. (2019). What does Brexit mean for the UK social care workforce? Perspectives from the recruitment and retention frontline. *Health and Social Care in the Community, 27*(3), 676–682. https://doi.org/10.1111/hsc.12684
Silarova, B., Brookes, N., Palmer, S., Towers, A.-M., & Hussein, S. (2022). Understanding and measuring the work-related quality of life among those working in adult social care: A scoping review. *Health and Social Care in the Community, 30*(5), 1637–1664. https://doi.org/10.1111/hsc.13718
Simmons, C., Rodrigues, R., & Szebehely, M. (2021). Working conditions in the long-term care sector: A comparative study of migrant and native workers in Austria and Sweden. *Health and Social Care in the Community, 30*(5), e2191–e2202. https://doi.org/10.1111/hsc.13657
Social Welfare Department. (2021, June 18). *Overview of residential care services for the elderly.* https://www.swd.gov.hk/en/index/site_pubsvc/page_elderly/sub_residentia/id_overviewon/
Strandell, R. (2020). Care workers under pressure—A comparison of the work situation in Swedish home care 2005 and 2015. *Health and Social Care in the Community, 28*(1), 137–147. https://doi.org/10.1111/hsc.12848
Trydegard, G.-B. (2012). Care work in changing welfare states: Nordic care worker's experiences. *European Journal of Ageing, 9*, 119–129. https://doi.org/10.1007/s10433-012-0219-7
Wei, Y.-P., Li, H., Chen, P., Li, J., Chen, H., & Chen, L.-L. (2015). Working experiences of nursing aides in nursing homes: A qualitative study. *International Journal of Nursing Science, 2*(4), 371–377. https://doi.org/10.1016/j.ijnss.2015.10.006
Yau, S. Y., Lee, Y. K., Li, S. Y., Lai, S. K., Law, S. P., & Huang S. (2022). The social construction of "dirty work" for working in residential care homes for the elderly. In V. T. S. Law & B. Y. F. Fong (Eds.), *Ageing with dignity in Hong Kong and Asia: Holistic and humanistic care* (pp. 53–64). Springer. https://doi.org/10.1007/978-981-19-3061-4_5

Chapter 32
Depressive Symptoms and the Associated Factors Among the Older People Living in Residential Care Home: A Case Report from Hong Kong

Mei Kuen Li, Karen K. M. Cheung, Sarah S. S. Wong, and Po Po Chung

Abstract Depression is a common mental health problem, but not easily be detected and resulting in under-treatment among the elderly residential care home (RCH) residents. This case study aimed to investigate the prevalence of depressive symptoms and its associated factors among the older people from four elderly RCHs in Hong Kong. Participants' depressive symptoms were assessed by Patient Health Questionnaire-8 (PHQ-8). Higher score indicates more severe depressive symptoms suffered. The data were collected by interview. A total of 242 eligible participants were recruited in this study. The overall mean score of PHQ-8 was 5.95. The prevalence rate of depressive symptoms was 58.2%. There were significant differences in depressive symptoms among participants with different educational levels, different length of stay in RCHs and total number of co-morbidities. No significant results were found with the age groups and gender. This study reported a high prevalence rate and the associated factors of depressive symptoms among the elderly RCH residents. Appropriate strategies should be implemented to address this mental health problem by prevention and early detection.

Keywords Depressive symptoms · Older people · Residential care home · PHQ-8

M. K. Li (✉) · K. K. M. Cheung · S. S. S. Wong · P. P. Chung
School of Nursing and Health Studies, Hong Kong Metropolitan University, Hong Kong, China
e-mail: mkli@hkmu.edu.hk

K. K. M. Cheung
e-mail: karencheung@twc.edu.hk

S. S. S. Wong
e-mail: ssswong@hkmu.edu.hk

P. P. Chung
e-mail: michelle.chung2@nhs.net

B. Y. F. Fong and W. C. W. Wong (eds.), *Gaps and Actions in Health Improvement from Hong Kong and Beyond*,
https://doi.org/10.1007/978-981-99-4491-0_32

Introduction

In the contemporary society, maintaining mental health and wellness is a challenge to achieve "Health for all". Depression is one of the most common mental conditions that deserves greater attention among elderly people (Elderly Commission, 2021). The World Health Organization has estimated that 10–20% of the elderly population of the world suffered from depression (Barua et al., 2011). Its prevalence ranged from 4 to 25% for major depressive disorder and 29% to 82% for minor depression or presence of depressive symptoms (Seitz et al., 2010). In Hong Kong, this was significantly higher with more than 10% of older people manifesting the signs of depression (Tsang, 2018). The overall prevalence of depressive symptoms in Chinese older adults reported in a meta-analysis study was 23.6% and an increasing trend over the years was noted (Li et al., 2014).

For elderly residential care home (RCH) residents, previous studies reported that the depressive symptoms affected 21.1% to 65.4% of the population (Chow et al., 2004; Santiago & Mattos, 2014; Tiong et al., 2013; Tsai et al., 2005; Ulbricht et al., 2017; Zhao et al., 2018). Sridevi and Swathi (2014) also reported that significant depression was found among the institutionalised elderly than the non-institutionalised ones. All these indicate that the prevalence of depressive symptoms in elderly RCH residents is comparatively higher than that of community-dwelling older people.

In Hong Kong, the elderly population increased continuously from 8.2% in 1988 to 17.9% in 2018 and 18.3% in 2020 (Healthy HK, 2020a; Wong & Yeung, 2019). Furthermore, it is expected to increase to 24% in 2025 and about 33% in 2034 (Lam & Kao, 2017). Nearly 5.8% of the elderly live in RCHs in 2020 (Social Welfare Department, 2021). There is an increasing demand for elderly RCHs due to factors such as reduced family size, the decrease of co-residence between adult children and their elderly parents, and the limited space available in residential flats in Hong Kong (Chui et al., 2009). Accordingly, the prevalence of depressive symptoms among the older people living in RCHs in Hong Kong is expected to increase.

Elderly Depression

Elderly depression has significantly adverse impact on both the elderly and society at large. Depression was proven to be associated with poor physical health (Li et al., 2011), reduced quality of life and increased suicide among older people (Greenberg, 2019). Depressive symptoms were also reported to be significantly associated with suicide in the elderly Chinese population in a dose-response pattern (Sun et al., 2012). This poses a great concern for Hong Kong since the majority of its population are people of Chinese descent. Financially, the medical expenditure for treating depression was significantly higher than other chronic diseases. This was due to more frequent Emergency Department attendance, hospital admissions and medication in comparison with other diseases (Unutzer et al., 2009).

Depression among older people is always correlated with negative life events such as the loss of a partner, history of depression and physical illness (Institute of Mental Health, n.d.). The signs and symptoms of depression may not be immediately recognised and depend on the types and severity. It can manifest as abnormal emotional, physical, cognitive and behavioural presentation such as loss of interest in ordinary activities, social withdrawal, forgetfulness, insomnia, persistent feeling of sadness, low self-esteem and inappropriate self-blame, poor concentration, failure to fulfil duties and inability to enjoy life (Elderly Health Service, 2016). For depressed elderly RCH residents, they also exhibit lower levels of social engagement, more behavioural and vocal disturbance, poorer quality of life, increased use of health care services and mortality rate (Dow et al., 2011). Depressive symptoms also manifest in various forms, but only major depression has significant symptoms (Centre for Health Protection, 2012). Older people, who are more likely to be affected by minor and chronic mild depression, are also more likely to be overlooked and leading to under-treatment (Institute of Mental Health, n.d.).

Currently, treatments for depressive symptoms and depression include pharmacotherapy such as anti-depressants, and non-pharmacological treatment such as psychotherapy and complementary and alternative medicine (Skolnik et al., 2016). However, anti-depressants may cause severe adverse reaction such as withdrawal syndromes and relapse of depression if discontinued after prolonged use. This is relevant in Hong Kong, where the waiting time of the Psychiatry Special out-patient clinic could be up to 127 weeks (Cheung, 2016; Tsang, 2018). The side effects of anti-depressants and subsequent long waiting times for psychiatric consultation are major barriers for proper treatment.

Previous studies have examined the relationship between depressive symptoms and other factors such as age, gender, educational level, length of stay in elderly RCH, number of co-morbidities, frequency of visiting and relationship with the visitors of the elderly RCH residents (Chow et al., 2004; Lee et al., 2014; Tsai et al., 2005). Findings, however, were inconclusive. It is anticipated that elderly depression is becoming a serious mental health problem among older people living in RCHs in Hong Kong. This case study aimed to investigate the pressing issue of the latest prevalence of depressive symptoms and its associated factors among the elderly living in RCHs in Hong Kong. It also sought to provide evidence-based information for staff working in RCHs to identify high-risk groups and implement strategies for prevention and early detection of depressive symptoms among older RCH residents in Hong Kong.

Case Study in Hong Kong

A cross-sectional design was adopted to assess the prevalence of depressive symptoms and examine its associated factors among older people living in RCHs in Hong Kong in 2021. Participants were recruited from four large elderly RCHs with a total of about 750 residents. As various degree of dementia is rather common among the elderly RCH residents, full sampling method was adopted in which all the residents were invited to participate in this study to increase the sample size. Residents were recruited if they were aged 65 or above, and were able to communicate in Cantonese. However, the residents suffering from either severe mental illness or disturbance of consciousness were excluded. Ethical approval had been granted from the Research Ethics Committee of the Hong Kong Metropolitan University. Study objectives and data collection procedures were explained to the participants. Verbal consent was obtained to ensure their voluntary participation. Participants were also be assured of anonymity in handling the data. They could withdraw from the study at any time without affecting the care they received in the RCHs.

Interviews were adopted for data collection, as most of the RCHs residents were either illiterate or were unable to read the questionnaire clearly. All eligible participants were invited to attend an individual face-to-face interview to complete a questionnaire. Each interview lasted for about 15 min and was conducted by the research assistants. The questionnaire comprised two sections: Section One on demographic data and Section Two on Patient Health Questionnaire-8 (PHQ-8). Demographic data included participants' age, gender, educational level, length of stay in the elderly RCH, visiting record (frequency of being visited, relationship with the visitors) and co-morbidities (diagnosed chronic diseases with regular follow-up), while PHQ-8 was used to assess the participants' depressive symptoms (Kroenke et al., 2009). This included eight questions with answers ranked through a 4-point Likert scale. Points 0 (not at all) to 3 (nearly every day) were assigned to each question and likewise summated to obtain the total score ranging from 0 to 24. A higher score indicated more severe affliction of depressive symptoms. A total score of 0 to 4 indicated no significant depressive symptoms, 5 to 9 indicated mild depressive symptoms, 10 to 14 indicated moderate, 15 to 19 indicated moderately severe and 20 indicated severe depressive symptoms (Kroenke et al., 2009). PHQ-8 was a validated assessment tool for measuring depressive symptoms. The χ^2 value was 24.75 with 18 degrees of freedom ($p = 0.13$), and the goodness-of-fit index was 0.98. Internal consistency reliability (Cronbach α) was 0.82 (Pressler et al., 2011).

Due to the COVID-19 pandemic in Hong Kong, visitors were not allowed to enter the RCHs under the enforcement of infection-preventive measures. Therefore, staff of the participating RCHs were recruited as research assistants, who had a recognised degree in social sciences or health care-related disciplines and good communication skills. An online briefing session was conducted with the research assistants to ensure the consistency in data collection and conducting the interviews. Eventually, the recruitment and data collection processes were successfully accomplished from June to August 2021 in the four selected elderly RCHs. The processes were smooth since the research assistants were the staff of the participating RCHs who had already established rapport with the residents. As visits were not allowed before and during data collection, information on visiting record (frequency and relationship with visitors) could not be collected.

The total number of eligible participants was 242 as one resident was excluded for not meeting the inclusion criteria of aged 65 or above. Data analysis was performed using SPSS version 26. The χ^2 test was used to compare the categorical data between participants with and without significant depressive symptoms. Independent t-test and one-way analysis of variance were used to examine the differences in depressive symptoms (PHQ-8 scores) with participants' demographic data. Level of significance was set at $p < 0.05$.

Characteristics of the Participants

The demographic characteristics of all participants are shown in Table 32.1. The participants were older adults with a mean age at 85.7 (SD 8.63, range: 66–103) and a median age at 87. Nearly 60% participants belonged to the oldest-old age group, with most of the participants being female (65.3%). Nearly 80% of them were of low educational level as they either received no formal education (38.4%) or received primary-level education or lower (39.7%). The length of stay in the RCHs among the participants was quite evenly distributed in three periods, including one year to three years (26.4%), more than three years to five years (22.7%) and more than five years to ten years (25.2%). Majority of the participants (95%) suffered from various types of chronic diseases with the mean number of co-morbidities suffered at 2.75 (SD = 1.38, median: 3, range: 1–6). More than half of them (58.3%) suffered from three to six co-morbidities. The top five commonly suffered chronic diseases were hypertension (n = 155, 64%), cerebrovascular disease (n = 86, 35.5%), diabetic mellitus (n = 86, 35.5%), mental illness (85, 35.1%) and heart disease (n = 80, 33.1%).

Prevalence and Severity of Depressive Symptoms Among Participants

The prevalence rate of depressive symptoms among elderly RCH residents was high, as more than half (58.2%) suffered from various degrees of depressive symptoms, ranging from mild to moderately severe (Table 32.2). Herein, a majority of them fell into the category of mild depressive symptoms (35.1%) or moderate depressive symptoms (21.9%). No participants suffered from severe depressive symptoms.

The severity of depressive symptoms suffered was reflected by the mean PHQ-8 scores. The overall mean score (PHQ-8) of all participants was 5.95 ± 4.11 (range

0–17) which corresponded with mild depressive symptoms. This indicated that the participants were most likely suffering from mild depressive symptoms. It also paralleled with the greatest percentage of residents identified under this category ($n = 85$, 35.1%).

Characteristics of Participants with or Without Significant Depressive Symptoms

All participants were categorised into two groups: those with and without significant depressive symptoms for ease of further analysis. Table 32.3 shows that participants suffering from depressive symptoms ($n = 141$) had an average age of 85.7 (SD = 8.80) while the average number of co-morbidities suffered was 3.26 (SD = 1.31). These most likely came from the oldest-old age group ($n = 83$, 58.9%), mostly female ($n = 94$, 66.7%), received no formal education ($n = 56$, 39.7%), stayed in RCH between three and five years ($n = 42$, 29.8%) and had three to six co-morbidities ($n = 106$, 75.2%). Statistical significances were found between the participants with and without significant depressive symptoms regarding their length of stay (χ^2 =

Table 32.1 Demographic characteristics of all participants ($N = 242$)

Demographic characteristics	Mean ± standard deviation (range)
Age (year)	85.7 ± 8.63 (66–103)
Number of co-morbidities	2.75 ± 1.38 (0–6)
	Frequency (percentage %)
Age group (year)	
65–74 (youngest-old)	32 (13.2)
75–84 (middle-old)	67 (27.7)
≥85 (oldest-old)	143 (59.1)
Gender	
Male	84 (34.7)
Female	158 (65.3)
Educational level	
No formal education	93 (38.4)
Primary or below	96 (39.7)
Secondary school or above	53 (21.9)
Duration of stay in RCH	
≤1 year	37 (15.3)
>1 to 3 years	64 (26.4)
>3 to 5 years	55 (22.7)

(continued)

Table 32.1 (continued)

Demographic characteristics		Mean ± standard deviation (range)
>5 to 10 years		61 (25.2)
>10 years		25 (10.3)
Co-morbidities		
Yes		(95%)
No		(5%)
Number of co-morbidities		
0–2		101 (41.7)
3–6		141 (58.3)
Co-existing chronic diseases		
Hypertension	Yes	155 (64.0)
	No	87 (36.0)
Cerebro-vascular disease	Yes	86 (35.5)
	No	156 (64.5)
Diabetic mellitus	Yes	86 (35.5)
	No	156 (64.5)
Mental illness	Yes	85 (35.1)
	No	157 (64.9)
Heart disease	Yes	80 (33.1)
	No	162 (66.9)
Arthritis	Yes	53 (21.9)
	No	189 (78.1)
Chronic lung disease	Yes	32 (13.2)
	No	210 (86.8)
Cancer	Yes	29 (12.0)
	No	213 (88.0)
Renal disease	Yes	28 (11.6)
	No	214 (88.4)
Liver disease	Yes	20 (8.3)
	No	222 (91.7)
Stomach disease	Yes	12 (5)
	No	230 (95)

25.086, $p = 0.000$), the number of co-morbidities suffered ($\chi 2 = 39.741, p = 0.000$) and the average number of co-morbidities suffered ($t = -6.756$, $p = 0.000$). There were no statistically significant differences for age groups and gender between these two groups.

Table 32.2 Prevalence of depressive symptoms among participants ($N = 242$)

PHQ-8 mean scores	Frequency (%)	
0–4 (No significant depressive symptoms)	101 (41.7)	
5–9 (Mild depressive symptoms)	85 (35.1)	141 (58.2%)
10–14 (Moderate depressive symptoms)	53 (21.9)	
15–19 (Moderately severe depressive symptoms)	3 (1.2)	
20–24 (Severe depressive symptoms)	0 (0)	

Factors Associated with the Depressive Symptoms Among the Participants

There were no statistically significant differences for age groups and gender with the depressive symptoms (PHQ-8 mean scores) (Table 32.4). Yet, the mean scores were found to be higher in females and at the young-old age group (aged at 65–74 years). Significant differences were found in depressive symptoms among participants with different total number of co-morbidities ($t = -7.983$, $p = 0.000$), different educational levels (F (2, 239) = 3.565, $p = 0.030$), and different lengths of stay in RCHs ($F(4, 237) = 4.058$, $p = 0.003$). In the post hoc test by Tukey HSD, it was found that participants who received secondary school-level education or above suffered from more depressive symptoms than those with primary school-level education or below ($p = 0.024$). Regarding the length of stay, the post hoc test by Tukey HSD revealed that statistical significances were found in participants that stayed in RCHs for three to five years where they were found to have suffered from more severe depressive symptoms than those stayed for less than one year ($p = 0.004$) or one to three years ($p = 0.042$).

Discussion

Characteristics of Subjects

The majority of the participants belonged to the oldest-old age group (59.1%), were predominately females (65.3%) and suffered from co-morbidities (95%). There was an under-representation of the youngest-old and middle-old age groups in the study. The participants being predominately female may be explained by the fact that females live longer than males in Hong Kong with a longer life expectancy at birth (87.7 years) than their male counterparts (83.4 years) (Healthy HK, 2020b). It is also no surprise that 95% of the participants had co-morbidities since they mostly belonged to "oldest-old" age group where they had increased incidence of suffering from various types of chronic diseases. In addition, those admitted to RCHs mainly because they needed professional care for their health problems (Mello et al., 2014).

Table 32.3 Characteristics of the participants with or without suffering from significant depressive symptoms ($N = 242$)

Demographic characteristics	All participants ($N = 242$)	With depressive symptoms ($n = 141$)	Without significant depressive symptoms($n = 101$)		
	Mean ± standard deviation (range)			t	p
Age (year)	85.7 ± 8.63 (66–103)	85.7 ± 8.80 (66–103)	85.7 ± 8.44 (66–102)	0.059	0.953
		Frequency (percentage %)		χ^2	p
Age group (year)					
65–74 (youngest-old)	32 (13.2)	20 (14.2)	12 (11.9)	0.305	0.859
75–84 (middle-old)	67 (27.7)	38 (27.0)	29 (28.7)		
≥85 (oldest-old)	143 (59.1)	83 (58.9)	60 (59.4)		
Gender					
Male	84 (34.7)	47 (33.3)	37 (36.6)	0.283	0.595
Female	158 (65.3)	94 (66.7)	64 (63.4)		
Educational level					
No formal education	93 (38.4)	56 (39.7)	37 (36.6)	4.239	0.120
Primary or below	96 (39.7)	49 (34.8)	47 (46.5)		
Secondary school or above	53 (21.9)	36 (25.5)	17 (16.8)		
Length of stay in RCH					
≤1 year	37 (15.3)	11 (7.8)	26 (25.7)	25.086	0.000**

(continued)

Table 32.3 (continued)

Demographic characteristics	All participants ($N = 242$)	With depressive symptoms ($n = 141$)	Without significant depressive symptoms($n = 101$)		
	Mean ± standard deviation (range)			t	p
>1 to 3 years	64 (26.4)	31 (22.0)	33 (32.7)		
>3 to 5 years	55 (22.7)	42 (29.8)	13 (12.9)		
>5 to 10 years	61 (25.2)	39 (27.7)	22 (21.8)		
>10 years	25 (10.3)	18 (12.8)	7 (6.9)		
Number of co-morbidities					
0–2	101 (41.7)	35 (24.8)	66 (65.3)	39.741	0.000**
3–6	141 (58.3)	106 (75.2)	35 (34.7)		
	Mean ± standard deviation (range)			T	p
Number of co-morbidities	2.75 ± 1.38 (0–6)	3.26 ± 1.31 (0–6)	2.05 ± 1.15 (0–5)	−6.756	0.000**

Note $*p < 0.05$; $**p < 0.001$

Table 32.4 Comparison between different demographic characteristics and the depressive symptoms (PHQ-8 mean scores) ($N = 242$)

Demographic characteristics	Mean ± SD	*t*	*p*	
Gender				
Male	5.93 ± 4.225	−0.060	0.952	
Female	5.96 ± 4.055			
Total number of co-morbidities suffered		−7.983	0.000**	
0–2	3.73 ± 3.569			
3–6	7.54 ± 3.720			
	Mean ± SD	*F*	*p*	*Post-hoc test (Tukey HSD)*
Age group (year)				
65–74 (youngest-old)	6.53 ± 4.243			
75–84 (middle-old)	6.24 ± 4.218	0.782	0.459	
≥85 (oldest-old)	5.69 ± 4.029			
Educational level		3.565	0.030*	Secondary school or above > Primary school or below ($p = 0.024$*)
No formal education	6.08 ± 3.976			
Primary school or below	5.22 ± 3.950			
Secondary school or above	7.06 ± 4.405			
Length of stay in RCH (Year)				3–5 years > Less than 1 year ($p = 0.004$*) 3–5 years > 1–3 years ($p = 0.042$*)
≤1 year	4.24 ± 4.867			
>1–3 years	5.22 ± 4.045			
>3–5 years	7.29 ± 3.715	4.058	0.003*	
>5–10 years	6.23 ± 3.671			
>10 years	6.72 ± 3.900			

Note *$p < 0.05$; **$p < 0.001$

Prevalence Rate of Depressive Symptoms Among Elderly RCH Residents

The overall prevalence rate of depressive symptoms is very high (58.2%). Such findings indicate the high occurrence of depression symptoms among the elderly RCH residents in Hong Kong. On the one hand, compared to other local studies in elderly nursing homes, this prevalence rate (58.2%) is doubled of that (29%) reported by Chow et al. (2004), but lower than the rate (65.4%) reported by Tsai et al. (2005). On the other hand, this prevalence rate (58.2%) is higher than those reported in the elderly nursing homes in other countries, including 48.7% in Brazil (Santiago & Mattos, 2014), 47.8% in India (Kumar et al., 2021), 43.3% in Taiwan

(Tsai et al., 2005), 42.5% in Indonesia (Pramesona & Taneepanichskul, 2018), 28.4% in Norway (Iden et al., 2014), 26.6% in China (Zhao et al., 2018), 26% in United States of America (Ulbricht et al., 2017) and 21.1% in Singapore (Tiong et al., 2013). There is difficulty in making comparisons as different screening instruments for depressive symptoms were used in these previous studies, and they include Patient Health Questionnaire-8 (which was used by the current study), Geriatric Depression Scale (Kumar et al., 2021; Pramesona & Taneepanichskul, 2018; Santiago & Mattos, 2014), Hospital Depression Scale (Zhao et al., 2018), Minimum Data Set version 3.0 (Ulbricht et al., 2017), International Classification of Diseases, Tenth Revision (ICD-10) (Iden et al., 2014) Diagnostic and Statistical Manual of Mental Disorders, fourth edition (DSM-IV) criteria (Tiong et al., 2013) and the Chinese version of the Geriatric Depression Scale in short form (Chow et al., 2004; Tsai et al., 2005).

The high prevalence rate of depressive symptoms reported in this study may be accounted by the sample characteristics and the timing of the data collection process. The sample was dominated by the oldest-old age group; females and those with co-morbidities Depressive symptoms were found to be associated with older people especially the oldest-old age group. This is probably related to the longer life expectancy leading to an increase in the population of this age group (Yu et al., 2012). Previous studies reported that women were more likely to develop depression than men (Chow et al., 2004; Kumar et al., 2021; Ulbricht et al., 2017) and chronic medical conditions increased the risk of moderate depression (Lee et al., 2014; Pramesona & Taneepanichskul, 2018). As mentioned, the data were collected during the period of the COVID-19 pandemic, and visitors were not allowed to enter the elderly RCHs under the enforcement of infection-preventive measures. The social support to RCH residents was adversely affected with the prohibition of visits. Lack of social support was one significant factor that led to the development of depression among institutionalised older people (Glaesmer et al., 2011; Santiago & Mattos, 2014; Tiong et al., 2013).

Factors Associated with the Depressive Symptoms Among Elderly RCH Residents

The findings revealed that there were statistically significant differences for the demographic characteristics, including educational level, length of stay in RCH and total number of co-morbidities with the depressive symptoms (PHQ-8 scores) except for the age group and gender. The non-significant results found in age and gender was consistent with the results reported by Kumar et al. (2021) and Tiong et al. (2013).

In this study, the significant results in educational level were not in agreement with those reported by Kumar et al. (2021), Pramesona and Taneepanichskul (2018), and Tiong et al. (2013). This study revealed that participants who received secondary school-level education or above suffered from more severe depressive symptoms than those with primary school-level education or below. In many previous studies, older people with lower education had higher prevalence rate of depressive symptoms in the nursing home or community settings (Jia et al., 2011; Mullick et al., 2018; Tsai et al., 2005; Yu et al., 2012). It was suggested that older people with higher education level had lower risk of depressive symptoms as they may be involved in more social activities (Li et al., 2014). However, the situation may be different when they were admitted into the elderly RCHs where the residents have limited autonomy in their social environment, activities and connectivity, thus leading to more depressive symptoms.

Participants who stayed in RCHs for three to five years were significantly found to suffer from more severe depressive symptoms than those who stayed for less than three years. Institutionalisation is considered as a significant determinant of depressive symptoms among older people (Stek et al., 2006). In addition, lack of friends and social contact in the institution was reported to be associated with depressive symptoms (Santiago & Mattos, 2014; Tiong et al., 2013). All these may explain the supposed positive relationship between the length of stay in RCHs and the likelihood to develop depressive symptoms among the elderly residents.

Significant findings were also found between depressive symptoms and the number of co-morbidities among participants, and they supported the findings of other research studies (Glaesmer et al., 2011; Lee et al., 2014). Chronic diseases are usually associated with polypharmacy and functional impairment. All these impose negative feelings that result in the onset of depressive symptoms for elderly people.

Furthermore, statistically significant findings were found between the length of stay and the number of co-morbidities suffered between the participants with and without significant depressive symptoms, with regard to its occurrence. These two demographic characteristics also demonstrated statistical significance with the severity of depressive symptoms (PHQ-8 scores) as discussed above. It indicates that the length of stay and number of co-morbidities are two significant factors associated with the likelihood of depressive symptoms among elderly RCH residents.

Limitations of the Study

The study has three limitations: firstly, the data collection process was conducted during the COVID-19 pandemic in Hong Kong. Visitors were not allowed to enter the RCHs under the enforcement of infection-preventive measures for nearly two years. The information on visiting (frequency and relationship with visitors) could not be collected even though visiting was a significant factor associated with depressive symptoms among the elderly in RCHs. Most importantly, restricted visiting arrangement was expected to be detrimental to the residents' depressive symptoms owing to the lack of or no direct social contact or support from visitors. Secondly, full sampling in four elderly RCHs was adopted to increase the chances of recruiting more eligible participants in this study. Despite this, only 242 eligible residents were recruited; hence, the studied sample was not representative of all Hong Kong nursing home residents. Lastly, comparisons may not be appropriate due to the differences in the screening instruments used. Accordingly, the generalisability of the results of the study should be interpreted with caution. For future studies, it is recommended to recruit a larger sample size from more elderly RCHs, collect data on visiting record related to the frequency and relationship with the visitors, and adopt a universal screening instrument for depressive symptoms to obtain more reliable results for generalisation and enhance comparison across studies.

Actions in Health in All Policies

Maintaining mental health and wellness is a challenge to achieve "Health for all". Depression is one of the most common mental conditions that deserves greater attention among elderly people. Elderly depression has significant adverse impact on both the elderly and society. Yet, it is not easily be detected and always resulting in under-treatment, especially for those living in the elderly RCHs. In Hong Kong, the elderly population was 18.3% in 2020 and is expected to further increase to about 33% in 2034. It is anticipated that elderly depression is becoming a serious mental health problem among older people living in RCHs in Hong Kong. This study aimed to investigate the pressing issue of the latest prevalence of depressive symptoms and its associated factors among the elderly living in RCHs in Hong Kong.

This study found a high prevalence rate of depressive symptoms among the elderly RCH residents. Residents who were female, belonging to the "oldest-old" age group, having secondary school or above educational level, having stayed in RCHs between three and five years, and having at least three co-morbidities were found to be the high-risk groups.

As reflected in the above case study in Hong Kong, three approaches are recommended in addressing this imminent problem of mental health in order to move forward to achieve health for all, especially the elderly people living in the RCHs. The first approach is aimed at health care policymakers who should devise appropriate health policies to promote the mental health of the elderly population from a global perspective. The second approach targets at the staff of RCHs that they should be equipped with updated knowledge related to depressive symptoms, characteristics of the high-risk groups, and channels of resources through leaflets and regular training programmes. The programmes should also include workshops on using the screening tool for depressive symptoms and sharpening observation skills to identify the development of depressive symptoms among residents in early stage. The third approach focuses on elderly RCH residents themselves. All residents should undergo an initial assessment for detecting any depressive symptoms on admission, along with regular monitoring by the screening tool. Once the resident is identified to have depressive symptoms, medical consultations should be arranged for further assessment and treatment.

Most importantly, regular mental health programmes are recommended to be organised for residents to prevent the occurrence of any depressive symptoms or consequent worsening of the condition once diagnosed. Special attention should be given to residents who have presented with depressive symptoms. Early detection and appropriate preventive measures should be targeted at the high-risk groups to address mental health problems among elderly RCH residents in Hong Kong.

Acknowledgements The work described in this paper was fully supported by a grant from the Katie Shu Sui Pui Charitable Trust—Research and Publication Fund (Project Reference No.: KS 2020/02). Heartfelt thanks are also conveyed to all participants and the supervisors of the four participating elderly residential care homes.

References

Barua, A., Ghosh, M. K., Kar, N., & Basilio, M. A. (2011). Prevalence of depressive disorders in the elderly. *Annals of Saudi Medicine, 31*(6), 620–624. https://doi.org/10.4103/0256-4947.87100

Centre for Health Protection. (2012). Depression: Beyond feeling blue. *Non-communicable Diseases Watch, 5*(9). https://www.chp.gov.hk/files/pdf/ncd_watch_sep2012.pdf

Cheung, K. (2016, June 26). *HKFP's comprehensive guide to mental health services in Hong Kong.* Hong Kong Free Press. https://www.hongkongfp.com/2016/06/26/hkfps-comprehensive-guide-to-mental-health-services-in-hong-kong/

Chow, E. S. L., Kong, B. M. H., Wong, M. T. P., Draper, B., Lin, K. L., Ho, S. K. S., & Wong, C. P. (2004). The prevalence of depressive symptoms among elderly Chinese private nursing home residents in Hong Kong. *International Journal of Geriatric Psychiatry, 19*(8), 734–740. https://doi.org/10.1002/gps.1158

Chui, W. T. E., Chan, K. S., Chong, M. L. A., Ko, S. F. L., Law, C. K. S., Law, C. K., Leung, M. F. E., Leung, Y. M. A., Lou, W. Q. V., & Ng, Y. T. S. (2009). *Elderly commission's study on residential care services for the elderly final report.* https://www.elderlycommission.gov.hk/en/download/library/Residential%20Care%20Services%20-%20Final%20Report(eng).pdf

Dow, B., Lin, X. P., Tinney, J., & Haralambous, B. (2011). Depression in older people living in residential homes. *International Psychogeriatric, 23*(5), 681–699. https://doi.org/10.1017/S1041610211000494

Elderly Commission. (2021). *Report on healthy ageing executive summary.* https://www.elderlycommission.gov.hk/en/library/Ex-sum.htm

Elderly Health Service. (2016). *Depression.* Department of Health. http://www.elderly.gov.hk/english/common_health_problems/mental_illness/depression.html

Glaesmer, H., Riedel-Heller, S., Braehler, E., Spangenberg, L., & Luppa, M. (2011). Age and gender specific prevalence and risk factors for depressive symptoms in the elderly: A population-based study. *International Psychogeriatrics, 23*(8), 1294–1300. https://doi.org/10.1017/s1041610211000780

Greenberg, S. A. (2019). *The geriatric depression scale (GDS).* The Hartford Institute for Geriatric Nursing. https://hign.org/sites/default/files/2020-06/Try_This_General_Assessment_4.pdf

Healthy HK. (2020a). *Age structure.* https://www.healthyhk.gov.hk/phisweb/en/chart_detail/11/

Healthy HK. (2020b). *Current situation.* https://www.healthyhk.gov.hk/phisweb/en/chart_detail/12/

Iden, K. R., Engedal, K., Hjorleifsson, S., & Ruths, S. (2014). Prevalence of depression among recently admitted long-term care patients in Norwegian nursing homes: Associations with diagnostic workup and use of antidepressants. *Dementia and Geriatric Cognitive Disorders, 37*, 154–162. https://doi.org/10.1159/000355427

Institute of Mental Health. (n.d.). *Elderly depression.* Castle Peak Hospital. http://www3.ha.org.hk/cph/imh/mhi/article_02_02_03.asp

Jia, L. N., Zhuang, H. L., Wang, X. Y., Liu, F. F., Chen, B. Y., & Lin, Y. J. (2011). Depression status of the elderly and its relationship with quality of life in community of Fuzhou city. *Chinese Journal of Geriatrics, 30*(11), 970–973. https://doi.org/10.3760/cma.j.issn.0254-9026.2011.11.024

Kroenke, K., Strine, T. W., Spitzer, R. L., Williams, J. B. W., Berry, J. T., & Mokdad, A. H. (2009). The PHQ-8 as a measure of current depression in the general population. *Journal of Affective Disorders, 114*(1–3), 163–173. https://doi.org/10.1016/j.jad.2008.06.026

Kumar, S., Joseph, S., & Abraham, A. (2021). Prevalence of depression amongst the elderly population in old age homes of Mangalore city. *Journal of Family Medicine and Primary Care, 10*(5), 1868–1872. https://doi.org/10.4103/jfmpc.jfmpc_1850_20

Lam, J., & Kao, E. (2017, June 27). Hong Kong's ageing time bomb a cause for concern. *South China Morning Post.* https://www.scmp.com/news/hong-kong/health-environment/article/2099749/hong-kongs-ageing-time-bomb-cause-concern

Lee, H., Lee, J., Brar, J. S., Rush, E. B., & Jolley, C. J. (2014). Physical activity and depressive symptoms in older adults. *Geriatric Nursing, 35*, 37–41. https://doi.org/10.1016/j.gerinurse.2013.09.005

Li, D., Zhang, D. J., Shao, J. J., Qi, X. D., & Tian, L. (2014). A meta-analysis of the prevalence of depressive symptoms in Chinese older adults. *Archives of Gerontology and Geriatrics, 59*(1), 1–9. https://doi.org/10.1016/j.archger.2013.07.016

Li, N., Pang, L., Chen, G., Song, X., Zhang, J., & Zheng, X. (2011). Risk factors for depression in older adults in Beijing. *Canadian Journal of Psychiatry, 56*(8), 466–473. https://doi.org/10.1177/070674371105600804

Mello, A. D. C., Engstrom, E. M., & Alves, L. C. (2014). Health-related and sociodemographic factors associated with frailty in the elderly: A systematic literature review. *Cadernos de Saúde Pública, 30*(6), 1143–1168. https://doi.org/10.1590/0102-311x00148213

Mullick, T. H., Samanta, S., Maji, B., & Sarangi, L. (2018). Pattern of morbidity and depression among the urban geriatric population: A community-based survey in Bhubaneswar, Orissa, India. *International Journal of Health and Allied Sciences, 7*(4), 233–239. https://www.ijhas.in/text.asp?2018/7/4/233/243269

Pramesona, B. A., & Taneepanichskul, S. (2018). Prevalence and risk factors of depression among Indonesian elderly: A nursing home-based cross-sectional study. *Neurology, Psychiatry and Brain Research, 30*, 22–27. https://doi.org/10.1016/j.npbr.2018.04.004

Pressler, S. J., Subramanian, U., Perkins, S. M., Gradus-Pizlo, I., Kareken, D., Kim, J., Ding, Y., Sauve, M. J., & Sloan, R. (2011). Measuring depressive symptoms in heart failure: Validity and reliability of the patient health questionnaire–8. *American Journal of Critical Care, 20*(2), 146–152. https://doi.org/10.4037/ajcc2010931

Santiago, L. M., & Mattos, I. E. (2014). Depressive symptoms in institutionalized older adults. *Revista de Saúde Pública, 48*(2), 216–224. https://doi.org/10.1590/s0034-8910.2014048004965

Seitz, D., Purandare, N., & Conn, D. (2010). Prevalence of psychiatric disorders among older adults in long-term care homes: A systematic review. *International Psychogeriatric, 22*, 1025–1039. https://doi.org/10.1017/S1041610210000608

Skolnik, N., Sutton, A., & Lcsw. (2016). Treatment of depression—Nonpharmacologic vs. pharmacologic. *Clinical Guidelines for Family Physicians. Family Practice.* https://www.mdedge.com/familypracticenews/article/115932/mental-health/treatment-depression-nonpharmacologic-vs

Social Welfare Department. (2021). *Overview of residential care services for the elderly.* https://www.swd.gov.hk/en/index/site_pubsvc/page_elderly/sub_residentia/id_overviewon/

Sridevi, G., & Swathi, P. (2014). Death anxiety, death depression, geriatric depression and suicidal ideation among institutionalized and non-institutionalized elders. *International Journal of Scientific and Research Publications, 4*(10), 1–8. https://www.ijsrp.org/research-paper-1014.php?rp=P343245

Stek, M. L., Vinkers, D. J., Gussekloo, J., Van der Mast, R. C., Beekman, A. T. F., & Westendorp, J. W. (2006). Natural history of depression in the oldest old population-based prospective study. *British Journal of Psychiatry, 188*(1), 65–69. https://doi.org/10.1192/bjp.188.1.65

Sun, W. J., Xu, L., Chan, W. M., Lam, T. H., & Schooling, C. M. (2012). Depressive symptoms and suicide in 56,000 older Chinese: A Hong Kong cohort study. *Social Psychiatry and Psychiatric Epidemiology, 47*(4), 505–514. https://doi.org/10.1007/s00127-011-0362-z

Tiong, W. W., Yap, P., Koh, G. C. H., Fong, N. P., & Luo, N. (2013). Prevalence and risk factors of depression in the elderly nursing home residents in Singapore. *Aging and Mental Health, 17*(6), 724–731. https://doi.org/10.1080/13607863.2013.775638

Tsai, Y. F., Chung, J. W. Y., Wong, T. K. S., & Huang, C. M. (2005). Comparison of the prevalence and risk factors for depressive symptoms among elderly nursing home residents in Taiwan and Hong Kong. *International Journal of Geriatric Psychiatry, 20*(4), 315–321. https://doi.org/10.1002/gps.1281

Tsang, E. (2018, January 31). Health and environment. *South China Morning Post*. https://www.scmp.com/news/hong-kong/health-environment/article/1907974/over-10-cent-hong-kong-elderly-persons-show-signs

Ulbricht, C. M., Rothschild, A. J., Hunnicutt, J. N., & Lapane, K. L. (2017). Depression and cognitive impairment among newly admitted nursing home residents in the USA. *International Journal of Geriatric Psychiatry, 32*(11), 1172–1181. https://doi.org/10.1002/gps.4723

Unutzer, J., Schoenbaum, M., Katon, W. J., Fan, M., Pincus, H. A., Hogan, D., & Taylor, J. (2009). Health care costs associated with depression in medically ill fee-for-service Medicare participants. *Journal of the American Geriatric Society, 57*(3), 506–510. https://doi.org/10.1111/j.1532-5415.2008.02134.x

Wong, K., & Yeung, M. (2019). Population ageing trend of Hong Kong. *Office of the Government Economist—Economic Letter*. https://www.hkeconomy.gov.hk/en/pdf/el/el-2019-02.pdf

World Health Organization. (2010). *Mental health and substance abuse: Fast and figure of depression*. http://www.searo.who.int/en/section1174/section1199/section1567_6741.htm

Yu, J., Li, J., Cuijpers, P., Wu, S., & Wu, Z. (2012). Prevalence and correlates of depressive symptoms in Chinese older adults: A population-based study. *International Journal of Geriatric Psychiatry, 27*(3), 305–312. https://doi.org/10.1002/gps.2721

Zhao, X., Zhang, D., Wu, M., Yang, Y., Xie, H., Li, Y., Jia, J., & Su, Y. (2018). Loneliness and depression symptoms among the elderly in nursing homes: A moderated mediation model of resilience and social support. *Psychiatry Research, 268*, 143–151. https://doi.org/10.1016/j.psychres.2018.07.011

Chapter 33
Residential Choices of the Elderly Under Medical and Aged Care Integration: Evidence from Shanghai

Ruixin Xing, Pi-Ying Yen, and Haoyu Liu

Abstract The population of the elderly is growing faster than ever due to substantial increases in life expectancy. One critical decision the elderly have to make is their residential choices, and nursing homes are one of their options. Recently, the integration of medical and aged care, a mode where nursing homes deliver both medical care and daily aged care to meet the needs of the elderly, is flourishing because of increasing health awareness. Though the integration mode is developing rapidly in the industry, little literature has documented this topic. This chapter examines the elderly's residential choices and preferences for nursing homes under the integration mode, by collecting data from residents and conducting an interview with a manager of a leading nursing home in Shanghai, China. Residents' demographics are comprehensively studied. Furthermore, we uncover that hospital visits may trigger a resident to leave the nursing home, even though his or her health remains unchanged. Hence, residents' decisions to return after hospital visits are also investigated, providing operational implications for nursing homes that adopt the integration mode.

Keywords Aged care · Chronic disease · Medical care · Nursing home · Residential choice

Background

The number and proportion of people aged 60 and above (the elderly hereafter) in the global population have both seen fast growth in recent times because of the substantial increase in life expectancy. According to the World Health Organization

R. Xing · P.-Y. Yen
School of Business, Macau University of Science and Technology, Macau, China
e-mail: pyyen@must.edu.mo

H. Liu (✉)
Faculty of Business, City University of Macau, Macau, China
e-mail: tonyliuhaoyu@gmail.com

B. Y. F. Fong and W. C. W. Wong (eds.), *Gaps and Actions in Health Improvement from Hong Kong and Beyond*,
https://doi.org/10.1007/978-981-99-4491-0_33

(WHO), the population of the elderly reached one billion in 2019 (World Health Organization, n.d.-a), and the WHO expects this number to reach 1.4 billion by 2030 and 2.1 billion by 2050. In developing countries, the population of the elderly is expanding at an unprecedented pace, and this drastic expansion will continue in the coming decades. Thus, a novel need has arisen to adapt to this significant change in the population structure. Making the world more ageing-friendly is an urgent issue, and efforts in health and social care deserve more attention.

In 2015, the WHO published the *World Report on Ageing and Health* and established the goal of healthy ageing as helping people develop and maintain the functional ability that enables well-being, which includes an individual's intrinsic capacity, the environment, and their interactions. In 2017, the WHO further launched the initiative Integrated Care for Older People (ICOPE) and released the *Guidelines on Community-Level Interventions to Manage Declines in Intrinsic Capacity* (World Health Organization, n.d.-g). The concept of "integrated care" in the context of the elderly requires that medical care and aged care, which were delivered separately in the past, be delivered together. This concept aims to fully meet the needs of the elderly in various aspects. Specifically, the guidelines provide recommendations on assessing health status, delivering integrated healthcare services to enable the elderly to maintain their physical and mental capacities, and performing effective interventions to manage declines in their intrinsic capacity. Notably, ICOPE not only benefits caregivers in the context of an ageing society but also meets the context of sustainable development. ICOPE well supports the third Sustainable Development Goal (SDG3: Good Health and Well-being), which is committed to ensuring healthy lives, promoting well-being for all at all ages, and making progress against leading causes of death and disease (United Nations, n.d.).

Countries around the world have also taken measures to combat issues raised by population ageing, and the integration of medical and aged care points out a pathway to do so. The United States (US) developed its mode of integrated care, the Programme of All-Inclusive Care for the Elderly (PACE). PACE stems from the "On Lok" mode in Chinese communities in San Francisco, which caters to the needs of the elderly who prefer to stay at home but whose families cannot offer adequate healthcare services (Cheng & Feng, 2015; Li et al., 2017). In PACE, Adult Day Health Centres (ADHCs) are the primary outlets for service provision, where daily aged care, physical examinations, health consultations, and various treatments are offered. In addition to ADHCs, PACE also provides interdisciplinary teams (IDTs) that consist of medical and aged care professionals, such as physicians, nurses, dentists, drivers, and social workers, who provide more innovative and flexible services. For example, though ADHCs can treat mosquito bites, they cannot prevent them. IDTs, however, can help the elderly to solve the problem at the source.

The United Kingdom (UK) is faced with an ageing society. In the UK, the number and percentage of people aged 65 and above were 12.5 million and 18.6%, respectively, in mid-2020, and these are expected to continue to increase (Office for National Statistics, 2021). In response to its ageing society, the UK government devoted itself to combining medical care and daily aged care (i.e. integrated care) by bridging the gap between the healthcare department and the social services department as early as the 1970s (Geng & Wang, 2016; Li et al., 2020). The current integrated care programme in the UK is Enhanced Health in Care Homes (EHCH). EHCH promotes the concept of "personalisation, prevention first and health first". It utilises social and voluntary power to provide personalised aged care to the elderly. It also advocates a proactive healthcare model, which actively assesses the needs of the elderly so that each of them can be taken good care of.

France has been an ageing society since 1985 and now has 15 million elderly people, making up 24% of the population (Liu & Luo, 2016). The country has established a relatively mature aged care system with three major components: (1) medical institutions, where geriatric specialists provide comprehensive healthcare services to ageing patients; (2) nursing homes, which receive the elderly with substandard health but without care from family; and (3) family-based care, where the elderly receive healthcare services at home to avoid over-utilisation of medical resources, crowdedness, or cross-infection in hospitals. In particular, the second component, nursing homes, incorporates medical care functions. They can provide general treatment to the elderly and transfer them to medical institutions for specialised treatment when needed. Among French nursing homes, EHPADs (les etablissements d'hebergement pour personnes agees dependants) receive disabled elderly and have a rather strong medical capacity, which can be recognised as integrated care.

Many countries in Asia have also moved towards ageing societies. For example, the proportion of the elderly is over 28% in Japan, and the country has explored and enhanced its related public policy since the 1960s (Yang & Wang, 2021; Zhou et al., 2018). After forty years of improvement, Japan has successfully transformed its mode from traditional aged care to modern integrated care. Homes and nursing homes are more popular residential choices for the elderly than medical institutions. Hospitals are encouraged to participate in healthcare services in homes and nursing homes, and preventive care services have prospered.

Medical and Aged Care Integration in China

China is one of the fastest-growing ageing populations in the world, and the WHO expects the elderly people of the population to reach 28% by 2040 (World Health Organization, n.d.-b). This considerable change in the population structure brings both unprecedented challenges and opportunities to China regarding public health and socioeconomic development. Establishing an integrated system to meet the health and social needs of the elderly is an urgent task.

Nursing homes are among the most popular residential choices for the elderly in China. In nursing homes, the integration of medical and aged care is prospering because of increasing health awareness. Medical and aged care integration is a mode where nursing homes deliver both medical care and daily aged care to meet the needs of the elderly. Notably, the integration mode is not only a business decision but also a public policy. In 2014, the term "medical and aged care integration" first appeared in the government document *Announcement about Accelerating the Construction of the*

Health and Aged Care Industry. In 2015, the *Outline for the Planning of the National Medical and Health Service System* defined the term as a collaboration of medical institutions and aged care institutions. The contents of the outline include establishing and enhancing the coordination between two parties, developing channels for aged care institutions to make appointments at medical institutions, and coordinating the provision of chronic care management and rehabilitation services for the elderly. Moreover, the outline also discusses how to promote transfers and collaborations between medical and aged care institutions, integrate medical care into daily aged care, and support aged care institutions to set up their own medical facilities. These policies combine the resources between medical and aged care institutions and point out the direction for creating a safe, convenient, and fully functional aged care service network.

As the integration mode has developed in China, it has significantly affected the elderly's residential choices since nursing homes now cover the needs of the elderly that they originally did not. However, little literature has documented this topic, and little research has been carried out. The elderly's residential choices are a critical decision for the well-being of their remaining years since they will face more and more physical and mental limitations as their age progresses. Whether their residence can provide adequate care and immediate support is thus critical. The elderly's residential choices and preferences for nursing homes under the integration mode were examined by the authors, by collecting data from residents and conducting interviews with a manager in a leading nursing home in Shanghai. The results were meaningful in the sense that the residents' decisions to return to the nursing homes after hospital visits were carefully investigated. The findings can provide operational implications for nursing homes that adopt the medical and aged care integration mode.

The Case Study

Data were collected from a leading nursing home in Shanghai, China. The nursing home had been selected as one of the top 10 medical and aged care integration brands in China for two consecutive years (2020 and 2021). The nursing home mainly focused on daily aged care, rehabilitation services, and health consultations, and it was committed to providing joint "medical-caring-health-nursing" professional service. The nursing home collaborated with a hospital established in 1985. The hospital served as a practical teaching base for a medical school and was chosen as one of Shanghai's most age-friendly hospitals in 2022. Therefore, choosing this nursing home as the sample fitted well with the research context and could provide rich and helpful operational insights for other nursing homes that would pursue a medical and aged care integration mode.

The data were collected from December 2021 to January 2022. Questionnaires were distributed to both residents with and without self-care ability, including former residents. Those who had self-care ability filled out the questionnaires by themselves, with assistance from the nursing home's staff if needed. For those without self-care ability, the questionnaires were completed by the staff based on known facts about the residents. Note that a person was included as long as he or she had once lived in the nursing home. For the elderly who had previously lived in the nursing home but had chosen to leave, the staff of the nursing home interviewed them by phone and helped them fill out the questionnaires.

The sample size was 319. In this nursing home, females ($N = 180$, 56.43%) outnumbered males ($N = 139$, 43.57%). The largest proportion of residents were 80–89 years old ($N = 138$, 43.26%), followed by 70–79 years old ($N = 81$, 25.39%), 90 and above years old ($N = 55$, 17.24%), 60–69 years old ($N = 42$, 13.17%), and 60 or below years old ($N = 3$, 0.94%). Regarding education level, 15 (4.7%) residents attended university, while 133 (41.69%) and 171 (53.61%), respectively, only attended high school or elementary school. Regarding monthly income, most of the residents ($N = 260$, 81.5%) earned 2590–5000 RMB (approximately 370–720 USD), followed by 2590 RMB (approximately 370 USD) or below ($N = 51$, 15.99%) and 5000 RMB (approximately 720 USD) and above ($N = 8$, 2.51%). To meet their expenses in the nursing home, most of the residents paid a certain portion themselves ($N = 209$, 65.52%), while 31.66% ($N = 101$) paid all costs, and 2.82% ($N = 9$) did not pay any costs themselves. Among all people who filled out the questionnaires, 92.16% ($N = 294$) were local residents of Shanghai, and 7.84% ($N = 25$) were non-local residents. Table 33.1 provides a summary of the demographics. Note that 2590 RMB is the threshold of Shanghai's monthly minimum wage standard.

To gain more insights into the topic, the manager of the operational department in the nursing home was interviewed. During the interview, the manager mentioned that keeping residents living in the nursing home was always an important issue for them since the medical facilities could not be fully utilised if residents left, and the social benefits that the nursing home could offer would therefore be limited. Regarding the triggers for withdrawing from the nursing home, the manager commented, "hospital visits may trigger a resident to leave the nursing home, even though his or her health remains unchanged before and after the visit". He also added, "we notice that residents' health, especially whether they already have chronic diseases or not, is a key indicator of their return after hospital visits". The observations from the manager showed a possible pathway to analyse the elderly's residential choices and motivated the following analysis. In the next section, attention was limited to the residents who had hospital visits. A preliminary analysis of this group of people is presented to display the big picture, and then, whether there is any relationship between chronic diseases and return decisions after hospital visits is investigated.

Analysis of the Elderly Who Visited Hospitals

The total number of the elderly who had hospital visits was 128, comprising 95 (74.22%) who returned to the nursing home after the visits and 33 (25.78%) who did not. Table 33.2 provides descriptive statistics about gender, age, education, monthly

Table 33.1 Descriptive statistics ($N = 319$)

Items	Frequency	Percentage
Gender		
Male	139	43.57
Female	180	56.43
Age (years)		
60 or below	3	0.94
60–69	42	13.17
70–79	81	25.39
80–89	138	43.26
90 and above	55	17.24
Education		
Elementary school or below	171	53.61
High school	133	41.69
College	15	4.70
Monthly income (RMB)		
2590 or below	51	15.99
2590–5000	260	81.50
5000 and above	8	2.51
Expenses		
Totally covered	101	31.66
Partially covered	209	65.52
Totally not covered	9	2.82
Residency		
Local	294	92.16
Non-local	25	7.84

income, expenses, and residency of the elderly who had hospital visits while residing in the nursing home.

Chi-squared tests were performed to analyse differences among the demographic groups. For groups with a number of observations less than five, Yates' Correction for Continuity was applied. In particular, a significant relationship was found between expenses and return decisions, with $p < 0.05$. Among the elderly who had hospital visit experiences, 95 returned to the nursing home and 33 did not. Of those who returned to the nursing home, 64 partially covered their expenses, 25 totally covered their expenses, and six totally did not. Of those who did not return to the nursing home, 30 partially paid their costs, one of them totally paid their costs, and two of them did not pay any costs themselves. Table 33.3 summarises these statistics.

Through Table 33.3, a tendency could be observed among the residents entirely responsible for their own expenses to return to the nursing home after hospital visits; specifically, 25 of these residents returned to the nursing home after hospital visits, but

Table 33.2 Descriptive statistics of the elderly who had hospital visits ($N = 128$)

Items	Frequency	Percentage
Gender		
Male	61	47.66
Female	67	52.34
Age (years)		
60 or below	1	0.78
60–69	21	16.41
70–79	39	30.47
80–89	44	34.38
90 and above	23	17.97
Education		
Elementary school or below	52	40.63
High school	68	53.13
College	8	6.25
Monthly income (RMB)		
2590 or below	20	15.63
2590–5000	102	79.68
5000 and above	6	4.69
Expenses		
Totally covered	26	20.31
Partially covered	94	73.44
Totally not covered	8	6.25
Residency		
Local	117	91.41
Non-local	11	8.59

Table 33.3 Cross table for expenses and return decisions ($N = 128$)

	Return to the nursing home after hospital visits		
Expenses	Yes	No	Total
Totally covered	25	1	26
Partially covered	64	30	94
Totally not covered	6	2	8
Total	95	33	128

only one decided not to return. A possible reason was that residents who fully cover their expenses themselves might lack care and support from their family members. Thus, returning to the nursing home might be their only choice. Another possible reason was that these people had the right to decide whether they wanted to go back to the nursing home or not because they paid for themselves. Other options, such as going back home and being taken care of by family members, might not have as satisfactory a level of medical services as the nursing home from their perspective.

Chronic Diseases and Return Decisions

It was noticed from the interview with the manager that the elderly's hospital visits are usually due to chronic diseases. Chronic diseases are diseases that last a relatively long time and are caused by a combination of genetic, physiological, environmental, and behavioural factors. The considerable costs of chronic diseases, such as lengthy and expensive treatments, combined with a loss of income, enmesh millions of people into poverty and stagnate a country's development and growth. There are four main types of chronic diseases: cardiovascular diseases (such as heart attacks and stroke), cancers, chronic respiratory diseases (such as chronic obstructive pulmonary disease and asthma), and diabetes. According to the WHO, cardiovascular diseases lead to the most deaths annually (17.9 million) among these four types, followed by cancers (9.3 million), respiratory diseases (4.1 million), and diabetes (1.5 million). Though evidence shows that more than 15 million of the annual deaths attributed to chronic diseases occur in those between the ages of 30 and 69, these conditions are more prevalent in older age groups (World Health Organization, 2021).

From the interview, some elderly people did not return to the nursing home after hospital visits, and hospital visits were often a result of chronic diseases. Therefore, it was expected that there might be a correlation between chronic diseases and return decisions, and the relationship between the two was analysed. Specifically, respective logistic regressions were performed to investigate the impact of cardiovascular diseases, cancers, chronic respiratory diseases, and diabetes on return decisions after hospital visits. For ease of exposition, cardiovascular diseases and chronic respiratory diseases were labelled as CVDs and CRDs, respectively. The dependent variable in this study was the return decision, which had two categories, "return to the nursing home after hospital visits" and "not return to the nursing home after hospital visits". The latter was set as the reference group. Four chronic disease variables (CVDs, cancers, CRDs, and diabetes) were set as the independent variable in each regression. They were translated into dummy variables: with such a chronic disease (1) and without a chronic disease (0).

The results for the CVDs are presented in Table 33.4. CVDs were significantly and negatively correlated with return decisions ($p = 0.089 < 0.1$); that is, the elderly who had CVDs were less likely to return to the nursing home after hospital visits than those without CVDs. CVDs are a leading cause of death, with 85% of such deaths due to heart attack and stroke (World Health Organization, n.d.-d). Elderly people with CVDs needed access to immediate treatments and appropriate related technology and medication, which were available only in hospitals but not nursing homes. For the elderly who had CVDs, leaving the nursing home and staying in the hospital was a likely decision, if the staff in the nursing home could not provide constant monitoring for in-time treatment or appropriate medical equipment was unavailable.

The results for cancer are shown in Table 33.5. The elderly who had cancer were also significantly less likely to return to the nursing home after hospital visits than those who did not have cancer ($p = 0.024 < 0.05$). As the second leading cause of death globally, cancer caused approximately 9.6 million deaths in 2018, equal to one in six deaths (World Health Organization, n.d.-c). The elderly who had cancer usually needed quality diagnosis and treatment. However, such services could be a tremendous burden for a nursing home, and the institution might not offer such services. Once the elderly with cancer visited hospitals, they might realise that the medical resources in their nursing home could not satisfy their needs, and better medical facilities might considerably extend their lives. Thus, the elderly would seek hospital care to manage their conditions.

Table 33.6 shows the results for CRDs. A significantly negative relationship was found between CRDs and return decisions ($p = 0.002 < 0.05$). In other words, the elderly who had CRDs were less likely to return to the nursing home after hospital visits. CRDs destroy the airways and other structures of the lungs (World Health Organization, n.d.-e). Though CRDs are not curable, various types of treatment can help control symptoms and improve comfort, such as helping open the air passages and improving shortness of breath. It is important to get these medical or physical treatments promptly and properly, as an unsatisfactory treatment may lead to death. Therefore, the elderly with CRDs might turn to more professional institutions if the level of the equipment in the nursing home could not fulfil their needs.

Unlike the other chronic diseases, there was no significant relationship between diabetes and return decisions. The possible reason is that the elderly with diabetes can usually manage their conditions with interventions that are relatively easy to obtain and can be given anywhere (World Health Organization, n.d.-f).

Table 33.4 Logistic regression of CVDs on return decisions

Predictor	β	SE	Wald's χ^2	df	p
CVDs	−0.778	0.457	2.900	1	0.089
Constant	1.584	0.388	16.658	1	0.000

Table 33.5 Logistic regression model of cancers on return decisions

Predictor	β	SE	Wald's χ^2	df	p
Cancers	−2.562	1.138	5.069	1	0.024
Constant	1.176	0.212	30.650	1	0.000

Table 33.6 Logistic regression model of CRDs on return decisions

Predictor	β	SE	Wald's χ^2	df	p
CRDs	−1.320	0.427	9.552	1	0.002
Constant	1.531	0.276	30.855	1	0.000

Solutions and Recommendations

From the study, it is essential to enhance the medical capability of nursing homes that adopt a medical and aged care integration mode to satisfy the residents' needs and keep them in the nursing home. In this way, nursing homes can effectively relieve the pressure on hospitals, and the elderly can receive comprehensive care and services that are unavailable in hospitals. The findings were shared with the manager, and some concrete recommendations came up.

The first recommendation is to raise financial support from the authorities. The central concept of the integration mode is to be responsible for both daily aged care and medical care of the elderly. The latter is tough to achieve as it requires different resources from those traditionally found in nursing homes. Particularly, CVDs, cancers, CRDs, and diabetes are the most common diseases that the elderly may have. If the nursing home's level of medical support cannot provide the proper treatments for these diseases, the residents will be triggered to leave. For nursing homes, professional medical equipment is usually a huge financial burden, and there will be a long way to achieve the integration mode on their own. More financial support from the authorities could thus accelerate the progress of the integration mode in nursing homes.

The second recommendation is to strengthen the staff's professional medical training. The staff in nursing homes that adopt the integration mode should understand how to monitor the residents' health and take care of them. Providing regular training and enhancing the staff's medical professionalism may be helpful.

Conclusion

An ageing population has become an unavoidable issue for many countries, and China is no exception. Nursing homes are one of the most common residential choices for the elderly in China, and many are adopting a medical and aged care integration mode in which they provide both medical care and daily aged care to residents. Despite the growth of this integration mode in practice, little literature has focused on this topic. In this chapter, a case study is presented in which data were collected from residents of a leading nursing home in Shanghai and its manager was interviewed. The elderly's residential choices and preferences for nursing homes under the integration mode were comprehensively studied.

From the interview, it was learned from the manager that hospital visits might trigger a resident to leave the nursing home, even though his or her health remained the same before and after the visit. Furthermore, residents' suffering from a chronic disease might impact return decisions after hospital visits. This insight was validated with the data of the elderly who had hospital visits while residing in the nursing home. The results showed significant negative relationships between three chronic disease types (CVDs, cancers, and CRDs) and return decisions. In other words, residents with CVDs, cancers, and CRDs were less likely to return to the nursing home once they visit hospitals compared to those without. The findings of this chapter provide operational implications for nursing homes that adopt a medical and aged care integration mode.

To conclude, caring the elderly is an essential element in achieving the goal of "health for all", and the development of "all for health" navigates endeavours towards the achievement of this goal. The medical and aged care integration mode, in which relevant functions are integrated and target the health delivery to the elderly, is a typical "all for health" effort. Nevertheless, in the process of implementing the integration mode, challenges and opportunities occur. The chapter has discussed the implementation of the integration mode and points out the directions of improving it. Hopefully, the example of the integration mode may inspire other studies and implementation of "all for health" so that the goal of "health for all" can eventually be attained.

References

Cheng, Q. X., & Feng, Z. Y. (2015). Mei guo PACE ji qi dui wo guo she qu yi yang jie he de qi shi [The program of all-inclusive care for the elderly (PACE) from the United States and its implications to develop medical-nursing combined community support mode in China]. *Yi xue yu zhe xue: A, 9*, 78–80. http://www.cqvip.com/QK/92694A/20159/665954850.html

Geng, A. S., & Wang, K. (2016). Ying guo "yi yang jie he "de jing yan yu qi shi [The implication of the experience of the integrated care in the United Kingdom]. *Hua Dong Li Gong Da Xue Xue Bao (she hui ke xue ban), 5*, 87–94. https://doi.org/10.3969/j.issn.1008-7672.2016.05.010

Li, A., Zhang, J. Y., Guo, Q., Wang, Q. Y., & Liu, Y. (2017). Mei guo PACE mo shi ji qi dui wo guo yi yang jie he de qi shi [PACE and its implications on the development of medical-nursing combination in China]. *Zhong guo yi yuan guan li, 2017*(10), 78–80. http://www.zgyygl.com/ch/reader/view_abstract.aspx?file_no=2201703164&flag=1

Li, L., Hu, J., & Zheng, Y. (2020). Ying guo EHCH yi yang jie he shi jian mo shi fen xi [Analysis of enhanced health in care homes in England]. *Zhong guo she hui yi xue za zhi, 37*(3), 245–248. https://doi.org/10.3969/j.issn.1673-5625.2020.03.006

Liu, Y. H., & Luo, J. K. (2016). Fa guo yi yang jie he mo shi dui wo guo yang lao ti xi jian she de qi shi [The enlightenment of the senior care in France to Chinese researchers]. *Zhong guo hu li guan li, 16*(7), 930–933. http://www.zghlgl.com/CN/Y2016/V16/I7/930

Office for National Statistics. (2021, June 25). *Population estimates for the UK, England and Wales, Scotland and Northern Ireland: Mid-2020.* https://www.ons.gov.uk/peoplepopulationandcommunity/populationandmigration/populationestimates/bulletins/annualmidyearpopulationestimates/mid2020

United Nations. (n.d.). *Do you know all 17 SDGs?* https://sdgs.un.org/goals

World Health Organization. (n.d.-a). *Ageing*. https://www.who.int/health-topics/ageing
World Health Organization. (n.d.-b). *Ageing and health in China.* https://www.who.int/china/health-topics/ageing
World Health Organization. (n.d.-c). *Cancer*. https://www.who.int/health-topics/cancer
World Health Organization. (n.d.-d). *Cardiovascular diseases.* https://www.who.int/health-topics/cardiovascular-diseases
World Health Organization. (n.d.-e). *Chronic respiratory diseases.* https://www.who.int/health-topics/chronic-respiratory-diseases
World Health Organization. (n.d.-f). *Diabetes*. https://www.who.int/health-topics/diabetes
World Health Organization. (n.d.-g). *Integrated Care for Older People (ICOPE).* https://www.who.int/teams/maternal-newborn-child-adolescent-health-and-ageing/ageing-and-health/integrated-care-for-older-people-icope
World Health Organization. (2021). *Noncommunicable diseases.* https://www.who.int/news-room/fact-sheets/detail/noncommunicable-diseases
Yang, Z., & Wang, M. F. (2021). Ri ben yi yang jie he yang lao fu wu de shi jian ji dui wo guo de qi shi [The practice of elderly service with combination of medical care and nursing in Japan and enlightenment to China]. *She hui bao zhang yan jiu za zhi, 1*, 93–102. https://doi.org/10.3969/j.issn.1674-4802.2021.01.010
Zhou, C., Weng, J., & Zhang, B. D. (2018). Ri ben yi yang jie he yang lao mo shi ji qi dui wo guo de qi shi [Pension mode of integrated medical and elderly care services in Japan and its implication for China]. *Yi xue yu zhe xue: A, 12*, 33–36. http://www.cqvip.com/QK/92694A/201812/6100066793.html

Chapter 34
Gender Differences in Maintaining Cleanliness and Hygiene in Public Toilets: New Evidence from Hong Kong

Yuk-sik Chong, Victor W. T. Zheng, and Po-san Wan

Abstract Public toilets have a significant impact on hygiene and infectious disease control, affecting the health of the community and arousing the concern about how to effectively maintain a clean environment. However, existing toilet management logics have paid scant attention to gender difference in interacting with toilet environments and facilities. The aim of this study was to explore the impacts of gender on the maintenance of cleanliness in public toilets. A telephone survey of randomised number was used to assess gender differences in interacting with toilet facilities. We applied ordinal logistic regression and multinominal logistic regression to analyse the gender impacts. The results showed that there was a difference between male and female users in: (1) the perception about toilet cleanliness; (2) the problems relating to the cleanliness; (3) the causes of poor hygiene; and (4) dealing with dirt on their own. Being a male or female affects how people use public toilets and their consciousness of the importance of maintaining the cleanliness of a facility, with a higher level of cleanliness being more important to females than to males. These findings provide important policy implications that different management of male and female toilets should be introduced which could improve the standard of toilet cleanliness and hygiene. Significant policy measures based on empirical conclusions are proposed. The study contributes to the sanitation sector in toilet design and management, and how this helps the prevention of infectious diseases and outbreaks.

Keywords Gender · Hong Kong · Public toilet · Sanitation · Toilet environmental management

---

Y. Chong (✉) · V. W. T. Zheng · P. Wan
Hong Kong Institute of Asia-Pacific Studies, The Chinese University of Hong Kong, Hong Kong, China
e-mail: yschong@cuhk.edu.hk

V. W. T. Zheng
e-mail: vzheng@cuhk.edu.hk

P. Wan
e-mail: shirleywan@cuhk.edu.hk

B. Y. F. Fong and W. C. W. Wong (eds.), *Gaps and Actions in Health Improvement from Hong Kong and Beyond*,
https://doi.org/10.1007/978-981-99-4491-0_34

Introduction

As a global metropolis in Asia, Hong Kong is praised for its unique blend of Western and Chinese culture and civilisation. It is not only well known as an international financial centre and as the world's freest economy, but also for its very high population density and for being one of the most popular tourist destinations in the world. As with most global cities, although some of the public toilets in Hong Kong are clean and comfortable, especially those located in places frequently visited by tourists, such as the airport, theme parks, and museums, many others are not.[1] Although excretion is a basic human activity, there are gender differences in toilet use behaviour, which might affect the cleanliness of public toilets. Based on empirical research, this paper examines how gender differences in interacting with toilet environments and facilities affect the consciousness of individuals of the importance of maintaining toilet cleanliness, an often-overlooked issue in public health and environmental hygiene.

With a per capita GDP of over US$48,756, Hong Kong is one of the wealthiest places in the world, ranking 15th out of 179 in 2019 (World Bank, 2020). The educational attainment of the population has continued to improve, with one-third of those aged 15 or above having received a post-secondary education as of 2019 (Census & Statistics Department, 2020). No one can deny that Hong Kong is a highly modernised and developed city, yet the cleanliness of its public toilets compares poorly with its levels of economic development and educational attainment. According to *The Travel & Tourism Competitiveness Report*, Hong Kong's Health and Hygiene pillar ranking (which includes accessibility to improved sanitation and drinking water) dropped from 15 to 45th between 2015 and 2019 (World Economic Forum, 2015, 2019).

The government has adopted a series of measures to improve public toilet cleanliness, including earmarking HK$600 million to refurbish 240 public toilets (one-third of public toilets maintained by the Food and Environmental Hygiene Department, the main department for managing government public toilets) between 2019–2020 and 2023–2024 (Audit Commission, 2019).[2] Refurbishment work has been undertaken continually since the early 1990s, and between the 1990s and 2024, a total of at least HK$1.53 billion could be spent (including the abovementioned work started in 2019–2020) (Audit Commission, 2019; Urban Council, 1994; The Government of the Hong Kong Special Administrative Region, 1998, 2002, 2011). Meanwhile, the outsourcing of cleansing services for a 2-year period (78% of the department's public toilets are maintained by outsourced service contractors) costs about HK$210 million as of April 2019 (Audit Commission, 2019). Expenditures on education and publicity on toilet hygiene and proper use of toilet facilities increased from HK$0.45 million in 2017–2018 to HK$1.66 million in 2019–2020 (Public Accounts

[1] Public toilets are defined as toilets that can be accessed by the general public and that are in a public area, regardless of whether they are provided by the government, the commercial sector or a public institution.

[2] The Hong Kong dollar has been pegged between 7.75 and 7.85 per US dollar.

Committee, 2020).[3] Despite these heavy investments, the number of complaints about public toilets has increased sevenfold from 328 in 2000–2001 to 2367 in 2019 (The Government of the Hong Kong Special Administrative Region, 2001, 2020).[4] The toilet governance logic is that the government believes self-regulating toilet behaviour can be fostered through refurbishment works and cleaning services, and that improved sanitary conditions will teach users to appreciate the clean toilet environment and the effort the toilet attendants put in, encouraging them to maintain toilet cleanliness. Clearly though, the poor toilet conditions indicate that the above governance logic does not work, and so the government should adopt an innovative approach to address this age-old problem of insanitary public toilets to mitigate public health risks to the community.

Many studies have also been conducted on the causes of poor sanitation in Hong Kong public toilets. In the first approach, the emphasis is on the potential for diseases to be transmitted in public toilets due to the particular environmental features of the toilets, such as a humid environment and the generation of airborne pathogens from the flushing of toilets (Lai et al., 2018; Suen et al., 2019). This is quite true that it is difficult to maintain cleanliness with regard to the salient features of public toilets as sanitary facilities. In the second, the focus is on investigating the implications of Chinese culture and practices, such as the habits of squatting on the toilet seat and spitting in the toilet bowl or urinal before urinating (Wu et al., 2019). In the third, attention is paid to investigating user-facility interactions, such as opening the toilet lid with one's foot or flushing without closing the lid, thereby lessening their risk of contagion from disease. It is argued by Siu (2006) that such interactions have an important influence on toilet cleanliness.

Little attention has been paid to another aspect, that is of equal importance, in the effort to maintain clean toilets, namely the issue of gender-related differences in the use of public toilet facilities, and how this might affect the level of consciousness and alertness of male and female users to the importance of maintaining the cleanliness of the facilities (Anthony & Dufresne, 2007; Greed, 1995). Generally, female toilets are cleaner than male ones (Jolanta et al., 2015; Siu, 2006). This difference in condition seems to be strongly correlated with the different behaviours of males and females, which arise from their different biological designs and needs, and their cultural caregiving roles, which impact their concern for cleanliness. Males do not need to sit down, squat or use a cubicle to urinate, while females have extra sanitary needs that males do not. A majority, about 90%, of away-from-home toilet usage is for urination rather than defecation (Electronic Connection Staff, 2011). It is self-evident that males are more likely to urinate in a urinal than in a toilet bowl, which means that they do not need to enter a cramped cubicle and, in doing so, touch the associated surfaces (the cubicle door and lock, toilet seat, seat lid, and flush handle). Females, on the other hand, can only relieve themselves (whether urinating or defecating) in

[3] The expense for the financial year 2019–2020 was as of January 2020.

[4] The figure for 2000–2001 included complaints about toilets provided by the Food and Environmental Hygiene Department and the Leisure and Cultural Services Department from January 2000 to March 2001.

a cubicle; thus, they are required to touch surfaces associated with using a cubicle which are potential places for the transmission of germs.

In terms of the duration to use a toilet facility, on average females spend twice as much time as males (Greed, 1995). Chinese females spend 70–73 s, compared to 30–35 s for Chinese males (Department of Environmental Protection, 2017). During pregnancy and menstruation, the amount of time that females spend in a public toilet increases. Moreover, females are in particular need of public toilets because they often take on family caregiving roles for infants, children, and the elderly; furthermore, some breastfeed or change diapers in public toilets, which need to be clean for both the mother and the baby (Anthony & Dufresne, 2007; Barcan, 2010). The different states of male and female toilets, and the gendered uses of such facilities, mean that a gendered understanding is required when approaching the issue of management and cleanliness of public toilets. The authors performed a hypothesis test to determine if different gendered practices of interacting with and using toilet facilities would influence the consciousness of males and females about the importance of maintaining cleanliness in toilets. The aim of this study was to identify user-facility interactions (toilet cleanliness, insanitary problems encountered, causes of poor cleanliness, and methods of dealing with dirt improperly left in toilets) as gendered phenomena and thereby develop insights for the effective management of specifically male or female toilets.

The Study

Cleanliness in public toilets is a long-term problem in Hong Kong. With the spread of COVID-19 around the world, the issue has become even more important, as toilets have potentially become sites for the transmission of viruses (Li et al., 2020). During the second wave of outbreaks in Hong Kong, the authors designed a questionnaire and commissioned the Hong Kong Institute of Asia-Pacific Studies to conduct a dual-frame telephone survey (landline and mobile) in the evening from the 12th to the 23rd of March 2020, to gauge public views on cleanliness in public toilets. A total of 1006 people aged 18 or above were successfully interviewed (542 respondents came from landline numbers and 464 from mobile numbers), with a response rate of 39.2% for landline numbers and 46.9% for mobile numbers. The aim of this study was to investigate the effects of gender in maintaining toilet cleanliness in Hong Kong. In doing so, the authors tested gender differences in the following five aspects: the types of public toilets frequently used, perceptions of the cleanliness of public toilets, problems relating to insanitary conditions encountered in public toilets, perceptions of the causes of poor cleanliness, and the methods that people would use to deal with their dirt left improperly in public toilet facilities. The correlation between gender and toilet cleanliness was analysed by ordinal logistic regression. Based on the ordinal logistic regression, we analysed the relationship between gender and perceptions of the cleanliness in different types of public toilets in order to identify the effect of gender on toilet cleanliness perception in different types of toilets. Aiming to differentiate the impacts of gender and toilet practices, we studied how males and females dealing with their dirt left in the toilets by the employment of multinomial logistic regression.

Perceptions of Toilet Cleanliness

The respondents were first asked what types of public toilets they had frequently used over the past three years and how clean they perceived the different types of toilets to be. The choices included the three most commonly used kinds of public toilets in Hong Kong: government toilets (stand-alone facilities accessed from the street, those in government-run indoor markets, and those in public libraries), commercial toilets (located in restaurants and recreational places), and public institution toilets (located in the airport, hospitals, and metro rail stations). Although only 15.2% of the respondents were frequent users of government toilets over the past three years, the survey showed that 57.7% of the respondents regarded these toilets to be insanitary (including very insanitary). This is a higher percentage than those who considered public toilets in the commercial sector and in public institutions to be insanitary. The results of a cross-tabulation analysis revealed no significant gender differences in patterns of public toilet usage or in perceptions of the cleanliness of government toilets. However, females held a more negative view than males of the cleanliness of both commercial toilets and public institution toilets (Table 34.1).

An ordinal logistic regression was performed to confirm the relationship between gender and perceptions of the cleanliness of the three types of public toilets. Gender (male = 0, female = 1) was the independent variable. The dependent variable was measured on a four-point scale (from "very insanitary" = 1 to "very sanitary" = 4). Since a number of socio-demographic factors like age, level of education, working status, and subjective social class might correlate with toilet behaviours and perceptions of the cleanliness of public toilets, these factors were added as control variables. As shown in Table 34.2, on the one hand, gender failed to pass the significance level of 0.05 in the regression of government toilets. This demonstrates that, after controlling for the effects of other socio-demographic variables, both genders had a similar perception of the cleanliness of government toilets. On the other hand, gender passed the level of significance with regard to commercial toilets ($p < 0.05$) and public institution toilets ($p < 0.001$), and its coefficients were negative. This suggests that females held a more negative view about the cleanliness of commercial toilets and public institution toilets than males.

Insanitary Problems Encountered in Toilets

It is important to note that toilet cleanliness and the problems of the insanitary conditions that are encountered can be different for different types of public toilets.

Table 34.1 Gender differences in usage and perceived cleanliness of public toilets (%)

	Total	Female	Male	χ^2 test
Public toilet usage				ns
Government toilets	15.2	13.3	17.3	
Commercial toilets	77.7	80.1	75.1	
Public institution toilets	7.0	6.6	7.6	
(*n*)	(911)	(486)	(424)	
Perceived cleanliness				
Government toilets				ns
Very insanitary/insanitary	57.7	56.7	58.8	
Very sanitary/sanitary	42.3	43.3	41.2	
(*n*)	(862)	(466)	(396)	
Commercial toilets				*
Very insanitary/insanitary	14.6	17.5	11.5	
Very sanitary/sanitary	85.4	82.5	88.5	
(*n*)	(871)	(456)	(415)	
Public institution toilets				**
Very insanitary/insanitary	13.2	16.6	9.4	
Very sanitary/sanitary	86.8	83.4	90.6	
(*n*)	(936)	(490)	(446)	

*$p < 0.05$, **$p < 0.01$, ns: not significant

The respondents were given a list of insanitary problems encountered in public toilets, which covered common environmental problems such as rubbish on the floor, slippery floors, and dirty toilet seats (Audit Commission, 2019; Siu, 2006; Wu et al., 2019). They were asked to identify whether they had encountered any of those problems and the question allowed for multiple responses. The three main insanitary problems mentioned by the respondents were bad odour, slippery floors, and no flushing water in all three types of public toilets.

Among those respondents who held a negative view of the sanitary condition of government toilets, 74.3% said that having no flushing water was the main issue related to the insanitary conditions that they encountered, 61.2% mentioned bad odour, while 55.0% indicated slippery floors. Furthermore, around a third of the respondents complained about issues such as dirty toilet seats, clogged urinals or toilet bowls, and rubbish on the floor. The results of the cross-tabulation revealed that most of the differences between the genders in the insanitary problems that they encountered in different types of toilets were statistically insignificant at the level of 0.05. However, males were more likely than females to encounter a clogged urinal or toilet bowl in government toilets, while females indicated that they encountered a dirty toilet seat in commercial toilets much more frequently than males (Table 34.3).

Table 34.2 Ordinal logistic regression on perceived cleanliness of public toilets

	Government toilets	Commercial toilets	Public institution toilets
Female	−0.063	−0.385*	−0.652***
Age (18–29)			
30–59	0.655**	−0.088	0.445
60 or above	0.976***	0.004	0.824**
Post-secondary education	−0.212	−0.326	0.206
Working	−0.139	−0.210	0.270
Subjective social class (Lower/Lower-middle)			
Middle	0.206	0.713***	0.247
Upper-middle/Upper	−0.097	0.938**	0.142
Threshold 1	−1.484	−5.444	−3.694
Threshold 2	0.803	−1.967	−1.476
Threshold 3	5.525	2.553	2.809
Nagelkerke R^2	0.055	0.040	0.044
(n)	(784)	(785)	(843)

$^*p < 0.05$, $^{**}p < 0.01$, $^{***}p < 0.001$

Causes of Poor Cleanliness

In order to further explore the factors contributing to poor cleanliness and conditions, we asked the respondents to give their perception of the causes, choosing from the following list: toilet users lacked civility, insufficient manpower and cleaning, high usage rate, and facility damage. Respondents could choose multiple causes. It was found that the top cause was perceived to be toilet users lacking civility, with a percentage of 80.1%, compared to 63.7% for insufficient cleaners and frequency of cleaning, 56.6% for high usage, and 35.0% for frequent facility damage. The results of the cross-tabulation indicated that males and females differed only slightly in their perceptions of the causes of poor cleanliness, with only one exception, which was that females (60.5%) were more likely than males (56.6%) to perceive high usage as a major cause ($p < 0.05$).

Methods of Cleaning Own Dirt

As males and females have different interactions with toilet environments and facilities, they may deal differently with the dirt that they leave in improper places (toilet floor, the seat, and edge of the toilet bowl), which would significantly affect the

Table 34.3 Gender differences in insanitary problems encountered in public toilets (%)

	Total	Female	Male		χ^2 test
Government toilets					
No flushing water	74.3	75.5	73.0		ns
Bad odor	61.2	61.1	61.3		ns
Slippery floor	55.0	55.5	54.4		ns
Dirty toilet seat	39.8	41.2	38.2		ns
Clogged urinal/toilet bowl	38.5	33.8	43.7		*
Rubbish on the floor	31.9	30.8	33.0		ns
Clogged sink	27.5	27.8	27.2		ns
(*n*)	(493)	(261)	(233)		
Commercial toilets					
No flushing water	68.5	71.8	63.0		ns
Bad odor	50.0	51.1	48.2		ns
Slippery floor	46.3	45.8	47.0		ns
Dirty toilet seat	44.1	51.6	32.0		*
Clogged urinal/toilet bowl	26.4	31.2	18.5		ns
Rubbish on the floor	45.4	49.5	38.8		ns
Clogged sink	24.0	29.7	14.6		ns
(*n*)	(123)	(76)	(47)		
Public institution toilets					
No flushing water	56.3	55.0	58.6		ns
Bad odor	49.5	43.3	60.9		ns
Slippery floor	62.3	65.5	56.4		ns
Dirty toilet seat	35.6	39.1	28.9		ns
Clogged urinal/toilet bowl	35.2	31.7	41.6		ns
Rubbish on the floor	45.9	43.3	50.7		ns
Clogged sink	37.7	40.3	32.9		ns
(*n*)	(120)	(78)	(42)		

*$p < 0.05$, ns: not significant
Note Only respondents who answered insanitary or very insanitary for each type of toilet were asked. Multiple responses were permitted

cleanliness of such facilities in a gendered manner. Thus, in this study, the respondents were asked to estimate what methods they and other users would employ in cleaning their dirt. The three methods were: do not clean up, clean up on their own, and ask a toilet attendant to clean up. In examining the methods used to deal with dirt, it was found that 78.8% of the respondents said they would clean up on their own, 11.1% would ask the toilet attendant to clean it up, and 10.1% would not clean up. Meanwhile, 73.3% of the respondents believed that other users would not clean up, 16.4% believed that others would ask an attendant to clean up, and only 10.4% said that others would clean it on their own (Table 34.4).

Males and females varied significantly in their responses ($p < 0.001$). While 90.4% of females said they would clean up their dirt, only 65.8% of males indicated they would do so. Moreover, 15.1% of males versus 5.6% of females were inclined not to deal with the dirt, and 19.1% of males versus 4.0% of females would ask an attendant to clean up. In sum, compared to females, males were less likely to clean up their dirt on their own and more likely to ask an attendant to clean it up. It is also interesting to note that females were more likely not to clean up their dirt themselves than to ask an attendant to clean it up. For females, the order of preference was: clean it up on their own, do not clean up, and then ask an attendant to clean up. For males, the order of preference was: clean it up on their own, ask an attendant to clean up, and do not clean up (Table 34.5).

We employed a multinomial logistic regression to ascertain the relationship between gender and the method of cleaning dirt. The dependent variable has three nominal categories, and thus, three sets of comparisons were made for both the respondents' view of the practices of other users and that of their own. Table 34.5 shows the results of the regression. There were no significant gender differences in the respondents' view of other users. However, in the respondents' own practices, the gender coefficients were negative and significant at the level of 0.001 in the comparisons of "do not clean up" and "ask an attendant to clean up" with "clean up on their own". The results suggest that females are more likely than males to clean up on their own than do not clean up or ask an attendant to clean up, when all other socio-demographic variables in the model are held constant.

Table 34.4 Gender differences in method of cleaning their dirt left improperly in public toilets (%)

	Total	Female	Male	χ^2 test
Respondents themselves				***
Do not clean up	10.1	5.6	15.1	
Clean up on their own	78.8	90.4	65.8	
Ask an attendant to clean up	11.1	4.0	19.1	
(*n*)	(936)	(495)	(440)	
Other users				ns
Do not clean up	73.3	73.8	72.6	
Clean up on their own	10.4	9.9	10.9	
Ask an attendant to clean up	16.4	16.3	16.5	
(*n*)	(833)	(446)	(387)	

***$p < 0.001$, ns: not significant

Table 34.5 Multinomial logistic regressions on methods of cleaning dirt

	Respondents' own practices			Respondents' view of other users		
	Do not clean up vs clean up on their own	Ask an attendant vs clean up on their own	Do not clean up vs ask an attendant	Do not clean up vs clean up on their own	Ask an attendant vs clean up on their own	Do not clean up vs ask an attendant
Female	−1.436***	−1.752***	0.316	0.326	0.608	−0.281
Age (18–29)						
30–59	−0.490	0.397	−0.887	−0.972*	−1.240*	0.268
60 or above	−0.037	0.041	−0.078	−0.782	−1.316*	0.534
Post-secondary education	0.303	−0.273	0.576	0.018	−1.048**	1.065***
Working	−0.218	−0.157	−0.61	0.282	0.340	−0.058
Subjective social class (Lower/ Lower-middle)						
Middle	0.313	−0.432	0.745*	−0.180	−0.061	−0.119
Upper-middle/ Upper	0.320	0.068	0.252	−0.378	0.226	−0.604
Constant	−1.417	−1.152	−0.265	2.642	1.528	1.114
Nagelkerke R^2			0.147			0.049
(*n*)			(842)			(750)

$^*p < 0.05$, $^{**}p < 0.01$, $^{***}p < 0.001$

Cleanliness and Hygiene in Public Toilets—Gender Differences

Existing public toilet management on cleanliness and hygiene in public toilets in Hong Kong pays little attention to the role of gender in interactions with toilet environments and facilities. This is surprising, as gender has important impacts on the use of toilet facilities. This study fills a research gap by examining toilet users' sensitivity to cleanliness and the methods that they use to deal with their own dirt, comparing the disparities between the two main anatomical genders. Thus, this study contributes to a fuller understanding of the role and effect of gender on public toilet use and public toilet maintenance.

Compared to males, the biology and cultural caregiving role of females greatly increases their need to use public toilet facilities and the amount of time that they spend in such facilities, which are at once public and private. This makes females more vulnerable to being adversely affected by the poor condition and cleanliness of such facilities (Barcan, 2010; Greed, 1995). It is impossible for females to avoid touching any surfaces in toilet facilities when using them. This increased requirement to use public toilets, and the fear of contamination, makes females more sensitive about the issue of cleanliness, leading to a higher level of consciousness about the condition of public toilet facilities. Therefore, females feel more obliged than males to maintain the sanitary condition of such facilities to protect their own health. In the following discussion, we will show how the major findings support our hypothesis that gendered practices of interacting with and using toilet facilities affect the consciousness of males and females about the importance of maintaining cleanliness in toilets.

Obviously, there was a gender difference in perceptions about the cleanliness of public toilets. Females held a more negative view than males about the cleanliness of commercial toilets and public institution toilets. This suggests that females were more sensitive to cleanliness and had a higher standard of cleanliness than males. This difference has an important implication: females might be more willing to maintain cleanliness in order to protect themselves from disease contamination.

The second finding is that there was a marked gender disparity in the two problems related to the cleanliness of public toilets. Females have to use the toilet bowl for urination, meaning that they have a greater chance than males of encountering a dirty toilet seat, while males are likely to use a urinal. While more males than females reported encountering a clogged urinal or toilet bowl, more females reported encountering a dirty toilet seat, which may have a more adverse effect on females, as they need to sit down or squat to urinate. This indicates that the problems encountered by females may have more of an impact on their health or comfort, leading females to have a greater concern for cleanliness.

The third finding regards the perceptions of the causes of poor cleanliness. It was found that more females than males blamed high usage, which is closely related to the toilet experiences of females. An insufficient number of female toilet cubicles and the fact that 54.4% of Hong Kong's population of 7.5 million are female make high usage a more acute problem for females than for males (Census & Statistics Department, 2020). The relationship between high usage and poor cleanliness implies improper use and inadequate cleaning services. This is a particular problem faced more by females than males, and hence arouses greater awareness among them of the sanitary condition of public toilets.

Furthermore, the majority of respondents perceived that a lack of civility on the part of other users was the major cause of poor cleanliness and conditions, compared to the other causes that were measured (damaged facilities and inadequate cleaning services), on which the government has recently been allocating more money and resources by refurbishing toilets and contracting out cleaning services. This signifies a policy gap between government and society in managing toilet cleanliness, which requires a new pattern of managing the habits of users through better management of toilet environments.

We also evaluated the gendered differences in dealing with dirt. Compared to females, males were more likely not to clean up dirt on their own and would rather ask an attendant to carry out this task. In comparison, females were more willing to clean up on their own. The above four findings support our hypothesis that males and females interact differently with public toilet environments and facilities. This affects their sensitivity towards toilet cleanliness and their consciousness of the maintenance of cleanliness, with a higher level of cleanliness being more important to females than to males.

Conclusion and Policy Implication

This study explored the effects of gender on the maintenance of cleanliness in public toilets. It was found that more females than males had a negative perception of the condition of the public toilets they had encountered over the prior three years. There were differences in the sanitary problems that males and females stated they had encountered, in their perceptions of the causes of poor cleanliness, and in the methods they commonly used to deal with dirt improperly left behind. This is of great significance in offering a scientific basis for improving cleanliness and hygiene in public toilets using gender-specific strategies to manage toilet environments, which will help to achieve clean and odourless public toilets while preventing disease infections and outbreaks. As our hypothesis suggested, the findings allow us to deduce gender differences in their consciousness of the importance of maintaining cleanliness in toilets, which were very much related to the different interactions with toilet environments and facilities that males and females typically have.

Public toilets are among the very few gender-segregated spaces remaining in society. The physical and cultural differences in caregiving roles between males and females remain central to their different interactions with toilet environments and facilities; therefore, the government should take a gender perspective in introducing methods of managing the environment in male and female toilets. Behaviours repeated in the same context (facility, location, and setting) easily develop into unconscious habits that are then performed with minimal explicit thought. This implies that changes to the environment may lead to changes in behaviour, and that any new behaviours are opportunities to form new habits through repetition (Curtis et al., 2009; Siu, 2006; Wood & Neal, 2007). From a gender perspective, we propose the application of nudge theory by integrating new contextual cues that might be implicated in the toilet environment, triggering more sanitary toilet behaviours and habits. In short, the correct contextual cues could disrupt the existing insanitary toilet habits of males and females, reshaping their respective interactions with public toilet environments and facilities.

The first cue to users should be from the posting of stickers which make better toilet habits easier for them to follow. Stickers depicting a small black fly could also be etched into each urinal, to motivate males to urinate inside the urinal and reduce spillage, as males urinating outside toilet bowls and urinals is a common cause of insanitary conditions (Thaler & Sunstein, 2009). To nudge users to wash their hands to reduce the transmission of diseases, the stickers shaped like arrows or handprints placed above hand basins could be targeted at males, who are less likely than females to wash their hands due to their minimal need to touch any surfaces inside public toilet facilities (Blackwell et al., 2018; Lawson & Vaganay-Miller, 2019; Thaler & Sunstein, 2009). Stickers encouraging people to put rubbish inside the waste bin could also be posted, especially in female toilets, to encourage women to properly dispose of used tissues and sanitary napkins (Kratzke et al., 2014). Finally, stickers reminding users to close the toilet lid before flushing could be posted in both male and female toilets to mitigate the transmission of diseases from splashing water.

The second cue could come from the installation of more infrared sensor facilities, such as automatic flush mechanisms. These sensors can minimise the chances of clogging in urinals or toilet bowls, which is important to reducing foul odours. Other sensors that could be used are automated water taps and hand-drying devices, which would encourage users to wash and dry their hands, thereby reducing the spread of disease and lowering humidity levels in toilets (Wu et al., 2019).

The third comes from the introduction of different toilet facility designs to cater to the different needs of different users (to reduce the need of touching facilities such as toilet seats). Including squat toilets and urinals (to enable urination while standing, with the help of a reusable urination device) in female toilets could better satisfy sanitary requirements (Cai & You, 1998; Electronic Connection Staff, 2011; Greed, 1995). Foot-operated flush mechanisms in both male and female toilets could encourage flushing, helping to reduce clogged toilet bowls and hence foul odours.

Fourth, with reference to painting walls with urine-repellent paint to discourage public urination (Winkless, 2016), painting the toilet seat and the edges of urinals and toilet bowls in male toilets with the paint could keep urine within bounds, encouraging males to urinate more carefully and reduce spillage. This could be an effective approach to reducing foul smells and stained floors in the male section of sanitary facilities.

Fifth, both cubicles and urinals could be included in the ratio of male-to-female toilet facilities,[5] in consideration of the longer duration that females need to use toilet facilities and the greater number of females in Hong Kong. To further enhance the female experience of using public toilets, cubicle sizes could be increased and alcohol for cleaning toilet seats could be provided (Anthony & Dufresne, 2007; Wu et al., 2019).

References

Anthony, K. H., & Dufresne, M. (2007). Potty parity in perspective: Gender and family issues in planning and designing public restrooms. *Journal of Planning Literature, 21*(3), 267–294. http://doi.org/10.1177/0885412206295846

Audit Commission. (2019). *Planning, provision and management of public toilets by the Food and Environmental Hygiene Department*. https://www.aud.gov.hk/pdf_e/e73ch01.pdf

[5] According to the Hong Kong government's Toilet Handbook, the ratio of male to female toilet facilities is 1:2. However, the ratio only includes cubicles, and so excludes male urinals, meaning that the sanitary facilities in male and female toilets as a whole are not evenly matched (Audit Commission, 2019: vii).

Barcan, R. (2010). Dirty spaces: Separation, concealment, and shame in the public toilet. In H. Molotch & L. Norén (Eds.), *Toilet: Public restrooms and the politics of sharing* (pp. 25–41). New York University Press. http://doi.org/10.18574/nyu/9780814759646.003.0006

Blackwell, C., Goya-Tocchetto, D., & Sturman, Z. (2018). Nudges in the restroom: How hand-washing can be impacted by environmental cues. *Journal of Behavioral Economics for Policy, 2*(2), 41–47. https://sabeconomics.org/wordpress/wp-content/uploads/JBEP-2-2-5.pdf

Cai, D., & You, M. (1998). An ergonomic approach to public squatting-type toilet design. *Applied Ergonomics, 29*(2), 147–153. http://doi.org/10.1016/S0003-6870(96)00023-3

Census and Statistics Department. (2020). *Hong Kong in figures: 2020 edition.* https://www.statistics.gov.hk/pub/B10100062020AN20B0100.pdf

Curtis, V. A., Danquah, L. O., & Aunger, R. V. (2009). Planned, motivated and habitual hygiene behaviour: An eleven country review. *Health Education Research, 24*(4), 655–673. http://doi.org/10.1093/her/cyp002

Department of Environmental Protection. (2017). *臺北市公廁之男女廁間比例* [Male-to-female toilet compartment ratio in Taipei]. https://www-ws.gov.taipei/Download.ashx?u=LzAwMS9VcGxvYWQvcHVibGljL0F0dGFjaG1lbnQvNzIyMzEwMjUxNzUucGRm&n=NzIyMzEwMjUxNzUucGRm

Electronic Connection Staff. (2011, February 25). *We know squat about female urinals.* Plumbing Connection. https://plumbingconnection.com.au/we-know-squat-about-female-urinals/

Greed, C. H. (1995). Public toilet provision for women in Britain: An investigation of discrimination against urination. *Women's Studies International Forum, 18*(5/6), 573–584. https://doi.org/10.1016/0277-5395(95)80094-6

Jolanta, M.-B., Wolny, M., & Krause, M. (2015). Hand washing practices of the residents of Silesia (Poland) based on observations in public toilets. *Journal of Water, Sanitation and Hygiene for Development, 5*(1), 107–114. https://doi.org/10.2166/washdev.2014.078

Kratzke, C., Short, M., & San Filippo, B. (2014). Promoting safe hygiene practices in public restrooms: A pilot study. *Journal of Environmental Health, 77*(4), 8–12.

Lai, A. C. K., Tan, T. F., Li, W. S., & Ip, D. K. M. (2018). Emission strength of airborne pathogens during toilet flushing. *Indoor Air, 28*(1), 73–79. https://doi.org/10.1111/ina.12406

Lawson, A., & Vaganay-Miller, M. (2019). The effectiveness of a poster intervention on hand hygiene practice and compliance when using public restrooms in a university setting. *International Journal of Environmental Research and Public Health, 16*(24), Article 5036. https://doi.org/10.3390/ijerph16245036

Li, Y. Y., Wang, J. X., & Chen, X. (2020). Can a toilet promote virus transmission? From a fluid dynamics perspective. *Physics of Fluids, 32*, Article 065107. https://doi.org/10.1063/5.0013318

Public Accounts Committee. (2020). *Report of the Public Accounts Committee on the Reports of the Director of Audit on the accounts of the government of the Hong Kong special administrative region for the year ended 31 march 2019 and the results of value for money audits* (Report No. 73). https://www.legco.gov.hk/yr19-20/english/pac/reports/73/73_rpt.pdf

Siu, K. W. M. (2006). Design quality of public toilet facilities. *International Journal of Reliability, Quality and Safety Engineering, 13*(4), 341–354. https://doi.org/10.1142/S021853930600229X

Suen, L. K. P., Siu, G. K. H., Guo, Y. P., Yeung, S. K. W., Lo, K. Y. K., & O' Donoghue, M. (2019). The public washroom—Friend or foe? An observational study of washroom cleanliness combined with microbiological investigation of hand hygiene facilities. *Antimicrobial Resistance & Infection Control, 8*, Article 47. https://doi.org/10.1186/s13756-019-0500-z

Thaler, R. H., & Sunstein, C. R. (2009). *Nudge: Improving decisions about health, wealth, and happiness.* Penguin Books. https://www.penguin.co.uk/books/56784/nudge-by-richard-h-thaler-cass-r-sunstein/9780141999937

The Government of the Hong Kong Special Administrative Region. (1998, May 20). *Improvement of toilet hygiene urged.* https://www.info.gov.hk/gia/general/199805/20/0520058.htm

The Government of the Hong Kong Special Administrative Region. (2001, May 16). *LCQ2: Hygienic conditions of public toilets* [Press release]. https://www.info.gov.hk/gia/general/200105/16/0516259.htm

The Government of the Hong Kong Special Administrative Region. (2002, May 22). *LCQ19: Cleansing and renovation of public toilets* [Press release]. https://www.info.gov.hk/gia/general/200205/22/0522210.htm

The Government of the Hong Kong Special Administrative Region. (2011, April 13). *LCQ9: Public toilet services* [Press release]. https://www.info.gov.hk/gia/general/201104/13/P201104130211.htm

The Government of the Hong Kong Special Administrative Region. (2020, May 27). *LCQ18: Management of public toilets* [Press release]. https://www.info.gov.hk/gia/general/202005/27/P2020052700250.htm?fontSize=1

Urban Council. (1994). *The development of public toilets in Hong Kong.*

Winkless, L. (2016, July 31). The science behind "the paint that pees back". *Forbes.* https://www.forbes.com/sites/lauriewinkless/2016/07/31/the-science-behind-the-paint-that-pees-back/?sh=5173f44701b3

Wood, W., & Neal, D. T. (2007). A new look at habits and the habit-goal interface. *Psychological Review, 114*(4), 843–863. https://doi.org/10.1037/0033-295X.114.4.843

World Bank. (2020). *GDP per capita (current US$): Hong Kong SAR, China.* https://data.worldbank.org/indicator/NY.GDP.PCAP.CD?locations=HK

World Economic Forum. (2015). *The travel & tourism competitiveness report 2015.* https://www3.weforum.org/docs/TT15/WEF_Global_Travel&Tourism_Report_2015.pdf

World Economic Forum. (2019). *The travel & tourism competitiveness report 2019.* https://www3.weforum.org/docs/WEF_TTCR_2019.pdf

Wu, D., Lam, T. P., Chan, H. Y., Lam, K. F., Zhou, X. D., Xu, J. Y., Sun, K. S., & Ho, P. L. (2019). A mixed-methods study on toilet hygiene practices among Chinese in Hong Kong. *BMC Public Health, 19*, Article 1654. https://doi.org/10.1186/s12889-019-8014-4

Index

B. Y. F. Fong and W. C. W. Wong (eds.), *Gaps and Actions in Health Improvement from Hong Kong and Beyond*,
https://doi.org/10.1007/978-981-99-4491-0

MIX
Papier aus verantwortungsvollen Quellen
Paper from responsible sources
FSC® C105338

If you have any concerns about our products,
you can contact us on
ProductSafety@springernature.com

In case Publisher is established outside the EU,
the EU authorized representative is:
Springer Nature Customer Service Center GmbH
Europaplatz 3, 69115 Heidelberg, Germany

Printed by Libri Plureos GmbH
in Hamburg, Germany